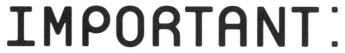

W9-BYK-892

IMPORTANT:

HERE IS YOUR REGISTRATION CODE TO ACCESS
YOUR PREMIUM McGRAW-HILL ONLINE RESOURCES.

For key premium online resources you need THIS CODE to gain access. Once the code is entered, you will be able to use the Web resources for the length of your course.

If your course is using **WebCT** or **Blackboard**, you'll be able to use this code to access the McGraw-Hill content within your instructor's online course.

Access is provided if you have purchased a new book. If the registration code is missing from this book, the registration screen on our Website, and within your WebCT or Blackboard course, will tell you how to obtain your new code.

Registering for McGraw-Hill Online Resources

TO gain access to your McGraw-Hill web resources simply follow the steps below:

1. USE YOUR WEB BROWSER TO GO TO: http://www.mhhe.com/corbin5e

2. CLICK ON **FIRST TIME USER**.

3. ENTER THE REGISTRATION CODE* PRINTED ON THE TEAR-OFF BOOKMARK ON THE RIGHT.

4. AFTER YOU HAVE ENTERED YOUR REGISTRATION CODE, CLICK **REGISTER**.

5. FOLLOW THE INSTRUCTIONS TO SET-UP YOUR PERSONAL UserID AND PASSWORD.

6. WRITE YOUR UserID AND PASSWORD DOWN FOR FUTURE REFERENCE.
   KEEP IT IN A SAFE PLACE.

TO GAIN ACCESS to the McGraw-Hill content in your instructor's **WebCT** or **Blackboard** course simply log in to the course with the UserID and Password provided by your instructor. Enter the registration code exactly as it appears in the box to the right when prompted by the system. You will only need to use the code the first time you click on McGraw-Hill content.

Thank you, and welcome to your McGraw-Hill online Resources!

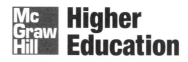

* YOUR REGISTRATION CODE CAN BE USED ONLY ONCE TO ESTABLISH ACCESS. IT IS NOT TRANSFERABLE.
0-07-292165-X TO ACCCOMPANY CORBIN: CONCEPTS OF FITNESS AND WELLNESS 5/E

MCGRAW-HILL
ONLINE RESOURCES

REGISTRATION CODE

FKRI-E3VF-HPWB-GR5F-4S0F

Mc Graw Hill Higher Education

Concepts of Fitness and Wellness

A COMPREHENSIVE LIFESTYLE APPROACH

Fifth Edition

Charles B. Corbin
Arizona State University

Gregory J. Welk
Iowa State University

Ruth Lindsey
California State University—Long Beach

William R. Corbin
Yale University

Boston   Burr Ridge, IL   Dubuque, IA   Madison, WI   New York   San Francisco   St. Louis
Bangkok   Bogotá   Caracas   Kuala Lumpur   Lisbon   London   Madrid   Mexico City
Milan   Montreal   New Delhi   Santiago   Seoul   Singapore   Sydney   Taipei   Toronto

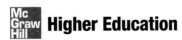

Higher Education

CONCEPTS OF FITNESS AND WELLNESS: A COMPREHENSIVE LIFESTYLE APPROACH, FIFTH EDITION

Published by McGraw-Hill, a business unit of The McGraw-Hill Companies, Inc., 1221 Avenue of the Americas, New York, NY 10020. Copyright © 2004, 2002, 2000, 1997, 1994 by The McGraw-Hill Companies, Inc. All rights reserved. No part of this publication may be reproduced or distributed in any form or by any means, or stored in a database or retrieval system, without the prior written consent of The McGraw-Hill Companies, Inc., including, but not limited to, in any network or other electronic storage or transmission, or broadcast for distance learning.

Some ancillaries, including electronic and print components, may not be available to customers outside the United States.

 This book is printed on recycled, acid-free paper containing 10% postconsumer waste.

Domestic   3 4 5 6 7 8 9 0 QPD/QPD 0 9 8 7 6 5 4

ISBN 0-07-255666-8

Vice president and editor-in-chief: *Thalia Dorwick*
Publisher: *Jane E. Karpacz*
Executive editor: *Vicki Malinee*
Senior developmental editor: *Michelle Turenne*
Senior marketing manager: *Pamela S. Cooper*
Project manager: *Christine Walker*
Production supervisor: *Enboge Chong*
Developmental editor for technology: *Lynda Huenefeld*
Media technology producer: *Lance Gerhart*
Design coordinator: *Mary Kazak*
Interior Design: *Ellen Pettengell*
Cover Design: *Asylum Studios*
Cover image: *Phillip & Karen Smith/ImageState*
Art editor: *Emma Ghiselli/Jennifer DeVere*
Photo research coordinator: *Alexandra Ambrose*
Senior supplement producer: *David A. Welsh*
Compositor: *Precision Graphics*
Typeface: *10/12 Janson*
Printer: *Quebecor World Dubuque, IA*

The credits section for this book begins on page C-1 and is considered an extension of the copyright page.

Library of Congress Cataloging-in-Publication Data

Concepts of fitness and wellness : a comprehensive lifestyle approach / Charles B. Corbin . . .
[et al.]. --5th ed.
    p. cm.
  Includes bibliographical references and index.
  ISBN 0-07-255666-8 (alk. paper) -- ISBN 0-07-121523-9 (alk. paper)
  1. Exercise. 2. Physical fitness. 3. Physical fitness--Problems, exercises, etc. I. Corbin,
Charles B.

RA781 .C644 2004
613.7--dc21   2003043209

The Internet addresses listed in the text were accurate at the time of publication. The inclusion of a website does not indicate an endorsement by the authors or McGraw-Hill, and McGraw-Hill does not guarantee the accuracy of the information presented at these sites.

www.mhhe.com

Contents

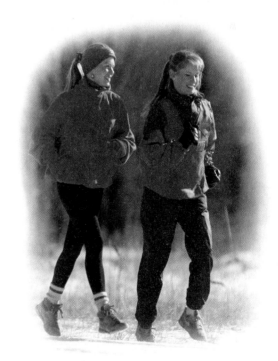

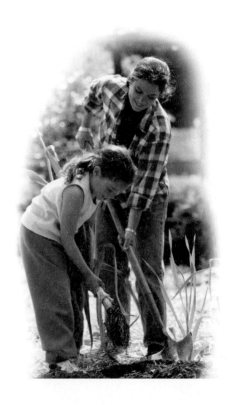

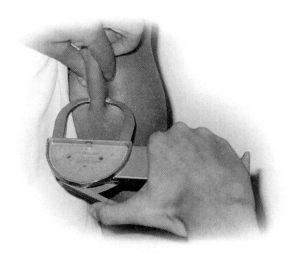

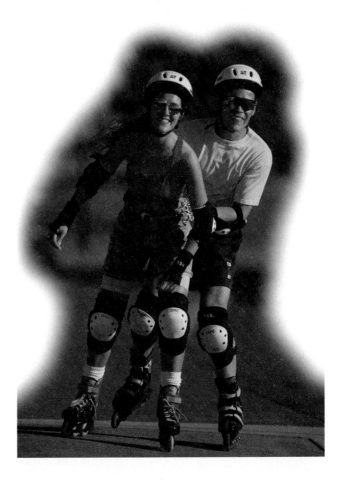

Section VII

Avoiding Destructive Behaviors 383

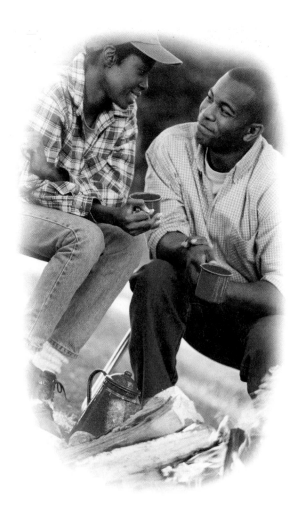

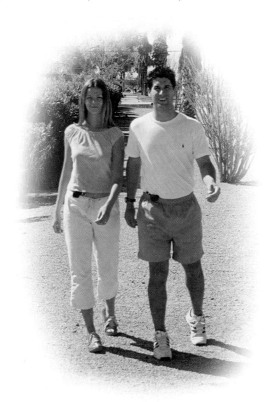

Preface

Fitness and Wellness: Evolving in the New Century

Although the fifth edition of *Concepts of Fitness and Wellness: A Comprehensive Lifestyle Approach* contains many of the same features that has made it so successful over the past thirty years, it also is considerably different. As you will see, the look of the book has evolved. The intent of the new design is to create an attractive look while incorporating several new pedagogical features.

Just as the look of the book has evolved, so has the authorship team. Greg Welk, because of his increased contribution, has been made second author. Will Corbin, the newest member of the team, has recently accepted an appointment in the Department of Psychology at Yale University. We think that the combination of older more experienced authors (Chuck Corbin and Ruth Lindsey) and younger energetic authors serves us well. The key is that each of the team members has different expertise allowing us to have expert and up-to-date coverage in all areas.

Our content continues to evolve as we learn more about fitness, wellness, and healthy lifestyles. In our early editions we focused on trying to get people fit and well. To be sure, fitness is an important product, as is wellness, another product of healthy lifestyle change. But scientific advances have shown that health, fitness, and wellness (all products) are not things you can "do" to people. You have to help people help themselves. Educating them and giving them the self-management skills that help them adopt healthy lifestyles can do this.

The focus of the new millennium is on the *process*. Healthy lifestyles, or what a person does, rather than what a person can do, constitutes process. If a person does the process (i.e., adopting a healthy lifestyle), positive changes will occur to the extent that change is possible for that specific person. As noted in the first concept of the book, lifestyles are the most important factors, influencing health, fitness, and wellness. Healthy lifestyles (the processes) are also within a person's individual control. *Any person* can benefit from lifestyle change, and any person can change a lifestyle. These lifestyle changes will make a difference in health, fitness, and wellness for all people.

The emphasis on lifestyle change in the fifth edition is consistent with the focus of national health objectives for the new millennium. Though the principal national health goals are to increase years and quality of life (products) for all people, the methods of accomplishing these goals focus on changing lifestyles. As we move into the new century, we must adopt a new way of thinking to help all people change their lifestyles to promote health, fitness, and wellness.

Our Basic Philosophy
The HELP Philosophy

Over time, the features of our book evolve. However the HELP philosophy on which the book is based remains sound. We believe that the "new way of thinking" based on the HELP philosophy serves us, the faculty who choose our book, and the students who use it. **H** is for *health*. Health and its positive component—wellness—are central to the philosophy. Health, fitness, and wellness are for all people. **E** is for *everyone*. **L** is for *lifetime lifestyle change*, and **P** is for *personal*. The goal is to HELP all people to make personal lifetime lifestyle changes that promote health, fitness, and wellness.

To assure that the book is consistent with the HELP philosophy and to be sure it is useful to everyone, we include discussions to adapt healthy lifestyles based on personal needs. Separate sections are *not* included for specific groups such as older people, women, ethnic groups, or those with special needs. Rather, we focus on healthy lifestyles *for all people* throughout the book.

Meeting Higher-Order Objectives

The "new way of thinking" based on the HELP philosophy suggests that each person must make decisions about healthy lifetime lifestyles if the goals of longevity and quality of life are to be achieved. What one person chooses may be quite different from what another chooses. Accordingly, our goal in preparing this edition is to help readers become good problem solvers and decision makers. Rather than focusing on telling them what to do, we offer information to help readers make informed choices about lifestyles. The stairway to lifetime fitness and wellness that we present helps readers understand the importance of "higher-order objectives" devoted to problem solving and decision making.

New Features

New features introduced in this fifth edition include the following.

New Content.   Every concept contains new content. New content highlights include the following.

- Concept 24 has been retitled "Cancer, Diabetes, and Other Health Threats" and revised to place greater emphasis on the discussion of cancer and how it spreads through the body. It provides additional information on some of the major types of cancer (breast, lung, prostate, colon-rectal, and skin). Revisions also include greater attention to diabetes and osteoporosis.
- Concept 26 also integrates new coverage of spirituality. This is presented in the context of physical, social, intellectual, work, and spiritual environments with suggestions for prayer, meditations, support, etc., rather than any emphasis on religiosity.
- In concept 16 the new Table 1 presents summary information on vitamins and minerals. Also, new Appendix E includes a table of fast food nutritive content values.
- Extensive new information on the environment and wellness.
- More coverage on the importance of social interactions to health and wellness.
- New information on health disparities.
- Additional information on self-management skills.
- Wind-chill chart based on new formula.
- New maximal heart rate formula.
- Material updated to new ACSM guidelines.
- Revised apparent temperature classifications.
- New information on HRT, HIV, and sedentary death syndrome.
- New information on dose response and exercise.
- New information on exercise and immune system.
- Swim test for cardiovascular fitness included.
- New information about micronutrients and new dietary intake terminology.
- Information on the healthy eating index and the glycemic index.
- New content on coping strategies, tobacco cessation, and strategies for dealing with alcohol problems.
- New information on food supplements.
- Several of the labs have been revised to provide easier organization for student completion. Two new labs include "Factors Influencing Fitness, Health, and Wellness" and "Evaluating Fast Food Options."

An All New Design.   As mentioned at the beginning of this preface, the fifth edition has a completely new design. The new design includes aesthetic features created with the intent of making the book attractive and pleasing to the eye. Some examples of these features include a new color scheme, new concept opener pages, new color tabs, new icons for various concept features, new lab format, and new presentation of the basic concept headers.

New Pedagogical Features of the Design.   While much of the new design was created to make the book look good, many of the features were created for educational reasons. For example, concepts within book sections are color coded as are Lab Resource Materials and tear out labs. Concept openers, labs, Lab Resource Materials, and exercise tables include color tabs that help students locate the materials they are looking for. Tables and charts are color-coded and have alternating bands to help students locate materials contained in them. Special features have an icon or logo with a special design and color code to make them easy to find. The tear-out labs can easily be identified by their unique color.

Online Labs.   The popular labs are now available online. To access the labs Visit the Online Learning Center at www.mhhe.com/corbin5e.

New Tables, Figures, and Photos.   More than 75 new tables, figures, and photos are included. Some of the figures and photos are done with a special treatment called text wrapping. This allows pictures to be integrated in the text. This method also helps us present complex information in an easy-to-understand way. Several new anatomical illustrations have been added.

Technology Today Features.   Over 20 new technology features are included in this fifth edition. These features describe technological advances relating to fitness, wellness, and healthy lifestyles. Examples include Global Positioning Systems, Heart Rate Watches, and Glucowatches.

In the News Features.   These features include information that is so current that much of it was added right before the book went to press.

New Web Materials.   Over the years we have prided ourselves on being current. We have provided Web icons in the book that allow students to access current information exclusively related to our book, as well as more generic information. Access to Web materials has been made easier by including the book Web address for the accompanying Online Learning Center at the top of each left hand page. As in the past, specific URLs appear in the body of the text as well as at the end of each concept.

Expanded Coverage for North America.   New statistics for all of North America have been added to those typically presented for the United States. Several Canadian websites have been included as have been new statistics, and a color version of the Canadian food guide is included.

Factual Updates.   As is true with all of our new editions, facts, statistics, references, and other information is updated throughout.

Deleted Content.· One of the problems that we have encountered over time has been the lengthening of the book because of the expansion of knowledge related to fitness, wellness, and health. In this edition, we made a conscious effort to cut words to save space and to allow new material to be added without lengthening the book. Also, the new design is more efficient allowing us to add new information.

Popular Continuing Features

The fifth edition retains many of the popular features that made the fourth edition so successful. Some of these features are as follows:

Pedagogically Sound Organization.   Planning and self-management strategies are presented early to familiarize students with basic principles and guidelines that will be used in later planning. Preparation strategies and basic activity principles follow. Each type of health-related fitness and the type of activity that promotes each component of fitness are included in the next section. This section is organized around the physical activity pyramid. Special considerations—including safe exercise, care of the back and neck, posture, and performance—are included in the next section. Other priority healthy lifestyles are the focus of nutrition, body composition, and stress management sections. The final section is designed to help students become good fitness, wellness, and health consumers.

Strategies for Action.   At the end of each concept, *strategies for action* are provided. These are suggestions for putting content into action. Many of these strategies require readers to perform or practice self-assessment or other self-management techniques.

Magazine Format.   The attractive new design supports student reading and studying with an appealing magazine format. This format has been shown to be educationally effective and has been well received by users.

Activity Features with Activity Labs.   Each of the exercises described in the book is contained in activity features using the magazine format. This format allows students to get immediately involved in activity and to keep activity logs. "Basic 8" tables feature easy to use exercises.

Web Icons.   The Web icons unique to this book allow learners to locate (at point of use) additional pictures, tables, and figures that illustrate concepts presented in the book. Web addresses to supplemental resource materials such as a self-study guide, sample exam questions, and definitions of terms, as well as other enrichment materials, are also provided on the Online Learning Center and in the Web Resources section at the end of each concept. The Web address for the Online Learning Center (www.mhhe.com/corbin5e) is included as a header at the top of each left facing page.

Attractive and Easy-to-Use Labs.   The attractive and popular labs are designed to get users involved in practicing self-management skills that will promote healthy lifestyle change. The labs are in a bright, attractive, and educationally effective format. They are easy to find and easy to use. In many cases, lab resource materials that aid the student in performing lab activities precede them. These resources are retained in the book even when the labs are torn out. This allows future use of such materials as fitness self-assessments. The physical activity labs are designed to get people active early in the course and ultimately to allow each user to plan his or her own personal activity program.

Focus on Self-Management Skills.   The educational effectiveness of a book depends on more than just presenting information. If lifestyle changes are to be implemented, there must be opportunities to learn how to make these changes. Research suggests that learning self-management skills is important to lifestyle change. A section on self-management skills is included early in the book, and additional discussions of how to practice and implement these skills is included throughout the book.

Health Goals for the Year 2010.   The health goals are based on the health goals for the new millennium (Health Goals for the Year 2010). These goals are provided at the beginning of each concept to help readers relate content to goals.

What's In This for You?   This student guide follows the Preface and is designed to help students use the features of the book more effectively. Instructors are encouraged to urge students to read this section prior to using the book.

Terms at Point-of-Use.   It greatly pleased us that the *Surgeon General's Report on Physical Activity and Health* adopted our physical fitness definitions in their report. Just as we have led the way in defining fitness, we now include state-of-the-art definitions related to wellness and quality of life. These—and all other definitions—are now included at the first point-of-use to make them easier to locate.

Continued Use of Conceptual Format.   We use concepts rather than chapters, and each concept contains factual statements that follow concise informational paragraphs. This tried-and-true method has proven to be educationally sound and well received by students and instructors.

Pedagogical Aids
Web Resources

Located at the end of every concept, additional websites are listed to provide students with additional online resources that supplements the content just learned.

Suggested Readings

Because students want to know more about a particular topic, a list of readings is given at the end of each chapter. Most suggested readings are readily available at bookstores or public libraries.

Appendices

Concepts of Fitness and Wellness: A Comprehensive Lifestyle Approach, fifth edition, includes six appendices that are valuable resources for the student. The metric conversion chart; metric conversions of selected charts and tables; calorie guide to common foods; calories of protein, carbohydrates, and fats in foods; calorie, fat, saturated fat, cholesterol, and sodium content of selected fast food items; and the Canadian food guide are included for your use.

Ancillaries
A Note for Instructors

As with past editions, you will see that we have updated this edition with the most recent scientific information. As noted earlier, we have included two new labs. We have designed experiences to promote higher-order thinking. There is another consideration we think to be important. As usual, we have worked to keep the price of the book low.

As always with our *Concepts* books, an extensive list of ancillary materials is available to help you provide the most effective instruction. Brief descriptions of these materials follow.

Instructor's Resource Materials
Course Integrator Guide

This manual includes all the features of a useful instructor's manual, such as learning objectives, suggested lecture outlines, suggested activities, media resources, and

Web links. It also integrates the text with all the health resources McGraw-Hill offers, such as the Online Learning Center, Image Presentation CD-ROM, HealthQuest CD-ROM, *Healthy Living* Video Clips CD-ROM, and the Health and Human Performances website, etc. The guide also includes references to relevant print and broadcast media. Instructors can access the guide at **www.mhhe.com/corbin5e.**

Computerized Test Bank CD-ROM

Brownstone's Computerized Testing is the most flexible, powerful, easy-to-use electronic testing program available in higher education. The Diploma system (for Windows users) allows the test maker to create a print version, an online version, (to be delivered to a computer lab), or an Internet version of each test. Diploma includes a built-in instructor gradebook, into which student rosters and files can be imported. The CD-ROM includes a separate testing program, Exam VI, for Macintosh users.

Image Presentation CD-ROM

The Image Presentation CD-ROM is an electronic library of visual resources. The CD-ROM comprises images from the test displayed in PowerPoint™, which allows the user to view, sort, search, use, and print catalog images. It also includes a complete, ready-to-use PowerPoint™ presentation, which allows users to play chapter-specific slideshows.

Instructional Videos

Video 1: Introduction to Physical Fitness.   This video includes a statement of fitness philosophy, a look at important fitness objectives, including the Stairway to Lifetime Fitness, and a description of the fitness tests included in the *Concepts* books. Test descriptions include estimated 1 RM for strength, the trunk rotation test for flexibility, and the curl-up test for muscular endurance. Other fitness test descriptions are also described. This video may be viewed by instructors or shown to students to help them understand the various tests. It has been proven popular with both students and instructors. The HELP philosophy is part of the flow of the video presentation of concepts.

Video 2: Introduction to Wellness.   This second instructional video defines wellness and puts wellness, health, and fitness in perspective for both students and instructors. The video helps establish common ground for the study of wellness. This proven video has helped provide the basic foundation for the study of wellness that is needed by many students.

Concepts Transparencies

Fifty-four color acetate transparencies illustrate anatomical and physiological concepts, and help instructors to describe the scientific concepts of physical fitness and health-related fitness.

Student Self-Assessment Materials

Fitsolve II Software. Fitsolve is educational software designed to facilitate the teaching of high-order physical fitness objectives such as self-evaluation, diagnosis, and problem-solving skills, which in turn enable the achievement of fitness independence, and a state of self-sufficiency in which individuals can design and implement their own fitness programs. Available for Windows.

Dietary Analysis Software. Available for Windows and Macintosh computers, this user-friendly diet analysis software allows students to track their food intake over a period of days and generate a variety of easy-to-read reports and graphs. The program tracks over thirty nutrient categories. Students can choose from nearly 8,000 foods or add their own to the database. Other features include a weight management function and a website devoted to diet analysis-related resources.

Internet Resources

Online Learning Center

 www.mhhe.com/corbin5e This website offers resources to students and instructors. It includes downloadable ancillaries, Web links, student quizzes, additional information on topics of interest, and more. Resources for the instructor include:

- Course Integrator Guide
- Downloadable PowerPoint Presentations
- Lecture outlines
- Discussion questions
- Concept summaries

Resources for the student include:

- Flashcards
- Online labs
- Interactive quizzes

Health and Human Performance Website

www.mhhe.com/hhp McGraw-Hill's Health and Human Performance Discipline Page provides a wide variety of information for instructors and students—including monthly articles that celebrate our diveristy, text ancillaries, a "how to" guide to technology, study tips, and athletic training exam preparation materials. It includes professional organization, convention, and career information, and information on how to become a McGraw-Hill author. Additional features of the website include:

- This Just In—This feature provides information on the latest hot topics, the best Web resources, and more—all updated monthly.
- Faculty Support—Access online course supplements, such as lecture outlines and PowerPoint™ presentations, and create your own website with PageOut!
- Student Success Center—Find online study guides and other resources to improve your academic performance. Explore scholarship opportunities and learn how to launch your career!
- Author Arena—Interested in writing a textbook or supplement for the college market? Read the McGraw-Hill proposal guidelines and links to the Editorial Marketing teams, and meet and converse with our current authors!

PageOut: The Course Website Development Center

www.pageout.net PageOut enables you to develop a website for your course. The site includes:

- A course home page
- An instructor home page
- A syllabus (interactive, customizable, and includes quizzing, instructor notes, and links to the Online Learning Center)
- Web links
- Discussions (multiple discussion areas per class)
- An online grade book
- Student Web pages
- Design templates

This program is now available to registered adopters of McGraw-Hill textbooks.

Primis Online

www.mhhe.com/primis/online Create content-rich textbooks, lab manuals, or readers right from our website. Choose the material you would like to include in your own customized book. A Primis e-book is a digital version of the text you created (and is sold directly to your students as a downloadable file to their computer, or it may be accessed online by a password). And Primis Online customized books are affordable for your students. Visit our website for further information.

Interactive CD-ROMs

HealthQuest *CD-ROM.* *HealthQuest* is designed to help students explore the behavioral aspects of personal health and wellness through a state-of-the-art interactive CD-ROM. Your students will be able to assess their current health and wellness status, determine their health risks, and explore options and make decisions to improve the behaviors that impact their health.

Interactive Personal Trainer CD-ROM. The Interactive Personal Trainer CD-ROM provides users with a variety of features. First, self-assessments for all parts of health-related fitness are provided. Still pictures and Quick-Time™ movies illustrate the assessments, and written statements describe each one. Second, a fitness profile allows users to input assessment results to get a rating profile. In many cases (e.g., skinfolds), calculations are made automatically. Third, physical activities and exercises are provided for each part of fitness and for care of the back and good posture. Users can select exercises for any part of fitness or for different body parts and get descriptions, still pictures, and real-time videos of each. Finally, pictures and descriptions of risky exercises are provided, followed by descriptions and real-time movies of appropriate alternatives. The CD-ROM is available in either Windows or Mac versions. Instructors may encourage use on a computer accessible to students.

Print Publications

Diet and Fitness Log by McGraw-Hill. This logbook helps students keep track of their diet and exercise programs, and it serves as a diary to help students log their behaviors.

Acknowledgments

The evolution of this book would not have been possible without the input of those who have used the book and those who have provided us with reviews. At the risk of inadvertently failing to mention someone, we want to acknowledge the following people for their role in the development of this book.

First, we would like to acknowledge a few people who have made special contributions over the years. Linus Dowell, Carl Landiss, and Homer Tolson, all of Texas A & M University, were involved in the development of the first *Concepts* book, and their contributions were also important as we helped start the fitness movement in the 1960s.

Other pioneers were Jimmy Jones of Henderson State University, who started one of the first *Concepts* classes in 1970 and has led the way in teaching fitness in the years that have followed; Charles Erickson, who started a quality program at Missouri Western; and Al Lesiter, a leader in the East at Mercer Community College in New Jersey. David Laurie and Barbara Gench (now at Texas Women's University) at Kansas State University, as well as others on that faculty, were instrumental in developing a prototype concepts program, which research has shown to be successful.

A special thanks is extended to Andy Herrick and Jim Whitehead, who have contributed to much of the development of various editions of the book, including excellent suggestions for change. Mark Ahn, Keri Chesney, Chris MacCrate, Guy Mullin, Stephen Hustedde, Greg Nigh, Doreen Mauro, Marc vanHorne, along with other employees of the Consortium for Instructional Innovation and the Micro Computer Resource Facility at Arizona State University, and Betty Craft and Ken Rudich and other employees at the Distance Learning Technology Program at Arizona State University, deserve special recognition.

Second, we wish to extend thanks to the following people who provided comments for the current editions of our *Concepts* books: Virginia L. Hicks, Unviersity of Wisconsin at Whitewater; Jon Kolb, University of Calgary; J. Dirk Nelson, LeTourneau University (TX); and Patricia A. Zezula, Huntington College (IN).

Third, we want to acknowledge the following people who have aided us in t he preparation of past editions: Craig Koppelman, University of Central Arkansas; Robert W. Rausch, Jr., Westfield State College; Amy P. Richardson, University of Central Arkansas; Terry R. Tabor, University of North Florida; Sharon Rifkin, Broward Community College; William B. Karper, University of North Carolina at Greensboro; Larry E. Knuth, Rio Hondo College; Maridy Troy, University of Alabama at Tuscaloosa; Kenneth L. Cameron, United States Military Academy at West Point; Thomas E. Temples, North Georgia College & State University; Bridget Cobb, Armstrong Atlantic State University; Tillman (Chuck) Williams, Southwest Missouri State University; Mary Jeanne Kuhar, Central Oregon Community College; Jennifer L. H. Lechner, St. Petersburg Junior College; Laura Switzer, Southwestern Oklahoma State University; Robert L. Slevin, Towson University; Karen (Pea) Poole, University of North Carolina at Greensboro; Paul Downing, Towson University; David Horton, Liberty University; Lindy S. Pickard, Broward Community College; Laura L. Borsdorf, Ursinus College; Frederick C. Surgent, Frostsburg State University; James A. Gemar, Moorhead State University; Vincent Angotti, Towson University; Judi Phillips, Del Mar College; Joseph Donnelly, Montclair State University; Harold L. Rainwater, Asbury College; Candi D. Ashley, University of South Florida; Dennis Docheff, United States Military Academy; Robin Hoppenworth, Wartburg College; Linda Farver, Liberty University; Peter Rehor, Montana State University; Martin W. Johnson, Mayville State University; Keri Lewis, North Carolina State University; J. D. Parsley, University of St. Thomas; Marika Botha, Lewis-Clark State College; Robert J. Mravetz, University of Akron; Debra A. Beal, Northern Essex Community College; Roger Bishop, Wartburg College; David S. Brewster, Indiana State University; Ronnie Carda, University of Wisconsin—Madison; Curt W. Cattau, Concordia University; Cindy Ekstedt Connelley, Catawaba College; J. Ellen Eason, Towson State University; Bridgit A. Finley, Oklahoma City Community College; Diane Sanders Flickner,

Bethel College; Judy Fox, Indiana Wesleyan University; Earlene Hannah, Hendrix College; Carole J. Hanson, University of Northern Iowa; John Merriman, Valdosta State College; Beverly F. Mitchell, Kennesaw State College; George Perkins, Northwestern State University; James J. Sheehan, Fitchburg State College; Mary Slaughter, University of Illinois; Paul H. Todd, Polk Community College; Susan M. Todd, Vancouver Community College—Langara Campus; Kenneth E. Weatherman, Floyd College; Newton Wilkes, Bridget Cobb, John Dippel, and Todd Kleinfelter of Northwestern State University of Louisiana and John R. Webster, Central Connecticut State University. A special thanks is extended to Patty Williams, Ann Woodard, Laurel Smith, Bill Carr (Polk Community College), James Angel, Jeanne Ashley, Stanley Brown, Ronnie Carda, Robert Clayton, Melvin Ezell Jr., Brigit Finley, Pay Floyd, Carole Hanson, James Harvey, John Hayes, David Horton, Sister Janice Iverson, Tony Jadin, Richard Krejei, Ron Lawman, James Marett, Pat McSwegin, Betty McVaigh, John Merriman, Beverly Mitchell, Sandra Morgan, Robert Pugh, Larry Reagan, Mary Rice, Roberts Stokes, Paul Tood, Susan Todd, Marjorie Avery Willard, Karen Cookson, Dawn Strout, Earlene Hannah, Ken Weatherman, J. Ellen Eason, William Podoll, John Webster, James Shebban, David Brewster, Kelly Adam, Lisa Hibbard, Roger Bishop, Mary Slaughter, Jack Clayton Stovall, Karen Watkins, Ruth Cohoon, Mark Bailey, Nena Amundson, Bruce Wilson, Sarah Collie, Carl Beal, George Perkins, Stan Rettew, Ragene Gwin, Judy Fox, Diane Flickner, Cindy Connelley, Curt Cattau, Don Torok, and Dennis Wilson.

Finally we want to acknowledge others who have contributed, including Virginia Atkins, Charles Cicciarella, Donna Landers, Susan Miller, Robert Pangrazi, Karen Ward, Darl Waterman, and Weimo Zhu. Among other important contributors are former graduate students who have contributed ideas, made corrections, and contributed in other untold ways to the success of these books. We wish to acknowledge Jeff Boone, Laura Borsdorf, Lisa Chase, Tom Cuddihy, Darren Dale, Bo Fernhall, Ken Fox, Connie Fye, Louie Garcia, Steve Feyrer-Melk, Sarah Keup, Guy LeMasurier, Kirk Rose, Jack Rutherford, Cara Sidman, Scott Slava, Dave Thomas, Min Qui Wang, Jim Whitehead, Bridgette Wilde, and Ashley Woodcock.

Author Acknowledgments

A very special thanks goes to David E. Corbin of the University of Nebraska at Omaha and Karen Welk of Ames, Iowa. Dr. Corbin is a health educator who has provided valuable assistance. Karen is a physical therapist who advised us concerning correct performance of the exercises in the book. We also want to thank Ron Hager and Lynda Ransdell for their assistance with the development of the Web resources and the development of the test bank materials for past editions and to Cara Sidman for developing the current test bank materials.

We would like to thank two excellent students—George Ritz, who provided excellent proofreading, and Tony Ericson, who assisted with locating valuable references. A special thanks goes to Jodi Hickman who spent many hours researching photos for this book and developed the index.

Finally, we would like to thank all past editors (there have been many) and our current editors Michelle Turenne, Christine Walker, and Vicki Malinee who do the tedious jobs that make these excellent books possible.

What's in This for You?

Students, are you looking for fitness and wellness information online? Working hard to get in shape? Trying to improve your grade? All the features in *Concepts of Fitness and Wellness: A Comprehensive Lifestyle Approach* will help you do this and more! Take a look....

Concept Statement

A concept statement is included at the beginning of each Concept. The content elaborates and expands on each concept statement.

Health Goals

The content of each concept is designed to help you meet national health goals outlined in Healthy People 2010.

Technology Update

The Technology Update features include information about a technological innovation that is related to the content of the concept.

Good health, wellness, fitness, and healthy lifestyles are important for all people.

Health Goals
for the year 2010

- Increase quality and years of healthy life.
- Eliminate health disparities.
- Increase incidence of people reporting "healthy days."
- Increase access to health information and services for all people.

National Health Goals

 t the beginning of each concept in this book is a section containing abbreviated statements of the national health goals from the document *Healthy People 2010: National Health Promotion and Disease Prevention Objectives.* These statements, established by expert groups representing more than 350 national organizations, are intended as realistic national health goals to be achieved by the year 2010. These objectives for the first decade of the new millennium are intended to improve the health of those in the United States, but they seem important for all people in North America and in other industrialized cultures throughout the world. The health objectives are designed to contribute to the current World Health Organization strategy of "Health for All." This book is written with the achievement of these important health goals in mind.

Introduction

www.mhhe.com/fit_well/web01 Click 01. The first national health goals were developed in 1979 to be accomplished by the year 1990. The focus of those objectives was on reduction in the death rate among infants, children, adolescents, young adults, and adults. Except for reducing death rates among adolescents, those goals were met and the average life expectancy was increased by more than two years by the 1990s. Those first national health objectives gave way to the *Healthy People 2000* objectives designed to be accomplished by the turn of the

century. The emphasis in these objectives shifted from reduction in premature death to disease prevention and health promotion. While many of these objectives have been achieved, others have yet to be accomplished.

For *Healthy People 2010*, achieving the vision of "healthy people in healthy communities" is paramount. Two central goals have been established. First, the goals emphasize quality of life, well-being, and functional capacity—all important wellness considerations. This emphasis is based on the World Health Organization statement that "It is counterproductive to evaluate development of programs without considering their impact on the quality of life of the community. We can no longer maintain strict, artificial divisions between physical and mental well-being" (World Health Organization, 1995). Second, the national health goals for 2010 take the "bold step" of trying to "eliminate" health disparities as opposed to reducing them. Consistent with national health goals for the new millennium, this book is designed to aid all people in adopting healthy lifestyles that will allow them to achieve lifetime health, fitness, and wellness.

Technology Update

This book provides a number of ways to help you access reliable health and wellness information from the Internet. The *On the Web* icons throughout the book include URLs that will provide additional information and links to informative sites on the Internet. The list of *Web Resources* at the end of each concept provide URLs for various organizations that provide high-quality health information. The *On the Web* and *Web Resources* features can be accessed electronically (without typing the URL) by visiting the Online Learning Center address that is featured at the top of every even numbered page of the book. This site also includes a number of study aids including concept outlines, concept terms, and sample quiz questions to help you apply the information in the book.

Health and Wellness

Good health is of primary importance to adults in our society. When polled about important social values, 99 percent of adults in the United States identified "being in good **health**" as one of their major concerns. Two other concerns expressed most often were good family life and good self-image. The 1 percent who did

---

Benign Tumor A slow-growing tumor that does not spread to other parts of the body.

Malignant Tumor Malignant means "growing worse." A malignant tumor is one that is considered to be cancerous and will spread throughout the body if not treated.

Carcinoma A malignant or invasive form of tumor.

Metastases The spread of cancer cells to other parts of the body.

Biopsy Removal of a tissue sample that can be checked for cancer cells.

Mammogram An x-ray of the breast.

Definition Boxes

All terms that are bold in your book are defined in an accompanying definition box to reinforce this information.

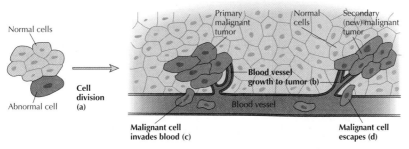

Figure 1 ► The spread of cancer (metastasis).

to take a **biopsy** of suspicious lumps in the breasts, testicles, or other parts of the body.

Cancer is a leading killer in our society. www.mhhe.com/fit_well/web24 Click 01. Cancer is the second leading cause of death in our society. One of every four deaths in the United States is caused by some form of cancer. Slightly more than one in three women

screening. Like colon-rectal and lung cancers, breast cancer is most prevalent among African Americans and least prevalent among Asians and Hispanics (more than twice as frequent).

Symptoms include lumps and/or thickening or swelling of the breasts. In many cases, lumps or tumors are present before they can be detected with self-exams. This is one reason for regular **mammograms** (breast x-

On the Web

Web icons appear to indicate supplemental materials that are available on the web. Look for the icons throughout your book. To access the information, simply type the Web address provided next to the icon and you will be taken directly to the supplementary information.

Strategies for Action

A self-assessment of risk factors can help you modify your lifestyle to reduce risk of heart disease. www.mhhe.com/fit_well/web06 Click 10. The Heart Disease Risk Factor Questionnaire in Lab 6A will help you assess your personal risk for heart disease. While this questionnaire considers the major risk factors, several recently identified factors are not included: C-reactive protein (CRP) homocysteine, an enzyme called MPO, and a substance called interleukin-6. Women with high CRP have four times the risk of having heart disease as those with low CRP. Used along with other blood tests, the CRP may prove to be useful in the future. Screening for CRP is currently available with regular blood lipid tests though data are lacking for men.

High levels of the amino acid homocysteine have also been associated with increased risk of heart disease

though the American Heart Association says it is too soon to do general screening for it. Adequate folic acid, vitamin B6, and vitamin B12 help prevent high homocysteine in the blood, so eating foods that insure adequate daily intake of these vitamins is recommended.

Both MPO and interleukin-6 are elevated in people with known heart disease and are associated with inflammation. They may damage artery walls causing fat build-up. Because evidence is only preliminary at this point, these four risk factors are not included in this questionnaire.

You can use your self-assessments on the questionnaire to determine your alterable, unalterable, and total risk scores. These scores should be useful in preparing a plan for lifestyle change to reduce risk.

Web Resources

American Cancer Society www.cancer.org
American Diabetes Association www.diabetes.org
American Heart Association www.americanheart.org
Canadian Diabetes Association www.diabetes.ca
Centers for Disease Control and Prevention www.cdc.gov
Healthy People 2010 www.health.gov/healthypeople
National Stroke Association www.stroke.org
National Osteoporosis Foundation www.nof.org

Suggested Readings

Additional reference materials for concept 6 are available at www.mhhe.com/fit_well/web06 Click 11.

Blair, S. N. 2001. Guest editorial to accompany physical fitness and activity as separate heart disease risk-factors. *Medicine and Science in Sports and Exercise* 33(5):762–764.
Booth, F. W., and M. W. Chakravarthy. 2002. Cost and consequences of sedentary living: New battleground for an old enemy. *President's Council on Physical Fitness and Sports Research Digest* 3(16):1–8.
Booth, F. W. et al. 2000. Waging war on modern chronic diseases: Primary prevention through exercise biology. *Journal of Applied Physiology* 88(2):774-787.
Brehm, B. A. 2000. Maximizing the psychological benefits of physical activity. *ACSM's Health and Fitness Journal* 4(6):7–11.
Brill, P. A. et al. 2000. Muscular strength and physical function. *Medicine and Science in Sports and Exercise* 32(2):412–416.
Chitnaadilok, J., and D. T. Lowenthal. 2002. Exercise in treating hypertension. *Physician and Sports Medicine* 30(3):11–28.
Colberg, S. R. 2001. Exercise: A diabetes "cure" for many. *ACSM's Health and Fitness Journal* 5(2):20–26.
Cotman, C. W., and C. Engesser-Cesar. 2002. Exercise enhances and protects brain function. *Exercise and Sport Sciences Reviews* 30(2):75–79.
Cooper, C. B. 2001. Diabetes mellitus and exercise. *ACSM's Health and Fitness Journal* 5(4):27–28.
Dembo, L., and K. M. McCormick. 2000. Exercise prescription to prevent osteoporosis. *ACSM's Health and Fitness Journal* 4(1):32–38.
Drezner, J. A., and S. A. Herring. 2001. Managing low back pain. *Physician and Sports Medicine* 29(8):37–43.
Durak, E. 2001. The use of exercise in the cancer recovery process. *ACSM's Health and Fitness Journal* 5(1):6–10.
Friedenreich, C. M. et al. 2001. Relation between intensity of physical activity and breast cancer risk reduction. *Medicine and Science in Sports and Exercise* 33(9):1538–1545.
Friedland, R. P. 2001. Activity and Alzheimer's. *Proceedings of the National Academy of Sciences* 98:3440–3445.
Lee, I. M., and S. N. Blair. 2002. Cardiorespiratory fitness and stroke mortality in men. *Medicine and Science in Sports and Exercise* 34(4):592–595.

Hyperkinetic Condition A disease/illness or health condition caused by or contributed to by too much physical activity.

Illustration Program

Concept 24 has been revised to place greater emphasis on the discussion of cancer and how it spreads though the body. Instructional full-color illustrations and photographs here and throughout the book enhance learning with an exciting visual appeal.

Strategies for Action

Located toward the end of each concept, these these strategies provide information and suggest Labs that can help promote self-management skills to achieve your healthy lifestyle goals.

Web Resources and Suggested Readings

At the end of each concept, URLs help you find quality online resources. Recent references are provided to help you read more about current topics.

Online Learning Center Resources

Want a better grade? This address appears throughout to remind you about the study aids and other resources available at our free Online Learning Center.

Tear-Out Labs

These are located at the end of each concept, and are designed to help you improve your skills to achieve a healthy lifestyle.

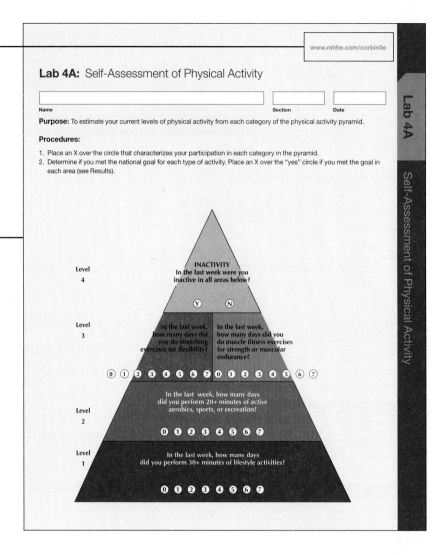

Lab 4A: Self-Assessment of Physical Activity

Name   Section   Date

Purpose: To estimate your current levels of physical activity from each category of the physical activity pyramid.

Procedures:

1. Place an X over the circle that characterizes your participation in each category in the pyramid.
2. Determine if you met the national goal for each type of activity. Place an X over the "yes" circle if you met the goal in each area (see Results).

Level 4

INACTIVITY
In the last week were you inactive in all areas below?

Ⓨ Ⓝ

Level 3

In the last week, how many days did you do stretching exercises for flexibility?

In the last week, how many days did you do muscle fitness exercises for strength or muscular endurance?

⓪ ① ② ③ ④ ⑤ ⑥ ⑦ ⓪ ① ② ③ ④ ⑤ ⑥ ⑦

Level 2

In the last week, how many days did you perform 20+ minutes of active aerobics, sports, or recreation?

⓪ ① ② ③ ④ ⑤ ⑥ ⑦

Level 1

In the last week, how many days did you perform 30+ minutes of lifestyle activities?

⓪ ① ② ③ ④ ⑤ ⑥ ⑦

Health, Wellness, Fitness, and Healthy Lifestyles: An Introduction

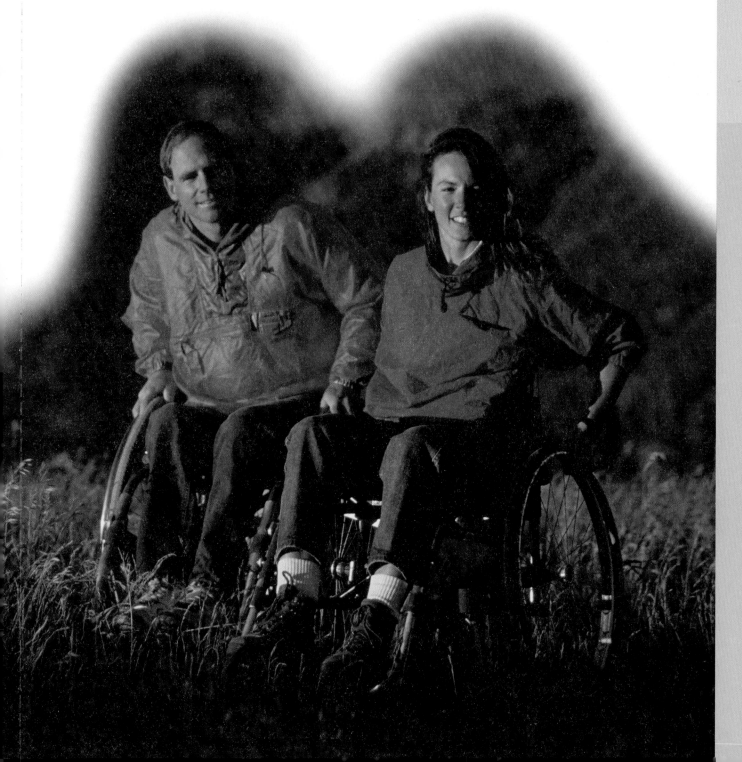

Good health, wellness, fitness, and healthy lifestyles are important for all people.

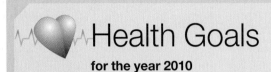

Health Goals

for the year 2010

- Increase quality and years of healthy life.
- Eliminate health disparities.
- Increase incidence of people reporting "healthy days."
- Increase access to health information and services for all people.

National Health Goals

At the beginning of each concept in this book is a section containing abbreviated statements of the national health goals from the document *Healthy People 2010: National Health Promotion and Disease Prevention Objectives.* These statements, established by expert groups representing more than 350 national organizations, are intended as realistic national health goals to be achieved by the year 2010. These objectives for the first decade of the new millennium are intended to improve the health of those in the United States, but they seem important for all people in North America and in other industrialized cultures throughout the world. The health objectives are designed to contribute to the current World Health Organization strategy of "Health for All." This book is written with the achievement of these important health goals in mind.

Introduction

 www.mhhe.com/fit_well/web01 Click 01. The first national health goals were developed in 1979 to be accomplished by the year 1990. The focus of those objectives was on reduction in the death rate among infants, children, adolescents, young adults, and adults. Except for reducing death rates among adolescents, those goals were met and the average life expectancy was increased by more than two years by the 1990s. Those first national health objectives gave way to the *Healthy People 2000* objectives designed to be accomplished by the turn of the

century. The emphasis in these objectives shifted from reduction in premature death to disease prevention and health promotion. While many of these objectives have been achieved, others have yet to be accomplished.

For *Healthy People 2010,* achieving the vision of "healthy people in healthy communities" is paramount. Two central goals have been established. First, the goals emphasize quality of life, well-being, and functional capacity—all important wellness considerations. This emphasis is based on the World Health Organization statement that "It is counterproductive to evaluate development of programs without considering their impact on the quality of life of the community. We can no longer maintain strict, artificial divisions between physical and mental well-being" (World Health Organization, 1995). Second, the national health goals for 2010 take the "bold step" of trying to "eliminate" health disparities as opposed to reducing them. Consistent with national health goals for the new millennium, this book is designed to aid all people in adopting healthy lifestyles that will allow them to achieve lifetime health, fitness, and wellness.

Technology Update

This book provides a number of ways to help you access reliable health and wellness information from the Internet. The *On the Web* icons throughout the book include URLs that will provide additional information and links to informative sites on the Internet. The list of *Web Resources* at the end of each concept provide URLs for various organizations that provide high-quality health information. The *On the Web* and *Web Resources* features can be accessed electronically (without typing the URL) by visiting the Online Learning Center address that is featured at the top of every even numbered page of the book. This site also includes a number of study aids including concept outlines, concept terms, and sample quiz questions to help you apply the information in the book.

Health and Wellness

Good health is of primary importance to adults in our society. When polled about important social values, 99 percent of adults in the United States identified "being in good **health**" as one of their major concerns. Two other concerns expressed most often were good family life and good self-image. The 1 percent who did

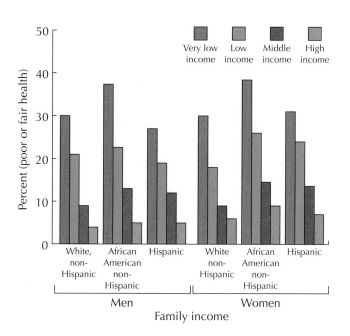

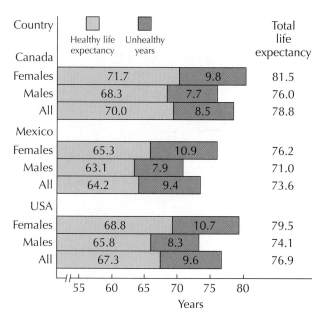

Figure 1 ▶ Fair or poor health among adults 18 and over by income, gender, and family origin.

Note: Percents are adjusted.

Source: Centers for Disease Control and Prevention.

Figure 2 ▶ Healthy life expectancy for North America.

Sources: World Health Organization & National Center for Health Statistics

not identify good health as an important concern had no opinion on any social issues. Among those polled, none felt that good health was unimportant. Results of surveys in Canada and other Western nations show similar commitments to good health.

Health varies greatly with income, gender, age, and family origin. Reducing health disparities among adults over eighteen is a major national health goal. We have some distance to go in accomplishing this goal because health varies widely depending on income, gender, age, and family origin. Self-ratings of health have been shown to be good general indicators of health status. When asked to rate health as excellent, good, fair, or poor, more than a few adults indicated that their health was only fair or poor (see Figure 1). It is evident that many more people in poor or near-poor income groups are considered to be fair or poor in health as opposed to good or excellent. African Americans and Hispanics are more often classified as fair or poor in health than white non-Hispanics. Minority women are also likely to be classified as fair or poor in health. Though not indicated in Figure 1, there is good evidence that older adults are especially likely to report poor health and wellness. An important national health goal is to increase the number of **healthy days** people have each month.

🌐 **Increasing the span of healthy life is a principal health goal.** www.mhhe.com/fit_well/web01 **Click 02.** The principal public health goal of Western

nations is to increase the healthy life span of all individuals. During this century, the life expectancy for the average person has increased by 60 percent. Currently, life expectancy is at a record high of nearly 76.9 years for all races in the United States. Among Whites, life expectancy is 77.4 years as opposed to 71.8 for African Americans. As illustrated in Figure 2, women live longer than men. Depending on where you live, males can expect 63 to 68 years of healthy life and females 65 to 72. For an average person, approximately 8 to 11 years of the total life span is considered as "unhealthy" or lacking in quality of life. Diseases and illnesses often associated with poor health limit the length of life and contribute to poor quality of life.

Health is more than freedom from illness and disease. Over fifty years ago, the World Health Organization defined health as being more than freedom from illness, disease, and debilitating conditions. In recent years, public

Health Health is optimal well-being that contributes to one's quality of life. It is more than freedom from disease and illness though freedom from disease is important to good health. Optimal health includes high-level mental, social, emotional, spiritual, and physical wellness within the limits of one's heredity and personal abilities.

Healthy Days A self-rating of the number of days (per week or month) a person considers himself or herself to be in good or better than good health.

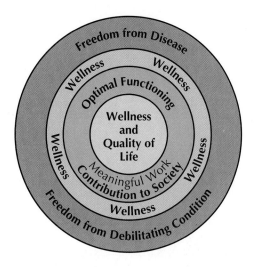

Figure 3 ► A model of optimal health including wellness.

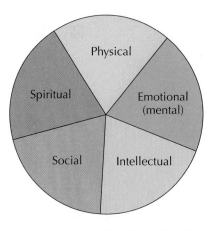

Figure 4 ► The dimensions of health and wellness.

health experts have identified **wellness** as "a sense of well-being" and **"quality of life."** *Healthy People 2010* objectives use the term health-related quality of life to describe the personal sense of physical and mental health as well as the general sense of happiness and satisfaction with life.

Many illnesses are manageable and have only limited effect on total health. Many **illnesses** are curable and may have only a temporary effect on health. Others, such as diabetes, are not curable but can be managed with proper eating, physical activity, and sound medical supervision. It should be noted that those possessing manageable conditions may be more at risk for other health problems, so proper management is essential. For example, unmanaged diabetes is associated with high risk for heart disease and other health problems.

Wellness is the positive component of optimal health. Death, disease, illness, and debilitating conditions are negative components that detract from optimal health. Death is the ultimate opposite of optimal health. Disease, illness, and debilitating conditions obviously detract from optimal health. Wellness has been recognized as the positive component of optimal health as evidenced by a sense of well-being reflected in optimal functioning, health-related quality of life, meaningful work, and a contribution to society (see Figure 3). Wellness allows the expansion of one's potential to live and work effectively and to make a significant contribution to society.

Health and wellness are multidimensional. The dimensions of health and wellness include the emotional (mental), intellectual, social, spiritual, and physical. Figure 4 illustrates the importance of each dimension to total wellness. Throughout this book, references will be

made to these wellness dimensions (see Table 1) to help reinforce their importance.

Wellness reflects how one feels about life as well as one's ability to function effectively. A positive total outlook on life is essential to wellness and each of the wellness dimensions. A "well" person is satisfied in work, is spiritually fulfilled, enjoys leisure time, is physically fit, is socially involved, and has a positive emotional-mental outlook. This person is happy and fulfilled. Many experts believe that a positive total outlook is a key to wellness (see Table 2).

The way one perceives each of the dimensions of wellness affects total outlook. Researchers use the term *self-perceptions* to describe these feelings. Many researchers believe that self-perceptions about wellness are more important than actual ability. For example, a person who has an important job may find less meaning and job satisfaction than another person with a much less important job. Apparently, one of the important factors for a person who has achieved high-level wellness and a positive outlook on life is the ability to reward himself/herself. Some people, however, seem unable to give themselves credit for their successes. The development of a system that allows a person to perceive the self positively is important. Of course, the adoption of positive **lifestyles** that encourage improved self-perceptions is also important. The questionnaire in the Lab 1A will help you assess your self-perceptions of the various wellness dimensions. For optimal wellness, it would be important to find positive feelings about each dimension.

Health and wellness are integrated states of being. The segmented pictures of health and wellness shown in Figure 5 and Table 2 are used only to illustrate the multidimensional nature of health and wellness. In reality, health, and its positive component (wellness), is an integrated

Table 1 ▶ Definitions of Health and Wellness Dimensions

Emotional-mental health—A person with emotional health is (1) free from emotional/mental-illnesses or debilitating conditions such as clinical depression and (2) possesses emotional wellness. The goals for the nation's health refer to mental rather than emotional health and wellness. In this book, mental health and wellness are considered to be the same as emotional health and wellness.

Emotional/mental wellness—Emotional wellness is a person's ability to cope with daily circumstances and to deal with personal feelings in a positive, optimistic, and constructive manner. A person with emotional wellness is generally characterized as happy instead of depressed.

Intellectual health—A person with intellectual health is free from illnesses that invade the brain and other systems that allow learning. A person with intellectual health also possesses intellectual wellness.

Intellectual wellness—Intellectual wellness is a person's ability to learn and to use information to enhance the quality of daily living and optimal functioning. A person with intellectual wellness is generally characterized as informed instead of ignorant.

Physical health—A person with physical health is free from illnesses that affect the physiological systems of the body such as the heart and the nervous system. A person with physical health possesses an adequate level of physical fitness and physical wellness.

Physical wellness—Physical wellness is a person's ability to function effectively in meeting the demands of the day's work and to use free time effectively. Physical wellness includes good physical fitness and the possession of useful motor skills. A person with physical wellness is generally characterized as fit instead of unfit.

Social health—A person with social health is free from illnesses or conditions that severely limit functioning in society, including antisocial pathologies.

Social wellness—Social wellness is a person's ability to interact with others successfully and to establish meaningful relationships that enhance the quality of life for all people involved in the interaction (including self). A person with social wellness is generally characterized as involved instead of lonely.

Spiritual health—Spiritual health is the one component of health that is totally comprised of the wellness dimension; for this reason, spiritual health is considered to be synonymous with spiritual wellness.

Spiritual wellness—Spiritual wellness is a person's ability to establish a values system and act on the system of beliefs, as well as to establish and carry out meaningful and constructive lifetime goals. Spiritual wellness is often based on a belief in a force greater than the individual that helps one contribute to an improved quality of life for all people. A person with spiritual wellness is generally characterized as fulfilled instead of unfulfilled.

Table 2 ▶ The Dimensions of Wellness

–	Wellness Dimensions	+
Depressed	Emotional-mental	Happy
Ignorant	Intellectual	Informed
Unfit	Physical	Fit
Lonely	Social	Involved
Unfulfilled	Spiritual	Fulfilled
Negative	Total outlook	Positive

state of being that is best depicted as many threads that can be woven together to produce a larger, integrated fabric. Each specific dimension relates to each of the others and overlaps all others. The overlap is so frequent and so great that the specific contribution of each thread is almost indistinguishable when looking at the total (Figure 5). The total is clearly greater than the sum of the parts.

Health and wellness are individual in nature. Each individual is different from all others. Health and wellness depend on each person's individual characteristics. Making comparisons to other people on specific individual characteristics may produce feelings of inadequacy that detract from one's profile of total health and wellness. Each of us has personal limitations and personal strengths. Focusing on strengths and learning to accommodate weaknesses are essential keys to optimal health and wellness.

Wellness Wellness is the integration of many different components (social, emotional-mental, spiritual, and physical) that expand one's potential to live (quality of life) and work effectively and to make a significant contribution to society. Wellness reflects how one feels (a sense of well-being) about life as well as one's ability to function effectively. Wellness, as opposed to illness (a negative), is sometimes described as the positive component of good health.

Quality of Life A term used to describe wellness. An individual with quality of life can enjoyably do the activities of life with little or no limitation and can function independently. Individual quality of life requires a pleasant and supportive community.

Illness Illness is the ill feeling and/or symptoms associated with a disease or circumstances that upset homeostasis.

Lifestyles Lifestyles are patterns of behavior or ways an individual typically lives.

P = Physical   I = Intellectual   Sp = Spiritual
S = Social   E = Emotional

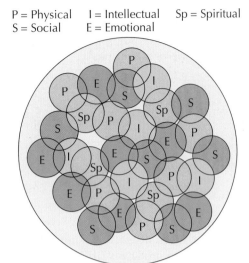

Figure 5 ▶ The integration of wellness dimensions.

It is possible to possess wellness while being ill or possessing a debilitating condition. All people can benefit from enhanced wellness. Wellness and an improved quality of life are possible for everyone, regardless of disease states. Evidence is accumulating to indicate that people with a positive outlook are better able to resist the progress of disease and illness than those with a negative outlook. Thinking positive thoughts has been associated with enhanced results from various medical treatments and better results from surgical procedures.

Because self-perceptions are important to wellness, positive perceptions of self are especially important to the wellness of people with disease, illness, and disability. The concepts of wellness and optimal health must be considered in light of one's heredity and personal disabilities and disease states.

Figure 6 illustrates the fact that the most desirable condition is buoyant health (*a*) including freedom from illness and a high level of wellness. However, a person with a physical illness but who possesses a good wellness (*b*) has a better overall health status than a person with no illness but poor wellness (*c*).

🌐 **Wellness is a useful term that may be used by quacks as well as experts. www.mhhe.com/ fit_well/web01 Click 03.** Unfortunately, some individuals and groups have tried to identify wellness with products and services that promise benefits that cannot be documented. Because well-being is a subjective feeling that is hard to document, it is easy for quacks to make claims of improved wellness for their product or service without facts to back them up.

Holistic health is a term that is similarly abused. Optimal health includes many areas, thus the term *holistic* (total) is appropriate. In fact, the word *health* originates from a root word meaning "wholeness." Unfortunately, many quacks include their questionable health practices under the guise of holistic health. Care should be used when considering services and products that make claims of wellness and/or holistic health to be sure that they are legitimate.

Physical Fitness

Physical fitness is a multidimensional state of being. **Physical fitness** is the body's ability to function efficiently and effectively. It is a state of being that consists of at least five health-related and six skill-related physical fitness components, each of which contributes to total quality of life. Physical fitness is associated with a person's ability to work effectively, enjoy leisure time, be healthy, resist **hypokinetic diseases,** and meet emergency situations. It is related to,

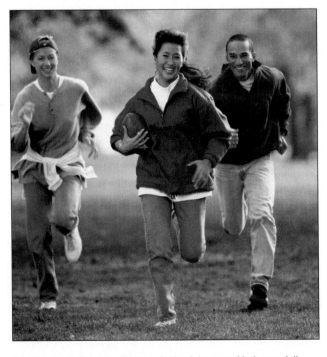

Possessing wellness includes enjoying leisure and being socially involved.

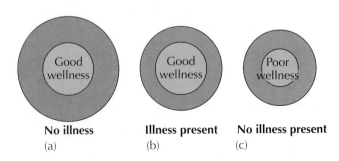

No illness   **Illness present**   **No illness present**
(a)   (b)   (c)

Figure 6 ▶ Wellness need not be limited by illness.

but different from, health and wellness. Although the development of physical fitness is the result of many things, optimal physical fitness is not possible without regular physical activity.

The health-related components of physical fitness are directly associated with good health. The five components of health-related physical fitness are body composition, cardiovascular fitness, flexibility, muscular endurance, and strength (see Figure 7). Each health-related fitness characteristic has a direct relationship to good health and reduced risk of hypokinetic disease.

Possessing a moderate amount of each component of health-related fitness is essential to disease prevention and health promotion, but it is not essential to have exceptionally high levels of fitness to achieve health benefits. High levels of health-related fitness relate more to performance than health benefits. For example, moderate amounts of strength are necessary to prevent back and posture problems, whereas high levels of strength contribute most to improved performance in activities such as football and jobs involving heavy lifting.

The skill-related components of physical fitness are more associated with performance than good health. The components of skill-related physical fitness are agility, balance, coordination, power, reaction time, and speed (see Figure 8). They are called skill-related because people who possess them find it easy to achieve high levels of performance in motor skills, such as those required in sports and in specific types of jobs. Skill-related fitness is sometimes called sports fitness or motor fitness.

There is little doubt that other abilities could be classified as skill-related fitness components. Also, each part of skill-related fitness is multidimensional. For example, coordination could be hand-eye coordination such as batting a ball, foot-eye coordination such as kicking a ball, or any of many other possibilities. The six parts of skill-related fitness identified here are those commonly associated with successful sports and work performance. It should be noted that each could be measured in ways other than those presented in this book. Measurements are provided to help the reader understand the nature of total physical fitness and to help the reader make important decisions about lifetime physical activity.

Metabolic fitness is a nonperformance component of total fitness. Research studies show that health benefits often occur even without dramatic improvements in traditional health-related physical fitness measures. **Metabolic fitness** is a state of being associated with lower risk of many chronic health problems but not necessarily associated with high performance levels of health-related physical fitness. Examples of nonperformance indicators of reduced risk are lowered blood pressure, lowered fat levels in the blood, and better regulation of blood sugar. Moderate physical activity has been shown to enhance metabolic fitness. Conventional wisdom classifies body composition as a component of health-related physical fitness, but some consider it to be a part of metabolic fitness because it is a nonperformance measure and it is highly related to nutrition as well as physical activity. You will learn how to assess your metabolic fitness in subsequent concepts.

Bone integrity is often considered to be a nonperformance measure of fitness. Traditional definitions do not include **bone integrity** as a part of physical fitness, but some experts feel that it should be. Like metabolic fitness, bone integrity cannot be assessed with performance measures as can most health-related fitness parts. Regardless of whether it is considered as a part of fitness or a component of health, there is little doubt that strong healthy bones are important to optimal health and are associated with regular physical activity and sound diet.

Physical Fitness Physical fitness is the body's ability to function efficiently and effectively. It consists of health-related physical fitness and skill-related physical fitness, which have at least eleven different components, each of which contributes to total quality of life. Physical fitness also includes metabolic fitness and bone integrity. Physical fitness is associated with a person's ability to work effectively, enjoy leisure time, be healthy, resist hypokinetic diseases, and meet emergency situations. It is related to but different from health, wellness, and the psychological, sociological, emotional, and spiritual components of fitness. Although the development of physical fitness is the result of many things, optimal physical fitness is not possible without regular exercise.

Hypokinetic Diseases or Conditions *Hypo-* means "under" or "too little," and *-kinetic* means "movement" or "activity." Thus, *hypokinetic* means "too little activity." A hypokinetic disease or condition is one associated with lack of physical activity or too little regular exercise. Examples of such conditions include heart disease, low back pain, adult-onset diabetes, and obesity.

Metabolic Fitness Metabolic fitness is a positive state of the physiological systems commonly associated with reduced risk of chronic diseases such as diabetes and heart disease. Metabolic fitness is evidenced by healthy blood fat (lipid) profiles, healthy blood pressure, healthy blood sugar and insulin levels, and other nonperformance measures. This type of fitness shows positive responses to moderate physical activity.

Bone Integrity Soundness of the bones is associated with high density and absence of symptoms of deterioration.

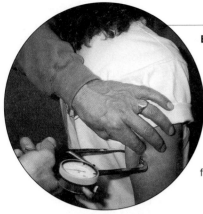

Body composition— The relative percentage of muscle, fat, bone, and other tissues that comprise the body. A fit person has a relatively low, but not too low, percentage of body fat (body fatness).

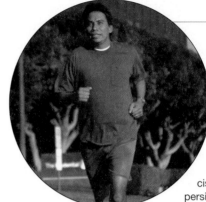

Cardiovascular fitness— The ability of the heart, blood vessels, blood, and respiratory system to supply fuel and oxygen to the muscles and the ability of the muscles to utilize fuel to allow sustained exercise. A fit person can persist in physical activity for relatively long periods without undue stress.

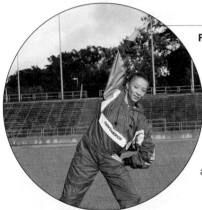

Flexibility— The range of motion available in a joint. It is affected by muscle length, joint structure, and other factors. A fit person can move the body joints through a full range of motion in work and in play.

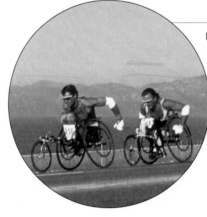

Muscular endurance— The ability of the muscles to exert themselves repeatedly. A fit person can repeat movements for a long period without undue fatigue.

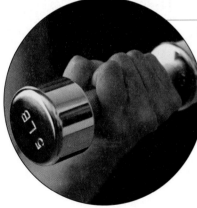

Strength— The ability of the muscles to exert an external force or to lift a heavy weight. A fit person can do work or play that involves exerting force, such as lifting or controlling one's own body weight.

Figure 7 ▶ Health-related physical fitness terms.

The many components of physical fitness are specific in nature but are also interrelated. Physical fitness is a combination of several aspects rather than a single characteristic. A fit person possesses at least adequate levels of each of the health-related, skill-related, and metabolic fitness components. People who possess one aspect of physical fitness do not necessarily possess the other aspects.

Some relationships exist among different fitness characteristics, but each of the components of physical fitness is separate and different from the others. For example, people who possess exceptional strength do not necessarily have good cardiovascular fitness, and those who have good coordination do not necessarily possess good flexibility. Lab 1B is designed to help you distinguish the different parts of health-related and skill-related physical

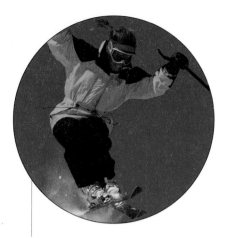

Agility—The ability to rapidly and accurately change the direction of the movement of the entire body in space. Skiing and wrestling are examples of activities that require exceptional agility.

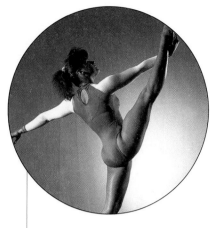

Balance—The maintenance of equilibrium while stationary or while moving. Water skiing, performing on the balance beam, or working as a riveter on a high-rise building are activities that require exceptional balance.

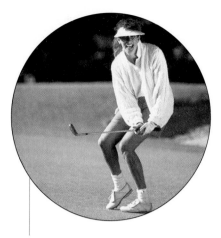

Coordination—The ability to use the senses with the body parts to perform motor tasks smoothly and accurately. Juggling, hitting a golf ball, batting a baseball, or kicking a ball are examples of activities requiring good coordination.

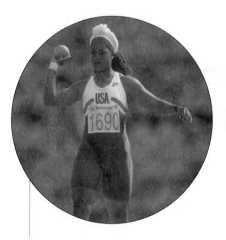

Power—The ability to transfer energy into force at a fast rate. Throwing the discus and putting the shot are activities that require considerable power.

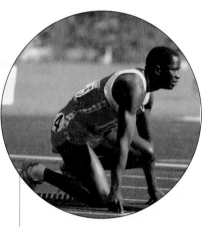

Reaction time—The time elapsed between stimulation and the beginning of reaction to that stimulation. Driving a racing car and starting a sprint race require good reaction time.

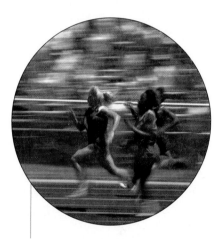

Speed—The ability to perform a movement in a short period of time. A runner on a track team or a wide receiver on a football team needs good foot and leg speed.

Figure 8 ► Skill-related physical fitness terms.

fitness. A separate questionnaire helps you estimate your current fitness levels.

Good physical fitness is important, but it is not the same as physical health and wellness. Good physical fitness contributes directly to the physical component of good health and wellness and indirectly to the other four components. Good fitness has been shown to be associated with reduced risk of chronic diseases such as coronary heart disease and has been shown to reduce the consequences of many debilitating conditions. In addi-

tion, good fitness contributes to wellness by helping us look our best, feel good, and enjoy life. Other physical factors can also influence health and wellness. For example, having good physical skills enhances quality of life by allowing us to participate in enjoyable activities such as tennis, golf, and bowling. While fitness can assist in performing these activities, regular practice is also necessary. Another example is the ability to fight off viral and bacterial infections. While fitness can promote a strong immune system, other physical factors can influence our susceptibility to these and other conditions.

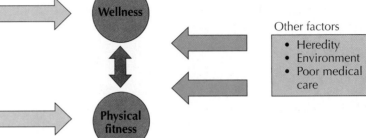

Healthy lifestyles

1. Regular physical activity
2. Eating well
3. Managing stress
4. Avoiding destructive habits
5. Practicing safe sex
6. Adopting good safety habits
7. Learning first aid
8. Adopting good personal health habits
9. Seeking and complying with medical advice
10. Being an informed consumer
11. Protecting the environment

Figure 9 ▶ Factors influencing health, wellness, and physical fitness.

For optimal health and wellness it is important to have good physical fitness *and* physical wellness. It is also important to strive for good emotional-mental, social, spiritual, and intellectual health and wellness. Each of the healthy lifestlyes described in Figure 9 will be discussed in greater detail later in this book.

Healthy Lifestyles

Lifestyle change, more than any other factor, is considered to be the best way of preventing illness and early death in our society. www.mhhe.com/fit_well/web01 Click 04. When people in Western society die before the age of sixty-five, the death is considered to be early or premature. The most important factors contributing to early death are unhealthy lifestyles. Based on the "leading health indicators" in *Healthy People 2010*, eleven healthy lifestyles have been associated with reduced disease risk and increased wellness. As shown in Figure 9, these lifestyles affect health, wellness, and physical fitness. The double-headed arrow between health and wellness and physical fitness illustrates the interaction between these factors. Physical fitness is important to health and wellness development and vice versa. Others factors, some not as much in your control as healthy lifestyles, also affect your health, fitness, and wellness. These factors include environmental factors (e.g., pollution, contaminants in the workplace), human biology (inherited conditions), and inadequacies in the health-care system, to name but a few.

The major causes of early death have shifted from infectious diseases to chronic lifestyle-related conditions. www.mhhe.com/fit_well/web01 Click 05. Scientific advances and improvements in medicine and health care have dramatically reduced the incidence of infectious diseases over the past 100 years (see Table 3).

For example, new drugs have dramatically reduced deaths from pneumonia and influenza. Small pox, a major cause of death less than a century ago, was globally eradicated in 1977 because of the advent of immunizations. Other examples are the virtual elimination of diphtheria and polio in the United States and Canada.

As infectious diseases have been eliminated, other illnesses have replaced them as the leading causes of early death in Western culture. HIV/AIDS, formerly eighth on the list, has dropped from the top fifteen, not because of fewer new cases, but because of new treatments that increase length of life among those who are infected. Many among the top ten are referred to as chronic lifestyle-related conditions because alteration of lifestyles can result in reduced risk for these conditions.

Table 3 ▶ **Major Causes of Death**

1900 Rank	Cause	Current Rank	Cause
1.	Pneumonia	1.	Heart disease
2.	Tuberculosis	2.	Cancer
3.	Diarrhea/enteritis	3.	Stroke
4.	Heart disease	4.	Bronchitis/emphysema
5.	Stroke	5.	Injuries
6.	Liver disease	6.	Pneumonia/influenza
7.	Injuries	7.	Diabetes
8.	Cancer	8.	Suicide
9.	Senility	9.	Kidney disease
10.	Diphtheria	10.	Chronic liver disease

Source: National Center for Health Statistics.

Healthy lifestyles are critical to wellness. Just as unhealthy lifestyles are the principal causes of modern-day illnesses such as heart disease, cancer, and diabetes, healthy lifestyles can result in an improved feeling of wellness that is critical to optimal health. In recognizing the importance of "years of healthy life," the Public Health Service also recognizes what it calls "measures of well-being." This well-being or wellness is associated with social, mental, spiritual, and physical functioning. Being physically active and eating well are two examples of healthy lifestyles that can improve well-being and add years of quality living. Many of the healthy lifestyles associated with good physical fitness and optimal wellness will be discussed in detail later in this book. The Healthy Lifestyle Questionnaire at the end of this concept gives you the opportunity to assess your current lifestyles.

Regular physical activity, sound nutrition, and stress management are considered to be priority healthy lifestyles. Three of the healthy lifestyles listed in Figure 9 are considered to be priority healthy lifestyles. These are regular **physical activity (exercise),** eating well, and managing stress. There are several reasons for placing priority on these lifestyles. First, they are behaviors that affect the lives of all people. Second, they are lifestyles in which large numbers of people can make improvement. Finally, modest changes in these behaviors can make dramatic improvements in individual and public health.

To be sure, the other healthy lifestyles listed in Figure 9 are important. For example people who use tobacco, abuse drugs (including alcohol), or practice unsafe sex can have immediate and dramatic health benefits by changing these behaviors. On the other hand, large segments of the population do not have problems in these areas. Obviously, these people cannot benefit from lifestyle changes in these areas. However, most people can benefit from increasing their activity levels, eating a better diet, and managing personal stress. For example, statistics suggest that modest changes in physical activity patterns and nutrition can prevent more than 200,000 premature deaths annually. Similarly, learning to manage daily stressors can result in significant reductions in more than a few health problems. Stress has a major impact on drug, alcohol, and smoking behavior so managing stress can help individuals minimize or avoid these behaviors. Many healthy lifestyles will be discussed in this book, but the focus is on the priority healthy lifestyles because virtually all people can achieve positive wellness benefits if they adopt them.

The change in causes of illness and the new emphasis on fitness, wellness, and healthy lifestyles have resulted in a shift toward prevention and promotion. Early medicine focused on treatment of

Table 4 ▶ The HELP Philosophy		
H	=	Health
E	=	Everyone
L	=	Lifetime
P	=	Personal

disease. Physicians were scarce and were consulted only when illness occurred. A shift toward prevention began with advancements in medical science (e.g., immunizations, antibiotics) and the development of public health efforts (e.g., safe water supplies). More than at any other time in history, efforts are being made to promote healthy lifestyles that lead to fitness and wellness. In this text, the emphasis will be on strategies for preventing chronic diseases and promoting fitness and wellness.

The HELP Philosophy

The HELP philosophy can provide a basis for making healthy lifestyle change possible. The four-letter acronym illustrated in Table 4 provides a basis for a philosophy that has helped thousands of people adopt healthy lifestyles. Each letter in the word *HELP* characterizes an important part of the philosophy. The twenty-six concepts in this book are based on the *HELP* philosophy. The forty-two lab experiences are designed to help all people (everyone) to develop personal programs for lifetime health, fitness, and wellness.

A personal philosophy that emphasizes Health can lead to behaviors that promote it. The **H** in HELP stands for health. One theory that has been extensively tested indicates that people who believe in the benefits of healthy lifestyles are more likely to

Exercise Exercise is defined as physical activity done for the purpose of getting physically fit.

Physical Activity Generally considered to be a broad term used to describe all forms of large muscle movements including sports, dance, games, work, lifestyle activities, and exercise for fitness. In this book, exercise and physical activity will often be used interchangeably to make reading less repetitive and more interesting.

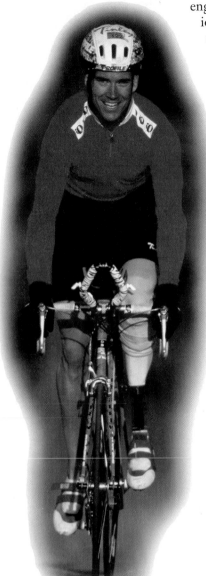

Physical activity is for everyone.

engage in healthy behaviors. The theory also suggests that people who state intentions to put their beliefs in action are likely to adopt behaviors that lead to health, wellness, and fitness.

Everyone can benefit from healthy lifestyles. The **E** in HELP stands for everyone. Accepting the fact that anyone can change a behavior or lifestyle means that *YOU* are included. Nevertheless, many adults feel ineffective in making lifestyle changes. Physical activity is not just for athletes—it is for all people. Eating well is not just for other people—you can do it too. All people can learn stress-management techniques. Healthy lifestyles can be practiced by everyone. As noted earlier in this concept, important health goals include eliminating health disparities and promoting "Health for All."

Healthy behaviors are most effective when practiced for a Lifetime. The **L** in HELP stands for lifetime. Young people sometimes feel immortal because the harmful effects of unhealthy lifestyles are often not immediate. As we grow older, we begin to realize that we are not immortal and that unhealthy lifestyles have cumulative negative effects. Starting early in life to emphasize healthy behaviors results in long-term health, wellness, and fitness benefits. One recent study shows that the longer healthy lifestyles are practiced, the greater the beneficial effects. This study also demonstrated that long-term healthy lifestyles can even overcome hereditary predisposition to illness and disease.

Healthy lifestyles should be based on Personal needs. The **P** in HELP stands for personal. No two people are exactly alike. Just as no single pill will cure all illnesses, no single lifestyle prescription exists for good health, wellness, and fitness. Each person must assess personal needs and make lifestyle changes based on those needs.

Strategies for Action

Self-assessments of lifestyles will help you determine areas in which you may need changes to promote optimal health, wellness, and fitness. As you begin your study of health, wellness, fitness, and healthy lifestyles, it is wise to make a self-assessment of your current behaviors. The Healthy Lifestyle Questionnaire in the lab resource materials will allow you to assess your current lifestyle behaviors to determine if they are contributing positively to your health, wellness, and fitness. Because this questionnaire contains some very personal information, answering all questions honestly will help you get an accurate assessment. As you continue your study, you may want to refer back to this questionnaire to see if your lifestyles have changed.

Initial self-assessments of wellness and fitness will provide information for self-comparison. www.mhhe.com/fit_well/web01 Click 06. The Healthy Lifestyle Questionnaire allows you to assess your lifestyles or behaviors. It is also important to assess your wellness and fitness at an early stage. These early assessments will only be estimates. As you continue your study, you will have the opportunity to do more comprehensive self-assessments that will allow you to see how accurate your early estimates were.

In Lab 1A, you will estimate your wellness using a Wellness Self-Perceptions Questionnaire, which assesses five wellness dimensions. Remember, wellness is a state of being that is influenced by healthy lifestyles. Because other factors such as heredity, environment, and health care affect wellness, it is possible to have good wellness scores even if you do not do well on the lifestyle questionnaire. However, over a lifetime, unhealthy lifestyles will catch up with you and have an influence on your wellness and fitness.

Lab 1B allows you to get a better understanding of the different components of health-related and skill-related physical fitness. You will perform some simple stunts to help you distinguish among the different fitness parts. You can use these as a basis for estimating your current fitness levels. Later, you will use more accurate tests to get a good assessment of your fitness. Like wellness, fitness is a state of being that is influenced by healthy lifestyles, especially regular physical activity. Young people sometimes have relatively good fitness—especially skill-related fitness—even if they have not been doing regular activity. Over a lifetime, inactivity greatly influences your fitness.

Web Resources

American Medical Association (AMA) www.ama-assn.org

Centers for Disease Control and Prevention (CDC)
     www.cdc.gov

Healthfinder www.healthfinder.gov

Health Canada www.hc-sc.ca

Healthy People 2010 www.health.gov/healthypeople

National Center for Chronic Disease Prevention and Health Promotion Publications www.cdc.gov/nccdphp/publicat.htm

National Center for Health Statistics www.cdc.gov/nchs/

President's Council on Physical Fitness and Sports
     www.fitness.gov

Suggested Readings

 Additional reference materials for Concept 1 are available at www.mhhe.com/fit_well/web01 Click 06.

Armbruster, B., and L. A. Gladwin. 2001. More than fitness for older adults: A whole-istic approach to wellness. *ACSM's Health and Fitness Journal* 5(2):6–10.

Blair, S. N. et al. 2001. *Active Living Every Day.* Champaign, IL: Human Kinetics.

*Booth, F. W. and M. V. Chakravarthy. 2002. Cost and consequences of sedentary living: new battleground for an old enemy. *President's Council on Physical Fitness and Sports Research Digest* 3(16):1–8.

Centers for Disease Control and Prevention. 2000. *Measuring Healthy Days.* Atlanta, GA: CDC.

Centers for Disease Control and Prevention. 2000. Ten great public health accomplishments—United States. *Morbidity and Mortality Weekly Reports* 48(12): 241–243. Also available at www.cdc.gov.

*Corbin, C. B., and R. P. Pangrazi 2001. Toward a uniform definition of wellness: A commentary. *President's Council on Physical Fitness and Sports Research Digest* 3(15): 1–8.

*Corbin, C. B., R. P. Pangrazi, and B. D. Franks. 2000. Definitions: Health, fitness, and physical activity. *President's Council on Physical Fitness and Sports Research Digest* 3(9):1–8.

Payne, W. A., and D. B. Hahn. 2002. *Understanding Your Health.* 7th ed. St. Louis: McGraw-Hill.

*Spain, C. G., and B. D. Franks. 2001. Healthy People 2010: Physical activity and fitness. *President's Council on Physical Fitness and Sports Research Digest* 3(13):1–16.

U.S. Department of Health and Human Services. 1996. *Physical Activity and Health: A Report of the Surgeon General.* Atlanta: U.S. Department of Health and Human Services.

U.S. Department of Health and Human Services. Nov. 2000. *Healthy People 2010.* 2nd ed. With *Understanding and Improving Health* and *Objectives for Improving Health.* 2 vols. Washington, DC: U.S. Government Printing Office.

*Also available at www.fitness.gov.

In the News

The tragic events of September 11, 2001, resulted in great stress for each of us. It caused us all to pause and consider what is important in our lives including family, friends, and personal safety. It is our hope that the information in this book will help you to cope with distressful events and to focus on wellness and quality of life issues important to you, your friends, and loved ones.

Though reports of bad news are common in the media, evidence suggests considerable good news exists regarding our fitness, health, and wellness.

Fitness, Health, and Wellness: The Good News

- The 20th century produced many great achievements in health. The Centers for Disease Control and Prevention (CDC) recently identified ten major achievements including vaccinations, safer workplaces, safer and healthier foods, and decline in heart disease deaths to name but a few. Evidence suggests many similar positive developments will occur this new century.
- Life expectancy is currently at an all-time high (see Figure 2).

- Eighty-one percent of adults rate their personal health as good or excellent.
- More than 78 percent of adults are satisfied with their standard of living.
- More adults use seat belts, have had adult vaccinations, and more women have had mammograms than in previous decades.
- Health and fitness club membership increased 100 percent from 1980 to 1990 and 63 percent to the present.
- Over 50 percent of all adults own home exercise equipment.
- We have more vacation time than previous generations.
- Smoking has decreased by 50 percent over the past five decades.

This "good news" provides optimism that we can overcome threats to our safety and health and make progress in meeting national health goals outlined in this book. We have placed special emphasis on the *Healthy People 2010* vision of helping "us all to make healthy lifestyle choices for ourselves and our families."

Lab Resource Materials: The Healthy Lifestyle Questionnaire

The purpose of this questionnaire is to help you analyze your lifestyle behaviors and to help you make decisions concerning good health and wellness for the future. Information on this Healthy Lifestyle Questionnaire is of a personal nature. For this reason, this questionnaire is not designed to be submitted to your instructor. It is for your information only. Answer each question as honestly as possible and use the scoring information to help you assess your lifestyle.

Directions: Place an X over the "yes" circle to answer yes. If you answer "no," make no mark. Score the questionnaire using the procedures that follow.

yes 1. I accumulate 30 minutes of moderate physical acitivty most days of the week (brisk walking, climbing stairs, yard work, or home chores.

yes 2. I do vigorous acitivity that elevates my heart rate for 20 minutes at least 3 days a week.

yes 3. I do exercises for flexibility at least 3 days a week.

yes 4. I do exercises for muscle fitness at least 2 days a week.

yes 5. I eat three regular meals each day.

yes 6. I select appropriate servings from the food guide pyramid each day.

yes 7. I restrict the amount of fat in my diet.

yes 8. I consume only as many calories as I expend ech day.

yes 9. I am able to identitfy sutuations in daily life that cause stress.

yes 10. I take time out during the day to relax and recover from daily stress.

yes 11. I find time for family, friends, and things I especially enjoy doing.

yes 12. I regularly perform exercises designed to relieve tension.

yes 13. I do not smoke or use other tobacco products.

yes 14. I do not abuse alcohol.

yes 15. I do not abuse drugs (prescription or illegal).

yes 16. I take over-the-counter drugs sparingly and use them only according to directions.

yes 17. I abstain from sex or limit sexual activity to a safe partner.

yes 18. I practice safe procedures for avoiding STDs.

yes 19. I use seat belts and adhere to the speed limit when I drive.

yes 20. I have a smoke detector in my house and check it regularly to see that it is working.

yes 21. I have had training to perform CPR if called on in an emergency.

yes 22. I can perform the Heimlich maneuver effectively if called on in an emergency.

yes 23. I brush my teeth at least 2 times a day and floss at least once a day.

yes 24. I get an adequate amount of sleep each night.

yes 25. I do regular self-exams, have regular medical check-ups, and seek medical advice when symptoms are present.

yes 26. When I receive advice and/or medication from a physician, I follow the advice and take the medication as prescribed.

yes 27. I read product labels and investigate their effectiveness before I buy them.

yes 28. I avoid using products that have not been shown by research to be effective.

yes 29. I recycle paper, glass, and aluminum.

yes 30. I practice environmental protection such as car pooling and conserving energy.

Overall Score—Total Yes Answers

15

Scoring: Give yourself one point for each yes answer. Add your scores for each of the lifestyle behaviors. To calculate your overall score, sum the totals for all lifestyles.

Physical Activity	Nutrition	Managing Stress	Avoiding Destructive Habits	Practicing Safe Sex	Adopting Safety Habits
1. ☐	5. ☐	9. ☐	13. ☐	17. ☐	19. ☐
2. ☐	6. ☐	10. ☐	14. ☐	18. ☐	20. ☐
3. ☐	7. ☐	11. ☐	15. ☐		
4. ☐	8. ☐	12. ☐	16. ☐		
3 Total +	*3* Total +	*3* Total +	*2* Total +	*2* Total +	*2*

Knowing First Aid	Personal Health Habits	Using Medical Advice	Being an Informed Customer	Protecting the Environment	Sum All Totals for Overall Score
21. ☐	23. ☐	25. ☐	27. ☐	29. ☐	
22. ☐	24. ☐	26. ☐	28. ☐	30. ☐	
2 Total +	*2* Total +	*2* Total +	☐ Total +	*2* Total =	*23*

Interpreting Scores: Scores of 3 or 4 on the four-item scales are indicative of generally positive lifestyles. For the two-item scales, a score of 2 would indicate the presence of positive lifestyles. An overall score of 26 or more would be a good indicator of healthy lifestyle behaviors. It is important to consider the following special note when interpreting scores.

Special Note: Your scores on the Healthy Lifestyle Questionnaire should be interpreted with caution. There are several reasons for this. First, all lifestyle behaviors do not pose the same risks. For example, using tobacco or abusing drugs has immediate negative affects on health and wellness, while others, such as knowing first aid, may have only occasional use. Second, you may score well on one item in a scale, but not on another. If one item indicates an unhealthy lifestyle in an area that poses a serious health risk, your lifestyle may appear to be healthier than it really is. For example, you could get a score of 3 on the destructive habits scale and be a regular smoker. For this reason, the overall score can be particularly deceiving.

Strategies for Change: In the space below, you may want to make some notes concerning the healthy lifestyle areas in which you could make some changes. You can refer to these notes later to see if you have made progress.

Lab 1A Wellness Self-Perceptions

Name	**Section**	**Date**

Purpose: To assess self-perceptions of wellness.

Procedures:

1. Place an X over the appropriate circle for each question (4 = strongly agree, 3 = agree, 2 = disagree, 1 = strongly disagree).
2. Write the number found in that circle in the box to the right.
3. Sum the three boxes for each wellness dimension to get your wellness dimension totals.
4. Sum all wellness dimension totals to get your comprehensive wellness total.
5. Use the rating chart to rate each wellness area.
6. Complete the Results section and the Conclusions and Implications section.

Question	Strongly Agree	Agree	Disagree	Strongly Disagree	Score
1. I am happy most of the time.	4	3	2	1	
2. I have good self-esteem.	4	3	2	1	
3. I do not generally feel stressed.	4	3	2	1	
			Emotional Wellness Total	=	
4. I am well informed about current events.	4	3	2	1	
5. I am comfortable expressing my views and opinions.	4	3	2	1	
6. I am interested in my career development.	4	3	2	1	
			Intellectual Wellness Total	=	
7. I am physically fit.	4	3	2	1	
8. I am able to perform the physical tasks of my work.	4	3	2	1	
9. I am physically able to perform leisure activities.	4	3	2	1	
			Physical Wellness Total	=	
10. I have many friends and am involved socially.	4	3	2	1	
11. I have close ties with my family.	4	3	2	1	
12. I am confident in social situations.	4	3	2	1	
			Social Wellness Total	=	
13. I am fulfilled spiritually.	4	3	2	1	
14. I feel connected to the world around me.	4	3	2	1	
15. I have a sense of purpose in my life.	4	3	2	1	
			Spiritual Wellness Total	=	
			Comprehensive Wellness (Sum of 5 wellness scores)		

Wellness Rating Chart:

Rating	Wellness Dimension Scores	Comprehensive Wellness Score
High-level wellness	10–12	50–60
Good wellness	8–9	40–49
Marginal wellness	6–7	30–39
Low wellness	below 6	below 30

Results:

Wellness Dimension	Score	Rating
Emotional		
Intellectual		
Physical		
Social		
Spiritual		
Comprehensive		

Conclusions and Implications: In the space provided below, use several paragraphs to describe your current state of wellness. Do you think the ratings are indicative of your true state of wellness? Are there areas in which there is room for improvement?

Lab 1B Fitness Stunts and Fitness Estimates

Name	Section	Date

Purpose: To help you better understand each of the eleven components of health-related and skill-related physical fitness and to help you estimate your current levels of physical fitness.

Special Note: The stunts performed in the lab are not intended as valid tests of physical fitness. It is hoped that the performance of the stunts will help you better understand each component of fitness so that you can estimate your current fitness levels. You should not rely primarily on the results of the stunts to make your estimates. Rather, you should rely on previous fitness tests you have taken and your own best judgment of your current fitness. Later in this book, you will learn how to perform accurate assessments of each fitness component and determine the accuracy of your estimates.

Procedures:

1. Perform each of the stunts described in Chart 1 on page 20.
2. Use past fitness test performances and your own judgment to estimate your current levels for each of the health-related and skill-related physical fitness parts. Low Fitness = improvement definitely needed, Marginal = some improvement necessary, Good = adequate for healthy daily living.
3. Place an X in the appropriate circle for your fitness estimate in the results section below.

Results:

Fitness Component	Low Fitness	Marginal Fitness	Good Fitness
Body composition	◯	◯	◯
Cardiovascular fitness	◯	◯	◯
Flexibility	◯	◯	◯
Muscular endurance	◯	◯	◯
Strength	◯	◯	◯
Agility	◯	◯	◯
Balance	◯	◯	◯
Coordination	◯	◯	◯
Power	◯	◯	◯
Reaction time	◯	◯	◯
Speed	◯	◯	◯

Conclusions and Implications: In several sentences, discuss the information you used to make your estimates of physical fitness. How confident are you that these estimates are accurate?

19

Directions: Attempt each of the stunts in the chart below. Place an X in the circle next to each component of physical fitness to indicate that you have attempted the stunt.

Chart 1 ▶ Physical Fitness Stunts

Balance ◯

1. *One-foot balance.* Stand on one foot; press up so that the weight is on the ball of the foot with the heel off the floor. Hold the hands and the other leg straight out in front for ten seconds.

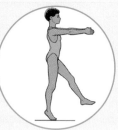

Power ◯

2. *Standing long jump.* Stand with the toes behind a line. Using no run or hop step, jump as far as possible. Men must jump their height plus 6 inches. Women must jump their height only.

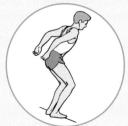

Agility ◯

3. *Paper ball pickup.* Place two wadded paper balls on the floor 5 feet away. Run until both feet cross the line, pick up the first ball, and return both feet behind the starting line. Repeat with the second ball. Finish in five seconds.

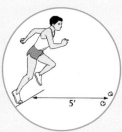

Reaction Time ◯

4. *Paper drop.* Have a partner hold a sheet of notebook paper so that the side edge is between your thumb and index finger, about the width of your hand from the top of the page. When your partner drops the paper, catch it before it slips through the thumb and finger. Do not lower your hand to catch the paper.

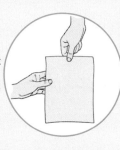

Speed ◯

5. *Double-heel click.* With the feet apart, jump up and tap the heels together twice before you hit the ground. You must land with your feet at least 3 inches apart.

Coordination ◯

6. *Paper ball bounce.* Wad up a sheet of notebook paper into a ball. Bounce the ball back and forth between the right and left hands. Keep the hands open and palms up. Bounce the ball three times with each hand (six times total), alternating hands for each bounce.

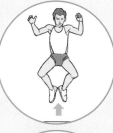

Cardiovascular Fitness ◯

7. *Run in place.* Run in place for one-and-a-half minutes (120 steps per minute). Rest for one minute and count the heart rate for 30 seconds. A heart rate of 60 (for 30 sec.) or lower passes. A step is counted each time the right foot hits the floor.

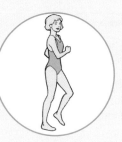

Flexibility ◯

8. *Backsaver toe touch.* Sit on the floor with one foot against a wall. Bend the other knee. Bend forward at the hips. After three warm-up trials, reach forward and touch your closed fists to the wall. Bend forward slowly; do not bounce. Repeat with the other leg straight. Pass if fists touch the wall with each leg straight.

Note: This is a stunt, not an exercise.

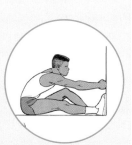

Body Composition ◯

9. *The pinch.* Have a partner pinch a fold of fat on the back of your upper arm (body fatness), halfway between the tip of the elbow and the tip of the shoulder.

Men: No greater than 3/4 of an inch.

Women: No greater than 1 inch.

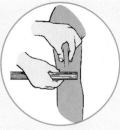

Strength ◯

10. *Push-up.* Lie face down on the floor. Place the hands under the shoulders. Keeping the legs and body straight, press off the floor until the arms are fully extended. Women repeat once; men, three times.

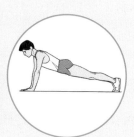

Muscular Endurance ◯

11. *Side leg raise.* Lie on the floor on your side. Lift your leg up and to the side of the body until your feet are 24 to 36 inches apart. Keep the knee and pelvis facing forward. Do not rotate so that the knees face the ceiling. Perform ten with each leg.

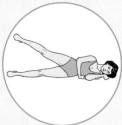

Using Self-Management Skills to Adhere to Healthy Lifestyle Behaviors

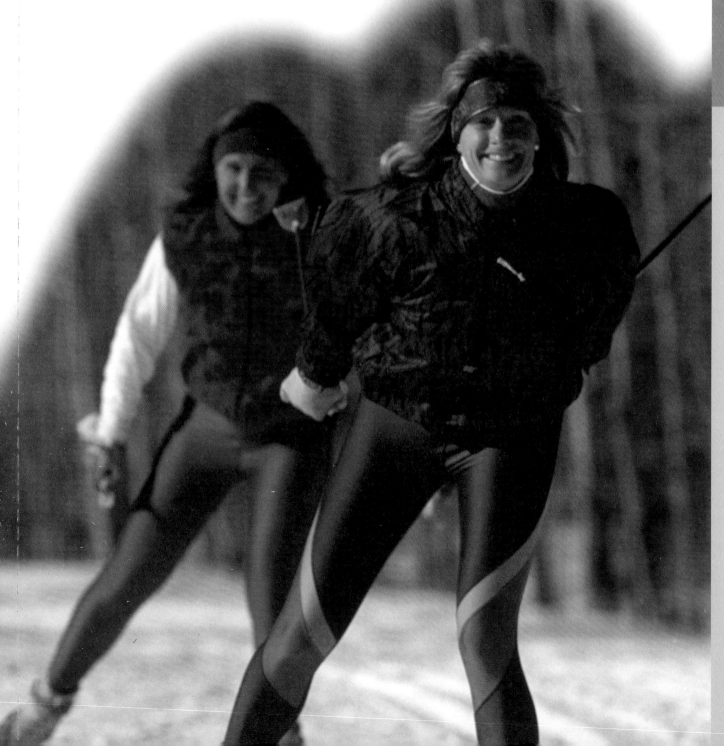

Learning and regularly using self-management skills can help you to adopt and maintain healthy lifestyles throughout life.

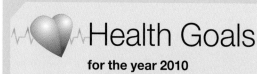

Health Goals
for the year 2010

- Increase quality and years of healthy life.
- Increase incidence of people reporting "healthy days."
- Increase the adoption and maintenance of daily physical activity.
- Increase the proportion of all people who eat well.
- Decrease personal stress levels and mental health problems.
- Modify determinants of good health.

Reducing illness and debilitating conditions and promoting wellness and fitness are important goals for all of us. Practicing lifelong healthy lifestyles is the key to health, wellness, and fitness. Yet, there is considerable evidence that many people are not effectively making lifestyle changes, even when they want to do so. Experts have determined that people who practice healthy lifestyles possess certain characteristics. These characteristics can be modified to improve health behaviors of all people. Researchers have also identified several special skills, referred to as self-management skills, that can be useful in helping you alter factors related to adherence and ultimately help you make lifestyle changes. Like any skill, self-management skills must be practiced if they are to be useful. In this concept, factors relating to healthy lifestyle adherence and self-management skills will be described.

Making Lifestyle Changes

Many adults want to make lifestyle changes but are unable to do so. The majority of adults (66 percent) would prefer to alter their diet to improve health rather than take medicine. Nine out of ten people indicate that regular physical activity is important to their health. Approximately two-thirds of adults feel "great stress" at least one day a week and would like to reduce their stress levels. In spite of these statistics, those who profess interest in dietary change are often unsuccessful in making lasting changes. Those who say they value physical activity often fail to adhere to even modest activity schedules. Though stress reduction is important, nearly half of all adults still feel that there is a stigma associated with seeking help for an emotional problem, yet they frequently lack the skills to help themselves. Changes in other lifestyles are frequently desired but often not accomplished.

Practicing one healthy lifestyle does not mean you will practice another, though adopting one healthy behavior often leads to the adoption of another. College students are more likely to participate in regular physical activity than older adults. However, they are also much more likely to eat poorly and abuse alcohol. Many young women adopt low-fat diets to avoid weight gain and also smoke because they have the mistaken belief that smoking will contribute to long-term weight maintenance. These examples illustrate the fact that practicing one healthy lifestyle does not insure **adherence** to another. However, there is evidence that making one lifestyle change often makes it easier to make other changes. For example, smokers who have started regular physical activity programs often see improvements in fitness and general well-being and decide to stop smoking.

People do not make lifestyle changes overnight. Rather, people progress forward and backward through several stages of change. www.mhhe.com/fit_well/web02 Click 01. When asked about a specific healthy lifestyle, people commonly respond with "yes" or "no" answers. If asked, "Do you exercise regularly?", the answer is "yes" or "no." When asked, "Do you eat well?", the answer is "yes" or "no." We now know that there are many different stages of lifestyle behavior.

Prochaska and colleagues developed a model for classifying **stage of change** as part of their Transtheoretical model (see Table 5 for more details). They suggest that lifestyle changes occur in at least five different stages. These stages are illustrated in Figure 1. The stages were originally developed to help understand negative lifestyles. Smokers were among the first studied. Smokers who are not considering stopping are at the stage of precontemplation. Those who are thinking about stopping

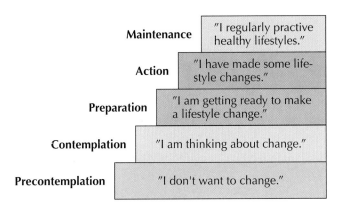

Figure 1 ▶ Stages of lifestyle change.

are classified in the contemplation stage. Those who have bought a nicotine patch or a book about smoking cessation are classified in the preparation stage. They have moved beyond contemplation and are preparing to take action. The action stage occurs when the smoker makes some change in behavior, even a small one. Cutting back on the number of cigarettes smoked is an example. The fifth stage is the stage of maintenance. When a person finally stops smoking for a relatively long period of time (six months), this stage has been reached.

The stages of change model (as illustrated in Figure 1), has now been applied to positive lifestyles as well as negative ones. Those who are totally sedentary are considered to be in the precontemplation stage. Contemplators are thinking about becoming active. A person at the preparation stage may have bought a pair of walking shoes and appropriate clothing for activity. Those who have started some activity, even if infrequent, are considered to be at the stage of action. Those who have been exercising regularly for at least six months are said to be at the stage of maintenance.

Whether the lifestyle is positive or negative, people move from one stage to another in an upward or downward direction. Individuals in action may move on to maintenance or revert back to contemplation depending on their attitudes and personal experiences. Smokers who succeed in quitting permanently report having stopped and started dozens of times before reaching lifetime maintenance. Similarly, those attempting to adopt positive lifestyles such as eating well often move back and forth from one stage to another depending on their life circumstances.

Once maintenance is attained, relapse is less likely to occur. While it is possible to relapse completely, it is generally less likely after the maintenance stage is reached. At this point, the behavior has been integrated into a personal lifestyle and it becomes easier to sustain. For example, a person who has been physically active for years does not

have to undergo the same thought processes as a beginning exerciser—the behavior becomes automatic and habitual. Similarly, a nonsmoker is not tempted to smoke in the same way as a person who is currently trying to quit. Some people have termed the end of this behavior change process as termination.

Factors That Promote Lifestyle Change

There are many factors associated with achieving advanced stages of healthy behavior. The ultimate goal for any health behavior is to reach the stage of maintenance (see Figure 1). Healthy People 2010 refers to these factors as **determinants,** which are factors that determine health behaviors. In fact, the national strategy is to help people change these factors so that an increased number of adults will reach and stay at the level of maintenance. These factors relate equally well to stages of change for other healthy lifestyles. For ease of understanding, they are classified as **personal, predisposing, enabling,** and **reinforcing factors.** Predisposing factors help precontemplators get going-to move them toward contemplation or even preparation. Enabling factors help those in contemplation or preparation take the step toward action. Reinforcing factors move people from action to maintenance and help those in maintenance stay there.

Adherence Adopting a healthy behavior such as regular physical activity or sound nutrition as part of your lifestyle.

Stage of Change A stage of change refers to the level of lifestyle behavior a given individual has for a specific health behavior.

Determinates Factors identified by health experts as responsible for healthy and unhealthy behaviors.

Personal Factor Factors such as age or gender related to healthy lifestyle adherence but are typically not under your personal control.

Predisposing Factor Anything that makes you more likely to decide that you should make a healthy lifestyle such as regular physical activity a part of your normal routine.

Enabling Factor Anything that helps you carry out your healthy lifestyle plan.

Reinforcing Factor Anything that provides encouragement to maintain healthy lifestyles such as physical activity for a lifetime.

Personal factors affect health behaviors but are often out of your personal control. Your age, gender, heredity, social status, and current health and fitness levels are all personal factors that affect your health behaviors. For example, there are significant differences in health behaviors among people of various ages. According to one survey, young adults between the ages of eighteen and thirty-four are more likely to smoke (30 percent) than those sixty-five and older (13 percent). On the other hand, young adults are much more likely to be physically active than older adults.

Gender differences are illustrated by the fact that women use health services more often than men. Women are more likely than men to have identified a primary care doctor and are more likely to participate in regular health screenings. As you will discover in more detail later in this book, heredity plays a role in health behaviors. For example, some people have a hereditary predisposition to gain weight, and this may affect their eating behaviors.

Age, gender, and heredity are factors you cannot control. Other personal factors that relate to health behaviors include social status and current health and fitness status. Evidence indicates that people of lower socioeconomic status and those with poor health and fitness are less likely to contemplate or participate in activity and other healthy behaviors. No matter what personal characteristics you have, you can change your health behaviors. If you have several personal factors that do not favor healthy lifestyles, it is important to do something to change your behaviors. Making an effort to modify the factors that predispose, enable, and reinforce healthy lifestyles is essential.

Predisposing factors are important in getting you started with the process of change. There are many predisposing factors that help you move from contemplation to preparation and taking action with regard to healthy behavior. A person who possesses many of the predisposing factors is said to have self-motivation (also called intrinsic motivation). If you are self-motivated, you will answer positively to two basic questions: "Am I able?" and "Is it worth it?"

Am I able to do regular activity? Am I able to change my diet or to stop smoking? Figure 2 includes a list of four different factors that help you say "Yes, I am able." Two of these factors are **self-confidence** and **self-efficacy**. Both have to do with having positive perceptions about your own ability. People with positive self-perceptions are more self-motivated and feel they are capable of making behavior changes for health improvement. Other factors that help you feel you are able to do a healthy behavior include easy access and a safe environment. For example, we know that people who have easy access to exercise equipment at home or the workplace or who have a place to exercise within ten minutes of home are more likely to be active than those who do not

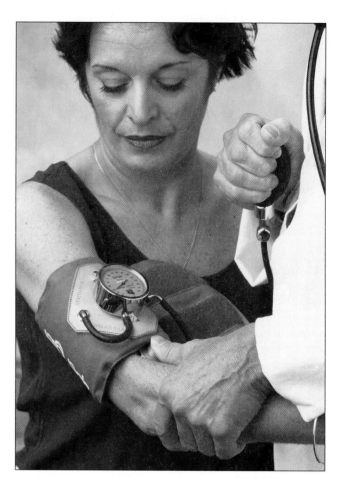

Women are more likely to use healh-care services than men.

have easy access. A safe environment such as safe neighborhoods or parks increases the chances that a person will be active.

Is it worth it? People who say "yes" to this question are willing to make an effort to change their behaviors. Predisposing factors that make it worth it to change behaviors include enjoying the activity, balancing attitudes, believing in the benefits of a behavior, and having knowledge of the health benefits of a behavior (see Figure 2). If you enjoy something and feel good about it (have positive attitudes and beliefs), you will be self-motivated to do it. It will be worth it. Taking steps to change the predisposing factors will help you become self-motivated and move toward effectively changing your health behaviors.

Enabling factors are important in moving you from the beginning stages of change to action and maintenance. Enabling factors include a variety of skills that help people follow through with decisions to make changes in behaviors. Eight of these most important skills are listed in Figure 2. A few examples of the skills that enable healthy lifestyle change include goal setting, self-assessment, and self-monitoring.

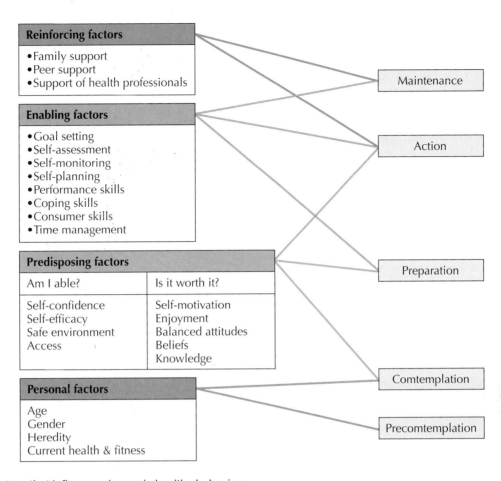

Figure 2 ▶ Factors that influence change in healthy behaviors.

Reinforcing factors are important in adhering to lifestyle changes. Once a person has reached the action or maintenance stages, it is important to stay at this high level. Reinforcing factors help people stick with a behavior change (see Figure 2).

Family, peer, and health professional influences are all reinforcing factors. If your family, friends, or a doctor encourage you, it may help you adhere. It is important, however, that support from others does not create unnecessary pressure. Though social support can be reinforcing, perhaps the most important reinforcing factor is success. If you change a behavior and have success, it makes you want to keep doing the behavior. If you fail, you may conclude that the behavior does not work and give up on it. Planning for success is very important in adhering to healthy lifestyle change.

Self-Management Skills

Learning self-management skills can help you alter factors that lead to healthy lifestyle change. Personal, predisposing, enabling, and reinforcing factors influence the way you live. These factors are of little practical significance, however, unless they can be altered to promote healthy lifestyles. Learning **self-management skills** (sometimes called self-regulation skills) can help you change the predisposing, enabling, and reinforcing factors described in Tables 1, 2, and 3. In fact, some of the enabling factors are self-management skills. It takes practice to learn these skills, but with effort anyone can learn them. There are many opportunities to learn self-management skills in this book. Many of the labs allow you to practice these skills.

Self-Confidence The belief that you can be successful at something (for example, the belief that you can be successful in sports and physical activities and can improve your physical fitness).

Self-Efficacy Confidence that you can perform a specific task. (A type of specific self-confidence.)

Self-Management Skills Skills that you can learn to help you change and adhere to healthy lifestyles such as regular physical activity and good nutrition (see Tables 1, 2, and 3 for examples).

Table 1 ▶ Self-Management Skills for Changing Predisposing Factors

Self-Management Skill	How Is It Useful?
Overcoming Barriers	**Lifestyle Example**
This involves developing skills that allow you to overcome problems such as lack of facilities, lack of equipment, and inconvenience. People who develop skills to overcome barriers can learn to rearrange schedules and acquire personal equipment and other skills to overcome these barriers.	People at work are often exposed to snack foods high in empty calories. For this reason his/her nutrition is not what it could be. Skills in overcoming barriers include planning, preparing, and selecting good foods.
Building Self-Confidence and Motivation	**Lifestyle Example**
This involves taking small steps that allow success. With each small step, confidence and motivation increase and you develop the feeling that "I can do that."	A person says, "I would like to be more active, but I have never been good at physical activities." Starting with a 10-minute walk, the person sees that "I can do it." Over time the person becomes confident and motivated to do more physical activity.
Balancing Attitudes	**Lifestyle Example**
This involves learning to balance positive and negative attitudes. To adhere to a healthy lifestyle, it is important to develop positive attitudes and reduce the negative attitudes.	A person does not do activity because he or she lacks support from friends, has no equipment, and does not like to get sweaty. These are negatives. Shifting the balance to positive things such as fun, good health, and looking good can help promote activity.
Building Knowledge and Changing Beliefs	**Lifestyle Example**
An educated person knows the truth and builds his or her beliefs on sound information. Knowledge does not always change beliefs, but awareness of the facts can play an important role in achieving good health.	A person says, "I don't think what I eat has much to do with my health and wellness." Acquiring knowledge is fundamental to being an educated person. Studying the facts about nutrition can provide the basis for changes in beliefs and modifications of lifestyles.

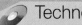

Technology Update

Many adults underestimate the number of calories they consume and overestimate the activity they perform each day. One important self-management skill that can help people be more realistic is self-monitoring. The development of hand-held computers can now make self-monitoring easier. These computers are also called Personal Digital Assistants (PDAs). Software is now available for PDAs that allow you to record and analyze calories consumed in food and expended in activity. For more information, consult the website in the Web Resources at the end of this concept.

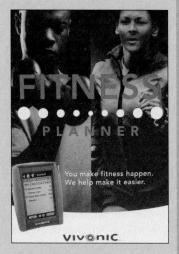

It takes time to change unhealthy lifestyles. People in Western cultures are used to seeing things happen quickly. We flip a switch, and the lights come on. We want food quickly, and thousands of fast food restaurants provide it. The expectation that we should have what we want when we want it has led us to expect instantaneous changes in health, wellness, and fitness. Unfortunately, there is no quick way to health. There is no pill that can reverse the effects of a lifetime of sedentary living, poor eating, or tobacco abuse. Changing your lifestyle is the key. But lifestyles that have been practiced for years are not easy to change. As you progress through this book, you will have the opportunity to learn how to implement self-management skills. Learning these skills is the surest way to make permanent lifestyle changes.

Table 2 ▶ Self-Management Skills for Changing Enabling Factors

Self-Management Skill	How Is It Useful?
Goal-Setting Skills	**Lifestyle Example**
This involves learning how to establish things that you want to achieve in the future. It is important that goals be realistic and achievable. Learning to set goals for behavior change is especially important for beginners.	A person wants to lose body fat. If he/she sets a goal of losing 50 pounds, success is unlikely. Setting a process goal of restricting 200 calories a day or expending 200 more a day for several weeks makes success more likely.
Self-Assessment Skills	**Lifestyle Example**
This involves how to assess your own fitness, health, and wellness. In addition it requires you to learn to interpret your own self-assessment results. It takes practice to become good at doing self-assessments.	A person wants to know his/her health strengths and weaknesses. The best procedure is to select good tests and self-administer them. Practicing the assessments in this book will help you become good at self-assessment.
Self-Monitoring Skills	**Lifestyle Example**
This involves monitoring behavior and recordkeeping. Many people think that they adhere to healthy lifestyles, but they do not. They have a distorted view of what they actually do. Self-monitoring helps give you a true picture of your own behavior and progress toward goals.	A person can't understand why he/she is not losing weight even though restricting calories. Keeping records may show that the person was eating more than he/she thought. Learning to keep records of progress is also important to adherence.
Self-Planning Skills	**Lifestyle Example**
This involves learning how to plan for yourself rather than having others do all the planning for you. Knowledge and practice in planning can help you develop these skills.	A person wants to be more active, to eat better, and to manage stress. Self-planning skills will help him/her plan a personal activity, nutrition, or stress-management program.
Performance Skills	**Lifestyle Example**
This involves learning skills necessary for performance of specific tasks, such as sport or relaxation. These skills can help you feel confident and enjoy activities.	A person avoids physical activity because he/she does not have the physical skills equal to peers. Learning sports or other motor skills allows this person to choose to be active anyway.
Coping Skills	**Lifestyle Example**
This involves developing a new way of thinking about things. People with this skill can see situations in more than one way and learn to think more positively about life situations.	A person is stressed and frequently anxious. Learning stress-management skills, such as relaxation, can help a person cope. Like all skills, stress-management skills must be practiced to be effective.
Consumer Skills	**Lifestyle Example**
This involves gaining knowledge about products and services. It also may require rethinking untrue beliefs that may lead to poor consumer decisions.	A person avoids seeking medical help when sick. Instead, the person takes an unproven remedy. Learning consumer skills provides knowledge for making sound medical decisions.
Time Management	**Lifestyle Example**
This involves recordkeeping similar to self-monitoring. It relates to total time use rather than monitoring specific behaviors. Skillful monitoring of time can help you plan and adhere to healthy lifestyles.	A person wants more quality time with family and friends. Monitoring time can help a person reallocate time to spend it in ways that are more consistent with personal priorities.

Strategies for Action

Many people feel that factors influencing health and wellness are out of their control. www.mhhe.com/ fit_well/web02 Click 02. A recent poll indicates that 91 percent of adults would like to change their lifestyles to make their lives more enjoyable and to change factors associated with wellness. Unfortunately, many people feel that they do not have personal control over good health and wellness. For example, one survey suggests that most of the lifestyle changes deemed important in our society remain in the realm of fantasies, just beyond realization. Experts have shown that people who feel that health is beyond personal control express such ideas as "Bad things [illness] can't happen to me and good things [wellness] are beyond my reach."

Many people can benefit from a new way of thinking about health, wellness, and fitness. Many people have unrealistic expectations about health and fitness. They compare their fitness to athletes and their appearance to models and movie stars, often setting standards for themselves that are impossible to achieve. Some say "I could never do that" when considering becoming physically active, altering eating patterns, or learning to manage stress. Many lack information about what is really possible concerning healthy lifestyles. Those who feel a lack of control set unrealistic standards for themselves and lack confidence in their own abilities to change.

Adopting a new way of thinking can have dramatic implications. A major purpose of this text is to help you adopt a new way of thinking toward health behaviors. This new way of thinking acknowledges that many of the factors that influence health, fitness, and wellness are largely within your control. Learning and practicing self-management skills can help you develop this new way of thinking.

With practice, you can improve the self-management skills that lead to acquiring and maintaining healthy lifestyles. Many opportunities are provided in this book for you to practice and learn self-management skills. Table 4 refers you to different labs in the text designed to enhance specific self-management skills.

Assessing self-management skills that influence healthy lifestyles provides a basis for changing your health, wellness, or fitness. Lab 2A allows you to assess predisposing, enabling, and reinforcing factors associated with regular physical activity. Lab 2B provides you with an opportunity to assess your current self-management skills for physical activity. In subsequent concepts, you will practice the self-management skills relating to a variety of different healthy lifestyles.

You can benefit from a critical analysis of the theories and models that help us understand the factors that lead to healthy living. www.mhhe.com/ fit_well/web02 Click 03. Table 5 describes some of the best-known theories and models used by researchers to study the factors associated with healthy living. Much of the information presented in this concept was derived from research using these theories and models. The suggested readings provide more information about the theories and models for those interested for studying them further.

Table 3 ▶ Self-Management Skills for Changing Reinforcing Factors	
Self-Management Skill	**How Is It Useful?**
Social Support	**Lifestyle Example**
This involves learning how to get the support of others for healthy lifestyles you want to adopt. You learn how to get support from family and friends. Support of an outside authority such as a doctor can help.	A person has gradually developed a plan to be active. Friends and loved ones encourage activity and help the person develop a schedule that will allow and encourage regular activity.
Relapse Prevention	**Lifestyle Example**
This involves staying with a healthy behavior once you have adopted it. It is sometimes easy to relapse to an unhealthy lifestyle. There are skills such as avoiding high-risk situations and learning how to say "no" that can help avoid relapse.	A person stops smoking. To stay at maintenance, the person can learn to avoid situations where there is pressure to smoke. The person can learn methods of saying "no" to those who offer tobacco.

Web Resources

ACSM's Fit Society Page **www.acsm.org/health%2Bfitness/fit_society.htm**

ACSM's Health and Fitness Journal **www.acsm-healthfitness.org**

Journal of Sport and Exercise Psychology **www.humankinetics.com/products/journals/journal.cfm?id=JSEP**

Personal Digital Assistant (PDA) Software **www.vivonic.com**

The Sport Psychologist **www.humankinetics.com/products/journals/journal.cfm?id=TSP**

Suggested Readings

 Additional reference materials for Concept 2 are available at **www.mhhe.com/fit_well/web02 Click 04.**

Table 4 ▶ Opportunities for Learning Self-Management Skills

Self-Management Skill	Lab Number
Overcoming Barriers	19C, 25A, 25B
Building Self-Confidence and Motivation	1A, 5A
Balancing Attitudes	5A
Building Knowledge and Beliefs	3B, 5A, 6A, 8A, 12A, 25A, 25B
Goal Setting	7A, 10B, 11C, 11D, 13C, 17A, 21A, 21B, 26C
Self-Assessment	1A, 1B, 2A, 3A, 4A, 6A, 8A, 10A, 11A, 11B, 13A, 13B, 14A, 15A, 15B, 15C, 16A, 16B, 18A, 18B, 18C, 19B, 20A, 21A, 21B, 22A, 23A, 24A, 24B, 26A
Self-Monitoring	7A, 9B, 10B, 11C, 11D, 13C, 16A, 16B, 17B, 26B, 26C
Self-Planning	7A, 9B, 10B, 11C, 11D, 13C, 26B, 26C
Performance Skills	3B, 9A, 12A, 19B, 19C
Adopting Coping Skills	19A, 19D
Learning Consumer Skills	16B, 25A, 25B
Managing Time	19C
Finding Social Support	19B
Preventing Relapse	17A, 21B, 26B, 26C

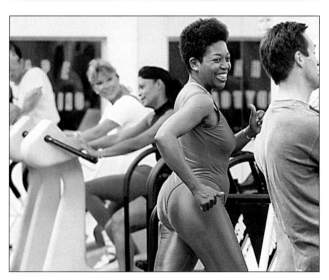

A new way of thinking can help you adopt healthy lifestyles.

Table 5 ▶ Theories and Models Associated with Healthy Lifestyle Adoption

Theory/Model and Brief Description

Transtheoretical model

This model is also referred to as the stages of change model. As described earlier in this concept, this model suggests five stages of change that characterize various health behaviors. The model suggests that doing the correct things (processes) at the right time (stage of change) is important to self-change in health behaviors.

Health beliefs model

This model suggests that a person's health behavior is related to the following five factors: the belief that a health problem will have harmful effects, the belief that a person is susceptible to the problem, the perceived benefits of changing a lifestyle to prevent the problem, the perceived barriers to overcoming the problem, and the confidence that he/she can do what is necessary to prevent it.

Social cognitive theory

Social cognitive theory is also referred to as social learning theory. Central to this theory are self-efficacy and positive expectations about behavior change. Also, the theory suggests that a person must value the outcomes of a behavior if he/she is likely to do that behavior.

Theory of reasoned action

This theory suggests that a person's behavior is most associated with the person's intention to do the behavior. The two factors most likely to influence a person's intentions are attitudes (beliefs) and the social environment (opinions of others).

Theory of planned behavior

This theory is often combined with the theory for reasoned action. It has the same basic tenets but adds the concept of "perceived control" over the environment. The person must believe that he/she has some control over the factors that allow performance of that behavior. Perceived control is in many ways similar to self-efficacy in social cognitive theory.

Self-determination theory

Central to self-determination theory is the importance of choice in a person's life (autonomy). Perceptions of competence at mastering life's tasks are also critical to the theory. Making personal choices in an attempt to master the tasks of daily living are emphasized rather than making choices based on external pressures to comply. Self-determination theory, and cognitive evaluation theory (its subtheory), emphasize intrinsic motivation. The intrinsic motivation inherent in behaviors that are exciting and/or fulfilling to do is important in making activity choices.

American College of Sports Medicine. 2000. Methods for changing exercise behaviors. In *ACSM's Guidelines for Exercise Testing and Prescription*. 6th ed. Philadelphia: Lippincott, Williams and Wilkins.

Bandura, A. 1986. *Social Foundations of Thought and Action: A Social-Cognitive Theory*. Englewood Cliffs, NJ: Prentice-Hall.

Deci, E. L., and R. M. Ryan, (eds.). 2002. *Handbook of Self-Determination Research*. Rochester, NY: University of Rochester Press.

Epstein, L. H., and J. N. Roemmich. 2001. Reducing sedentary behavior: Role in modifying physical activity. *Exercise and Sport Sciences Reviews* 29(3):103–108.

Gill, D. L. 2000. *Psychological Dynamics of Sport and Exercise*. 2nd ed. Champaign, IL: Human Kinetics.

Haussenblas, H. A. et al. 1997. Applications of the theories of reasoned action and planned behaviors: A meta analysis. *The Journal of Sport and Exercise Psychology* 19:36.

Juniu, S. 2002. Implementing handheld computing technology in physical education. *Journal of Physical Education, Recreation and Dance* 73(3):43–48.

Maddux, J. E. 2002. Self-efficacy: The power of believing you can. In Snyder, C. R., and S. J. Lopez. *Handbook of Positive Psychology*. Oxford, UK: University Press.

Marcus, B. H. et al. 2000. Physical activity behavior change: Issues in adoption and maintenance. *Health Psychology* 19(1):32–41.

McAuley, E., and B. Blissmer. 2000. Self-efficacy determinants and consequences of physical activity. *Exercise and Sport Sciences Reviews* 28:85–88.

Prochaska, J. O., and B. H. Markus. 1994. The transtheoretical model: Applications to exercise." In Dishman, R. K. (ed.), *Advances in Exercise Adherence*. Champaign, IL: Human Kinetics.

Rhodes, R. E. et al. 2002. Extending the theory of planned behavior to the exercise domain. *Research Quarterly for Exercise and Sport* 73(2):193–199.

Roberts, G. 2001. *Advances in Motivation in Sport and Exercise*. Champaign, IL: Human Kinetics.

Rosenstock, I. M. 1990. The health belief model: Explaining health behavior through expectancies." In Glantz, K., F. M. Lewis, and B. K. Riner, *Health Behavior and Education*. San Francisco: Jossey-Bass.

Ryan, R. M., and E. L. Deci. 2000. Self-determination theory and the facilitation of intrinsic motivation, social development, and well-being. *American Psychologist* 55:68–78.

Sallis, J. F., and N. Owen. 1999. *Physical Activity and Behavioral Medicine*. Chapter 7. Thousand Oaks, CA: Sage.

Whitehead, J. R. 1999. Physical activity and intrinsic motivation. In Corbin, C. B., and R. P. Pangrazi, (eds.), *Towards a Better Understanding of Physical Fitness and Activity*. Scottsdale, AZ: Holcomb-Hathaway.

 In the News

One-third of all adult men do NOT have a regular physician. Fewer than 20 percent of women have no regular doctor. Over half of young men (eighteen to twenty-nine) do not have a doctor compared to 33 percent of women in this age range. Three times as many men (24 percent) have not visited a doctor in the past year as compared to women (8 percent). This is interesting since women outlive men by six years and have much lower rates of chronic disease such as heart disease. Other interesting facts include the following:

- Fewer than one in five men visit a doctor in the first few days of sickness.
- Two in five say they wait at least one week or as long as possible.
- Many men do not know whom to see if a problem arises.
- Men often fail to get important health screenings (e.g., prostate, testicular, and blood lipids).

Experts have suggested several reasons why men, especially young men, avoid seeing a physician:

- Sickness is seen as a weakness, seen as unmanly.
- Pain is considered normal, not a symptom of a problem.
- Men may deny possible illness.
- I don't have time. I will do it later.

Experts offer some suggestions as to why women are more willing to see a doctor and take preventive action:

- Have established a relationship with physicians early because of family health care, child-bearing, or women's health issues.
- Awareness of women's health issues from media.
- More open to health discussions with friends.

Married men are more likely to seek medical consultation than single men. Studies show that wives may prompt their husbands to take better care of themselves. For good health it is important for all people to do regular self-screening such as described in this book and to have regular medical check-ups.

Source: Commonwealth Fund and American Medical News.

Lab 2A: The Physical Activity Adherence Questionnaire

Name	Section	Date

Purpose: To help you understand the factors that influence physical activity adherence and to see which factors you might change to improve your chances of achieving the action or maintenance level for physical activity.

Procedures:

1. The factors that predispose, enable, and reinforce adherence to physically active living are listed below. Read each statement. Place an X in the circle under the most appropriate response for you: very true, somewhat true, or not true.
2. When you have answered all of the items, determine a score by summing the four numbers for each type of factor. Then sum the three scores (predisposing, enabling, reinforcing) to get your total score.
3. Record your scores in the Results section and answer the questions in the Conclusions and Implications section.

	Very True	Somewhat True	Not True	
Predisposing Factors				
1. I am very knowledgeable about physical activity.	3	2	1	
2. I have a strong belief that physical activity is good for me.	3	2	1	
3. I enjoy doing regular exercise and physical activity.	3	2	1	
4. I am confident of my abilities in sports, exercise, and other physical activities.	3	2	1	
		Predisposing Score	**=**	
Enabling Factors				
5. I possess good sport skills.	3	2	1	
6. I know how to plan my own physical activity program.	3	2	1	
7. I have a place to do physical activity near my home or work.	3	2	1	
8. I have the equipment I need to do physical activities I enjoy.	3	2	1	
		Enabling Score	**=**	
Reinforcing Factors				
9. I have the support of my family for doing my regular physical activity.	3	2	1	
10. I have many friends who enjoy the same kinds of physical activities that I do.	3	2	1	
11. I have the support of my boss and my colleagues for participation in activity.	3	2	1	
12. I have a doctor and/or employer who encourages me to exercise.	3	2	1	
		Reinforcing Score	**=**	
		Total Score (Sum 3 Scores)	**=**	

Classification	Predisposing Score	Enabling Score	Reinforcing Score	Total Score
Adherence likely	11–12	11–12	11–12	33–36
Adherence possible	9–10	9–10	9–10	25–32
Adherence unlikely	<8	<8	<8	<24

Results: Record your scores and ratings in the spaces below.

Adherence Category	Score	Rating
Predisposing		
Enabling		
Reinforcing		
Total		

Conclusions and Implications: In several sentences, discuss your ratings from this questionnaire. Also discuss the predisposing, enabling, and reinforcing factors that you may need to alter to increase your prospects for lifetime activity.

In several sentences, speculate about adherence factors for other healthy lifestyles such as eating well and managing stress. Do you think you need more or less work in these areas as compared to physically active living?

Lab 2B: The Self-Management Skills Questionnaire

Name		Section		Date	

Purpose: To help you assess your self-management skills that are important to adhering to physically active lifestyles.

Procedures:

1. Each question reflects one of the self-management skills described earlier. Read each statement. After each statement, place an X over the circle indicating whether you think the item is very true, somewhat true, or not true.
2. When you have answered all of the items, score the questionnaire using the information in the Results section. Determine your ratings and answer the questions in the Conclusions and Implications section.

		Very True	Somewhat True	Not True	Score
1.	I regularly assess my health-related fitness and rate my fitness test results using health-fitness standards.	3	2	1 (X)	
2.	I keep regular physical activity logs to monitor current physical activity levels.	3	2	1 (X)	
3.	I set realistic and attainable fitness and activity goals and monitor progress in meeting these goals.	3	2 (X)	1	
4.	I have planned a personal program that includes activities for all parts of fitness and for optimal health benefits.	3	2	1 (X)	
5.	I have the motor skills necessary to perform several physical activities on a regular basis.	3 (X)	2	1	
6.	I have more positive than negative attitudes about physical activity.	3 (X)	2	1	
7.	I find a way to do my activity even when the weather is bad or my time is limited.	3 (X)	2	1	
8.	I know how to identify fitness misinformation and quackery.	3 (X)	2	1	
9.	I know how to get others to do exercise with me and to get the support of others for doing my own activity program.	3	2 (X)	1	
10.	I know and use strategies to stick with it especially when I have not been active for a while.	3 (X)	2	1	
11.	I participate in activities that I am not very good at because I am able to enjoy them even if I don't excel.	3	2 (X)	1	
12.	I manage my time to allow regular performance of my physical activity program.	3	2 (X)	1	

Total Score (Sum 12 Scores)

Rating	Individual Scores	Total Score
Good	3	30–36
Marginal	2	24–29
May need improvement	1	< 24

Results: Record your score for each skill as well as the rating in the chart below. There is one question for each self-management skill. Your score for each self-management skill is the number inside the circle for that question. The number of the question for each skill is noted in the chart below. To get your total score, sum the scores for all of the self-management skills.

Self-Management Skill	Item	Score	Rating
Self-assessment	1		
Self-monitoring	2		
Goal setting	3		
Self-planning	4		
Performance skills	5		
Balancing attitudes	6		
Overcoming barriers	7		
Learning consumer skills	8		
Finding social support	9		
Preventing relapse	10		
Adopting coping strategies	11		
Time management	12		
Total			

Conclusions and Implications: In several sentences, discuss your ratings regarding self-management skills. In which areas do you think you need to learn more to be able to be a better self-manager?

In several sentences, speculate about your self-management skills for other healthy lifestyles such as eating well and managing stress. Do you think you need more or less work in these areas as compared to managing for physically active living?

Preparing for Physical Activity

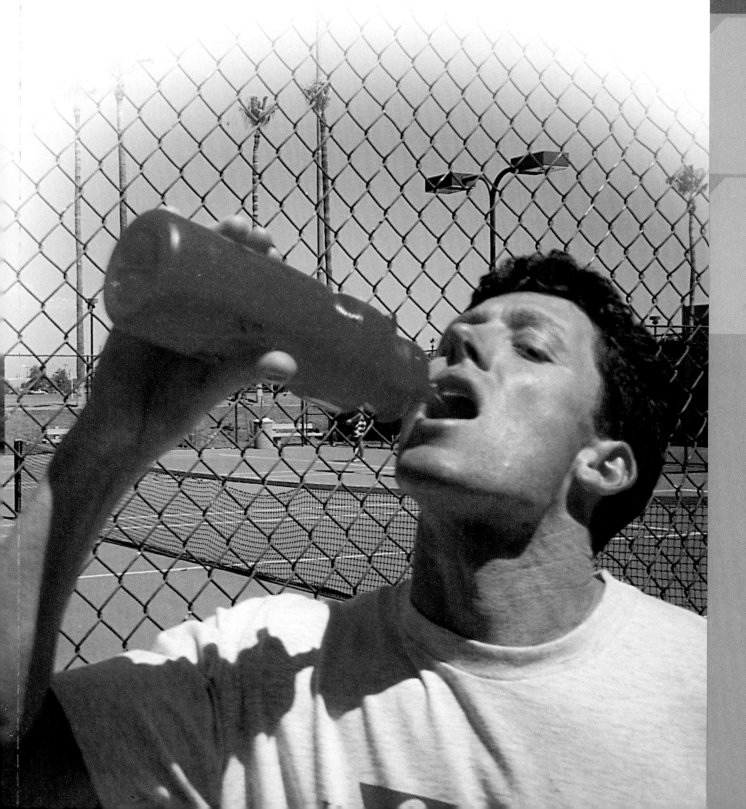

Proper preparation can help make physical activity enjoyable, effective, and safe.

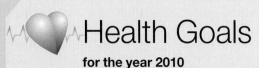

Health Goals

for the year 2010

- Improve the health, fitness, and quality of life through daily physical activity.
- Increase leisure time physical activity.

For people just beginning a physical activity program, adequate preparation may be the key to persistence. For those who have been regularly active for some time, sound preparation can help reduce risk of injury and make activity more enjoyable. It is hoped that a person armed with good information about preparation will become involved and stay involved in physical activity for a lifetime. For long-term maintenance, physical activity must be something that is a part of a person's normal lifestyle. Some factors that will help you prepare for and make physical activity a part of your normal routine are presented in this concept.

Factors to Consider before Beginning Physical Activity

Before beginning regular physical activity, it is important to establish medical readiness. www.mhhe.com/fit_well/web03 **Click 01.** Physical activity requires the cardiovascular system to work harder. While this level of stress can promote positive adaptations, the stress on the heart can be unsafe and dangerous for certain individuals. The British Columbia (Canada) Ministry of Health conducted extensive research to devise a procedure that would help people know when it was advisable to seek medical consultation prior to beginning or altering an exercise program. The goal was to prevent unnecessary medical examinations, while at the same time helping people to be reasonably assured that regular exercise was appropriate. The research resulted in the development of the Physical Activity Readiness Questionnaire **(PAR-Q)** questionnaire. The most recent revision of the PAR-Q consists of seven simple questions you can ask yourself to determine if medical consultation is necessary prior to exercise involvement.

The American College of Sports Medicine (ACSM) has developed additional guidelines to help determine if medical consultation or if a **clinical exercise test** is necessary prior to participation in physical activity programs. The ACSM divides people into three general categories (see Table 1). Apparently healthy young adults classified with low risk and who give no yes answers to the PAR-Q are generally cleared for moderate and vigorous physical activity without a medical exam or clinical exercise testing. For those with moderate risk, moderate exercise is generally appropriate without a medical exam or an exercise test, but both are recommended prior to undertaking vigorous physical activity. For those in the high risk category, a medical exam and exercise testing are recommended for moderate and vigorous activity. When resuming physical activity after an injury or illness, consultation with a physician is always wise no matter what your age or medical condition.

Table 1 ▶ American College of Sports Medicine Risk Stratification Categories and Criteria

Stratification Category	Criteria
Low Risk	Younger people (less than forty-five for men and fifty-five for women) are considered at low risk when they have no heart disease symptoms and have no more than one of the risk factors listed below.
Moderate Risk	People without heart disease symptoms but who are older (men forty-five or more and women fifty-five and older) OR who have two or more of the risk factors listed below.
High Risk	People with one or more of the signs or symptoms listed below OR who have known cardiovascular, pulmonary, or metabolic disease.

Risk Factors

Family history of heart disease; smoker; high blood pressure (hypertension); high cholesterol; abnormal blood glucose levels; obesity (BMI of >30 or waist girth of >100 cm); sedentary lifestyle; low HDL cholesterol level.

Signs and Symptoms

Chest, neck, or jaw pain from lack of oxygen to the heart; shortness of breath at rest or in mild exercise; dizziness or fainting; difficult or labored breathing when lying, sitting, or standing; ankle swelling; fast heart beat or heart palpitations; pain in the legs from poor circulation; heart murmur; unusual fatigue or shortness of breath with usual activities.

Source: American College of Sports Medicine.

Technology Update

Ideally it would be possible to screen all exercisers to assure that they are free from cardiovascular disease risk. Inevitably, however, there will be those for whom disease goes undetected resulting in heart problems in or after exercise. One form of new technology for saving lives is the Automated External Defibrillator (AED). After identifying cardiac arrest and performing CPR, if ventricular fibrillation (chaotic electrical activity to heart muscle) occurs it may be necessary to "shock" the heart back to a normal rhythm. The AED has a heart rhythm analysis system that advises

the operator when a "shock" is appropriate. The operator must then make the final action to deliver the shock. A recent position statement of the American College of Sports Medicine and the American Heart Association advises health and fitness clubs—especially those that have a large member base, those with older members, or those with members known to have disease—to have the AED system available. The AED should be used as part of an emergency plan that includes training of all exercise personnel. Federal law and "Good Samaritan Laws" in forty-seven states extend protection to AED users.

Table 2 ▶ Dressing for Activity

Clothing
- Avoid clothing that is too tight or that restricts movement.
- Material in contact with skin should be porous.
- Clothing should protect against wind and rain but allow for heat loss and evaporation, e.g., Gortex.
- Wear layers so that a layer can be removed if not needed.
- Wear socks for most activities to prevent blisters, abrasions, odor, and excessive shoe wear.
- Socks should be absorbent and fit properly (too tight causes ingrown toenails; too loose causes blisters).
- Do not use nonporous clothing that traps sweat in an attempt to lose weight; these garments prevent evaporation and cooling.

Special Clothing
- Women should consider an exercise bra.
- Men should consider an athletic supporter.
- Wear helmets and padding for activities with risk of falling such as biking or inline skating.
- Wear reflective clothing for night activities.
- Wear water shoes for some aquatic activities.
- Consider lace-up ankle braces to prevent injury.
- Consider a mouthpiece for basketball and other contact sports.

Shoes
- Heel counter and stabilizer for stability and movement control.
- Heel notch to protect Achilles tendon.
- Adequate heel width for stability and to prevent ankle injury.
- Some cushion prevents shock to the foot; too much cushion inhibits the reflexes that protect the foot.
- Lightweight shoes reduce energy cost in activity.
- Use soles (Out and Mid) with good traction to reduce risk of falling.
- Wear shoes of adequate size (about one-half size larger than normal).
- The toe box should have adequate room to wiggle toes and to allow space if you wear two pairs of socks.
- Replace shoes periodically if heels and soles break down—even if the fabric is still good.
- Wear shoes made of material that can breathe, such as nylon mesh, to help sweat evaporation and reduce shoe weight gain.
- Consider high tops for basketball.
- Cross trainers are the best all-purpose choice.

There is no way to be absolutely sure that you are medically sound to begin a physical activity program. Even a thorough exam by a physician cannot guarantee that a person does not have some limitations that may cause a problem during exercise. Use of the PAR-Q and adherence to the ACSM guidelines are advised to help minimize the risk while preventing unnecessary medical cost. However, if you are unsure about your readiness for activity, a medical exam and a clinical exercise test are the surest ways to make certain that you are ready to participate.

Those who plan to do intensive training (particularly for sports) may want to answer some additional questions concerning whether a medical exam is necessary before beginning (see Lab 3A).

🌐 **It is important to dress properly for physical activity.** www.mhhe.com/fit_well/web03 Click 02. The clothing and footwear you choose should be appropriate for the specific activity you plan to perform. Though appearance is important, comfort is more

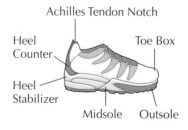

Figure 1 ▶ Characteristics of a good activity shoe.

PAR-Q An acronym for Physical Activity Readiness Questionnaire; designed to help you determine if you are medically suited to begin an exercise program.

Clinical Exercise Test A test typically administered on a treadmill in which exercise is gradually increased in intensity while the heart is monitored by an EKG. Symptoms not present at rest, such as an abnormal EKG, may be present in an exercise test.

important than looks. Table 2 provides guidelines for dressing for activity, including Figure 1 for shoes.

Factors to Consider during Daily Physical Activity

There are three key components of the daily activity program: the warm-up exercise, the workout, and the cool-down exercise. The key component of a fitness program is the daily workout. Experts agree, however, that the workout should be preceded by a warm-up and followed by a cool-down. The **warm-up** prepares the body for physical activity, and the **cool-down** returns the body to rest and promotes effective recovery by aiding the return of blood from the working muscles to the heart (see Figure 2).

The cardiovascular warm-up prior to the workout is recommended to prepare the muscles and heart for the workout. www.mhhe.com/ fit_well/web03 Click 03. There are two good reasons for warming up prior to activity. The first is to prepare the heart muscle and circulatory system. When you start physical activity, blood flow is not immediately available to the heart and muscles. A proper warm-up decreases the risk of irregular heart beats associated with poor coronary circulation. A proper warm-up can also improve performance since it minimizes the premature formation of **lactic acid** at the start of physical activity (for more information see Concept 14). Research suggests that two minutes of walking, jogging, or mild exercise is adequate for moderate activities; however, some experts recommend five minutes or more of moderate activity as a warm-up for vigorous activity.

The second reason for a warm-up is to stretch the skeletal muscles. When you begin exercise, muscles and joints are usually cold and stiff. By gradually warming up the body, the muscles become more elastic and extensible. The skeletal muscle warm-up should include static stretching of the major muscle groups involved in the exercise that is to follow. It should be emphasized that even though warming up prior to an activity may help reduce the chance of muscle injury, it is not a substitute for a regular program of exercise designed to improve flexibility.

A warm-up that is suitable for walking, jogging, running, cycling, and even basketball is illustrated in Figure 3. This warm-up can be used for other activities provided stretching exercises for the major muscle groups involved in the activities are added. Additional exercises that are appropriate for inclusion in a stretching warm-up are illustrated in the flexibility concept. The cardiovascular warm-up is suitable for most activities, but other mild exercise (such as a slow swim for swimmers or a slow ride for cyclists) can be substituted.

Many experts recommend that the stretching portion of the warm-up be done after the cardiovascular portion. Some experts believe that the cardiovascular portion of the warm-up should precede the stretching portion because warm muscles are less likely to be injured by the stretch. Warm muscles also stretch farther. Some experts are concerned that the stretch warm-up may be abandoned by people who feel that they do not have time to do the cardiovascular and stretching warm-up before doing their activity program. In this case, it is better to do stretching without the cardiovascular warm-up than do nothing at all. If you choose to stretch before the warm-up, make certain it is a gentle, static stretch. This is not the time for a flexibility workout in which you try to increase your normal range of motion. Rather, it should be for the purpose of limbering up or loosening.

A cool-down after the workout is important to promote an effective recovery from physical activity. The cool-down is done immediately after the workout. Like the warm-up, there are two principal components of a cool-down: static muscle stretching and an activity for the cardiovascular system. Although not all experts agree, some believe that static muscle stretching *after* the workout is

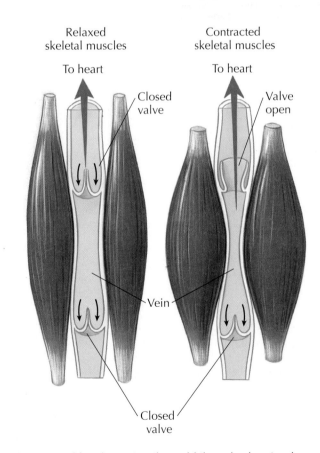

Figure 2 ▶ Muscle contractions aid the veins in returning blood to the heart.

Cardiovascular Exercise

Before you perform a vigorous workout, walk or jog slowly for two minutes or more. After exercise, do the same. If possible do this portion of the warm-up prior to muscle stretching.

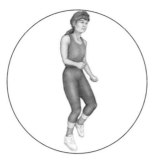

Calf Stretcher

This exercise stretches the calf muscles (gastrocnemius and soleus). Face a wall with your feet 2 or 3 feet away. Step forward on left foot to allow both hands to touch the wall. Keep the heel of your right foot on the ground, toe turned in slightly, knee straight, and buttocks tucked in. Lean forward by bending your front knee and arms and allowing your head to move nearer the wall. Hold. Repeat with the other leg.

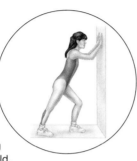

Hamstring Stretcher

This exercise stretches the muscles of the back of the upper leg (hamstrings) as well as those of the hip, knee, and ankle. Lie on your back. Bring the right knee to your chest and grasp the toes with the right hand. Place the left hand on the back of the right thigh. Pull the knee toward the chest, push the heel toward the ceiling, and pull the toes toward the shin. Attempt to straighten the knee. Stretch and hold. Repeat with the other leg.

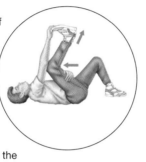

Leg Hug

This exercise stretches the hip and back extensor muscles. Lie on your back. Bend one leg and grasp your thigh under the knee. Hug it to your chest. Keep the other leg straight and on the floor. Hold. Repeat with the opposite leg.

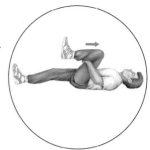

Seated Side Stretch

This exercise stretches the muscles of the trunk. Begin in a seated position with the legs crossed. Stretch the left arm over the head to the right. Bend at the waist (to right), reaching as far as possible to the left with the right arm. Hold. Do not let the trunk rotate. Repeat to the opposite side. For less stretch the overhead arm may be bent. This exercise can be done in the standing position but is less effective.

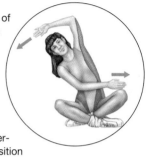

Zipper

This exercise stretches the muscle on the back of the arm (triceps) and the lower chest muscles (pecs). Lift right arm and reach behind head and down the spine (as if pulling up a zipper). With the left hand, push down on right elbow and hold. Reverse arm position and repeat.

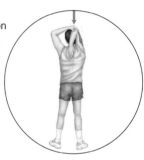

The exercises shown here can be used before a moderate workout as a warm-up, or after a workout as a cool-down. Perform these exercises slowly, preferably after completing a cardiovascular warm-up. Do not bounce or jerk against the muscle. Hold each stretch for at least 15 seconds. Perform each exercise at least once and up to three times. Other stretching exercises are presented in the concept on flexibility that can be used in a warm-up or cool-down.
Figure 3 ▶ Sample warm-up and cool-down exercises.

more important than stretching before because it may help relieve spasms in fatigued muscles. Stretching as part of the cool-down may be more effective for lengthening the muscles than stretching at other times because the muscle temperature is elevated and, therefore, the stretching is more likely to produce optimal flexibility improvements.

A cardiovascular portion of the cool-down is also important. During physical activity, the heart pumps a large amount of blood to supply the working muscles with the oxygen necessary to keep moving. The muscles squeeze the veins (see Figure 2), which forces the blood back to the heart. Valves in the veins prevent the blood from flowing backward. As long as exercise continues, the blood is moved by the muscles back to the heart, where it is once again pumped to the body. If exercise is stopped abruptly, the blood is left in the area of the working muscles and has

Warm-Up Light to moderate activity done prior to the workout. Its purpose is to reduce the risk of injury and soreness and possibly improve performance in a physical activity.

Cool-Down Light to moderate activity done after a workout to help the body recover; often consisting of the same exercises used in the warm-up.

Lactic Acid A byproduct of the metabolic processes that occurs during vigorous physical activity; a cause of muscle fatigue.

no way to get back to the heart. In the case of the runner, the blood pools in the legs. Because the heart has less blood to pump, blood pressure may drop. This can result in dizziness and can even cause a person to pass out. The best way to prevent this problem is to taper off or slow down gradually after exercise. A cardiovascular cool-down should include approximately 2 minutes of walking, slow jogging, or any nonvigorous activity that uses the muscles involved in the workout.

Physical Activity in the Heat

Physical activity in hot and humid environments challenges the body's heat loss mechanisms. www.mhhe.com/fit_well/web03 Click 04. The normal human body temperature is 98.6°F. During vigorous activity, the body produces large amounts of heat, which must be dissipated to keep the body temperature regulated. The body has several ways to dissipate heat. Conduction is the transfer of heat from a hot body to a cold body. Convection is the transfer of heat through the air or other medium. Fans and wind can facilitate heat loss by convection and help regulate temperature. The primary method of cooling is through evaporation of sweat. The chemical process involved in evaporation transfers heat from the body and reduces the body temperature. When conditions are humid, the effectiveness of evaporation is reduced since the air is already saturated with moisture. This is why it is difficult to regulate body temperature when conditions are both hot and humid.

Heat-related illness can occur if proper hydration is not maintained. Maximum sweat rates during physical activity in the heat can approach 1–2 liters per hour. If this fluid is not replaced, **dehydration** can occur. If dehydration is not corrected with water or other fluid-replacement drinks, it becomes increasingly more difficult for the body to maintain normal body temperatures. At some point, the rate of sweating decreases as the body begins to conserve its remaining water. It shunts blood to the skin to transfer excess heat directly to the environment, but this is less effective than evaporation, and various heat-related problems including heat stroke and **hyperthermia** can result (see Table 3).

One way to monitor the amount of fluid loss is to monitor the color of your urine. The American College of Sports Medicine indicates that clear (almost colorless) urine produced in large volumes indicates that you are hydrated and ready for activity. Dark yellow urine produced in small volume is a good indicator of dehydration and need for fluid replacement.

Acclimatization improves the body's tolerance in the heat. Individuals with good fitness will respond better to activity in the heat than individuals with poor fitness.

Table 3 ▶ Types of Heat-Related Problems

Problem	Symptoms	Severity
Heat cramps	Muscle cramps, especially in muscles most used in exercise	Least severe
Heat exhaustion	Muscle cramps, weakness, dizziness, headache, nausea, clammy skin, paleness	Moderately severe
Heat stroke	Hot, flushed skin, dry skin (lack of sweating), dizziness, fast pulse, unconsciousness, high temperature	Extremely severe

This is because the ability to sweat improves with training. With regular exposure to the heat, the body becomes conditioned to sweat earlier, to sweat more profusely, and to distribute sweat more effectively around the body. This process of acclimatization makes it easier for the body to maintain a safe body temperature.

When doing physical activity in hot and humid environments, special precautions should be taken to prevent heat-related problems. www.mhhe.com/fit_well/ web03 Click 05.

- Limit or avoid physical activity in hot or humid environments. The **apparent temperature** (also refered to as the heat index) is an index that combines temperature and humidity. Physical activity is safe when the apparent temperature is below 80°F (26.7°C). Above this temperature there are four zones (see Table 4) that illustrate the danger of doing physical activity when the apparent temperature is high. When apparent temperatures reach the Danger Zones, activity should be limited or canceled. With extreme care, experienced exercisers who have become acclimatized to the heat may be able to perform at higher apparent temperatures than those who are less experienced. However, care should be used by all people who perform physical activity in hot and humid environments.

- Replace fluids regularly. Drink water before (2 cups or 16 ounces) and during activity (1 cup or 5–10 ounces every 15 to 20 minutes). After activity, replacing 16 ounces of fluid for each pound of weight lost is a good rule. For exercise lasting more than one hour, fluid-replacement drinks containing simple carbohydrates (glucose, fructose, or sucrose) and electrolytes are considered beneficial to performance and body cooling. If the concentration of sugars is no more than 4–8 percent, they can replace fluids as quickly as water.

- Gradually expose yourself to physical activity in hot and humid environments. Too much at once is especially dangerous.

Table 4 ▶ Exercise in the Heat (Apparent Temperatures)

To read the table, find air temperature on the top, then find the humidity on the left.
Find the apparent temperature where the columns meet.

Relative Humidity (%)	Air Temperature (Degrees F)										
	70	75	80	85	90	95	100	105	110	115	120
100	72	80	91	108	132						
95	71	79	89	105	128						
90	71	79	88	102	122						
85	71	78	87	99	117	141					
80	71	78	86	97	113	136					
75	70	77	86	95	109	130					
70	70	77	85	93	106	124	144				
65	70	76	83	91	102	119	138				
60	70	76	82	90	100	114	132	149			
55	69	75	81	89	98	110	126	142			
50	69	75	81	88	96	107	120	135	150		
45	68	74	80	87	95	104	115	129	143		
40	68	74	79	86	93	101	110	123	137	151	
35	67	73	79	85	91	98	107	118	130	143	
30	67	73	78	84	90	96	104	113	123	135	148
25	66	72	77	83	88	94	101	109	117	127	139
20	66	72	77	82	87	93	99	105	112	120	130
15	65	71	76	81	86	91	97	102	108	115	123
10	65	70	75	80	85	90	95	100	105	111	116
5	64	69	74	79	84	88	93	97	102	107	111
0	64	69	73	78	83	87	91	95	99	103	107

"Apparent Temperatures" (Heat Index)

■ = Exreme Danger Zone
■ = Danger Zone
□ = Extreme Caution Zone
■ = Caution Zone
□ = Safe

Source: Data from National Oceanic and Atmospheric Administration.

- When possible, do your activity in the morning or evening.
- Dress properly for exercise in the heat and humidity. Wear white or light colors that reflect rather than absorb heat. Porous clothing allows the passage of air to cool the body. Rubber, plastic, or other nonporous clothing is especially dangerous. A porous hat or cap can help when exercising in direct sunlight.
- Do not change your wet shirt for a dry one. A wet shirt cools the body better.
- Rest at regular intervals, preferably in the shade.
- Watch for signs of heat stress. If signs are present, stop immediately.

If overheating occurs, take immediate steps to cool the body. Take these steps: stop physical activity, get out of the heat and into the shade, remove excess clothing, drink cool water, and immerse the body in cool water. If symptoms of heat stroke are present, seek immediate medical attention; and statically stretch cramped muscles.

Physical Activity in Other Environments

Physical activity in exceptionally cold and windy weather can be dangerous. www.mhhe.com/fit_well/web03 Click 06. Physical activity in the cold presents the opposite problems as exercise in the heat. In

Dehydration Excessive loss of water from the body, usually through perspiration, urination, or evaporation.

Hyperthermia Excessively high body temperature caused by excessive heat production or impaired heat loss capacity. Heat stroke is an example of a hyperthermic condition.

Apparent Temperature A combination of temperature and humidity used to determine if it is dangerous to perform physical activity (also called heat index).

the cold, the primary goal is to retain the body's heat and avoid **hypothermia** and frostbite. Early signs of hypothermia include shivering and cold extremities caused by blood shunted to the body core to conserve heat. As the core temperature continues to drop, heart rate, respiration, and reflexes are depressed. Subsequently, cognitive functions decrease, speech and movement become impaired, and bizarre behavior may occur. Frostbite results from water crystallizing in the tissues causing cell destruction.

A combination of cold and wind (**windchill**) poses the greatest danger. Recent research conducted in Canada, in cooperation with the U.S. National Weather Service, produced new tables for determining windchill and the time of exposure necessary to get frostbite (see Table 5). The old method of measurement overestimated the impact of cold weather. Consider the following guidelines for performing physical activity in cold and windy environments.

- Limit or cancel activity if the time to frostbite is 30 minutes or less (see Table 5).
- Dress properly in the wind and cold. Wear light clothing in several layers rather than one heavy garment. The layer of clothing closest to the body should ideally help to transfer (wick) moisture away from the skin and transfer it to a second, more absorbent layer. Fabric such as polypropylene and capilene are examples of wickable fabrics. A porous windbreaker will keep wind from cooling the body and will allow the release of body heat. The hands, feet, nose, and ears are most susceptible to frostbite so they should be covered. Wear a hat or cap, mask, and mittens. Mittens are warmer than gloves. A light coating of petroleum jelly on exposed body parts can be helpful.
- Keep from getting wet in cold weather.

High altitude and/or air pollution may limit performance and require adaptation of normal physical activity. www.mhhe.com/fit_well/web03 Click 07. The ability to do vigorous physical tasks is diminished as altitude increases. Breathing rate and heart rates are more elevated at high altitude. With proper acclimation (gradual exposure), the body adjusts to the lower oxygen pressure found at high altitude, and performance improves. Nevertheless, performance ability at high altitudes, especially for activities requiring cardiovascular fitness, is usually less than would be expected at sea level. At extremely high altitudes, the ability to perform vigorous physical activity may be impossible without an extra oxygen supply. When moving from sea level to a high altitude, vigorous exercise should be done with caution. Acclimation to high altitudes requires a minimum of two weeks and may not be complete for several months. Care should be taken to drink adequate water at high altitude.

www.mhhe.com/fit_well/web03 Click 08. Various pollutants such as ozone, carbon monoxide, pollens, and particulates can also cause poor physical performance, and in some cases, health problems. Ozone, a pollutant produced primarily by the sun's reaction to car

Table 5 ▶ Windchill Factor Chart

Actual Temperature Reading (Degrees F)	Estimated Wind Speed (mph)									Zones
	Calm	5	10	15	20	25	30	35	40	
50	50	48	40	36	32	30	28	27	26	Relatively safe with proper clothing
40	40	37	28	22	18	16	13	11	10	
30	30	27	16	9	4	0	-2	-4	-6	
20	20	16	4	-5	-10	-15	-18	-20	-21	
10	10	6	-9	-18	-25	-29	-33	-35	-37	Danger to exposed skin
0	0	-5	-24	-32	-39	-44	-48	-51	-53	
-10	-10	-15	-33	-45	-40	-59	-63	-67	-69	
-20	-20	-26	-46	-58	-67	-74	-79	-82	-85	Unsafe— postpone exercise
-30	-30	-36	-58	-72	-82	-88	-94	-98	-100	
-40	-40	-47	-70	-85	-96	-104	-109	-113	-116	

*NOTE: Wind speeds above 40 mph do not seem to add to danger of cold.

Source: National Weather Service.

exhaust, can cause symptoms including headache, coughing, and eye irritation. Similar symptoms result from exposure to carbon monoxide, a tasteless and odorless gas, caused by combustion of oil, gasoline, and/or cigarette smoke. Most news media in metropolitan areas now provide updates on ozone and carbon monoxide levels in their weather reports. When levels of these pollutants reach moderate levels, some people may need to modify their exercise. When levels are high, some may need to postpone exercise. Exercisers wishing to avoid ozone and carbon monoxide may want to exercise indoors early in the morning, or later in the evening. It is wise to avoid areas with a high concentration of motor vehicles.

Pollens from certain plants may cause allergic reactions for certain people. Some people are allergic to dust or other particulates in the air. Weather reports of pollens and particulates may help exercisers determine the best times for their activities and when to avoid vigorous activities.

Soreness and Injury

Understanding soreness can help you persist in physical activity and avoid problems. www.mhhe.com/fit_well/web03 Click 09. Some people avoid physical activity because they remember earlier experiences such as team practices or training for special events that led to soreness 24 to 48 hours after the intense exercise. They feel that all activity will make them sore, and they want to avoid this unpleasant experience. It is true that intense exercise, especially to muscle groups that are not normally exercised, can cause what is called delayed-onset muscle soreness **(DOMS).** Some people mistakenly believe that lactic acid is the cause of muscle soreness. Lactic acid, however, returns to normal levels 30 minutes after exercise, whereas DOMS occurs at least 24 hours following exercise. DOMS results from microscopic muscle tears, not a build-up of lactic acid. In some cases, DOMS is accompanied by swelling and pain, but in general, the condition has no long-term consequences.

Several steps can be taken to avoid DOMS and to make activity more enjoyable. Starting gradually (not doing too much after being inactive) is perhaps the most important thing you can do. Lengthening contractions (eccentric) are more likely to cause DOMS than shortening muscle contractions (concentric contractions). For this reason, you should phase walking or running downhill or downstairs into your program. Of course, a regular warm-up is also advised. Fortunately, DOMS lasts only a day or so. Doing moderate exercise when you have soreness does not seem to put you at risk of muscle injury. DOMS is only temporary and is uncommon for those who exercise regularly and consistently.

Being able to treat minor injuries will help reduce their negative effects. Minor injuries such as muscle sprains and strains are common to those who are persistent in their exercise. If a serious injury should occur, it is important to get immediate medical attention. However, for minor injuries, following the **RICE** formula will help you reduce the pain or the injury and will speed recovery. In this acronym, **R** stands for *rest*. Muscle sprains and strains heal best if rested, and rest also helps you avoid further damage to the muscle. **I** stands for *ice*. The quick application of cold (ice or ice water) to a minor injury minimizes swelling and speeds recovery. Cold should be applied to as large a surface area as possible (soaking is best). If ice is used, it should be wrapped to avoid direct contact with the skin. Apply cold for 20–30 minutes, three times a day for several days. **C** stands for *compression*. Wrapping or compressing the injured area also helps minimize swelling and speeds recovery. Elastic bandages are good for applying compression. For a sprained ankle, wearing a tied high top shoe until a bandage can be located provides good compression. Elastic socks may also be useful. Care should be taken to avoid wrapping an injury too tightly because this can result in loss of circulation to the area. **E** stands for *elevation*. Keeping the injured area elevated (above the level of the heart) is effective in minimizing swelling. If pain or swelling persists, or if there is any doubt about the seriousness of an injury, seek medical help.

Taking over-the-counter pain remedies can help reduce the pain of muscle strains and sprains. Aspirin and ibuprofen (e.g., Motrin, Excedrin) have anti-inflammatory properties. However, acetaminophen (e.g., Tylenol) does not have anti-inflammatory properties, so it may reduce the pain but it will not reduce the inflammation. Any over-the-counter remedy should be taken only as directed unless otherwise indicated by a physician.

Hypothermia Excessively low body temperature (less than 95°F) characterized by uncontrollable shivering, loss of coordination, and mental confusion.

Windchill Factor An index that uses air temperature and wind speed to determine the chilling effect of the environment on humans.

DOMS An acronym for delayed-onset muscle soreness; a common malady that follows relatively vigorous activity especially among beginners.

RICE An acronym for rest, ice, compression, and elevation; a method of treating minor injuries.

The most common injuries incurred in physical activity are sprains and strains. www.mhhe.com/fit_well/web03 Click 10. A strain occurs when the fibers in a muscle are injured. Common activity-related injuries are hamstring strains that occur after a vigorous sprint. A good example would be the occasional athlete who sprints to first base without warming up and after not playing for a long time. Other commonly strained muscles include the muscles in the front of the thigh, the low back, and the calf muscles. A sprain is an injury to a ligament—the connective tissue that connects bones to bones. The most common sprain is to the ankle. It frequently occurs when the ankle is rolled to the outside when jumping or running. Evidence suggests that lace-up ankle braces made of non-elastic material are effective in reducing ankle sprains. Other common sprains are to the knee, the shoulder, and the wrist. Sprains and strains respond well to RICE.

Tendonitis is an inflammation of the tendon and is most often a result of overuse rather than trauma. Tendonitis can be painful but often does not swell to the extent that sprains do. For this reason, elevation and compression are not especially effective, but ice and rest are especially useful.

Muscle cramps can be relieved by statically stretching a muscle. Muscle cramps are pains in the large muscles of the body that result when the muscle contracts vigorously for a continued period of time. Muscle cramps are usually not considered to be an injury, but they are painful and may seem like an injury. They are usually short in duration and can often be relieved with proper treatment. Cramps can result from lack of fluid replacement (dehydration), from fatigue, and from a blow directly to a muscle. A true cramp is not the same as a muscle tear, sprain, or strain. A cramp can be relieved by statically stretching the cramped muscle. For example, the calf muscle, which often cramps among runners, football players, and other sports participants, can be relieved using the calf stretcher exercise, which is part of the warm-up in this concept. Other stretching exercises from the concept on flexibility can be used to relieve cramps to other muscles or muscle groups. If stretching causes persistent pain, stop the stretching—you may have a muscle injury rather than a cramp. Of course, replacing fluids regularly during exercise helps avoid cramps, as does the development of flexibility.

Web Resources

ACSM's Health and Fitness Journal www.acsm-healthfitness.org
ACSM's Fit Society Page www.acsm.org/health%2Bfitness/fit_society.htm

American Alliance for Health, Physical Education, Recreation and Dance www.aahperd.org
American College of Sports Medicine www.acsm.org
National Athletic Trainers Association www.nata.org
Med Watch www.fda.gov/medwatch/
The Physician and Sports Medicine www.physsportsmed.com

Suggested Readings

Additional reference materials for Concept 3 are available at www.mhhe.com/fit_well/web03 Click 11.

American College of Sports Medicine. 2000. *ACSM's Guidelines for Exercise Testing and Prescription.* 6th ed. Philadelphia, PA: Lippincott, Williams and Wilkins.

American College of Sports Medicine. 1996. Position stand on exercise and fluid replacement. *Medicine and Science in Sports and Exercise* 28(1):i.

American College of Sports Medicine. 1996. Position stand on heat and cold illness during distance running. *Medicine and Science in Sports and Exercise* 28(12):i.

American College of Sports Medicine and American Heart Association. 2002. Automated external defibrillators in health/fitness facilities. *Medicine and Science in Sports and Exercise* 34(3):561–564.

Couture, C. J., and K. A. Karlson. 2002. Tibial stress injuries. *Physician and Sports Medicine* 30(6):29–36.

Eickhoff-Shemek, J. 2002. Exercise equipment injuries: Who's at fault? *ACSM's Health and Fitness Journal* 6(1):27–30.

Frankovich, R. J. et al. 2001. Inline skating injuries. *Physician and Sports Medicine* 29(4):57–64.

Hockenbury, R., and G. Sammarco. 2001. Evaluation and treatment of ankle sprains. *The Physician and Sports Medicine* 29(2):57–64.

Hootman, J. M. et al. 2002. Epidemiology of musculoskeletal injuries among sedentary and physically active adults. *Medicine and Science in Sports and Exercise* 34(5):838–844.

Shepard, R. J. 2001. Exercise in the heat: Double threat to immune system. *Physician and Sports Medicine* 29(6):21–31.

Shephard, R. J. 1999. Preparing for physical activity. In Corbin, C. B., and R. P. Pangrazi, (eds.), *Towards a Better Understanding of Physical Fitness and Activity.* Scottsdale, AZ: Holcomb-Hathaway.

Shirreffs, S. M., and R. J. Maughan. 2000. Rehydration and recovery of fluid balance after exercise. *Exercise and Sport Sciences Reviews* 28(1):27–32.

Stoike, P. J. Automated external defibrillators: Purchasing and staff training considerations. *ACSM's Health and Fitness Journal* 5(4):20–25.

Lab 3A: Readiness for Physical Activity

Name	Section	Date

Purpose: To help you determine your physical readiness for participation in a program of regular exercise.

Procedures:

1. Read the directions on the "PAR-Q & You" on page 46.
2. Answer each of the seven questions on the form.
3. If you answered "yes" to one or more of the questions, follow the directions just below the PAR-Q questions regarding medical consultation.
4. If you answered "no" to all seven questions, follow the directions at the lower left-hand corner of the PAR-Q.
5. Answer the five questions about Physical Readiness for Sports or Vigorous Training in Chart 1 below.
6. Record your score below and answer the question in the Conclusions and Implications section.

Results:

Chart 1 ▶ Physical Readiness for Sports or Vigorous Training

Answer the PAR-Q before using this chart. If your answer to any of these questions is "yes" then you should consult with your personal physician by telephone or in person to determine if you have a potential problem with sports or vigorous training.

Yes   No

☐ ☐ 1. Do you plan to participate on an organized team that will play intense competitive sports (i.e., varsity team, professional team)?

☐ ☐ 2. If you plan to participate in a collision sport (even on a less organized basis), such as football, boxing, rugby, or ice hockey, have you been knocked unconscious more than one time?

☐ ☐ 3. Do you currently have symptoms from a previous muscle injury?

☐ ☐ 4. Do you currently have symptoms from a previous back injury, or do you experience back pain as a result of involvement in physical activity?

☐ ☐ 5. Do you have any other symptoms during physical activity that give you reason to be concerned about your health?

Place an X over the circle that includes the number of yes answers that you had for the PAR-Q.

⓪ ① ② ③ ④ ⑤ ⑥ ⑦

Place an X over the number of yes answers that you had for the Physical Readiness for Sports or Vigorous Training questionnaire.

⓪ ① ② ③ ④ ⑤

Conclusions and Implications:

In several sentences, discuss your readiness for physical activity. Base your comments on your questionnaire results and the types of physical activities you plan to perform in the future.

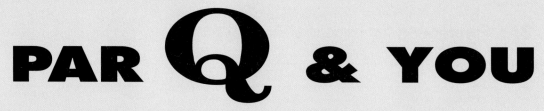

PAR Q & YOU

Regular physical activity is fun and healthy, and increasingly more people are starting to become more active every day. Being more active is very safe for most people. However, some people should check with their doctor before they start becoming much more physically active.

If you are planning to become much more physically active than you are now, start by answering the seven questions in the box below. If you are between the ages of fifteen and sixty-nine, the PAR-Q will tell you if you should check with your doctor before you start. If you are over sixty-nine years of age, and you are not used to being very active, check with your doctor.

Common sense is your best guide when you answer these questions. Please read the questions carefully and answer each one honestly: check YES or NO.

YES	NO	
☐	☐	1. Has your doctor ever said that you have a heart condition and that you should only do physical activity recommended by a doctor?
☐	☐	2. Do you feel pain in your chest when you do physical activity?
☐	☐	3. In the past month, have you had chest pain when you were not doing physical activity?
☐	☐	4. Do you lose your balance because of dizziness or do you ever lose consciousness?
☐	☐	5. Do you have a bone or joint problem that could be made worse by a change in your physical activity?
☐	☐	6. Is your doctor currently prescribing drugs (for example, water pills) for your blood pressure or heart condition?
☐	☐	7. Do you know of any other reason why you should not do physical activity?

If You Answered

Yes →

YES to one or more questions

Talk with your doctor by phone or in person BEFORE you start becoming much more physically active or BEFORE you have a fitness appraisal. Tell your doctor about the PAR-Q and which questions you answered YES.

- You may be able to do any activity you want—as long as you start slowly and build up gradually. Or, you may need to restrict your activities to those that are safe for you. Talk with your doctor about the kinds of activities you wish to participate in and follow his/her advice.
- Find out which community programs are safe and helpful for you.

No →

NO to all questions

If you answered NO honestly to all PAR-Q questions, you can be reasonably sure that you can:

- start becoming much more physically active—begin slowly and build up gradually. This is the safest and easiest way to go.
- take part in a fitness appraisal—this is an excellent way to determine your basic fitness so that you can plan the best way for you to live actively.

DELAY BECOMING MUCH MORE ACTIVE:

- if you are not feeling well because of a temporary illness such as a cold or a fever—wait until you feel better; or
- if you are or may be pregnant—talk to your doctor before you start becoming more active.

Please note: If your health changes so that you then answer YES to any of the above questions, tell your fitness or health professional. Ask whether you should change your physical activity plan.

Informed Use of the PAR-Q: The Canadian Society for Exercise Physiology, Health Canada, and their agents assume no liability for persons who undertake physical activity, and if in doubt after completing this questionnaire, consult your doctor prior to physical activity.

You are encouraged to copy the PAR-Q but only if you use the entire form

*Developed by the British Columbia Ministry of Health.
Produced by the British Columbia Ministry of Health and the Department of National Health & Welfare

Physical Activity Readiness
Questionnaire • PAR-Q
(revised 2002)

Note: It is important that you answer all questions honestly. The PAR-Q is a scientifically and medically researched pre-exercise selection device. It complements exercise programs, exercise testing procedures, and the liability considerations attendant with such programs and testing procedures. PAR-Q, like any other pre-exercise screening device, will misclassify a small percentage of prospective participants, but no pre-exercise screening method can entirely avoid this problem.

Lab 3B: The Warm-Up and Cool-Down

Name	**Section**	**Date**

Purpose: To familiarize you with a sample group of warm-up or cool-down exercises.

Procedures:

1. Perform a 2 to 5 minute cardiovascular warm-up (walk, jog, slow jump rope, swim).
2. Perform the exercises in the chart on the back of this lab page three times each. Hold the stretch for 15 to 30 seconds.
3. Complete the chart in the Results section and answer the questions in the Conclusions and Implications section.

Results: In the chart below, put an X over the circle that represents the amount of tightness you felt when performing each of the stretching warm-up and cool-down exercises. Tightness indicates that you may have shortness of a specific muscle group and that stretching exercises at times other than the warm-up or cool-down are needed.

	None	Moderate	Severe
Calf stretcher	◯	◯	◯
Hamstring stretcher	◯	◯	◯
Leg hug	◯	◯	◯
Sitting side stretch	◯	◯	◯
Zipper	◯	◯	◯

Conclusions and Implications: In several sentences, discuss the warm-up and cool-down. Include in the discussion your feelings about the adequacy of the warm-up and cool-down for you personally. Those who plan to do vigorous sports will need to supplement this group of exercises.

Sample warm-up and cool-down exercises.

The exercises shown here can be used before a moderate workout as a warm-up, or after a workout as a cool-down. Perform these exercises slowly, preferably after completing a cardiovascular warm-up. Do not bounce or jerk against the muscle. Hold each stretch for at least 15 seconds. Perform each exercise at least once and up to three times. Other stretching exercises are presented in the concept on flexibility that can be used in a warm-up or cool-down.

Cardiovascular Exercise
Before you perform a vigorous workout, walk or jog slowly for two minutes or more. After exercise, do the same. If possible do this portion of the warm-up prior to muscle stretching.

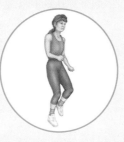

Calf Stretcher
This exercise stretches the calf muscles (gastrocnemius and soleus). Face a wall with your feet 2 or 3 feet away. Step forward on left foot to allow both hands to touch the wall. Keep the heel of your right foot on the ground, toe turned in slightly, knee straight, and buttocks tucked in. Lean forward by bending your front knee and arms and allowing your head to move nearer the wall. Hold. Repeat with the other leg.

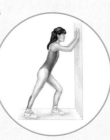

Hamstring Stretcher
This exercise stretches the muscles of the back of the upper leg (hamstrings) as well as those of the hip, knee, and ankle. Lie on your back. Bring the right knee to your chest and grasp the toes with the right hand. Place the left hand on the back of the right thigh. Pull the knee toward the chest, push the heel toward the ceiling, and pull the toes toward the shin. Attempt to straighten the knee. Stretch and hold. Repeat with the other leg.

Leg Hug
This exercise stretches the hip and back extensor muscles. Lie on your back. Bend one leg and grasp your thigh under the knee. Hug it to your chest. Keep the other leg straight and on the floor. Hold. Repeat with the opposite leg.

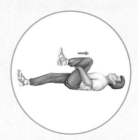

Seated Side Stretch
This exercise stretches the muscles of the trunk. Begin in a seated position with the legs crossed. Stretch the left arm over the head to the right. Bend at the waist (to right), reaching as far as possible to the left with the right arm. Hold. Do not let the trunk rotate. Repeat to the opposite side. For less stretch the overhead arm may be bent. This exercise can be done in the standing position but is less effective.

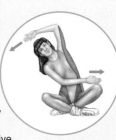

Zipper
This exercise stretches the muscle on the back of the arm (triceps) and the lower chest muscles (pecs). Lift right arm and reach behind head and down the spine (as if pulling up a zipper). With the left hand, push down on right elbow and hold. Reverse arm position and repeat.

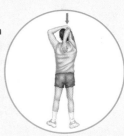

How Much Physical Activity Is Enough?

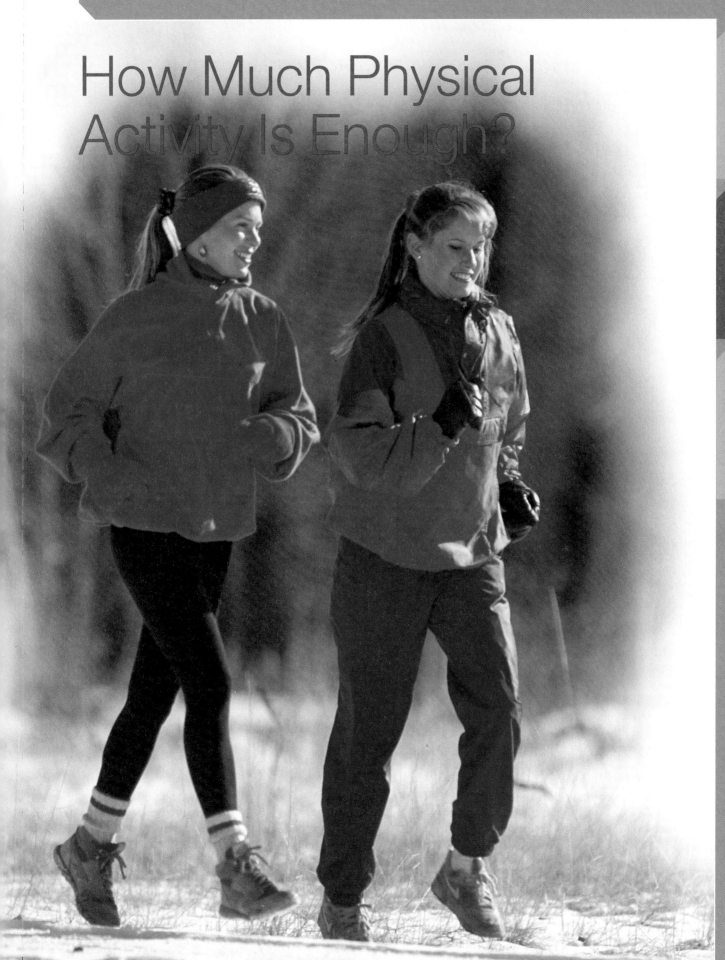

There is a minimal and an optimal amount of physical activity necessary for developing and maintaining good health, wellness, and fitness.

Health Goals

for the year 2010

- Improve the health, fitness, and quality of life of all people through the adoption and maintenance of regular, daily physical activity.

- Increase the proportion of people who do moderate daily activity for 30 minutes.

- Increase the proportion of people who do vigorous physical activity three days a week.

- Increase the proportion of people who do regular exercises for muscle fitness.

- Increase the proportion of people who do regular exercise for flexibility.

Just as there is a correct dosage of medicine for treating an illness, there is a correct dosage of physical activity for promoting health benefits and developing physical fitness. Several important principles of physical activity provide the basis for determining the correct dose or amount of physical activity. In this concept, a formula for implementing the important physical activity principles will be presented. This formula and the concepts of "threshold of training" and "target zones" will be described to help you determine how much physical activity is enough. New evidence indicates that the amount of physical activity necessary for developing metabolic fitness, and its associated health benefits, is different from the amount of physical activity necessary for developing health-related fitness and other performance benefits. Research also shows that the amount of activity or exercise necessary for maintaining fitness may differ from the amount needed to develop it. The guidelines presented in this concept, and throughout this book, are consistent with the most recent guidelines of the American College of Sports Medicine (see Suggested Readings). The guidelines were developed over time by many different experts. However, the research and writings of Dr. Michael L. Pollock (1936–1998) were instrumental in the creation and evolution of the guidelines.

The authors of this book would like to acknowledge Dr. Pollock's contribution to our knowledge and understanding of the amount of physical activity necessary for good health, fitness, and wellness.

The Principles of Physical Activity

Overload is necessary to achieve health, wellness, and fitness benefits of physical activity. The **overload principle** is the most basic of all physical activity principles. This principle indicates that doing "more than normal" is necessary if benefits are to occur. In order for a muscle (including the heart muscle) to get stronger, it must be overloaded, or worked against a load greater than normal. To increase flexibility, a muscle must be stretched longer than is normal. To increase muscular endurance, muscles must be exposed to sustained exercise for a longer than normal period. The health benefits associated with metabolic fitness seems to require less overload than for health-related fitness improvement, but overload is required just the same.

Physical activity should be increased progressively for safe and effective results. The **principle of progression** indicates that overload should not be increased too slowly or too rapidly if benefits are to result. A simple example relates to working with your hands. If you have not done anything for a while and you do too much work with your hands, you develop blisters. You are less able to work the next day. A day or more of recovery may be necessary before you are back to normal. If, however, you begin gradually and increase the work you do each day, you develop calluses. The calluses make your hands tougher, and you are able to work long, or longer without injury or soreness. The benefits of all forms of physical activity are best when you gradually increase overload. Doing too much too soon is counterproductive.

The benefits of physical activity are specific to the form of activity performed. The **principle of specificity** states that to benefit from physical activity, you must overload specifically for that benefit. For example, strength-building exercises may do little for developing cardiovascular fitness, and stretching exercises may do little for altering body composition or metabolic fitness.

Overload is specific to each component of fitness and each health or wellness benefit desired. Overload is also specific to each body part. If you exercise the legs, you build fitness of the legs. If you exercise the arms, you build fitness of the arms. For this reason, some people can have disproportionate fitness development. Some gymnasts, for example, have good upper body development but poor leg development, whereas some soccer players have well-developed legs but lack upper body development.

Specificity is important in designing your warm-up, workout, and cool-down programs for specific activities. Training is most effective when it closely resembles the activity for which you are preparing. For example, if your goal is to improve your skill in putting the shot, it is not enough to strengthen the arm muscles. You should perform a training activity requiring overload that closely resembles the motion you use in the actual sport.

The benefits achieved from overload last only as long as overload continues. The **principle of reversibility** is basically the overload principle in reverse. To put it simply, if you don't use it, you will lose it. It is an important principle because some people have the mistaken impression that if they achieve a health or fitness benefit, it will last forever. This, of course, is not true. There is evidence that you can maintain health benefits with less physical activity than it took to achieve them. Still, if you do not adhere to regular physical activity, any benefits attained will gradually erode away.

In general, the more physical activity you do the more benefits you receive. However, there are exceptions to this rule. A recent report of an international symposium (see *Medicine and Science in Sports and Exercise*, Suggested Readings) provides evidence to suggest that the larger the dose of physical activity the greater the benefits (response). This is called the **dose-response** relationship. This relationship is illustrated by the fact that people who do moderate amounts of regular activity (a moderate dose) have a lower overall death rate compared to those who are sedentary (who do no doses of activity). People who do vigorous activity or moderate activity of longer duration (a bigger dose) have an even greater reduction in risk of early death.

In general, the evidence supports a dose-response relationship for physical activity. It

Doing lifestyle activities can benefit your health.

is important, however, to recognize that more is not always better. As the principle of progression indicates, beginners will benefit most from small doses of activity. For them, doing too much too soon is a bad idea. Also, the **principle of diminishing returns** indicates that as you get fitter and fitter you may not get as big a benefit for each additional amount of activity that you perform. When improvements become more difficult and performance levels off, maintenance may become most important. In some cases, excessive amounts of activity can be counterproductive.

Health, wellness, and fitness benefits occur as you increase your physical activity. But it is important to understand that if you keep increasing physical activity by equal increments, each additional amount of activity will yield less benefit. At some point, improvements will plateau and if activity is overdone, may actually decrease.

The FIT Formula

The acronym FIT can help you remember the three important variables for applying the overload principle and its corollaries. www.mhhe.com/fit_well/web04 Click 01. For physical activity to be effective, it must be done with enough frequency and intensity and

Overload Principle A basic principle that specifies that you must perform physical activity in greater than normal amounts (overload) to get an improvement in physical fitness or health benefits.

Principle of Progression A corollary of the overload principle that indicates the need to gradually increase overload to achieve optimal benefits.

Principle of Specificity A corollary of the overload principle that indicates a need for a specific type of exercise to improve each fitness component or fitness of a specific part of the body.

Principle of Reversibility A corollary of the overload principle that indicates that disuse or inactivity results in loss of benefits achieved as a result of overload.

Dose-Response A term adopted from medicine. With medicine it is important to know what response (benefit) will occur from taking a specific dose. When studying physical activity it is important to know what dose provides the best response (most benefits). The contents of this book are designed to help you choose the best doses of activity for the responses (benefits) you desire.

Principle of Diminishing Returns A corollary of the overload principle indicating that the more benefits you gain as a result of activity, the harder additional benefits are to achieve.

for a long enough time. The first letter from these three words spells **FIT** and can be considered as the formula for achieving health, wellness, and fitness benefits.

Frequency (how often)—Physical activity must be performed regularly to be effective. The number of days a person does activity in a week is used to determine frequency. Most benefits require at least three days and up to six days of activity per week but frequency ultimately depends on the specific benefit desired.

Intensity (how hard)—Physical activity must be intense enough to require more exertion (overload) than normal to produce benefits. The method for determining appropriate intensity varies with the desired benefit. For example, metabolic fitness and associated health benefits require only moderate intensity; cardiovascular fitness for high-level performance requires vigorous activity that elevates the heart rate well above normal.

Time (how long)—Physical activity must be done for an adequate length of time to be effective. The length of the activity session depends on the type of activity and the expected benefit (see various levels of Figure 1).

Some people add a second T to create the acronym FITT. This is done to illustrate the fact that there is a FIT formula for each different **T**ype or mode of physical activity. In this book, the acronym FIT formula will be used to describe the amount of activity necessary to produce benefits for each type of activity from the physical activity pyramid described later in this concept. The FIT formula provides a practical means of applying the overload principle progressively for each specific type of activity and for each of the specific benefits expected.

The threshold of training and target zone concepts help you use the FIT formula. The **threshold of training** is the minimum amount of activity (frequency, intensity, and time) necessary to produce benefits. Depending on the benefit expected, slightly more than normal activity may not be enough to promote health, wellness, or fitness benefits. The **target zone** begins at the threshold of training and stops at the point where the activity becomes counterproductive. Figure 1 illustrates the threshold of training and target zone concepts.

Some people incorrectly associate the concepts of threshold of training and target zones with only cardiovascular fitness. As the principle of specificity suggests, each component of fitness, including metabolic fitness, has its own FIT formula and its own threshold and target zone. The target and threshold levels for **health benefits** are different from those for achieving **performance benefits** associated with high levels of physical fitness. Details of the different FIT formula, threshold levels, and target zones for the various benefits of activity are presented later in this book.

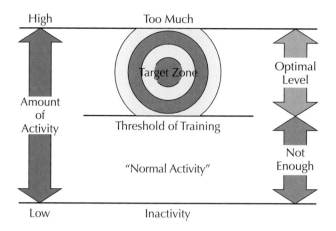

Figure 1 ▶ Physical activity target zone.

It takes time for physical activity to produce health, wellness, and fitness benefits even when the FIT formula is properly applied. **www.mhhe.com/fit_well/web04 Click 02.** Sometimes people just beginning a physical activity program expect to see immediate results. They expect to see large losses in body fat or great increases in muscle strength in just a few days. Evidence shows, however, that improvements in health-related physical fitness and the associated health benefits take several weeks to become apparent. Though some people report psychological benefits, such as "feeling better" and a "sense of personal accomplishment" almost immediately after beginning regular exercise, the physiological changes will take considerably longer to be realized. Proper preparation for physical activity includes learning not to expect too much too soon, and not to do too much too soon. Attempts to overdo it and to try to get fit fast will probably be counterproductive, resulting in soreness and even injury. The key is to start slowly, stay with it, and enjoy yourself. Benefits will come to those who persist.

The Physical Activity Pyramid

The physical activity pyramid classifies activities by type and associated benefits. The **physical activity pyramid** (see Figure 1) is a good way to illustrate different types of activities and how each contributes to the development of health, wellness, and physical fitness. The pyramid evolved from a pyramid of activity emphasis developed more than twenty years ago and from the food guide pyramid developed by the U.S. Department of Agriculture to help people understand appropriate servings of foods. Like the food guide pyramid, the physical activity pyramid has four different levels. Each level includes one or two types of activity and characterizes the "portions" of physical activity necessary to produce different health, wellness, and fitness benefits.

The four levels of the pyramid are based on the beneficial health outcomes associated with regular physical activity. Activities having broad general health and wellness benefits for the largest number of people are placed at the base of the pyramid. Significant national health and economic benefits will occur if we can get inactive people, especially those who are totally sedentary, to do some type of activity. The activities at the lower levels can provide these benefits, and because they are relatively low in intensity, they may appeal to the large number of people who can most benefit from beginning an activity program. The activities at the lower levels of the pyramid typically require greater frequency than those at higher levels.

Lifestyle activities are at the base of the physical activity pyramid. www.mhhe.com/fit_well/web04 Click 03. Lifestyle physical activity is encouraged as a part of everyday living and can contribute significantly to good health, fitness, and wellness. Lifestyle activities include walking to or from work, climbing the stairs rather than taking an elevator, working in the yard, or doing any other type of exercise as part of your normal daily activities. The *Surgeon General's Report on Physical Activity and Health* suggests the accumulation of 30 minutes of physical activity equal to brisk walking on most, if not all, days of the week (see Figure 2, level 1).

Studies that track active versus inactive adults over long periods of time show that lifestyle activities provide many health and wellness benefits. Metabolic fitness and modest gains in some parts of health-related physical fitness are associated with lifestyle activities. However, health-related fitness improvement as evidenced by high scores on performance tests are not generally considered to be a major benefit of this type of activity. The fact that lifestyle activities are moderate in intensity may encourage sedentary people to be more active. Some moderate sports and recreation such as golf, bowling, and fishing are appropriately considered to be lifestyle activities (level 1) because they are similar in intensity to other activities at this level. A summary of the FIT formula for this type of activity is illustrated in level one of Figure 2. While additional activity is encouraged, lifestyle activity is a baseline target that most people can achieve.

Active aerobics and sports and recreation are at the second level of the pyramid. Aerobic activities (level 2) include those that are of such an intensity that they can be performed for relatively long periods of time without stopping but that also elevate the heart rate significantly. Lifestyle activities (level 1), also known as **moderate activity,** are technically aerobic in nature but are not especially vigorous and are, therefore, not considered to be "active aerobics." More **vigorous activities** such as jogging, biking, and aerobic dance are commonly classified as "active aerobic" activities. This type of activity is included in the second level of the pyramid because benefits can be accomplished in as few as three days a week and is especially good for building cardiovascular fitness and helping to control body fat. This type of activity can provide metabolic fitness and health benefits similar to lifestyle activities.

Active sports and recreation are also included at level 2 of the pyramid. Examples of active sports include basketball, tennis, and racquetball, and active recreation includes hiking, backpacking, skiing, and rock climbing. Some active sports and recreational activities involve short bursts of physical activity followed by rests and, therefore, may not be considered to be aerobic in nature. If done for relatively long periods of time without stopping, active sports and recreation activities can have the same benefits of active aerobic activities. As noted earlier, sports such as golf and bowling may be classified as lifestyle activities rather than active sports since they are done at more moderate intensities. Activities at level 2 of the pyramid may substitute for activities at level 1 if done according to the FIT formula, but many experts encourage activities from both levels. They reason that people who develop active lifestyles from level 1 will be more likely to stay active later in life when they are less likely to participate in activities from level 2. Others argue that if you are active at level 2 you will be fit enough to continue active aerobics and sports as you grow older. A summary of the FIT formula for level 2 activities is included in Figure 2.

FIT A formula used to describe the frequency, intensity, and length of time for physical activity to produce benefits. (When "FITT" is used, the second T refers to the type of physical activity you perform.)

Threshold of Training The minimum amount of physical activity that will produce benefits.

Target Zone Amounts of physical activity that produce optimal benefits.

Health Benefit A result of physical activity that provides protection from hypokinetic disease or early death.

Performance Benefit A result of physical activity that improves physical fitness and physical performance capabilities.

Physical Activity Pyramid This pyramid illustrates how different types of activities contribute to the development of health and physical fitness. Activities lower in the pyramid require more frequent participation, whereas activities higher in the pyramid require less frequency.

Flexibility and muscle fitness exercises are at level 3 of the pyramid. Flexibility (stretching) exercises are a type of physical activity that is planned specifically to develop flexibility. This type of exercise is necessary because activities lower in the pyramid often do not contribute to flexibility development. The muscle fitness category includes exercises that are planned specifically to build strength and muscular endurance. This type of exercise is necessary because activities lower in the pyramid often do not contribute to these parts of fitness. A general description of the FIT formula for level 3 exercises is included in Figure 2.

Some rest is necessary, but with the exception of sleep, long periods of inactivity are discouraged. Rest or inactivity can be important to good health. Some time off just to relax is important to us all, and of course proper amounts of rest and eight hours of uninterrupted sleep help us recuperate. But sedentary living (too much inactivity) results in low fitness as well as poor health and wellness.

Rest and inactivity are placed at the top of the pyramid (see Figure 2) because they should be done sparingly compared to other types of activity in the pyramid.

🌐 **Some important guidelines should be considered when using the physical activity pyramid.** www.mhhe.com/fit_well/web04 Click 04. The physical activity pyramid is a useful model for describing different types of activity and their benefits. The pyramid is also useful in summarizing the FIT formula for each of the different benefits of activity. But as the American College of Sports Medicine pointed out, physical activity guidelines ". . . cannot be implemented in an overly rigid fashion . . . and . . . recommendations presented should be used with careful attention to the goals of the individual." This important point should be considered when using the pyramid. The following guidelines for using the pyramid should also be considered.

- *No single activity provides all of the benefits.* Many people have asked the question, "What is the perfect form of physical activity?" It is now evident that there is no single activity

Level 4

Rest or Inactivity
Watching TV
Reading

F = Infrequent
I = Low
T = Short

Level 3

Exercise for flexibility
Stretching

Exercise for strength & muscular endurance
Weight training
Calisthenics

F = 3–7 days/week
I = Stretching
T = 15–60 sec., 1–3 sets

F = 2–3 days/week
I = Muscle overload
T = 8–12 reps, 1–3 sets

Level 2

Active aerobic activity
Aerobics
Jogging
Biking

Active sports and recreation
Tennis
Basketball
Racquetball

F = 3–6 days/week   I = Moderate to vigorous   T = 20+ min

Level 1

Lifetime physical activity

Play golf
Go bowling
Go fishing

Walk rather than ride
Climb the stairs
Do yard work

F = All or most days/week   I = Moderate   T = 30+ min that can provide all of the health, wellness, and fitness benefits. For optimal benefits to occur, it is desirable to perform activities from all levels of the pyramid because each type of activity has quite different benefits. As other guidelines will indicate, care should be used not to overgeneralize this recommendation.

- *In some cases, one type of activity can substitute for another.* If a person does appropriate activity of either type at level 2 of the pyramid, similar benefits can result. Both types are not required. Also, if a person does adequate activity of either type at level 2, the activity can provide similar benefits to those at level 1 of the pyramid. Selecting activities from more than one category does provide variety and may aid in adherence for some people.

- *Something is better than nothing.* Some people may look at the pyramid and say, "I just don't have time to do all of these activities." This could lead some to throw up their hands in despair, resulting in the conclusion "I just won't do anything at all." The best evidence indicates that something is better than nothing. If you do nothing or feel that you can't do it all, performing a lifestyle physical activity is a good start. Additional activities from different levels of the pyramid can be added as time allows.

- *Activities from level 3 are useful even if you are limited in performing activities at other levels.* Though flexibility and muscle fitness exercises do not produce all of the benefits associated with regular physical activity, they will produce benefits even if you are unable to perform as much activity from other levels as you like.

- *Good planning will allow you to schedule activities from all levels in a reasonable amount of time.* In subsequent concepts, you will learn more about each level of the pyramid as well as more information about planning a total physical activity program.

Physical Activity Patterns

The proportion of adults meeting national health goals varies with activity type and gender. www.mhhe.com/fit_well/web04 Click 05. National health goals have been established for each of the different types of activity illustrated in the physical activity pyramid. The proportion of adults eighteen years of age and older meeting these goals is shown in Table 1. While lifestyle physical activities are recommended for 30+ minutes on most, if not all, days of the week, an adult is considered to be active if he or she does activity at least five days a week. The *Healthy People 2010* report shows that only 15 percent of adults meet this standard, with more men being active than women. The national goal is to increase this to 30 percent by the year 2010.

It is interesting that in recent years moderate activity has decreased and vigorous activity has increased among

adults (vigorous activity at least three days a week for 20 minutes). In the past more adults did moderate activity than vigorous activity, but the recent *Healthy People 2010* report indicates that more adults now do vigorous activity—mostly young adults—than moderate activity. The type of activity most practiced by adults is flexibility exercise (stretching), performed by 30 percent of all adults, though this statistic may be deceiving because of the frequency of doing the stretching exercises in days per week was not specified. Stretching is one form of exercise performed more frequently by women than men. Males are considerably more likely than females to do muscle fitness exercises at least two days per week. A total of 40 percent of adults do no regular leisure time physical activity, up considerably from previous years. Women are more likely than males to be sedentary (do no leisure time activity).

The proportion of people meeting national health goals varies based on age. www.mhhe. com/fit_well/web04 Click 06. Because it is difficult to measure physical activity among young children, the evidence concerning activity levels of children under age twelve is not as prevalent as for adolescents and adults. It is clear, however, that children are the most active group in western society, though they are active in different ways from adults. Young children are not likely to perform activity

Moderate Activity For the purposes of this book, moderate activity refers to activity equal in intensity to a brisk walk. Level 1 activities from the activity pyramid are included in this category.

Vigorous Activity For the purposes of this book, vigorous activity refers to activities that elevate the heart rate and are greater in intensity than brisk walking. It is also referred to as moderate to vigorous activity. Those activities from level 2 of the pyramid are included in this category.

Table 1 ▶ The Percentage of Adults Meeting Activity Goals

Characteristic	Moderate Activity	Vigorous Activity	Muscle Fitness Exercise	Flexibility Exercises	No Leisure Activity
Sex					
Female	13%	20%	16%	31%	43%
Male	16%	26%	23%	29%	36%
All	15%	23%	19%	30%	40%
Age					
18–24	17	32	28	36	31
25–44	15	27	21	32	34
45–64	14	21	14	28	42
65–74	16	13	10	24	51
75+	12	6	7	22	65
Education					
Grades 9–11	11	12	8	16	59
HS graduate	14	18	11	23	46
Some college	17	24	19	36	35
College graduate	17	32	26	no data	24
Ethnicity					
Native/Indian Alaskan	13	19	18	26	46
Asian or Pacific Islander	15	17	17	34	42
Black/African American	10	17	16	26	52
Hispanic/Latino	11	16	13	22	54
White/non-Hispanic	16	25	19	31	36
Geographic Location					
Urban	15	24*	19	32	39
Rural	15	21	15	24	43
Disability Status					
With	12	13	14	29	56
Without	16	25	20	31	36

Source: From *Healthy People 2010.*

continuously but rather do intermittent bouts of activity followed by short rests. Recent guidelines indicate that this type of activity is appropriate for children and attempts to get children to be active in ways similar to adults are inappropriate. For children, 60+ minutes and up to several hours of physical activity is recommended per day.

During adolescence, activity decreases with each year in school. Lack of physical education in the upper grades, TV watching, and video game-playing are thought to be reasons for the decline with age. Nevertheless, teens are considerably more vigorously active than adults in their twenties. As indicated, physical activity of all types decreases from ages eighteen to seventy-five with 50 percent or more of adults sixty-five and older performing no leisure activity at all (see Table 1).

The proportion of adults meeting national health goals varies based on a variety of characteristics. Among the major characteristics associated with different levels of physical activity are age, education level, ethnicity, geographic location, and disability status. Some statistics for various groups' characteristics are illustrated in Table 1.

Based on the data presented in Table 1, a variety of characteristics affect the amount and type of physical activities adults perform. Also of importance is the influence of social class and economic status. As a recent report indicates, social and economic factors are related to differences in activity levels among ethnic groups and those from urban versus rural areas. Clearly, education level is also a factor that contributes to inactivity and social/economic class. Adults identified as having one or more of a wide variety of physical disabilities have an especially high probability of being inactive. One of the two major goals of *Healthy People 2010* is to eliminate health disparities among different segments of the population. Education in general, and educating the public about the value of physical activity and other health issues in specific, would appear to be important if we are to achieve this goal.

Strategies for Action

A self-assessment of your current activity at each level of the pyramid can help you determine future activity goals. Lab 4A provides you with the opportunity to assess your physical activity at each level of the pyramid. Later you will be developing a program of activity, and these assessments will provide a basis for program planning.

Web Resources

American College of Sports Medicine **www.acsm.org**

Centers for Disease Control and Prevention (CDC)
    www.cdc.gov

Health Canada **www.hc-sc.gc.ca**

Healthy People 2010 **www.health.gov/healthypeople**

Morbidity and Mortality Weekly Reports **www.cdc.gov/mmwr**

Surgeon General's Report on Physical Activity and Health
    www.cdc.gov/nccdphp/sgr/sgr.htm

Suggested Readings

Additional reference materials for Concept 4 are available at **www.mhhe.com/fit_well/web04 click 07**.

American College of Sports Medicine. 2000. *ACSM's Guidelines for Exercise Testing and Prescription*. 6th ed. Philadelphia: Lippincott, Williams and Wilkins.

Crespo, C. J. et al. 1999. Prevalence of physical inactivity and its relation to social class in U.S. adults. *Medicine and Science in Sports and Exercise* 31(12):1821–1826.

Franks, B. D. E. T. Howley, and Y. Iyriboz. 1999. *The Health and Fitness Handbook*. Champaign, IL: Human Kinetics.

Medicine and Science in Sports and Exercise. 2001. Dose-response issues concerning physical activity and health: An evidence based symposium. *Medicine and Science in Sports and Exercise* 33(6): entire issue.

Roitman, J. L. (ed.). 2001. *ACSM's Resource Manual for Guidelines for Exercise Testing and Prescription*. 4th ed. Philadelphia: Lippincott, Williams and Wilkins.

Spain, C. G., and B. D. Franks. 2001. Healthy people 2010: Physical activity and fitness. *President's Council on Physical Fitness and Sports Research Digest* 3(13):1–16.

U.S. Department of Health and Human Services. Nov. 2000. *Healthy People 2010*. 2nd ed. With *Understanding and Improving Health* and *Objectives for Improving Health*. 2 vols. Washington, DC: U.S. Government Printing Office.

U.S. Department of Health and Human Services. 1996. *Physical Activity and Health: A Report of the Surgeon General*. Atlanta: U.S. Department of Health and Human Services.

In the News

In the fall of 2002, the Food and Nutrition Board of the National Institute of Medicine (NIM) released a report offering targets for nutrition and physical activity. The targets were widely disseminated in the news media. Some news reports indicated that the recommendations of this group superceded the physical activity recommendations of the Surgeon General, endorsed by the Centers for Disease Control and Prevention (CDC), the American College of Sports Medicine (ACSM), and other groups.

The fact that many different groups make recommendations on both nutrition and physical activity often leads to confusion. In fact, different guidelines are often compatible. As you will learn in this book, there are many reasons for doing physical activity. The benefits you expect to receive will dictate the type of activity you do. This is illustrated in Figure 2, the physical activity pyramid. Moderate lifestyle activities from the lower level of the pyramid, as recommended by the Surgeon General, provide substantial health benefits for a reasonable amount of activity.

While the NIM recommendation (60 minutes of daily moderate activity) was also made to reduce disease risk, its primary purpose was to recommend how much energy is necessary to "maintain a healthy weight." This report is by a private, non-governmental organization that focuses on nutrition. There is no doubt that some people will need to do more than 30 minutes of activity to achieve or maintain a healthy body weight. More time spent in activity and/or selection of more vigorous activities from the upper levels of the pyramid can also result in improved fitness, improved performance, added health benefits, and can be helpful in achieving desirable body fatness. This does not negate the fact that the Surgeon General's recommendation is a sound one. Daily activity for 30 minutes is a good start and is better than no activity at all.

Lab 4A: Self-Assessment of Physical Activity

Name		Section	Date

Purpose: To estimate your current levels of physical activity from each category of the physical activity pyramid.

Procedures:

1. Place an X over the circle that characterizes your participation in each category in the pyramid.
2. Determine if you met the national goal for each type of activity. Place an X over the "yes" circle if you met the goal in each area (see Results).

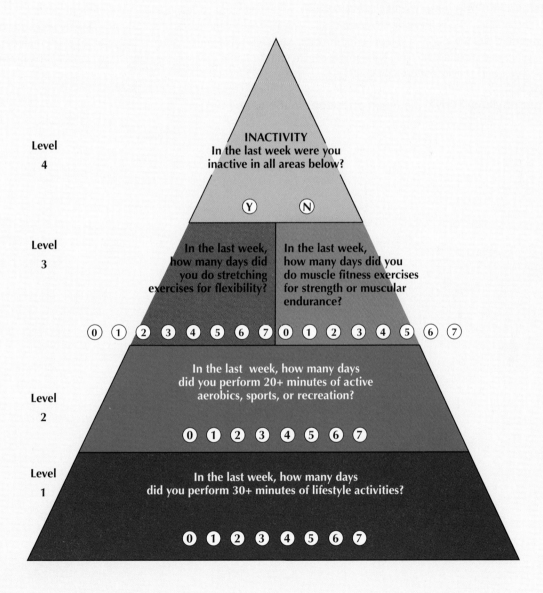

Level 4

INACTIVITY
In the last week were you inactive in all areas below?

Ⓨ   Ⓝ

Level 3

In the last week, how many days did you do stretching exercises for flexibility?

In the last week, how many days did you do muscle fitness exercises for strength or muscular endurance?

⓪ ① ② ③ ④ ⑤ ⑥ ⑦   ⓪ ① ② ③ ④ ⑤ ⑥ ⑦

Level 2

In the last week, how many days did you perform 20+ minutes of active aerobics, sports, or recreation?

⓪ ① ② ③ ④ ⑤ ⑥ ⑦

Level 1

In the last week, how many days did you perform 30+ minutes of lifestyle activities?

⓪ ① ② ③ ④ ⑤ ⑥ ⑦

Results

Activity Type	Level	National Goal	Did You Meet the National Health Goal?	
Lifestyle activity	1	5 days or more	Yes	No
Active aerobics/sports	2	3 days or more	Yes	No
Flexibility exercises	3	3 days or more	Yes	No
Muscle fitness	3	2 days or more	Yes	No
Inactivity	4	Avoid total inactivity	Yes	No

Conclusions and Implications: In the space below, write a brief paper describing your current physical activity patterns. Do you meet the national health goals in all areas? If not, in what types of activity from the pyramid do you need to improve? Are the answers you gave for the past week typical of your regular activity patterns? If you meet all national health goals, explain why you think this is so. Do you think that meeting the goals in the table on the previous page indicates good activity patterns for you?

Write your physical activity assessment paper in the space below.

Learning Self-Planning Skills for Lifetime Physical Activity

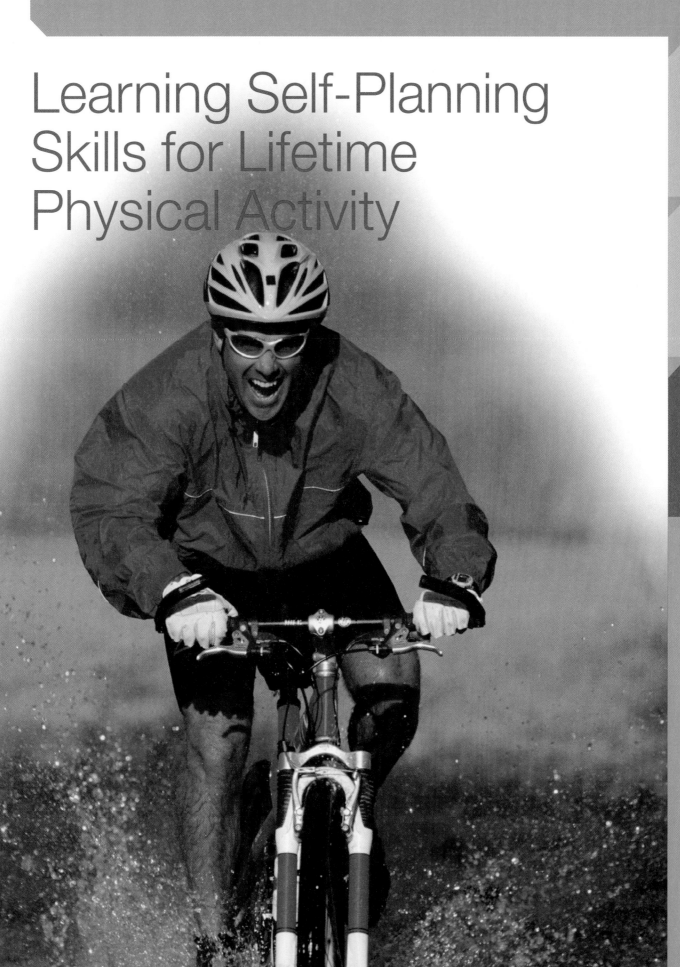

Planning for physically active living is essential to optimal health, wellness, and physical fitness

Health Goals
for the year 2010

- Improve the health, fitness, and quality of life through regular, daily physical activity.

- Increase leisure time physical activity.

- Increase proportion of people who do moderate daily activity for 30 minutes.

- Increase proportion of people who do vigorous physical activity three days a week.

- Increase proportion of people who do regular muscle fitness exercise.

- Increase proportion of people who do regular exercise for flexibility.

- Increase prevalence of a healthy weight.

Knowing the most common reasons for inactivity can help you avoid sedentary living. Some of the common reasons given by those who do not do regular physical activity are outlined in Table 2. Many of the reasons for not being active are considered by experts to be barriers that can be overcome. Overcoming barriers is a self-management skill. Using the strategies for change in Table 2 helps inactive people to become more active.

Knowing the reasons people give for being active can help you adopt positive attitudes. www.mhhe.com/fit_well/web05 Click 01. Table 3 describes some of the major reasons why people choose to be active. It also offers strategies for changing behavior if you have more than one or two negative attitudes. Active people have more positive than negative attitudes. This is referred to by experts as a positive "balance of attitudes." The questionnaire in Lab 5A gives you the opportunity to assess your balance of attitudes. If you have a negative balance score, you can analyze your attitudes and determine how you can change them to view activity more favorably.

There is no single physical activity program that is best suited for all people. In this concept you will learn about the six steps for effective personal program planning. Each of these six steps (see Table 1) will be discussed in detail. You will use many of the self-management skills described in Concept 2. Program planning is discussed early in the book to allow you to understand the planning process before you read more about various activities that you can select for your personal program. In the final concept of the book, you will have the opportunity to prepare a comprehensive lifetime program of physical activity as well as to do planning for other healthy lifestyle change.

STEP 1: Clarifying Reasons

Clarifying your reasons for participating in physical activity is an important step in self-planning. As you continue your study in this book, you will be presented with a wide variety of physical activity choices. Your personal reasons for choosing to participate or not to participate should be clarified prior to planning your program. Over time, attitudes change, so periodic reassessment is recommended.

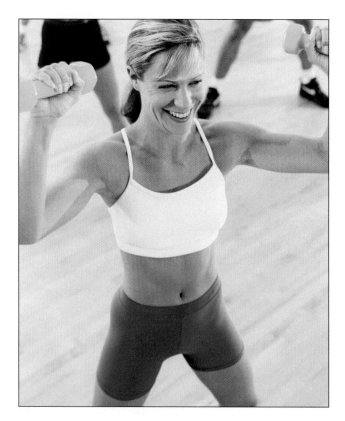

Active people have more positive than negative feelings about physical activity.

Table 1 ▶ Self-Planning Skills		
Self-Planning	**Description**	**Self-Management Skill**
1. **Clarifying reasons**	Knowing the general reasons why you might benefit helps you select activities that you will enjoy and adhere to for a lifetime.	Balancing Attitudes: Sections of this concept and Lab 5A help you determine if you have more positive than negative attitudes and help clarify your reasons for doing physical activity.
2. **Identifying needs**	If you know your strengths and weaknesses, you can plan to build on your strengths and overcome weaknesses.	Self-Assessment: In the concepts that follow, you will learn how to assess different health, wellness, and fitness characteristics. Learning these self-assessments will help you identify needs.
3. **Setting personal goals**	Goals are more specific than reasons (see above). Establishing specific things that you want to accomplish can provide a basis for feedback that your program is working.	Goal Setting: Guidelines in this concept will help you set goals. In subsequent concepts, you will establish goals for different types of activity from the pyramid.
4. **Selecting personal activities**	A personal plan should include activities that meet your needs and goals (see steps above) and provide fun and enjoyment. Having skill improves enjoyment.	Performance Skills: In subsequent concepts, you will learn how to enhance your performance skills. Self-assessments will also help you match your abilities to specific activities.
5. **Writing your plan**	Once you have determined which activities you will perform, you should put your plan in writing. This establishes your intentions and increases your chances of adherence.	Self-Planning: This includes writing down the time of day, day of the week, and length of exercise session for each activity you will include in your plan.
6. **Evaluating progress**	Keeping records including self-monitoring of activities performed and periodic self-assessment of fitness status helps you adhere to your program.	Self-Monitoring: Used as the basis for keeping activity records (logs) and determining if activity goals are met. Self-Assessment: Used as a basis for determining if fitness goals are met.

STEP 2: Identifying Needs

Self-assessments are useful in establishing personal needs, planning your program, and evaluating your progress. You have already done some self-assessments of wellness, current activity levels, and current lifestyles. In the lab for this concept and others that follow, you will make additional assessments. The results of these assessments help you build a personal profile that can be used as the basis for program planning. With practice, self-assessments become more accurate. It is for this reason that it is important to repeat self-assessments more than one time and to pay careful attention to the procedures for performing them. If questions arise, get a professional opinion rather than making an error.

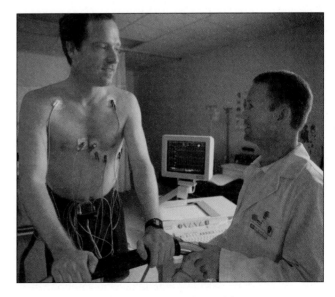

A fitness assessment by an expert can be useful.

Table 2 ▶ Common Reasons People Give for Not Being Active

Reason	Description	Strategy for Change
I don't have the time.	This is the number one reason people give for not exercising. Invariably, those who feel they don't have time know they should do more exercise. They say they plan to do more in the future when "things are less hectic." Young people say that they will have more time to exercise in the future. Older people say that they wish they had taken the time to be active when they were younger.	Planning a daily schedule can help you find the time for activity and avoid wasting time on things that are less important. Learning the facts in the concepts that follow will help you see the importance of activity and how you can include it in your schedule with a minimum of effort and with time efficiency.
It's too inconvenient.	Many who avoid physical activity do so because it is inconvenient. They are procrastinators. Specific reasons for procrastinating include: "It makes me sweaty" and "It messes up my hair."	If you have to travel more than ten minutes to do activity or if you do not have easy access to equipment, you will avoid activity. Locating facilities and finding a time when you can shower is important.
I just don't enjoy it.	Many do not find activity to be enjoyable or invigorating. These people may assume that all forms of activity have to be strenuous and fatiguing.	There are many activities to choose from. If you don't enjoy vigorous activity, try more moderate forms of activity such as walking.
I'm no good at physical activity.	"People might laugh at me," "Sports make me nervous" and "I am not good at physical activities" are reasons some people give for not being active. Some people lack confidence in their own abilities. This may be because of past experiences in physical education or sports.	With properly selected activities, even those who have never enjoyed exercise can get hooked. Building skills can help, as can changing your way of thinking. Avoiding comparisons to others can help you feel successful.
I am not fit so I avoid activity.	Some people avoid exercise because of health reasons. Some who are unfit lack energy. Starting slowly can build fitness gradually and help you realize that you can do it.	There are good medical reasons for not doing activity, but many people with problems can benefit from exercise if it is properly designed. If necessary, get help adapting activity to meet your needs.
I have no place to be active, especially in bad weather.	Regular activity is more convenient if facilities are easy to reach and the weather is good. Opportunities have increased considerably in recent years. Some of the most popular activities require little equipment, can be done in or near home, and are inexpensive.	If you cannot find a place, if it is not safe or if it is too expensive, consider using low-cost equipment at home such as rubber bands or calisthenics. Lifestyle activity can be done by anyone at almost any time.
I am too old.	As people grow older, many begin to feel that activity is something they cannot do. For most people, this is simply not true! Properly planned exercise for older adults is not only safe but also has many health benefits, e.g., longer life, fewer illnesses, an improved sense of well-being, and optimal functioning.	Older people who are just beginning activity should start slowly. Lifestyle activities are a good choice. Setting realistic goals can help, as can learning to do resistance training and flexibility exercises.

Periodic self-assessments can aid in determining if a person is meeting health and fitness standards and is making progress toward personal goals. www.mhhe.com/fit_well/web05 Click 02. At some point, it is wise to have an expert test your fitness. This helps you get an accurate assessment of your current fitness level and helps you determine if your self-assessment results are accurate. Expert tests are often expensive and require time and effort on your part. When possible, you should learn to perform self-assessments so that you can continue to assess your fitness for a lifetime without dependence on someone else. Tests such as skinfold measures are hard to administer

to yourself, but you can learn to teach a friend or relative to assist you with the measurement.

For many components of physical fitness, multiple assessments are provided in this book. For example, four different cardiovascular fitness assessments are included for your selection. You are encouraged to try several assessments for each component of fitness and then decide which one best meets your personal needs.

Self-assessments have the advantage of consistent error rather than variable error. As noted previously, the best type of assessments are done by highly qualified experts using precise instruments. Eliminating error is

Table 3 ▶ Common Reasons for Doing Regular Physical Activity

Reason	Description	Strategy for Change
I do activity for my health, wellness, and fitness.	Surveys show this is the number one reason for doing regular physical activity. Unfortunately, many adults say that a "doctor's order to exercise" would be the most likely reason to get them to begin a program. For some, however, waiting for a doctor's order may be too late.	Gaining information contained in this book will help you see the value of regular physical activity. Performing the self-assessments in the various concepts will help you determine the areas in which you need personal improvement.
I do activity to improve my appearance.	In our society, looking good is highly valued, thus physical attractiveness is a major reason why people participate in regular exercise. Regular activity can contribute to looking your best.	Some people have failed in past attempts to change their appearance through activity. Setting realistic goals and avoiding comparisons to others can help you to be more successful.
I do activity because I enjoy it.	A majority of adults say that enjoyment is of paramount importance in deciding to be active. Statements include experiencing the "peak experience," the "runner's high," or "spinning free." The sense of fun, well-being, and general enjoyment associated with physical activity are well-documented.	Those people who do not enjoy activity often lack performance skills or feel that they are not competent in activity. Improving skills with practice, setting realistic goals, and adopting a new way of thinking can help you to be successful and to enjoy activities.
I do activity because it relaxes me.	Relaxation and release from tension rank high as reasons why people do regular activity. It is known that activity in the form of sports and games provides a catharsis, or outlet, for the frustrations of daily activities. Regular exercise can help reduce depression and anxiety.	Activities, such as walking, jogging, or cycling are ways of getting some quiet time away from the job or the stresses of daily living. In a later concept, you will learn about exercises that you can do to reduce stress.
I like the challenge and sense of personal accomplishment I get from physical activity.	A sense of personal accomplishment is frequently a reason for people doing activity. In some cases, it is learning a new skill, such as racquetball or tennis; in other cases, it is running a mile or doing a certain number of crunches. The challenge of doing something you have never done before is apparently a powerful experience.	Some people get little sense of accomplishment from activity. Taking lessons to learn skills or attempting activities new to you can provide the challenge that makes activity interesting. Also, adopting a new way of thinking allows you to focus on the task rather than competition with others.
I like the social involvement I get from physical activities.	"Why am I physically active?": "It is a good way to spend time with members of my family." "It is a good way to spend time with close friends." "Being part of the team is satisfying." Activity settings can also provide an opportunity for making new friends.	If you find activity to be socially unrewarding you may have to find activities that you, friends, or family enjoy. Taking lessons together can help. Also finding a friend with similar skills can help. Focus on the activity rather than the outcome.
Competition is the main reason I enjoy physical activity.	"The thrill of victory" and "sports competition" are two reasons given for being active. For many, the competitive experience is very satisfying.	Some people simply do not enjoy competing. If this is the case for you, select noncompetitive individual activities.
Physical activity helps me feel good about myself.	For many people, participation in physical activity is an important part of their identity. They feel better about themselves when they are regularly participating.	Physical activity is something that is self-determined and within your control. Participation can help you feel good about yourself, build your confidence, and increase your self-esteem.
Physical activity provides opportunities to get fresh air.	Being outside and experiencing nature are reasons that some people give for being physically active.	Many activities provide opportunities to be outside. If this is an important reason for you, seek out parks and outdoor settings for your activities.

always desirable. Following directions and practicing sound assessment techniques will reduce error significantly. Still, errors will occur. One advantage of a self-assessment is that the person doing the assessment is always the same—you. Even if you make an error in a self-assessment, it is likely to be consistent over time, especially if you use the same equipment each time you make the assessment. For exam-

ple, if you measure your own weight using a home scale and your measurement shows your weight to be two pounds higher than it really is, you have made a consistent error. You can determine if you are making improvement because you know the error exists, but it is a consistent error. When different people using different instruments assess your fitness, the errors they make may be quite variable.

Results of fitness assessments are influenced by heredity. Heredity plays an important role in the amount of physical fitness a person can attain. More than a few people have become discouraged after completing an exercise program only to find that they have scored lower on fitness tests than friends who are less active. Though it is clear that regular exercise is critical to optimal physical fitness, each person also has a hereditary predisposition to fitness. Although achieving good scores on fitness tests is a desirable goal, it is important to understand that a person's hereditary predisposition to fitness limits one's potential for achieving exceptionally high scores.

 Health-based criterion-referenced standards are recommended for rating your fitness. www.mhhe.com/fit_well/web05 Click 03. Most experts now recommend **health-based criterion-referenced standards** to rate your current fitness. These standards help you determine "how much fitness is enough" for health and wellness. In the past, norms or percentiles have been used to rate physical fitness. These types of ratings compare an individual to a group. Knowing how you compare to someone else is not particularly important. In fact, such comparisons have been shown to be discouraging to many people. Determining if your fitness is adequate to enhance your health and wellness is much more relevant.

In this book, four categories are provided for you to rate each part of fitness. These are illustrated and described in Table 4. Your first goal should be to be sure that you do not rate low on any health-related fitness part. Ultimately, you should achieve the good fitness

zone for all parts of fitness. You may, for personal reasons, wish to achieve the high performance zone for some fitness components, but this choice has more to do with personal preference than health and wellness. The fitness ratings used in this book help you determine "how much fitness is enough" for your good health and wellness. They do not require you to compare yourself to others or set unrealistic standards.

Technology Update

Computer programs provide an effective way to track and monitor your fitness results over time. A customized software program called the "Interactive Personal Trainer" is available to users of the book. Go to the "On the Web" site for this concept www.mhhe.com/fit_well/web05 and click on the second link labeled Self-Testing and Self-Evaluation to learn how to download and use the program. Once you install it, you can enter your scores for the various fitness self-assessments in the book. The program will generate a personal **Fitness Profile** that rates each component of fitness testing using the criterion referenced standards in this book.

A comprehensive fitness profile can help you set program goals. Compiling all of your self-assessments in one comprehensive profile can help you determine your strengths and weaknesses. The profile will help you get a picture of the components of fitness in which you need improvement. This information can be used to help you establish personal program goals. In Lab 26C you will have the opportunity to prepare a fitness profile as part of the process of preparing a personal activity plan.

STEP 3: Setting Personal Goals

Learning to set realistic goals is useful as a basis for physical activity self-planning. If any lifestyle change is to be of value, it is important to determine—ahead of time—what you hope to accomplish. Goals are specific objectives you hope to accomplish as a result of a lifestyle change. To be effective, goals must be realistic—neither too hard nor too easy. If the goal is too hard, failure is likely. Failure is discouraging. By setting realistic and attainable goals, you will have a greater chance of being successful.

Beginners are encouraged to focus on short-term goals. Focus on **short-term goals** first. Short-term goals are easier to accomplish than **long-term goals.**

Table 4 ▶ The Four Fitness Zones
High Performance Zone It is not necessary to reach this level to experience good health benefits. Achievement of high performance scores has more to do with performance than it does with good health. In some cases, extreme fitness scores can increase health risk, e.g., very low body fatness.
Good Fitness Zone If you reach the good fitness zone, you have enough of a specific fitness component to help reduce health risk. However, even reaching the good fitness zone may not result in optimal health benefits for inactive people.
Marginal Zone Marginal scores indicate that some improvement is in order, but you are nearing minimal health standards set by experts.
Low Fit Zone If you score low in fitness, you are probably less fit than you should be for your own good health and wellness.

Realistic short-term goals make you successful because one success leads to another. When you meet short-term goals, establish new ones. Long-term goals take a long time to accomplish and may be discouraging to beginners. After a series of short-term goals have been successfully accomplished, set long-term goals. In fact, setting and achieving a series of short-term goals is the best way to achieve long-term goals.

Short-term goals should be specific. Many individuals make the mistake of setting vague or nebulous goals such as "be more active" or "eat less." While these may be your long-term objectives, goals should be more specific. Setting specific goals helps you commit to what you want to accomplish. It is also easier to assess whether you are making progress.

Short-term goals should be behavioral goals rather than outcome goals. A **behavioral goal** is associated with something you do. Performing physical activity for a specific period of time is something you do, so a **physical activity goal** is a type of behavioral goal. An example of a specific short-term behavioral goal would be "to perform 30 minutes of brisk walking six days a week for the next two weeks." It is specific because you specify how long and how often you expect to do the exercise. It is short-term because you can accomplish it in a few weeks or less. The principal factor associated with success is your willingness to give effort. No matter who you are, you can accomplish this behavioral goal if you give a daily effort. In addition, behavioral goals are easy to self-monitor. Keeping an activity log of your weekly participation in brisk walking will reveal your compliance with the goal.

An **outcome goal** is associated with something you "can do." For example, **fitness goals** such as being able to do ten push-ups or to run a mile in seven minutes are examples of outcome goals. Outcome or fitness goals are not recommended for beginners. Three reasons for this are listed below:

- *Typically, it takes time (weeks or months) to reach fitness and other outcome goals.* For this reason, short-term or fitness goals are often not achieved in the designated time, resulting in a perception of failure.
- *Outcome goals depend on many things other than your lifestyle behavior.* For example, your heredity affects your body fat and muscle development. Setting a goal of achieving a certain percentage of body fat or lifting a certain weight is influenced by heredity as well as your physical activity program. This makes it hard for beginners to set realistic fitness goals. Too often the tendency is to set the goal based on a comparative standard rather than on a standard that is

possible for the individual to achieve in a short period of time. Those more experienced in physical activity learn to set more realistic outcome goals and learn that these goals often take time to achieve.

- *Different people progress at different rates.* People not only inherit a predisposition to fitness and body composition, they inherit a predisposition to benefit from training. In other words, if ten people do the exact same physical activities, there will be ten different results. One may improve performance by 60 percent while another improves only 10 percent. Until you gain enough experience to see how you respond to physical activity, it is not wise to set fitness or outcome goals. You need experience to determine the areas of fitness in which you respond quickly and those areas in which your response to activity is slower. It is at this time that fitness or outcome goals become more appropriate.

Long-term goals can be either behavioral or outcome goals. Long-term goals can be of a behavioral nature similar to short-term goals. If you set as a goal participation in regular physical activity and meet the goal over a long period of time, fitness and other health

---

Health-Based Criterion-Referenced Standards The amount of a specific type of fitness necessary to gain a health or wellness benefit.

Fitness Profile A summary of results of self-assessments of physical fitness.

Short-Term Goal A statement of intent to change a behavior or outcome in a period of days or weeks.

Long-Term Goal A statement of intent to change behavior or achieve a specific outcome in a period of months or years.

Behavioral Goal A statement of intent to perform a specific behavior (changing a lifestyle) for a specific period of time. An example would be, "I will walk for 15 minutes each morning before work."

Physical Activity Goal An exercise or physical activity goal is a behavioral goal with exercise as the intended behavior.

Outcome Goal A statement of intent to achieve a specific test score (attainment of a specific standard) associated with good health, wellness, or fitness. An example would be, "I will lower my body fat level by 3 percent."

Fitness Goal A fitness goal is an outcome goal with a specific fitness score as the intended outcome.

benefits will occur to the extent that they are possible given your genetics and body type. For this reason, behavioral or physical activity goals are appropriate. This type of goal is easy to monitor, and self-assessments of fitness will provide feedback of program success.

Outcome or fitness goals can also be useful to the person experienced in physical activity. If realistic, these goals will be met with appropriate physical activity and provide evidence of success. When establishing long-term fitness goals, be careful not to base them on what other people can do. You may be setting yourself up for failure. Be sure that the fitness outcomes you expect are based on health standards or scores slightly above what you can currently perform, rather than on performance scores of other people.

It is appropriate to consider maintenance goals. There is a limit to the amount of fitness any person can achieve. You cannot improve forever. Limits on physical activity goals are appropriate. At some point, it is reasonable to set maintenance goals to help you to stay active and fit when improvement goals have already been met.

Set goals that you can maintain for a lifetime. Physical activity and fitness for a lifetime mean maintaining your program forever. If you set exercise or fitness goals that are excessive, you may burn out and quit exercising entirely. Consider the long term in setting your goals.

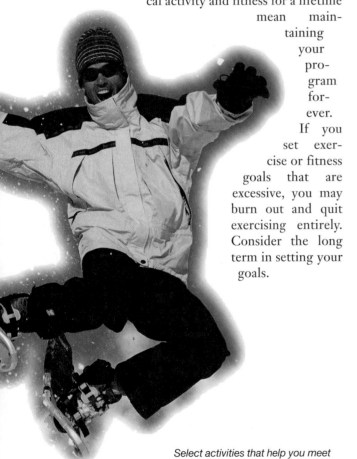

Select activities that help you meet personal goals.

Putting your goals in writing helps formalize them. Put your goals in writing. Otherwise, your goals will be easy to forget. Writing them helps establish a commitment to yourself and clearly establishes your goals. You can revise them if necessary. Written goals are not cast in concrete.

STEP 4: Selecting Activities

There are many activities from which you can choose to meet your goals. www.mhhe.com/ fit_well/web05 Click 04. A good lifetime physical activity program will include a wide variety of activities. In the concepts that follow you will learn more about activities from each level of the physical activity pyramid, including the benefits you can expect from each type of activity. The more you learn about each type of activity, the greater likelihood that you will select activities that meet your goals. Consider the following guidelines as you learn more about each type of activity.

- Choose activities you enjoy or find ways to make activity enjoyable.
- Choose activities that match your abilities.
- Practice to improve your performance skills or find activities that do not require a lot of skill.
- Choose activities that build all parts of fitness.

STEP 5: Writing Your Plan

Preparing a written plan can improve your adherence to the plan. A written plan is a pledge or a promise to be active. Research shows that intentions to be active are more likely to be acted on when put in writing. In the concepts that follow, you will be given the opportunity to prepare written plans for all of the activities in the physical activity pyramid. This will be done one activity at a time. When you have developed a plan for each type of activity, you can then develop a comprehensive physical activity plan.

In Lab 26C you will write a comprehensive lifetime activity plan. By then you will have learned more about a variety of activities. You will also have learned more about a variety of self-management skills that will assist you.

STEP 6: Evaluating Progress

Self-monitoring of physical activity can help you evaluate progress. www.mhhe.com/fit_well/ web05 Click 05. Once you have written a plan it is important to asses your effectiveness in sticking with your plan. Keeping written records is one type of self-monitoring.

You can monitor your physical activity goals by keeping daily records of the activities you perform. Keeping records in the form of physical activity logs is the preferred method of self-monitoring for beginners. Activity logs help you comply with physical activity goals. In the concepts that follow, you will prepare a plan for different types of physical activity from the pyramid and keep activity logs to chart progress.

Advanced exercisers can evaluate progress by keeping records of fitness improvement. By the time you complete your studies associated with this book, you should have the experience necessary to establish and self-monitor fitness goals. Many of you may already have the experience necessary but you are encouraged to focus on physical activity recordkeeping as you perform the lab experiences presented early in this book.

Periodic self-assessments allow you to monitor progress toward fitness and other outcome goals. If fitness has improved the results can be motivational. If done too frequently, monitoring improvements can be discouraging, since it takes time for fitness to improve. Also, changes that occur from day to day may not be representative of true changes in fitness. Fatigue, time of testing, and nutritional status are but a few of the factors that account for fitness differences from day to day. For example, strength test results may be low if done after a hard day's work, and your weight can vary from day to day or even hour to hour based on nutritional factors such as water loss from physical activity.

Fitness recordkeeping is important. Periodic self-assessment of each of the different fitness dimensions is encouraged as long as it is not too often. Doing self-assessments under the same conditions including the same time of the day is important if self-monitoring is to be meaningful.

Strategies for Action

A self-assessment of your attitudes about physical activity is a good first step in planning for lifelong physical activity. The physical activity attitudes questionnaire included in Lab 5A allows you the opportunity to consider your reasons for participating in physical activity. You will calculate a score for each of the nine attitudes described in Table 3. You will also calculate a balance of attitudes score that will indicate whether you have more positive than negative attitudes about physical activity. If you have low scores for certain attitudes, you should consider the strategies for change outlined in Table 3. Efforts to change attitudes are especially important for people with a negative balance of attitudes (poor or very poor ratings).

Self-planning skills can be used for each of the different types of activity in the physical activity pyramid. In subsequent concepts, you develop your own plans for each of the types of activity in the physical activity pyramid. As you develop those plans, it will be useful to refer to the self-planning skills outlined in this concept.

Web Resources

American College of Sports Medicine **www.acsm.org**
The Fitness Jumpsite **www.primusweb.com/fitnesspartner**
Health Canada-Physical Activity Guide **www.hc-sc.qc.ca/ hppb/paguide**
Planning Workouts **www.thriveonline.com**

Suggested Readings

 Additional reference materials for Concept 5 are available at **www.mhhe.com/fit_well/web05 Click 06**.

American College of Sports Medicine. 2000. *ACSM's Guidelines for Exercise Testing and Exercise Prescription.* 6th ed. Philadelphia: Lippincott, Williams and Wilkins.

Blair, S. N. et al. 2001. *Active Living Every Day.* Champaign, IL: Human Kinetics.

Brehm, B. A. 2000. Maximizing the psychological benefits of physical activity. *ACSM's Health and Fitness Journal* 4(6):7–11.

Corbin, C. B., and R. P. Pangrazi, (eds.) 1999. *Towards a Better Understanding of Physical Fitness and Activity.* Scottsdale, AZ: Holcomb-Hathaway.

Locke, E. A. 2002. Setting goals for happiness. In Snyder, C. R., and S. J. Lopez, (eds.), *Handbook of Positive Psychology.* Oxford, UK: University Press.

Roitman, J. L. (ed.). 2001. *ACSM's Resource Manual for Guidelines for Exercise Testing and Prescription.* 4th ed. Philadelphia: Lippincott, Williams and Wilkins.

U.S. Department of Health and Human Services. 1996. *Physical Activity and Health: A Report of the Surgeon General.* Atlanta: U.S. Department of Health and Human Services.

Lab 5A: Physical Activity Attitude Questionnaire

Name		Section	Date

Purpose: To evaluate your feelings concerning physical activity and to determine the specific reasons why you do or do not participate in regular physical activity.

The Physical Activity Attitude Questionnaire

Directions: The term *physical activity* in the following statements refers to all kinds of activities, including sports, formal exercises, and informal activities, such as jogging and cycling. Make an X over the circle that best represents your answer to each question.

	Strongly Disagree	Disagree	Undecided	Agree	Strongly Agree	Item Score	Attitude Score
1. I should do physical activity regularly for my health.	1	2	3	4	5		Health Fitness Score
2. Doing regular physical activity is good for my fitness and wellness.	1	2	3	4	5	+ =	
3. Regular exercise helps me look my best.	1	2	3	4	5		Appearance Score
4. I feel more physically attractive when I do regular physical activity.	1	2	3	4	5	+ =	
5. One of the main reasons I do regular physical activity is because it is fun.	1	2	3	4	5		Enjoyment Score
6. The most enjoyable part of my day is when I am exercising or doing a sport.	1	2	3	4	5	+ =	
7. Taking part in physical activity helps me to relax.	1	2	3	4	5		Relaxation Score
8. Physical activity helps me get away from the pressures of daily living.	1	2	3	4	5	+ =	
9. The challenge of physical training is one reason why I do physical activity.	1	2	3	4	5		Challenge Score
10. I like to see if I can master sports and activities that are new to me.	1	2	3	4	5	+ =	
11. I like to do physical activity that involves other people.	1	2	3	4	5		Social Score
12. Exercise offers me the opportunity to meet other people.	1	2	3	4	5	+ =	
13. Competition is a good way to make physical activity fun.	1	2	3	4	5		Competition Score
14. I like to see how my physical abilities compare to others.	1	2	3	4	5	+ =	
15. When I do regular exercise, I feel better than when I don't.	1	2	3	4	5		Feeling Good Score
16. My ability to do physical activity is something that makes me proud.	1	2	3	4	5	+ =	
17. I like to do outdoor activities.	1	2	3	4	5		Outdoor Score
18. Experiencing nature is something I look forward to when exercising.	1	2	3	4	5	+ =	

Procedures:

1. Read and answer each question in the questionnaire.
2. Write the number in the circle of your answer in the box labeled "item score."
3. Add scores for each pair of scores and record in the "attitude score" box.
4. Record each attitude score and a rating for each score (use Rating Chart) in the chart below. Place a + after scores that are good or excellent and a − after scores that are fair, poor, or very poor.
5. Subtract the number of negative ratings from the number of positive ratings to determine your "balance of feelings" score.

Results: Record your results as indicated in the procedures above.

The Physical Activity Attitude Questionnaire Results

Attitude	Score	Rating
Health and Fitness		
Appearance		
Enjoyment		
Relaxation		
Challenge		
Social		
Competition		
Feeling Good		
Outdoor		

Attitude Rating Chart

Rating Category	Attitude Score
Excellent	9–10
Good	7–8
Fair	5–6
Poor	3–4
Very Poor	2

+ scores [ ] minus scores [ ] = [ ]
Balance of Feeling Score

Balance of Feelings Rating Chart

Excellent	+5 to +9
Good	+2 to +4
Fair	0 to +1
Poor	−1 to −2
Very Poor	more than −2

1. In a few sentences, discuss your "balance of feelings" rating. Having more positive than negative scores (positive balance of feelings) increases the probability of being active. Include comments on whether you think your ratings suggest that you will be active or inactive and whether your ratings are really indicative of your feelings. Do you think that the scores on which you were rated poor or very poor might be reasons why you would avoid physical activity? Explain.

The Health Benefits of Physical Activity

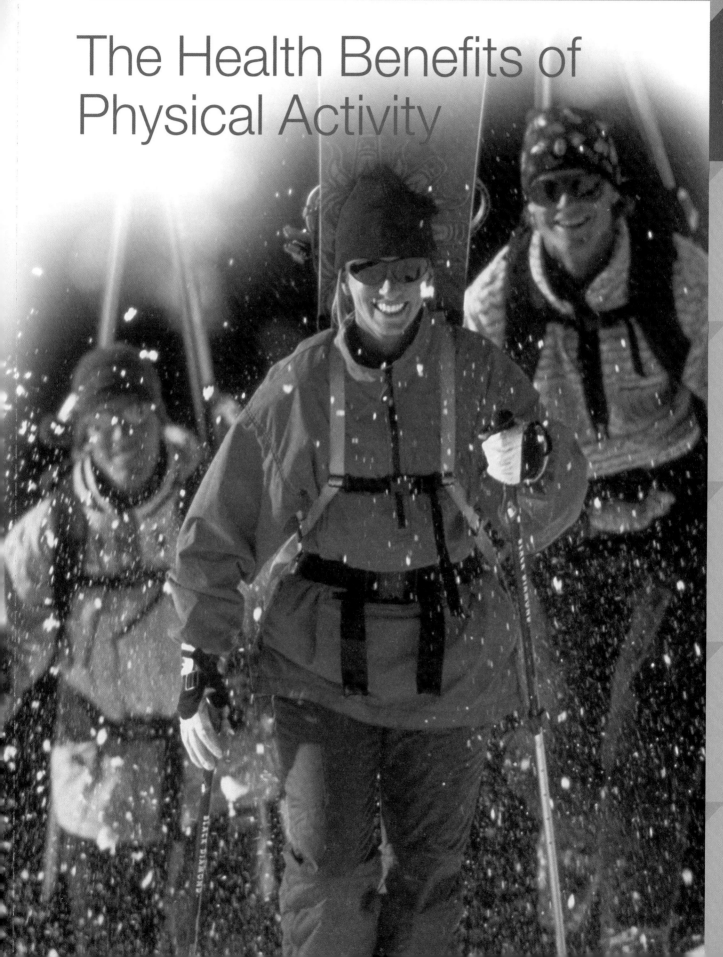

Physical activity and good physical fitness can reduce risk of illness and contribute to optimal health and wellness.

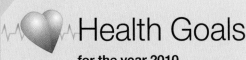

Health Goals

for the year 2010

- Increase quality and years of healthy life.

- Increase incidence of "healthy days."

- Increase daily physical activity.

- Increase prevalence of a healthy weight and reduce prevalence of overweight.

- Reduce days with pain for those with arthritis, osteoporosis, and chronic back problems.

- Reduce activity limitations, especially among older adults.

- Reduce incidence of and deaths from cancer.

- Increase diagnosis of and reduce incidence of Type II diabetes.

- Decrease incidence of depression.

- Decrease incidence of heart diseases including stroke and high blood pressure.

- Decrease incidence of high cholesterol levels among adults.

The *Surgeon General's Report on Physical Activity and Health* was an especially important document that informed the general public of the risks of sedentary living and the health benefits of physical activity. Since that document was published, more evidence has accumulated supporting the health benefits of an active lifestyle. One recent study has shown that exercise capacity measured on a treadmill is a more powerful predictor of longevity than any other risk factor including smoking, heart problems, high blood pressure, high cholesterol, or diabetes. The evidence has led to reports such as *Healthy People 2010* in the United States and *Achieving Health for All* in Canada that establish health goals designed to promote active healthy living in the 21st century. In this concept, the health benefits of regular physical activity will be summarized.

Physical Activity and Hypokinetic Diseases

Regular physical activity and good fitness can promote good health, help prevent disease, and be a part of disease treatment. www.mhhe.com/ fit_well/web06 Click 01. There are three major ways in which regular physical activity and good fitness can contribute to optimal health and wellness.

First, they can aid in disease/illness prevention. There is considerable evidence that the risk of **hypokinetic conditions** can be greatly reduced among people who do regular physical activity and achieve good physical fitness. Virtually all **chronic diseases** that plague society are considered to be hypokinetic, though some relate more to inactivity than others. Nearly three-quarters of all deaths among those eighteen and older are a result of chronic diseases. Leading public health officials have suggested that physical activity reduces the risk for several of these diseases. Physical activity also stimulates positive changes with respect to other risk factors and may produce a shortcut for the control of chronic diseases, much like immunization controlled infectious diseases.

Second, physical activity and fitness can be significant contributors to disease/illness treatment. Even with the best disease prevention practices, some people will become ill. Regular exercise and good fitness have been shown to be effective in alleviating symptoms and aiding rehabilitation after illness for such hypokinetic conditions as diabetes, heart attack, and back pain.

Finally, physical activity and fitness are methods of health and wellness promotion. They contribute to quality living associated with wellness, the positive component of good health. In the process they aid in meeting many of the nation's health goals.

Too many adults suffer from hypokinetic disease and the economic cost is high. www.mhhe. com/fit_well/web06 Click 02. In 1961, Kraus and Raab coined the term "hypokinetic disease." They pointed out that recent advances in medicine had been quite effective in eliminating infectious diseases but that chronic or degenerative diseases, characterized by sedentary or "take-it-easy" living, had increased in recent decades. In fact, heart disease is the leading cause of death in North America. High blood pressure, stroke, and coronary artery disease (including heart attack) afflict millions each year. The second leading medical complaint (headache is number one) is low back pain, and as many as one-half of all adults are considered to be obese. Studies show that the symptoms of hypokinetic conditions begin in youth. This suggests that the incidence of hypokinetic disease in our culture will not be reduced without considerable lifestyle change in people of all ages.

Experts use the term **sedentary death syndrome** (SeDS) to describe a group of symptoms associated with sedentary living. Included are weak skeletal muscles, low bone density, poor metabolic fitness (high blood sugar and fat levels, obesity, and high blood pressure at rest), and low cardiovascular fitness. As you will learn in this concept, these are all symptoms of hypokinetic diseases and sedentary people often have more than one.

The originators of the SeDS concept have suggested that our society must declare war on hypokinetic diseases and SeDS. They indicate that more than 250,000 Americans will die prematurely as a result of sedentary lifestyles and that the cost is in excess of $150 billion annually.

Regular physical activity over a lifetime may overcome the effects of inherited risk. Some people with a family history of disease may conclude they can do nothing because their heredity works against them. There is no doubt that heredity significantly affects risk of early death from hypokinetic diseases. New studies of twins, however, suggest that active people are less likely to die early than inactive people with similar genes. This suggests that long-term adherence to physical activity can overcome other risk factors such as heredity, at least for some people.

Hypokinetic diseases and conditions have many causes. Regular physical activity and good physical fitness are only two of the preventative factors associated with the conditions described in this concept as hypokinetic diseases. Other healthy lifestyle factors cannot be overlooked in the prevention of these diseases.

Physical Activity and Cardiovascular Diseases

The many types of cardiovascular diseases are the leading killers in automated societies. There are many forms of **cardiovascular diseases (CVD).** Some are classified as **coronary heart disease (CHD)** because they affect the heart muscle and the blood vessels inside the heart. **Coronary occlusion** (heart attack) is a type of CHD. **Atherosclerosis** and **arteriosclerosis** are two conditions that increase risk of heart attack and are also considered to be types of CHD. **Angina pectoris** (chest or arm pain), which occurs when the oxygen supply to the heart muscle is diminished, is sometimes considered to be a type of CHD though it is really a symptom of poor circulation.

Hypertension (high blood pressure), **stroke** (brain attack), **peripheral vascular disease,** and **congestive heart failure** are other forms of CVD. Inactivity relates in some way to each of these types of disease.

In the United States, CHD accounts for approximately 31 percent of all premature deaths. Stroke accounts for an

Hypokinetic Conditions *Hypo-* means "under" or "too little" and *-kinetic* means "movement" or "activity." Thus, *hypokinetic* means "too little activity." A hypokinetic disease or condition is associated with lack of physical activity or too little regular exercise. Examples of such conditions include heart disease, low back pain, adult-onset diabetes, and obesity.

Chronic Disease A disease or illness that is associated with lifestyle or environmental factors as opposed to infectious diseases; hypokinetic diseases are considered to be chronic diseases.

Sedentary Death Syndrome (SeDS) A group of symptoms associated with sedentary living including weak skeletal muscles, low bone density, poor metabolic fitness (high blood sugar and fat levels, obesity, and high blood pressure at rest), and low cardiovascular fitness.

Cardiovascular Disease (CVD) A broad classification of diseases of the heart and blood vessels that include CHD, as well as high blood pressure, stroke, and peripheral vascular disease.

Coronary Heart Disease (CHD) Diseases of the heart muscle and the blood vessels that supply it with oxygen, including heart attack.

Coronary Occlusion The blocking of the coronary blood vessels.

Atherosclerosis The deposition of materials along the arterial walls; a type of arteriosclerosis.

Arteriosclerosis Hardening of the arteries due to conditions that cause the arterial walls to become thick, hard, and nonelastic.

Angina Pectoris Chest or arm pain resulting from reduced oxygen supply to the heart muscle.

Hypertension High blood pressure.

Stroke (Cerebrovascular Accident or CVA) A condition in which the brain, or part of the brain, receives insufficient oxygen as a result of diminished blood supply; sometimes called apoplexy.

Peripheral Vascular Disease Lack of oxygen supply to the working muscles and tissues of the arms and legs resulting from decreased blood flow.

Congestive Heart Failure The inability of the heart muscle to pump the blood at a life-sustaining rate.

additional 7 percent. Men are more likely to suffer from heart disease than women. African American, Hispanic, and Native American populations are at higher-than-normal risk. Heart disease and stroke death rates are similar in the United States, Canada, Great Britain, Australia, and other automated societies.

There is a wealth of statistical evidence that physical inactivity is a primary risk factor for CHD. Much of the research relating inactivity to heart disease has come from occupational studies that show a high incidence of heart disease in people involved only in sedentary work. Even with the limitations inherent in these types of studies, the findings of more and more occupational studies present convincing evidence that the inactive individual has an increased risk of coronary heart disease. A study summarizing all of the important occupational studies shows a 90 percent reduced risk of coronary heart disease for those in active versus inactive occupations.

Studies also indicate that adults who expend a significant number of calories per week in strenuous sports and other activities have reduced risk of coronary heart disease. In fact, improving activity levels is among the best ways to reduce the risk of heart disease among adults.

The American Heart Association, after carefully examining the research literature, elevated sedentary living from a secondary to a primary risk factor comparable to high blood pressure, high blood cholesterol, obesity, and cigarette smoke. The reason for this change is that inactivity increases risk in multiple ways and large numbers of adults are sedentary and vulnerable to these risks. After reviewing hundreds of studies on exercise and heart disease, the *Surgeon General's Report on Physical Activity and Health* concluded that "physical inactivity is causally linked to atherosclerosis and coronary heart disease."

Physical Activity and the Healthy Heart

Regular physical activity will increase the ability of the heart muscle to pump blood as well as oxygen. A fit heart muscle can handle extra demands placed on it. Through regular exercise, the heart muscle gets stronger, contracts more forcefully and, therefore, pumps more blood with each beat. This results in a slower heart rate (especially during physical activity), and greater heart efficiency. The heart is just like any other muscle—it must be exercised regularly to stay fit. The fit heart has open, clear arteries free of atherosclerosis. (See Figure 1.)

The hypothetical "normal" resting heart rate is said to be 72 beats per minute (bpm). However, resting rates of 50 to 85 bpm are common. People who regularly do physical activity will typically have lower resting heart

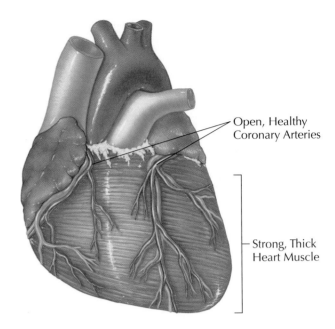

Open, Healthy Coronary Arteries

Strong, Thick Heart Muscle

Figure 1 ▶ The fit heart muscle.

rates than people who do no regular activity. Some endurance athletes have heart rates in the 30 and 40 bpm range, which is considered healthy or normal. While resting heart rate is *not* considered to be a good measure of health or fitness, decreases in individual heart rate following training reflect positive adaptations. Low heart rates in response to a standard amount of physical activity *are* a good indicator of fitness. The bicycle and step tests presented later in this book use your heart rate response to a standard amount of exercise to estimate your cardiovascular fitness.

Physical Activity and Atherosclerosis

 Atherosclerosis, which begins early in life, is implicated in many cardiovascular diseases. www.mhhe.com/fit_well/web06 Click 03. Atherosclerosis is a condition that contributes to heart attack, stroke, hypertension, angina pectoris, and peripheral vascular diseases. Deposits on the walls of arteries restrict blood flow and oxygen supply to the tissues. Atherosclerosis of the coronary arteries, the vessels that supply the heart muscle with oxygen, is particularly harmful. If these arteries become narrowed, the blood supply to the heart muscle is diminished, and angina pectoris may occur. Atherosclerosis increases the risk of heart attack because a fibrous clot is more likely to obstruct a narrowed artery than a healthy, open one.

Current theory suggests that atherosclerosis begins when damage occurs to the cells of the inner wall or

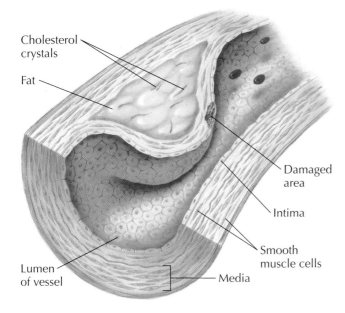

Cholesterol crystals

Fat

Damaged area

Intima

Smooth muscle cells

Lumen of vessel

Media

Figure 2 ▶ Atherosclerosis.

	Total Cholesterol	LDL-C	HDL-C	TC/HDL-C
Optimal	—	<100	—	3.5 or less
Near Optimal	—	100–129	—	—
Desirable	<200	—	>60	—
Borderline	200–240	130–160	39–59	3.6–5.0
High Risk	>240	>160	40	5.0+

Table 1 ▶ Cholesterol Classifications (mg/dL)

Source: Third Report of the National Cholesterol Education Program.

intima of the artery (see Figure 2). Substances associated with blood clotting are attracted to the damaged area. These substances seem to cause the migration of smooth muscle cells, commonly found only in the middle wall of the artery (media), to the intima. In the later stages, fats (including cholesterol) and other substances are thought to be deposited, forming plaques or protrusions that diminish the internal diameter of the artery. Research indicates that the first signs of atherosclerosis begin in early childhood.

Regular physical activity can help prevent atherosclerosis. www.mhhe.com/fit_well/web06 Click 04. All of the ways in which regular exercise helps prevent atherosclerosis are not yet known. However, three of the most plausible theories are discussed here.

Lipid Deposit Theory

There are several kinds of **lipids** in the bloodstream, including **lipoproteins,** phospholipids, triglycerides, and cholesterol. Cholesterol is the most well-known, but it is not the only culprit. Many blood fats are manufactured by the body itself, while others are ingested in high-fat foods, particularly saturated fats. Saturated fats are fats that are solid at room temperature.

As noted earlier, blood lipids are thought to contribute to the development of atherosclerotic deposits on the inner walls of the artery. One substance, called **low-density lipoprotein (LDL),** is considered to be a major culprit in the development of atherosclerosis. LDL is basically a core of cholesterol surrounded by protein and

another substance that makes it water soluble. The theory is that regular exercise can reduce blood lipid levels, including LDL-C (the cholesterol core of LDL). People with high total cholesterol and LDL-C levels have been shown to have a higher-than-normal risk of heart disease (see Table 1). New evidence indicates that there are subtypes of LDL cholesterol (characterized by their small size and high density) that pose even greater risks. These subtypes are hard to measure and not included in most current blood tests, but future research will no doubt help us better understand and measure them. Recently, the FDA approved a skin cholesterol test that, when combined with traditional tests, may help in predicting future heart disease.

Triglycerides are another type of blood lipid. Elevated levels of triglycerides are positively related to heart disease. Triglycerides lose some of their ability to predict heart disease with the presence of other risk factors, so high levels are more difficult to interpret than other blood lipids. Normal levels are considered to be 150 mg/dL or less. Values of 151 to 199 are borderline, 200 to 499 are high, and above 500 are very high. It would be wise to include triglycerides in a blood lipid profile. Physical activity is often prescribed as part of a treatment for high triglyceride levels.

Lipids All fats and fatty substances.

Lipoprotein Fat-carrying protein in the blood.

Low-Density Lipoprotein (LDL) A core of cholesterol surrounded by protein; the core is often called "bad cholesterol."

Triglyceride A type of blood fat associated with increased risk of heart disease.

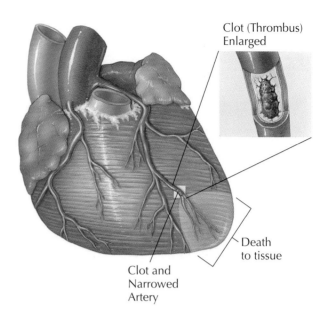

Figure 3 ▶ Heart attack.

Technology Update

Recent medical research and technology has led to the development of a new set of drugs called *statins*. Statins are effective in reducing blood fat levels, especially LDL. They are also thought to help promote blood flow in the heart and stabilize plaque that has already deposited as atherosclerosis. Of course, the preferred method of lowering high blood fat levels is through lifestyle change including regular physical activity and good nutrition. However, for those with high LDL levels statins provide a medical option. Statins are available from a number of manufacturers under several different names and require a prescription from a physician. Research suggests that the use of statins to reduce blood cholesterol levels can help reduce risk of stroke and Alzheimer's disease as well as heart disease.

Protective Protein Theory

Whereas LDLs carry a core of cholesterol that is involved in the development of atherosclerosis, **high-density lipoprotein (HDL)** picks up cholesterol (HDL-C) and carries it to the liver, where it is eliminated from the body. For this reason, it is often called the "protective protein." High levels of HDL are considered to be desirable. When you have a blood test, it is wise to ask for information about total cholesterol, LDL, and HDL levels. A recent report has provided new information about healthy levels for each (see Table 1). Individuals who do regular physical activity have lower total cholesterol, lower LDL, and higher HDL levels.

Other Theories

At least two other theories relate to the build-up of atherosclerosis in the arteries. The blood coagulant theory suggests that **fibrin** and platelets (types of cells involved in blood coagulation) deposit at the site of an injury on the wall of the artery contributing to the process of plaque build-up or atherosclerosis. Regular physical activity has been shown to reduce fibrin levels in the blood. The breakdown of fibrin seems to reduce platelet adhesiveness and the concentration of platelets in the blood. The immune system theory suggests that physical activity may influence the immune system in a positive way by lowering atherosclerosis promoting immune cells in the blood and by protecting the lining of the artery.

Physical Activity and Heart Attack

Regular physical activity reduces the risk of heart attack, the most prevalent and serious of all cardiovascular diseases. A heart attack (coronary occlusion)

occurs when a coronary artery is blocked (see Figure 3). A clot or thrombus is the most common cause, reducing or cutting off blood flow and oxygen to the heart muscle. If the blocked coronary artery supplies a major portion of the heart muscle, death will occur within minutes. Occlusions of lesser arteries may result in angina pectoris or a nonfatal heart attack.

People who perform regular sports and physical activity have half the risk of a first heart attack compared to those who are sedentary. Possible reasons are less atherosclerosis, greater diameter of arteries, and less chance of a clot forming.

Regular exercise can improve coronary circulation and, thus, reduce the chances of a heart attack or dying from one. Within the heart, many tiny branches extend from the major coronary arteries. All of these vessels supply blood to the heart muscle. Healthy arteries can supply blood to any region of the heart as it is needed. Active people are likely to have greater blood-carrying capacity in these vessels, probably because the vessels are larger and more elastic. Also, the active person may have a more profuse distribution of arteries within the heart muscle (see Figure 4), which results in greater blood flow. A few studies show that physical activity may promote the growth of "extra" blood vessels, which are thought to open up to provide the heart muscle with the necessary blood and oxygen when the oxygen supply is diminished, as in a heart attack. Blood flow from extra blood vessels is referred to as **coronary collateral circulation.**

Improved coronary circulation may provide protection against a heart attack because a larger artery would require more atherosclerosis to occlude it. In addition, the development of collateral blood vessels supplying the

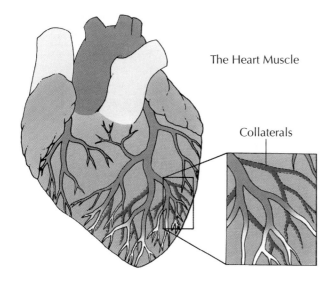

The Heart Muscle

Collaterals

Figure 4 ▶ Coronary collateral circulation.

heart may diminish the effects of a heart attack if one does occur. These extra (or collateral) blood vessels may take over the function of regular blood vessels during a heart attack.

The heart of the inactive person is less able to resist stress and is more susceptible to an emotional storm that may precipitate a heart attack. The heart is rendered inefficient by one or more of the following circumstances: high heart rate, high blood pressure, and excessive stimulation. All of these conditions require the heart to use more oxygen than is normal and decrease its ability to adapt to stressful situations.

The inefficient heart is one that beats rapidly because it is dominated by the **sympathetic nervous system,** which speeds up the heart rate. Thus, the heart continuously beats rapidly, even at rest, and never has a true rest period. A study of one college basketball coach who was under considerable stress indicated that his lowest resting heart rate during the day was 88 bpm. High blood pressure also makes the heart work harder and contributes to its inefficiency.

Research indicates five things concerning physical activity and the inefficient heart.

1. Regular activity leads to dominance of the **parasympathetic nervous system** rather than to sympathetic dominance; thus, the heart rate is reduced and the heart works efficiently.
2. Regular activity helps the heart rate return to normal faster after emotional stress.
3. Regular activity strengthens the heart muscle, making it better able to weather an **emotional storm.**
4. Regular activity decreases sympathetic dominance and its associated hormonal effects on the heart, thus lessening the chances of altered heart contractility

and the likelihood of the circulatory problems that accompany this state.
5. Regular activity reduces the risk of sudden death from ventricular fibrillation (arrhythmic heartbeat).

Regular physical activity is one effective means of rehabilitation for a person who has coronary heart disease or who has had a heart attack. Not only does regular physical activity seem to reduce the risk of developing coronary heart disease, those who already have the condition may reduce the symptoms of the disease through regular exercise. For people who have had heart attacks, regular and progressive exercise can be an effective prescription when carried out under the supervision of a physician. Remember, however, that exercise is not the treatment of preference for all heart attack victims. In some cases, it may be contraindicated.

Physical Activity and Other Cardiovascular Diseases

Regular physical activity is associated with a reduced risk of high blood pressure (hypertension). www.mhhe.com/fit_well/web06 Click 05. Approximately 30 percent of adults have borderline or high-risk hypertension. More men than women are likely to be hypertensive, as are more blacks than whites. Native Americans and Hispanics have a higher-than-normal incidence of hypertension, and the incidence for all groups increases as people grow older. A recent research summary indicates that the effects of physical activity on

High-Density Lipoprotein (HDL) A blood substance that picks up cholesterol and helps remove it from the body; often called "good cholesterol."

Fibrin A sticky threadlike substance that in combination with blood cells forms a blood clot.

Coronary Collateral Circulation Circulation of blood to the heart muscle associated with the blood-carrying capacity of a specific vessel or development of collateral vessels (extra blood vessels).

Sympathetic Nervous System Branch of the autonomic nervous system that prepares the body for activity by speeding up the heart rate.

Parasympathetic Nervous System Branch of the autonomic nervous system that slows the heart rate.

Emotional Storm A traumatic emotional experience that is likely to affect the human organism physiologically.

blood pressure are more dramatic than previously thought and are independent of age, body fatness, and other factors. Inactive, less-fit individuals have a 30 to 50 percent greater chance of being hypertensive than active, fit people. Regular physical activity can also be one effective method of reducing blood pressure for those with hypertension. Physical inactivity in middle age is associated with risk of high blood pressure later in life. The most plausible reason is a reduction in resistance to blood flow in the blood vessels, probably resulting from dilation of the vessels.

The hypothetical "goal" blood pressure is 120 mm Hg (**systolic blood pressure**) over 80 mm Hg (**diastolic blood pressure**). However, systolic pressures as low as 100 mm Hg and up to 130 mm Hg are considered in the normal range. Diastolic pressures of 60 to 85 mm Hg are also considered to be in the normal range. Exceptionally low blood pressures (below 100 systolic and 60 diastolic) do not pose the same risks to health as high blood pressure but can cause dizziness, fainting, and lack of tolerance to change in body positions. Classifications for blood pressure are shown in Table 2. Stage 1 hypertension is sometimes called "mild," Stage 2 "moderate," and Stage 3 "severe." Some experts do not like these terms because people with "mild" or "moderate" hypertension may not feel the need to seek medical help. All stages of hypertension should be taken seriously.

Regular physical activity can help reduce the risk of stroke. Stroke is a major killer of adults. People with high blood pressure and atherosclerosis are susceptible to stroke. Since regular exercise and good fitness are important to the prevention of high blood pressure and atherosclerosis, exercise and fitness are considered helpful in the prevention of stroke.

Regular physical activity is helpful in the prevention of peripheral vascular diseases. People who exercise regularly have better blood flow to the working muscles and other tissues than inactive, unfit people. Since peripheral vascular disease is associated with poor circulation to the extremities, regular exercise can be considered one method of preventing this condition.

Physical Activity and Other Hypokinetic Conditions

Physical activity reduces the risk of some forms of cancer. www.mhhe.com/fit_well/web06 **Click 06.** Cancer is the second leading cause of death in the United States. According to the American Cancer Society, cancer is a group of diseases characterized by uncontrollable growth and spread of abnormal cells. The first editions of this book did not include any form of cancer as a hypokinetic disease. We now know, however, that overall death rates from cancer are lower among active people than those who are sedentary (50 to 250 percent) and that some specific forms of cancer are related to sedentary living. These cancers are described in Table 3 with possible reasons for the cancer/inactivity link (if known). The entries in Table 3 are listed in order based on the strength of evidence supporting the cancer/inactivity link. For more information on cancer refer to concept 24.

The American Cancer Society recently released new guidelines designed to help reduce risk of cancer as a result of eating well and doing regular activity. The document places a special emphasis on maintaining a healthy body fatness level as one method of reducing cancer risk. Physical activity is also considered to be important to the wellness of the cancer patient. Patients can benefit from activity in many ways including: improved quality of life,

---

Table 2 ▶ Blood Pressure Classifications for Adults*

Category	Systolic Blood Pressure (mm Hg)	Diastolic Blood Pressure (mm Hg)
Goal	<120	<80
Normal	<130	<85
High Normal	130–139	85–89
Stage 1 Hypertension	140–159	90–99
Stage 2 Hypertension	160–179	100–109
Stage 3 Hypertension	≥180	≥110

*Not taking antihypertensive drugs and not acutely ill. When the systolic and diastolic blood pressure categories vary, the higher reading determines the blood pressure classification.

Source: National Institutes for Health.

Table 3 ▶ Cancer and Sedentary Living

Cancer Type	Link to Sedentary Living
Colon	Exercise speeds movement of food and cancer-causing substances through the digestive system.
Breast	Exercise decreases the amount of exposure of breast tissue to circulating estrogen. Lower body fat is also associated with lower estrogen levels. Early life activity is deemed important for both reasons.
Rectal	Similar to colon cancer.
Prostate	Limited evidence, no established link.
Testicular	Limited evidence, no established link.
Pancreatic	Limited evidence, no established link.

physical functioning, and self-esteem as well as less dependence on others, and reduced risk of other diseases. *Guidelines for Physical Activity and the Cancer Patient* and a *Complete Guide to Nutrition and Physical Activity* are available at the Society website (see Web Resources, also see Canadian Cancer Society).

Physical activity plays an important role in the management and treatment of diabetes. www.mhhe.com/fit_well/web06 Click 07. Diabetes mellitus (diabetes) is a group of disorders that results when there is too much sugar in the blood. It occurs when the body does not make enough **insulin** or when the body is not able to use insulin effectively. Diabetes is the seventh leading cause of death among people over forty. It accounts for at least 10 percent of all short-term hospital stays and has a major impact on health-care costs in Western society. According to the American Diabetes Association (ADA) there are 17 million people in the United States who have diabetes. Unfortunately, 5.9 million of those don't know it. An estimated additional 10 million are pre-diabetic; they have metabolic profiles characteristic of those with diabetes (see Web Resources, ADA or Canadian Diabetes Association for more statistics).

Type I diabetes or insulin dependent diabetes, accounts for a relatively small number of the diabetes cases and is not considered to be a hypokinetic condition. Type II diabetes (often not insulin dependent) was formerly called "adult onset diabetes." In recent years, Type II diabetes has become common in children and is associated with high levels of body fat.

People who perform regular physical activity are less likely to suffer from Type II diabetes than sedentary people. For people with Type II diabetes, regular physical activity can help reduce body fatness, decrease **insulin resistance,** improve **insulin sensitivity,** and improve the body's ability to clear sugar from the blood in a reasonable time. All of these factors contribute to controlling the disease. With sound nutritional habits and proper medication, physical activity can be useful in the management of both types of diabetes. For more information on diabetes refer to concept 24.

Regular physical activity is important to maintaining bone density and decreasing risk of osteoporosis. www.mhhe.com/fit_well/web06 Click 08. As noted in concept 1, bone integrity is considered by some experts as a health-related component of physical fitness. Healthy bones are dense and strong. When bones lose calcium and become less dense they become porous and are at risk of fracture. The bones of young children are not especially dense, but during adolescence (see Figure 5) bone density increases to a level higher than at any other time in life (peak bone density). Though bone density often begins to decrease in young adulthood, it is not until

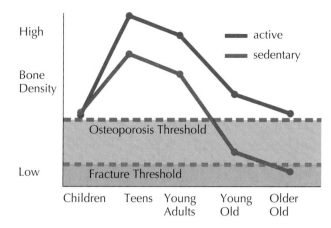

Figure 5 ► Changes in bone density with age.

older adulthood that bone loss becomes dramatic. As illustrated in Figure 5, many older adults have lost enough bone density to have a condition called **osteoporosis** (when bone density drops below the osteoporosis threshold). Some will have crossed the fracture threshold, putting them at risk of fractures especially to the hip, vertebrae, and other "soft" or "spongy" bones of the skeletal system. Active people have a higher peak bone mass and are more resistant to osteoporosis (see blue line in Figure 5) than sedentary people (see red line in Figure 5).

Women, especially post-menopausal women, have a higher risk of osteoporosis than men. Males typically

Systolic Blood Pressure The upper blood pressure number often called working blood pressure. It represents the pressure in the arteries at its highest level just after the heart beats.

Diastolic Blood Pressure The lower blood pressure number often called "resting pressure." It is the pressure in the arteries at its lowest level occurring just before the next beat of the heart.

Insulin A hormone secreted by the pancreas that regulates levels of sugar in the blood.

Insulin Resistance A condition that occurs when insulin becomes ineffective or less effective than necessary to regulate sugar levels in the blood.

Insulin Sensitivity A person with insulin resistance (see above) is said to have decreased insulin sensitivity. The body's cells are not sensitive to insulin so they resist it and sugar levels are not regulated effectively.

Osteoporosis A condition associated with low bone density and subsequent bone fragility leading to high risk of fracture.

have a higher peak bone mass than females and for this reason can lose more bone density over time without reaching the osteoporosis or fracture thresholds. More women reach the osteoporosis and fracture thresholds at earlier ages than men. Other risk factors for osteoporosis are northern European ancestry, smoking, alcohol use, current or previous eating disorders, early menstruation, and low dietary calcium intake. People who are confined to bed rest are especially at risk of osteoporosis because regular exercise is necessary for good bone health.

Guidelines for building bone integrity and preventing osteoporosis include the following:

- Do regular weight-bearing exercise and resistance training that stresses the bones of the body. The load bearing and pull of the muscles in these types of exercises builds bone density.
- Eat a diet rich in calcium. Calcium is necessary to build strong bones. At-risk groups should consider a calcium supplement.
- Post-menopausal women, after consultation with a physician, should consider a calcium supplement and special medications such as raloxifene (sold as Evista) and alendronate (sold as Fosomax) that help prevent bone loss. Another drug, zoledronic acid, that was originally approved to stop calcium loss from the bones of cancer patients shows promise for treatment of osteoporosis in the future.
- Hormone replacement therapy (HRT), also called estrogen replacement therapy (ERT), has been shown to reduce risk of osteoporosis among post-menopausal women. However, results of a long-term study (Women's Health Initiative) suggest that HRT can increase risk of breast cancer, stroke, and heart disease. Many women, and their doctors, are reevaluating their medication based on this recent evidence.
- Start early in life to build strong bones because peak bone mass is developed in the teen years.
- It is never too late to start. Following these guidelines has been shown to help people of all ages, including those eighty and over.
- Older people with osteoporosis should consider protective pads shown to prevent fractures from falls.

Active people who possess good muscle fitness are less likely to have back and musculoskeletal problems than inactive, unfit people. Because few people die from it, back pain does not receive the attention given to such medical problems as heart disease and cancer. But back pain is considered to be the second leading medical complaint in the United States, second only to headaches. Only the common cold and the flu cause more days lost from work. At some point in our lives, approximately 80 percent of all adults will experience back pain that limits their ability to function normally.

Recent National Safety Council data indicate that the back was the most frequently injured of all body parts, and the injury rate was double that of any other part of the body.

Many years ago, medical doctors began to associate back problems with the lack of physical fitness. It is now known that the great majority of back ailments are the result of poor muscle strength, endurance, and poor flexibility. Tests on patients with back problems show weakness and lack of flexibility in key muscle groups.

Though lack of fitness is probably the leading reason for back pain in Western society, there are many other factors that increase the risk of back ailments, including poor posture, improper lifting and work habits, heredity, and disease states, such as scoliosis and arthritis.

Physical activity is important in maintaining a healthy body weight and avoiding the numerous health conditions associated with obesity. Recently the Surgeon General issued a *Call to Action to Prevent and Decrease Overweight and Obesity*. This report notes that one-third of adults are obese and 61 percent are classified as overweight based on the body mass index. Approximately 13 percent of children and 14 percent of teens are classified as obese, dramatically up from twenty years ago. Obesity is not a disease state in itself but is a hypokinetic condition associated with a multitude of far-reaching complications. Research has shown that fat people who are fit are not at especially high risk of early death. However, when high body fatness is accompanied by low cardiovascular and low metabolic fitness, risk of early death increases substantially. Obesity contributes to sedentary death syndrome described earlier in this concept. For more information on obesity and overfatness consult concept 15.

Physical activity reduces the risk and severity of a variety of common mental (emotional) health disorders. Such disorders can be considered hypokinetic conditions. Some mental (emotional) health conditions are prevalent in modern society. Nearly one-half of adult Americans will report having a mental health disorder at some point in life. A recent summary of studies revealed that there are several emotional/mental disorders that are associated with inactive lifestyles.

Depression is a stress-related condition experienced by many adults. Thirty-three percent of inactive adults report that they often feel depressed. For some, depression is a serious disorder that physical activity alone will not cure; however, recent research does indicate that activity, combined with other forms of therapy, can be effective.

Anxiety is an emotional condition characterized by worry, self-doubt, and apprehension. More than a few studies have shown that symptoms of anxiety can be reduced by regular activity. Low-fit people who do regular aerobic activity seem to benefit the most. In one study, one-third of active people felt that regular activity helped them to better cope with life's pressures.

Physical activity is also associated with better and more restful sleep. People with insomnia (the inability to sleep) seem to benefit from regular activity if it is not done too vigorously right before going to bed. A recent study indicates that 52 percent of the population feel that physical activity helps them sleep better. Regular aerobic activity is associated with reduced brain activation that can result in greater ability to relax or fall asleep.

Even more common than depression and insomnia is the condition called Type A behavior. Type A personalities are stress-prone individuals with a greater than normal incidence of diseases. A Type A person is tense, overcompetitive, and worried about meeting time schedules. Apparently, all Type A personalities are not equally stressed. It has been suggested that aggressive Type A personalities are most likely to be prone to negative consequences of stress. Regular physical activity can benefit the Type A person, especially the aggressive Type A. Noncompetitive activities would probably be best for this stress-prone personality type.

A final benefit of regular physical activity is increased self-esteem. Improvements in fitness and appearance can improve self-confidence and self-esteem. The ability to regulate behavior and perform new tasks can also promote higher self-esteem.

Regular physical activity can have positive effects on some non-hypokinetic conditions. Some non-hypokinetic conditions that can benefit from physical activity are:

- Arthritis. Many, if not most, arthritics are in a deconditioned state resulting from a lack of activity. The traditional advice that arthritics should avoid physical activity is now being modified in view of the findings that carefully prescribed exercise can improve general fitness and, in some cases, reduce the symptoms of the disease.
- Asthma. Asthmatics often have physical activity limitations. New evidence suggests that, with proper management, activity can be part of their daily life. In fact, when done properly, activity can reduce airway reactivity and medication use. Because exercise can trigger bronchial constriction, it is important to choose appropriate types of activity and to use inhaled medications to prevent bronchial constriction caused by exercise or other triggers such as cold weather. Asthmatics should avoid cold weather exercise.
- Immune system disorders. Recent evidence suggests that regular moderate physical activity can enhance immune system function and help people resist infections. However, vigorous training can temporarily reduce immune function, so people with systemic infections such as colds or flu should avoid heavy training. There is evidence that regular activity for immune system disorders such as HIV can enhance quality of life.
- Premenstrual syndrome (PMS). PMS, a mixture of physical and emotional symptoms that occurs prior to menstruation, has many causes. However, current evidence suggests that changes in lifestyle, including regular exercise, may be effective in relieving PMS symptoms.
- Other conditions. Low to moderate intensity aerobic activity and resistance training are currently being prescribed for some people who have chronic pain (persistent pain without relief) and or fibromyalgia (chronic muscle pain). Evidence also suggests that active people have a 30 percent lesser chance of having gallstones than inactive people and activity may decrease risk of impotence.

Physical Activity and Aging

Regular physical activity can improve fitness and improve functioning among older adults. www.mhhe.com/fit_well/web06 Click 09. Approximately 30 percent of adults age seventy and over have difficulty with one or more activities of daily living. Women have more limitations than men, and low-income groups have more limitations than higher-income groups. Nearly one-half get no assistance with the activity in which they are limited.

The inability to function effectively as you grow older is associated with lack of fitness and inactive lifestyles. This loss of function is sometimes referred to as "acquired aging" as opposed to "time-dependent" aging. Because so many people experience limitations in daily activities and often find it difficult to get assistance, it is especially important for older people to stay active and fit. In Africa, Asia, and South America, where older adults

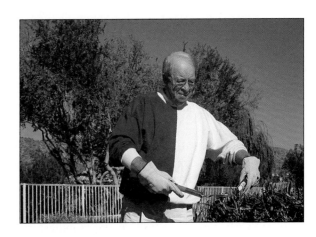

Fitness improves work efficiency.

maintain an active lifestyle, individuals do not acquire many of the characteristics commonly associated with aging in North America.

In general, older adults become much less active than younger adults. Losses in muscle fitness are associated with loss of balance, greater risk of falling, and less ability to function independently. Studies also show that exercise can enhance cognitive functioning and perhaps reduce risk of dementia. Though the amount of activity performed must be adapted as people grow older, fitness benefits discussed in the next section and throughout this book apply to people of all ages.

Regular physical activity can compress illness into a shorter period of our life. An important national health goal is to increase the years of healthy life. Living longer is important, but being able to function effectively during all years of life is equally—if not more—important. "Compression" refers to shortening the total number of years that illnesses and disabilities occur. Compressing the illness means dramatically decreasing the years of illness. Healthy lifestyles, including regular physical activity, have been shown to compress illness and increase years of effective functioning.

Health, Fitness, and Wellness Promotion

Good health-related physical fitness and regular physical activity are important to health promotion and feeling well. Regular physical activity and good fitness not only help prevent illness (see Table 4) and disease but also promote quality of life and wellness. Good health-related physical fitness can help you look good, feel good, and enjoy life. Some of the specific benefits of wellness that are associated with good fitness are listed below.

- *Good physical fitness can help an individual enjoy leisure time.* A person who is lean, has no back problems, does not have high blood pressure, and has reasonable skills in a lifetime of sports is more likely to get involved and stay regularly involved in leisure-time activities than one who does not have these characteristics. Enjoying your leisure time may not add years to your life but can add life to your years.
- *Good physical fitness can help an individual work effectively and efficiently.* A person who can resist fatigue, muscle soreness, back problems, and other symptoms associated with poor health-related fitness is capable of working productively and having energy left over at the end of the day. Surveys of employees who are involved with employee fitness programs indicate that 75 percent ▶ have an improved sense of well-being.

Employers indicate that absenteeism decreased by up to 50 percent among program participants. People with good skill-related fitness may be more effective and efficient in performing specific motor skills required for certain jobs.

- *Good physical fitness is essential to effective living.* Although the need for each component of physical fitness is specific to each individual, every person requires enough fitness to perform normal daily activities without undue fatigue. Whether it be walking, performing household chores, or merely feeling good and enjoying the simple things in life without pain or fear of injury, good fitness is important to all people.
- *Good physical fitness may help you function safely and assist you in meeting unexpected emergencies.* Emergencies are never expected, but when they do arise, they often demand performance that requires good fitness. For example, flood victims may need to fill sandbags for hours without rest, and accident victims may be required to walk or run long distances for help. Also, good fitness is required for such simple tasks as safely changing a spare tire or loading a moving van without injury.
- *Physical fitness is the basis for dynamic and creative activity.* Though the following quotation by former President John F. Kennedy is more than thirty years old, it clearly points out the importance of physical fitness.

The relationship between the soundness of the body and the activity of the mind is subtle and complex. Much is not yet understood, but we know what the Greeks knew: that intelligence and skill can only function at the peak of their capacity when the body is healthy and strong, and that hardy spirits and tough minds usually inhabit sound bodies. Physical fitness is the basis of all activities in our society; if our bodies grow soft and inactive, if we fail to encourage physical development and prowess, we will undermine our capacity for thought, for work, and for the use of those skills vital to an expanding and complex America.

President Kennedy's belief that activity and fitness are associated with intellectual functioning has now been backed up with research. A recent research summary suggests that, though modest, the effect of activity and fitness on intellectual functioning is positive. One study shows activity to foster new brain cell growth. Time taken to be active during the day has been shown to help children learn more, even though less time is spent in intellectual pursuits.

Many economic benefits are associated with employee physical activity. A comprehensive review of the literature indicates that worksite physical activity programs can improve health, wellness, and fitness;

Table 4 ▶ Health and Wellness Benefits of Physical Activity and Fitness

Improved cardiovascular

- Stronger heart muscle fitness and health
- Lower heart rate
- Better electric stability of heart
- Decreased sympathetic control of heart
- Increased O_2 to brain
- Reduced blood fat, including low-density lipids (LDLs)
- Increased protective high-density lipids (HDLs)
- Delayed development of atherosclerosis
- Increased work capacity
- Improved peripheral circulation
- Improved coronary circulation
- Resistance to "emotional storm"
- Reduced risk of heart attack
- Reduced risk of stroke
- Reduced risk of hypertension
- Greater chance of surviving a heart attack
- Increased oxygen-carrying capacity of the blood

Improved strength and muscular endurance

- Greater work efficiency
- Less chance of muscle injury
- Reduced risk of low back problems
- Improved performance in sports
- Quicker recovery after hard work
- Improved ability to meet emergencies

Resistance to fatigue

- Ability to enjoy leisure
- Improved quality of life
- Improved ability to meet some stressors

Other health benefits

- Decreased diabetes risk
- Quality of life for diabetics
- Improved metabolic fitness
- Extended life
- Decrease in dysfunctional years
- Aids some people who have arthritis, PMS, asthma, chronic pain, fibromyalgia, and impotence
- Improved immune system

Enhanced mental health and function

- Relief of depression
- Improved sleep habits
- Fewer stress symptoms
- Ability to enjoy leisure and work
- Improved brain function

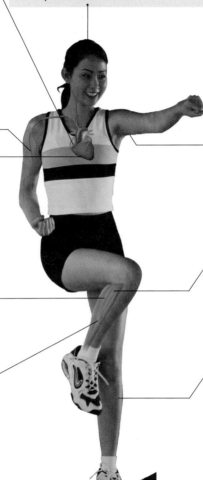

Improved wellness

- Improved quality of life
- Leisure time enjoyment
- Improved work capacity
- Ability to meet emergencies
- Improve creative capacity

Opportunity for successful experience and social interactions

- Improved self-concept
- Opportunity to recognize and accept personal limitations
- Improved sense of well-being
- Enjoy life and have fun
- Improved quality of life

Improved appearance

- Better figure/physique
- Better posture
- Fat control

Greater lean body mass and less body fat

- Greater work efficiency
- Less susceptibility to disease
- Improved appearance
- Less incidence of self-concept problems related to obesity

Improved flexibility

- Greater work efficiency
- Less chance of muscle injury
- Less chance of joint injury
- Decreased chance of low back problems
- Improved sports performance

Bone development

- Greater peak bone density
- Less chance of osteoporosis

Reduced cancer risk

- Reduced risk of colon and breast cancer
- Possible reduced risk of rectal, testicular, prostate, and pancreatic cancers

Reduced effect of acquired aging

- Improved ability to function in daily life
- Better short-term memory
- Fewer illnesses
- Greater mobility
- Greater independence
- Greater ability to operate an automobile
- Lower risk for dementia

Table 5 ▶ Hypokinetic Disease Risk Factors

Factors That Cannot Be Altered

1. **Age**—As you grow older, your risk of contracting hypokinetic diseases increases. For example, the risk of heart disease is approximately three times as great after sixty as before. The risk of back pain is considerably greater after forty.

2. **Heredity**—People who have a family history of hypokinetic disease are more likely to develop a hypokinetic condition such as heart disease, hypertension, back problems, obesity, high blood lipid levels, and other problems. African Americans are 45 percent more likely to have high blood pressure than Caucasians; therefore, they suffer strokes at an earlier age with more severe consequences.

3. **Gender**—Men have a higher incidence of many hypokinetic conditions than women. However, differences between men and women have decreased recently. This is especially true for heart disease, the leading cause of death for both men and women. Post-menopausal women have a higher heart disease risk than pre-menopausal women.

Factors That Can Be Altered

4. **Body fatness**—Having too much body fat is now a primary risk factor for heart disease and is a risk factor for other hypokinetic conditions as well. For example, loss of fat can result in relief from symptoms of Type II diabetes, can reduce problems associated with certain types of back pain, and can reduce the risks of surgery.

5. **Diet**—A clear association exists between hypokinetic disease and certain types of diets. The excessive intake of saturated fats, such as animal fats, is linked to atherosclerosis and other forms of heart disease. Excessive salt in the diet is associated with high blood pressure.

6. **Diseases**—People who have one hypokinetic disease are more likely to develop a second or even a third condition. For example, if you have diabetes,* atherosclerosis, or high blood pressure, your risk of having a heart attack or stroke increases dramatically. People with poor posture have a high risk of experiencing back pain, and those with too much body fat have a greater-than-normal risk of diabetes. Although you may not be entirely able to alter the extent to which you develop certain diseases and conditions, reducing your risk and following your doctor's advice can improve your odds significantly.

7. **Regular physical activity**—As noted throughout this book, regular exercise can help reduce the risk of hypokinetic disease.

8. **Tobacco use**—Smokers have a much higher risk of developing and dying from heart disease than nonsmokers. Smokers have five times the risk of heart attack as nonsmokers. Most striking is the difference in risk between older women smokers and nonsmokers. Tobacco use is also associated with the increased risk of high blood pressure, cancer, and several other medical conditions. Apparently, the more you use, the greater the risk. Stopping tobacco use even after many years can significantly reduce the hypokinetic disease risk.

9. **Stress**—People who are subject to excessive stress are predisposed to various hypokinetic diseases including heart disease and back pain. Statistics indicate that hypokinetic conditions are common among those in certain high-stress jobs and those having type A personality profiles.

*Some types of diabetes cannot be altered.

reduce health-care costs; and decrease absenteeism. The costs associated with providing physical activity for employees more than offsets the cost of medical care and lost days of work associated with inactivity. Nearly one-half of worksites offer some type of program. A national goal is to increase this to 75 percent.

Hypokinetic Disease Risk Factors

There are many different positive lifestyles that can reduce the risk of disease. Many of the factors that contribute to optimal health and quality of life are also considered risk factors. Changing these risk factors can dramatically reduce the risk of hypokinetic diseases such as heart disease, back pain, diabetes, and cancer. Lack of physical activity, poor nutrition, smoking, and inability to cope with stress are all risk factors associated with various diseases (see Table 5).

Not all risk factors are under your personal control. Some factors that can contribute to the increased risk of disease are not under your personal control. Three uncontrollable risk factors are age, heredity, and gender. These factors that cannot be altered by lifestyle changes are presented in Table 5.

Altering risk factors can help reduce the risk of more than one adverse condition at the same time. By altering the controllable risk factors, you can reduce the risk of several hypokinetic conditions. For example, controlling body fatness reduces the risk of diabetes, hypertension, and back problems. Altering your diet can reduce the chances of developing high levels of blood lipids, and reduce the risk of atherosclerosis.

Risk reduction does not guarantee freedom from disease. Reducing risk alters the probability of disease but does not assure disease immunity.

Too much activity can lead to hyperkinetic diseases or conditions. The information presented in this concept points out the health benefits of physical activity performed in appropriate amounts. When done in excess or incorrectly, physical activity can result in **hyperkinetic conditions.** The most common hyperkinetic condition is overuse injury to muscles, connective tissue, and bones. Recently, anorexia nervosa and body neurosis have been identified as conditions associated with inappropriate amounts of physical activity. These conditions will be discussed in the concept on performance.

Strategies for Action

 A self-assessment of risk factors can help you modify your lifestyle to reduce risk of heart disease. www.mhhe.com/fit_well/web06 Click 10. The Heart Disease Risk Factor Questionnaire in Lab 6A will help you assess your personal risk for heart disease. While this questionnaire considers the major risk factors, several recently identified factors are not included: C-reactive protein (CRP) homocysteine, an enzyme called MPO, and a substance called interleukin-6. Women with high CRP have four times the risk of having heart disease as those with low CRP. Used along with other blood tests, the CRP may prove to be useful in the future. Screening for CRP is currently available with regular blood lipid tests though data are lacking for men.

High levels of the amino acid homocysteine have also been associated with increased risk of heart disease though the American Heart Association says it is too soon to do general screening for it. Adequate folic acid, vitamin B6, and vitamin B12 help prevent high homocysteine in the blood, so eating foods that insure adequate daily intake of these vitamins is recommended.

Both MPO and interleukin-6 are elevated in people with known heart disease and are associated with inflammation. They may damage artery walls causing fat build-up. Because evidence is only preliminary at this point, these four risk factors are not included in this questionnaire.

You can use your self-assessments on the questionnaire to determine your alterable, unalterable, and total risk scores. These scores should be useful in preparing a plan for lifestyle change to reduce risk.

Web Resources

American Cancer Society **www.cancer.org**
American Diabetes Association **www.diabetes.org**
American Heart Association **www.americanheart.org**
Canadian Diabetes Association **www.diabetes.ca**
Centers for Disease Control and Prevention **www.cdc.gov**
Healthy People 2010 **www.health.gov/healthypeople**
National Stroke Association **www.stroke.org**
National Osteoporosis Foundation **www.nof.org**

Suggested Readings

Additional reference materials for concept 6 are available at www.mhhe.com/fit_well/web06 Click 11.

Blair, S. N. 2001. Guest editorial to accompany physical fitness and activity as separate heart disease risk-factors. *Medicine and Science in Sports and Exercise* 33(5):762–764.

Booth, F. W., and M. W. Chakravarthy. 2002. Cost and consequences of sedentary living: New battleground for an old enemy. *President's Council on Physical Fitness and Sports Research Digest* 3(16):1–8.

Booth, F. W. et al. 2000. Waging war on modern chronic diseases: Primary prevention through exercise biology. *Journal of Applied Physiology* 88(2):774-787.

Brehm, B. A. 2000. Maximizing the psychological benefits of physical activity. *ACSM's Health and Fitness Journal* 4(6):7–11.

Brill, P. A. et al. 2000. Muscular strength and physical function. *Medicine and Science in Sports and Exercise* 32(2):412–416.

Chintanadilok, J., and D. T. Lowenthal. 2002. Exercise in treating hypertension. *Physician and Sports Medicine* 30(3):11–28.

Colberg, S. R. 2001. Exercise: A diabetes "cure" for many. *ACSM's Health and Fitness Journal* 5(2):20–26.

Cotman, C. W., and C. Engesser-Cesar. 2002. Exercise enhances and protects brain function. *Exercise and Sport Sciences Reviews* 30(2):75–79.

Cooper, C. B. 2001. Diabetes mellitus and exercise. *ACSM's Health and Fitness Journal* 5(4):27–28.

Dembo, L., and K. M. McCormick. 2000. Exercise prescription to prevent osteoporosis. *ACSM's Health and Fitness Journal* 4(1):32–38.

Drezner, J. A., and S. A. Herring. 2001. Managing low back pain. *Physician and Sports Medicine* 29(8):37–43.

Durak, E. 2001. The use of exercise in the cancer recovery process. *ACSM's Health and Fitness Journal* 5(1):6–10.

Friedenreich, C. M. et al. 2001. Relation between intensity of physical activity and breast cancer risk reduction. *Medicine and Science in Sports and Exercise* 33(9):1538–1545.

Friedland, R. P. 2001. Activity and Alzheimer's. *Proceedings of the National Academy of Sciences* 98:3440–3445.

Lee, I. M., and S. N. Blair. 2002. Cardiorespiratory fitness and stroke mortality in men. *Medicine and Science in Sports and Exercise* 34(4):592–595.

Hyperkinetic Condition A disease/illness or health condition caused by or contributed to by too much physical activity.

Lee, I., and R. S. Paffenbarger. 2001. Preventing coronary heart disease: The role of physical activity. *The Physician and Sports Medicine* 29(2):37–52.

Manilow, M. R., A. G. Bostom, and R. M. Krauss. 1999. Homocysteine, diet and cardiovascular disease: A statement for health care professionals from the nutrition committee of the American Heart Association. *Circulation* 99(1):178–182.

McGill, S. M. 2001. Low back stability. *Exercise and Sports Science Reviews* 29(1):26–31.

Metcalf, L. et al. 2001. Postmenopausal women and exercise for prevention of osteoporosis. *ACSM's Health and Fitness Journal* 5(3):6–14.

Modlesky, C. M., and R. D. Lewis. 2002. Does exercise during growth have a long-term effect on bone health? *Exercise and Sport Sciences Reviews* 30(4):171–176.

National Cholesterol Education Program. 2001. Executive summary of the third report of the national cholesterol education program expert panel on detection, evaluation, and treatment of high blood cholesterol in adults. *Journal of the American Medical Association* 285:2486–2497.

National Institutes of Health. 2002. Osteoporosis prevention, diagnosis, and therapy. *NIH Consensus Statements* 17(1):1–45.

Nieman, D. C. 2001. Does exercise alter immune function and respiratory infections? *President's Council on Physical Fitness and Sports Research Digest* 3(13):1–8.

Nieman, D. C. 2000. Exercise soothes arthritis: Joint effects. *ACSM's Health and Fitness Journal* 4(3):20–28.

Rosenfeld, I. February 13, 2000. What women can do about PMS. *Parade Magazine* pp. 14–16.

Short, K. R., and M. J. Joyner. 2002. Activity, obesity, and type II diabetes *Exercise and Sport Sciences Reviews* 30(2):51–52.

Slattery, M. L., and J. D. Potter. 2002. Physical activity and colon cancer. *Medicine and Science in Sports and Exercise* 34(6):913–919.

Smith, J. K. 2001. Exercise and atherogenesis. *Exercise and Sports Sciences Reviews* 29(2): 49–53.

Taylor, A. J. et al. 2002. Physical activity and the presence and extent of calcified coronary atherosclerosis. *Medicine and Science in Sports and Exercise* 34(2):228–233.

Thompson. P. D. 2001. Exercise rehabilitation for cardiac patients. *Physician and Sports Medicine* 29(1):69–75.

U.S. Department of Health and Human Services. November 2000. *Healthy People 2010.* 2nd ed. With *Understanding and Improving Health* and *Objectives for Improving Health.* 2 vols. Washington, DC: U.S. Government Printing Office.

U.S. Department of Health and Human Services. 1996. *Physical Activity and Health: A Report of the Surgeon General.* Atlanta: U.S. Department of Health and Human Services.

Williams, P. T. 2001. Physical fitness and activity as separate heart disease risk factors: A meta analysis. *Medicine and Science in Sports and Exercise* 33(5):754–761.

In the News

Until recently, infectious disease and other diseases of the immune system were not considered to be hypokinetic in nature. Recent evidence indicates that regular moderate to vigorous activity can actually aid the immune system in fighting disease. Each of us is born with "an innate immune system" that includes anatomical and physiological barriers such as skin, mucous membranes, body temperature, and chemical mediators that help prevent and resist disease. We also develop an "acquired immune system" in the form of special disease fighting cells that help us resist disease. There is a J-shaped curve that illustrates the benefits of exercise to acquired immune function. Sedentary people have more risk than those who do moderate activity, but with very high and sustained vigorous activity such as extended high performance training, immune system function actually decreases.

Regular moderate and reasonable amounts of vigorous activity have been shown to reduce incidence of colds and days of sickness from infection. The immune system benefit may extend to other immune system disorders as well. However, as the figure here indicates, too much exercise may cause problems rather than solve them.

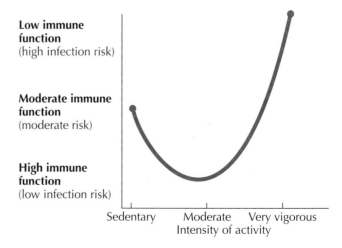

Lab 6A: Assessing Heart Disease Risk Factors

| Name | | | | Section | | Date | |

Purpose: To assess your risk of developing coronary heart disease.

Heart Disease Risk Factor Questionnaire

Risk Points

	1	2	3	4	Score
Unalterable Factors					
1. How old are you?	30 or less	31–40	41–54	55+	2
2. Do you have a history of heart disease in your family?	none	Grandparent with heart disease	Parent with heart disease	More than one with heart disease	2
3. What is your gender?	Female		Male		3
				Total Unalterable Risk Score	
Alterable Factors					
4. What is your percent of body fat?	F = 17–28% M = 10–20%	29–31% 21–23%	32–35% 24–30%	35+% 30+%	1
5. Do you have a high-fat diet?	No	Slightly high in fat	Above normal in fat	Eat a lot of meat, fried, and fatty foods	2
6. What is the systolic number in your blood pressure?	120	121–140	141–160	160+	3
7. Do you have other diseases?	No	Ulcer	*Diabetes	Both	1
8. Do you get regular physical activity?	4–5 days a week	3 days a week	Less than 3 days a week	No	1
9. Do you use tobacco?	No	Cigar or pipe	Less than 1/2 pack a day or use smokeless tobacco	More than 1/2 pack a day	4
10. Are you under much stress?	Less than normal	Normal	Slightly above normal	Quite high	3
				Total Alterable Risk Score	15
				Grand Total Risk Score	22

*Diabetes is a risk factor that is often not alterable.

Adapted from CAD Risk Assessor, William J. Stone. Reprinted by permission.

Procedures:

1. Complete the ten questions on the Heart Disease Risk Factor Questionnaire by circling the answer that is most appropriate for *you* (see front of this lab).
2. Look at the top of the column for each of your answers. In the box provided at the right of each question, write down the number of risk points for that answer.
3. Determine your unalterable risk score by adding the risk points for questions 1, 2, and 3.
4. Determine your alterable risk score by adding the risk points for questions 4 through 10.
5. Determine your total heart disease risk score by adding the scores obtained in steps 3 and 4.
6. Look up your risk ratings on the Heart Disease Risk Rating Scale and record them in the Results section. Answer the questions in the Conclusions and Implications section.

Results: Write your risk scores and risk ratings in the appropriate boxes below.

	Score	Rating
Unalterable risk		
Alterable risk		
Total heart disease risk		

Heart Disease Risk Rating Scale:

Rating Chart			
Rating	**Unalterable Score**	**Alterable Score**	**Total Score**
Very high	9 or more	21 or more	31 or more
High	7–8	15–20	26–30
Average	5–6	11–14	16–25
Low	4 or less	10 or less	15 or less

Conclusions and Implications: The higher your score on the Heart Disease Risk Factor Questionnaire, the greater your heart disease risk. In several sentences, discuss your risk for heart disease. Which of the risk factors do you need to control to reduce your risk of heart disease? Why?

Lifestyle Physical Activity

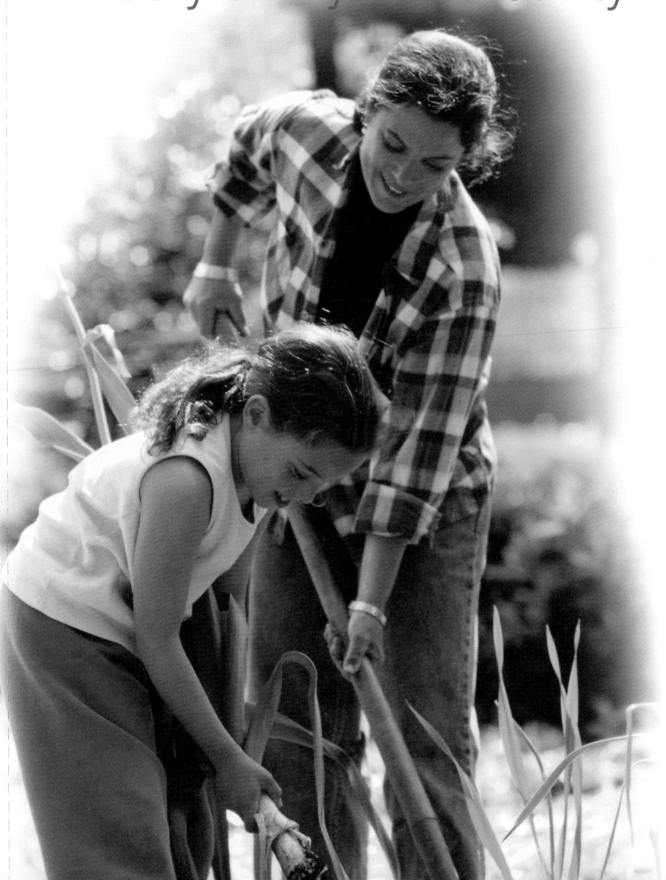

Moderate intensity physical activity done as a regular part of daily living has many health and wellness benefits.

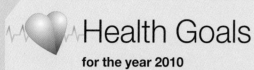

Health Goals

for the year 2010

- Increase the adoption and maintenance of daily physical activity.
- Increase leisure time physical activity.
- Increase proportion of people who do daily activity for 30 minutes.
- Increase travel by walking and by bicycle.

The heatlh benefits of lifestyle activities are now well documented. Governmental agencies and professional organizations in the United States, Canada, and other industrialized countries have developed guidelines describing these activities, detailing their benefits, and outlining the frequency, intensity, and time of activity necessary to achieve benefits. In this concept, lifestyle physical activity will be explained in detail.

Adopting an Active Lifestyle

Lifestyle activities include activities of daily living as well as some less intense sports and recreational activities. During rest, the body is able to meet all of its energy needs. This is done by the aerobic system that allows the body to produce energy by breaking down a food in the presence of oxygen. Thus, sedentary activities like sitting, playing a musical instrument, or even watching television can technically be considered "aerobic" in nature. To improve our health and fitness, activities must challenge the body to work above this resting level on a regular basis. One of the best ways to do this is to perform physical activity as part of your daily routine. Moderate intensity lifestyle physical activities that involve the larger muscle groups of the body are **aerobic physical activities** that are often referred to as lifestyle activities. Lifestyle activities include daily living activities such as walking to work or to the store, housework, gardening or yard work, and climbing the stairs.

Some light- to moderate-intensity sports can be classified as lifestyle physical activities. Golf, shuffleboard, bocci ball, table tennis, and bowling are examples. Recreational activities of light and moderate intensity can also be classified as lifestyle physical activities. Examples are fishing, canoeing, horseback riding, and gardening.

For children, play is considered to be a lifestyle physical activity because play is a normal activity for this age group. For retired adults, light- to moderate-intensity sports and recreational activities are lifestyle activities because they are a part of normal daily living.

Light- to moderate-intensity sports and recreational activities are very popular among adults, especially older adults. A recent Gallup poll indicated that fishing was the second most popular lifetime activity, bowling the fourth, and camping fifth. Though golf is not one of the top ten participation activities, it is a popular activity among older adults. More people over sixty-five play golf than those in the eighteen to thirty group, perhaps because older people have more time for activities that take several hours and because its intensity is more appropriate for older adults.

Lifestyle physical activities should expend more energy than normally expended at rest. www.mhhe.com/fit_well/web07 **Click 01.** Scientists have devised a method to classify levels of activity by intensity. With this system, all activities are compared against the amount of activity needed at rest. The amount of energy expended at rest (oxygen used) is referred to as one metabolic equivalent (1 **MET**). Activities listed as two METs require twice the energy of rest, and activities listed as four METs require four times the energy required for rest. Table 1 defines different intensity levels so that the reader can distinguish among the various terms used later in this book. For a person with good cardiovascular fitness, moderate-intensity activities typically require 4.7–7.0 METs. Fit people can perform moderate activity aerobically. This means that the aerobic system can meet the energy demands for this activity, and the activity can be performed for relatively long periods of time without stopping.

www.mhhe.com/fit_well/web07 **Click 02. Anaerobic physical activities** are so vigorous that your body cannot supply adequate oxygen to meet the energy demand using the aerobic system. The body must rely on short-term energy provided by the anaerobic metabolic system. Activities classified in Table 1 as hard, very hard, or maximum may be anaerobic, or at least partially anaerobic, and are not considered lifestyle physical activities.

Table 1 ▶ Classification of Physical Activity Intensities for a Person with Good Cardiovascular Fitness

Classification	Description	Examples
Very light	Activity that is about 2 to 2 1/2 times as intense as lying or sitting at rest	Washing your face, dressing yourself, typing, driving a car (2 to 2.5 METs)
Light	Activity that is 2 1/2 to 4 2/3 times as intense as rest (2.5 to 4.7 METs)	Normal walking, walking downstairs, bowling, mopping
Moderate	Activity about 4 2/3 to 7 times as intense as rest (4.7 to 7 METs)	Brisk walking, lawn mowing, shoveling, social dancing
Hard	Activities more than 7 and up to 10 times as intense as rest (7 to 10 METs)	Digging, level jogging (5 mph, 12 min. mile), cycling (13 mph), skiing, fencing
Very hard	Activities more than 10 and up to 12 times as intense as rest (10 to 12 METs)	Running (8.5 mph, 7 min. mile), handball, full-court competitive basketball
Maximum	Activities more than 12 times as intense as rest (12+ METs)	Running (10 mph, 6 min. mile)

selecting appropriate lifestyle physical activities. For example, activities considered very light to light for young fit people are equal to moderate activity for many people eighty and over. For many people over sixty-five, activities typically classified as light are equal to moderate activities.

Because lifestyle activities are relatively easy to perform, they are popular among adults. www.mhhe.com/fit_well/web07 Click 04. Walking is the most popular of all leisure time activities among adults eighteen years of age and over. Approximately 39 percent of all men and 48 percent of all women walked for exercise in the past two weeks. Also, among the ten most popular activities among adults is gardening (including yard work), which is done by 34 percent of all male and 25 percent of all female adults. Approximately 10 percent of men and 12 percent of women report that they regularly use the stairs to increase their activity levels.

Interestingly, the number of people participating in lifestyle physical activities increases with age. For example, only 33 percent of men eighteen to twenty-nine walk regularly, but 50 percent of men over sixty-five walk for exercise. Among young women, 47 percent walk, while 50 percent over sixty-five are walkers. Nearly twice as many

Activity classifications vary depending on one's level of fitness. www.mhhe.com/fit_well/web07 Click 03. Normal walking is considered as light activity for a person with good fitness (see Table 1), but for a person with low to marginal fitness the same activity is considered moderate. For a very low fit person, brisk walking is considered to be hard. Table 2 helps you determine the type of lifestyle activity that would be considered moderate for you. Beginners with low fitness should start with normal rather than brisk walking for example. Older people often have lower fitness levels than younger people and may find Table 2 useful in

Aerobic Physical Activity or Exercise Aerobic means "in the presence of oxygen." Aerobic activity is activity or exercise for which the body is able to supply adequate oxygen to sustain performance for long periods of time.

MET One MET equals the amount of energy a person expends at rest. METs are multiples of resting activity (two METS equals twice the resting energy expenditure).

Anaerobic Physical Activity or Exercise Anaerobic means "in the absence of oxygen." Anaerobic exercise is performed at an intensity so great that the body's demand for oxygen exceeds its ability to supply it.

Table 2 ▶ Classification of Lifestyle Physical Activities for People of Different Fitness Levels

Sample Lifestyle Activities	Activity Classification by Fitness Level			
	Low Fitness	Marginal Fitness	Good Fitness	High Performance
Washing your face, dressing, typing, driving a car	Light	Very Light/Light	Very Light	Very Light
Normal walking, walking downstairs, bowling, mopping	Moderate	Moderate	Light	Light
Brisk walking, lawn mowing, shoveling, social dancing	Hard	Moderate/Hard	Moderate	Light/Moderate

older men than young men do gardening, and the difference among women is almost as dramatic. As lifetime physical activity participation increases with age, involvement in sports dramatically decreases.

 Lifestyle physical activities can easily be performed by most people regardless of fitness level. www.mhhe.com/fit_well/web07 Click 05. Prior to the last two decades, the conventional wisdom concerning physical activity was that it had to be vigorous to provide health and fitness benefits. Long-term studies of large populations were conducted with a variety of groups showing that moderate activity produced many benefits. For example, postal carriers who delivered mail showed benefits not present in the postal workers who sorted the mail, and bus drivers in England did not get the benefits found for conductors who climbed the stairs in double-deck buses many times during the day. More recently, a study in Finland showed that people who do gardening are much less likely to have health problems than sedentary people, and people who hunt and hike in the forest have even more dramatic reductions in health conditions. A recent study found that people who commuted to work by bicycle had fewer health problems and fewer early deaths than those who drove. These are only a few of the studies that show the benefits of lifestyle physical activity.

Because lifestyle activities are moderate, most people can easily perform them. This is one reason lifestyle physical activities are placed at the bottom of the pyramid (see Figure 1). They are basic and provide a foundation for other activities.

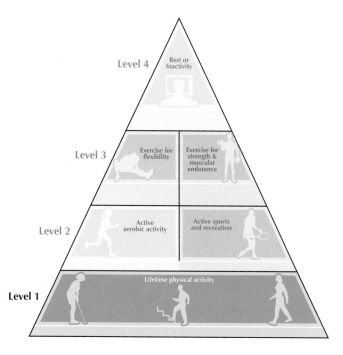

Figure 1 ▶ The physical activity pyramid: Level 1.

Technology Update

www.mhhe.com/fit_well/web07 Click 06. Digital pedometers are a technological innovation that allows a person to self-monitor physical activity by counting steps taken during the day. Mechanical pedometers have been around for centuries but were less accurate. Digital pedometers that are battery powered are much more accurate. Some pedometers offer features other than step counting including time in activity, calories expended in activity, and distance covered. These pedometers are more expensive and calorie and distance counts have been shown to be less accurate. Most experts suggest that simple step counts are most useful in monitoring activity. Time in activity can be useful in helping you monitor total minutes of activity in a day.

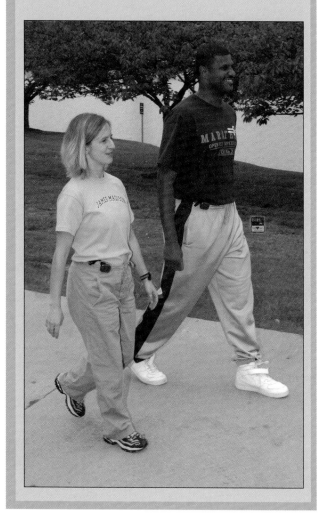

Moderate activity is more attractive than vigorous activity to many people. As the intensity of physical activity increases, it becomes less enjoyable to many people. Studies show that vigorous physical activity is a deterrent for more than a few people. This is another reason why lifestyle physical activities are placed at the base of the physical activity pyramid. Not only does this type of activity provide many health benefits, its intensity level makes it especially attractive to the people who most need to be active.

About 40 percent of all adult Americans do no leisure-time physical activity at all. They are totally sedentary. Statistics indicate that hundreds of thousands of premature deaths could be prevented if sedentary people would become active. Moderate physical activity is an alternative to vigorous activity that may be especially attractive to sedentary and/or less-fit adults.

The Health Benefits of Lifestyle Physical Activity

Many health benefits can be achieved as a result of participation in lifestyle physical activities. Figure 2 illustrates that disease risk and early death decrease with moderate lifestyle physical activity. This figure, based on several large studies done worldwide, shows that a great proportion of the **health benefits** of physical activity described in this book result from participation in moderate lifestyle physical activities. Though additional benefits occur with more vigorous activity, they do not produce the proportional gain resulting from moderate activity.

The benefits of moderate or lifestyle physical activities are illustrated by the long arrow in Figure 2. The shorter arrow shows the additional benefits that result from more vigorous activity. The principle of diminishing returns applies. Even modest increases in physical activity are better than doing no activity at all. Clearly, the adage that "something is better than nothing" applies to physical activity.

Lifestyle activity builds some components of fitness more than others. Metabolic fitness has been previously defined as fitness of the systems that provide the energy for effective daily living. Indicators of good metabolic fitness include normal blood lipid levels, normal blood pressure, normal blood sugar levels, and healthy body fat levels. Though lifestyle physical activity does not promote high-level cardiovascular fitness, commonly referred to as a **performance benefit,** it effectively promotes metabolic fitness associated with health and wellness benefits. This type of activity can produce enough cardiovascular fitness to help unfit people escape from the low-fit category.

Lifestyle physical activity has wellness benefits. Reduction in disease risk and early death are important. But equally important is quality of life. Many of the wellness benefits previously described result from moderate lifestyle physical activity. For example, people who do moderate exercise have been shown to take less time to go to sleep and sleep nearly an hour longer. A recent study shows that functional limitations are much lower in moderately active people than those who are sedentary. Lifestyle activity and its accompanying metabolic fitness benefits are also associated with enhanced self-esteem and less incidence of depression and anxiety.

How Much Lifestyle Physical Activity Is Enough?

The Surgeon General and the American College of Sports Medicine have outlined a basic recommendation for lifestyle physical activity. The recommendation for lifestyle physical activity is that adults accumulate 30 minutes or more of moderate-intensity physical activity on most, preferably all, days of the week. Brisk walking is an example of activity that typifies moderate activity. Table 3 provides some other examples of activities that meet the activity recommendation.

Near-daily activity is recommended because each activity session actually has short-term benefits that do

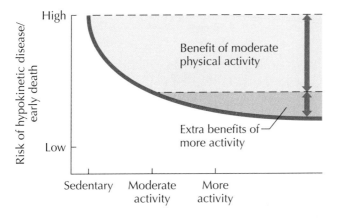

Figure 2 ▶ The benefits of moderate lifestyle physical activity.

Health Benefits Health benefits refer to reduction in hypokinetic disease risk, decreased risk of early death, and improved quality of life.

Performance Benefits Performance benefits refer to improved ability to score well on physical fitness tests or to perform well in athletic or work activities requiring high-level performance.

Table 3 ▶ Examples of Lifestyle Physical Activities

Activity	Time (min)	Less intense More time
Washing and waxing a car	45–60	
Washing windows or floors	45–60	
Gardening	30–45	
Wheeling self in wheelchair	30–40	
Social dancing	30	
Pushing a stroller (1 1/2 miles)	30	
Raking leaves	30	
Walking (2 miles)	30	More intense Less Time

Adapted from the *Surgeon General's Report on Physical Activity and Health.*

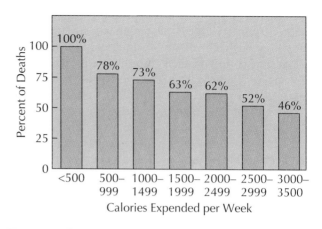

Figure 3 ▶ Deaths decrease as caloric expenditure increases.

not occur if activity is not relatively frequent. This is sometimes referred to as the **last bout effect**. Activity is beneficial only if you do the next bout before the effect of the last bout wears off.

🌐 **Many ways exist to determine if a person is doing enough to receive the health benefits of physical activity.** www.mhhe.com/fit_well/web07 Click 07. The threshold of training (minimum amount of activity) for producing many of the health benefits can be determined in several ways. Much of the early research was done based on calories expended per day or per week. As illustrated in Figure 3, people who expend as few as 500 to 1,000 calories per week can greatly reduce the risk of early death compared to those who do no regular physical activity. Expending 1,000 to 2,000 calories per week decreases risk even more and people who expend this number of calories meet the national health goal of performing 30 minutes of moderate activity per day (see Table 4).

The easiest method for beginners is to keep track of lifestyle activities performed with a goal of accumulating

at least 30 minutes each day of the week. More sophisticated methods for determining if activity is likely to produce health benefits include counting heart rate and using ratings of perceived exertion. You will learn more about these methods in the concept on cardiovascular fitness that follows. As you begin monitoring your lifestyle physical activity it is best to keep track of all of the activities that you perform, and try to accumulate at least 30 minutes in lifestyle activities per day (Lab 7A). Using METs (see Table 1) or calories expended per week (Table 5) are alternative methods that may be useful. Later you can use heart rate or RPE methods as you gain more experience.

There is a FIT formula for lifestyle physical activity. Table 4 summarizes the FIT formula for lifestyle physical activity. Threshold of training (minimum amounts to get a benefit) and target zones (optimal activity levels) are presented.

Last Bout Effect Some of the benefits of physical activity are short-term in nature. If the benefit of a bout of exercise lasts 24 hours, it is beneficial only if the last bout of activity was done before 24 hours elapsed.

Table 4 ▶ The FIT Formula for Lifestyle Physical Activity

	Threshold of Training	Target Zone
Frequency	Most days of the week	All, or most, days of the week
Intensity*	• Equal to brisk walking** • Approximately 150 calories accumulated per day • 3 to 5 METs**	• Equal to brisk to fast walking** • Approximately 150–300 calories accumulated per day • 3.0 to 7 METs**
Time (duration)	30 minutes or three 10-minute sessions per day	30–60 minutes accumulated in sessions of at least 10 minutes

*Heart rate and relative perceived exertion can also be used to determine intensity (see Concept 8).
**Depends on fitness level (see Table 2).

Table 5 ▶ Calories Expended in Lifestyle Physical Activities

Activity Classification / Description	METs*	Calories Used per Hour for Different Body Weights				
		100 lb. (45 kg)	120 lb. (55 kg)	150 lb. (70 kg)	180 lb. (82 kg)	200 lb. (91 kg)
Gardening Activities						
Gardening (general)	5.0	227	273	341	409	455
Mowing lawn (hand mower)	6.0	273	327	409	491	545
Mowing lawn (power mower)	4.5	205	245	307	368	409
Raking leaves	4.0	182	218	273	327	364
Shoveling snow	6.0	273	327	409	491	545
Home Activities						
Child care	3.5	159	191	239	286	318
Cleaning, washing dishes	2.5	114	136	170	205	227
Cooking / food preparation	2.5	114	136	170	205	227
Home / auto repair	3.0	136	164	205	245	273
Painting	4.5	205	245	307	368	409
Strolling with child	2.5	114	136	170	205	227
Sweeping / vacuuming	2.5	114	136	170	205	227
Washing / waxing car	4.5	205	245	307	368	409
Leisure Activities						
Bocci ball / croquet	2.5	114	136	170	205	227
Bowling	3.0	136	164	205	245	273
Canoeing	5.0	227	273	341	409	455
Cross-country skiing (leisure)	7.0	318	382	477	573	636
Cycling (<10 mph)	4.0	182	218	273	327	364
Cycling (12–14 mph)	8.0	364	436	545	655	727
Dancing (social)	4.5	205	245	307	368	409
Fishing	4.0	182	218	273	327	364
Golf (riding)	3.5	159	191	239	286	318
Golf (walking)	5.5	250	300	375	450	500
Horseback riding	4.0	182	218	273	327	364
Swimming (leisure)	6.0	273	327	409	491	545
Table tennis	4.0	182	218	273	327	364
Walking (4 mph)	4.0	182	218	273	327	364
Walking (3 mph)	3.5	159	191	239	286	318
Occupational Activities						
Bricklaying / masonry	7.0	318	382	477	573	636
Carpentry	3.5	159	191	239	286	318
Construction	5.5	250	300	375	450	500
Electrical work / plumbing	3.5	159	191	239	286	318
Digging	7.0	318	382	477	573	636
Farming	5.5	250	300	375	450	500
Store clerk	3.5	159	191	239	286	318
Waiter / waitress	4.0	182	218	273	327	364

Note: MET values and caloric estimates are based on values listed in the Compendium of Physical Activities (see Suggested Readings).
*Based on values of those with "good fitness" ratings.

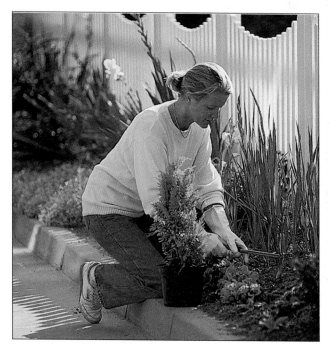
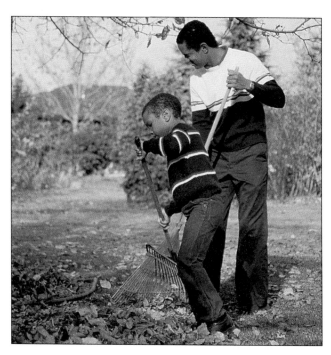

Moderate lifestyle physical activity can be accumulated in several activity sessions.

You can accumulate lifestyle physical activity to meet the recommendation. www.mhhe.com/fit_well/web07 Click 08. Previous recommendations suggested that physical activity had to be continuous to be effective. The evidence now indicates that all of the activity need not be done in one session to be effective. To achieve the health benefits you can "accumulate activity" throughout the day. While the bulk of the energy or calories expended should be in moderate activities, some light activity can also be beneficial. When some of the accumulated activity is in light activity, the duration of the activity must be increased (e.g., washing windows and floors as seen in Table 3). Some lifestyle physical activities, such as shoveling snow and climbing the stairs, are actually considered to be vigorous in nature. These activities can be counted in the accumulation of daily activities. Performing some of these activities can offset the performance of light activity and make it possible to expend adequate calories in a 30-minute period.

If the goal is to build cardiovascular fitness activity, sessions need to be at least moderate in nature, and activity sessions should probably be at least ten minutes in length. You will learn more about this in the concept on cardiovascular fitness.

A combination of several different activities can be used to accumulate lifestyle physical activity. www.mhhe.com/fit_well/web07 Click 09. A variety of different activities can be performed to expend the calories necessary to meet the guidelines for lifestyle physical activity. You may decide to walk to work, do some gardening after work, and do some social dancing in the evening to accumulate the activity for the day. Table 5 provides a general idea of the number of calories expended in a variety of lifestyle physical activities (including moderate-intensity sports and leisure activities). The table helps you account for your body weight when estimating calories expended in activity. This is

Table 6 ▶ Walking Time for Expending 1,000 Calories per Week

Days per Week	Pace	Minutes per Day		
		100 lb.* (45 kg)	150 lb.* (68 kg)	200 lb.* (90 kg)
5	2 mph (3.2 kph)	96	62	46
	3 mph (4.8 kph)	63	48	38
	4 mph (6.4 kph)	48	36	24
6	2 mph	80	52	40
	3 mph	62	40	32
	4 mph	40	26	20
7	2 mph	68	44	34
	3 mph	54	36	26
	4 mph	34	24	18

*Body weight

necessary because bigger people expend more calories than smaller people doing the same activity.

It is also important to account for the intensity of the activity you perform. For example, walking at different speeds results in less time needed to expend the same number of calories. Table 6 illustrates this point for walking. Just as there are a variety of speeds of walking, each of the activities in Table 5 can be performed at different intensi-

ties. This walking example shows you how important body weight and intensity level are to expending 1,000 calories in one week. It is impossible to include all activities and their different intensities. You can use the calories in Table 5 as a basis for making decisions about lifestyle physical activity. You may need to adjust them up or down based on the speed or intensity of the activities you perform.

Strategies for Action

A regular plan of lifestyle physical activity is a good place to start. Lifestyle physical activity is something that virtually anyone can do. In Lab 7A you can set lifestyle physical activity goals and plan a one-week lifestyle physical activity program. In the plan, you can indicate the lifestyle activities you plan to do on all, or most days, of the week. For some, this plan may be the main component of a lifetime plan. For others, it may be only a beginning that leads to the selection of activities from other levels of the physical activity pyramid. Even the most active people should consider regular lifestyle physical activity because it is a type of activity that can be done throughout life.

Self-monitoring lifestyle physical activity can help you stick with it. Self-monitoring is a self-management

skill that can be valuable in encouraging long-term activity adherence. A self-monitoring chart is provided in Lab 7A to help you keep a log of the lifestyle activities (or step counts) you perform during a one-week time period. This is a short-term record sheet. However, charts such as this can be copied to make a log book to allow long-term activity self-monitoring.

Because lifestyle physical activity is moderate in nature, a specific warm-up may not be necessary. Lifestyle activities are similar to the cardiovascular portion of the warm-up described in the concept on preparing for physical activity. For this reason, it may not be necessary to perform a special warm-up prior to doing activities such as walking. It would be wise to perform the stretching activities after the walk as a cool-down.

Web Resources

American College of Sports Medicine **www.acsm.org**
ACSM's Health and Fitness Journal
   www.acsm-healthfitness.org
Centers for Disease Control and Prevention **www.cdc.gov**
National Coalition for Promoting Physical Activity
   www.ncppa.org
Ordering Information for Pedometers **www.walk4life.com**
Surgeon General's Report on Physical Activity and Health
   www.cdc.gov/nccdphp/sgr/sgr.htm
Websites for Lifestyle Physical Activities
   www.mhhe.com/fit_well/web08 Click 10

Suggested Readings

 Additional reference materials for concept 7 are available at **www.mhhe.com/fit_well/web07 Click 11**.

Ainsworth, B. E. et al. 1993. Compendium of physical activities: Classification of energy costs of human activities. *Medicine and Science in Sports and Exercise* 25:71–80.

American College of Sports Medicine. 2000. *ACSM's Guidelines for Exercise Testing and Prescription.* 6th ed. Philadelphia: Lippincott, Williams and Wilkins.

Bassett, D. R., A. L. Cureton, and B. E. Ainsworth. 2000. Measurement of daily walking distance-questionnaire versus pedometer. *Medicine and Science in Sports and Exercise* 32(5):1018–1023.

Blair, S. N. et al. 2001. *Active Living Every Day.* Champaign, IL: Human Kinetics.

Franklin, B. A. 2001. Lifestye activity: A new paradigm for exercise prescription. *ACSM's Health and Fitness Journal* 5(4):33–35.

Katsanos, C. S. et al. 2001. Exercise expenditure relative to perceived exertion: Stationary cycling and treadmill walking. *Research Quarterly for Exercise and Sport.* 72(2):176–181.

Manson, W. C. et al. 1999. A prospective study of walking as compared with vigorous exercise in the prevention of coronary heart disease in women. *New England Journal of Medicine* 341(9):650–658.

Public Health Service. 1996. *Surgeon General's Report on Physical Activity and Health.* Washington, DC: U.S. Government Printing Office.

Quittner, J. 24 July 2000. "High-tech walking." *Time* 77.

Schniffing, L. 2001. Can exercise gadgets motivate patients? *The Physician and Sports Medicine* 29(1):15–18.

Sidman, C. L. 2002. Count your steps to health & fitness. *ACSM's Health and Fitness Journal* 6(1):13–17.

Steiger, L. H., and J. L. Hesson. 2001. *Walking for Fitness.* 4th ed. St. Louis, MO: McGraw-Hill.

Talbot, L. A., E. J. Metter, and J. L. Fleg. 2000. Leisure-time physical activities and their relationship to cardio-vascular fitness in healthy men and women 18–95 years. *Medicine and Science in Sports and Exercise* 32(2):417–425.

U.S. Department of Health and Human Services. Nov. 2000. *Healthy People 2010.* 2nd ed. With *Understanding and Improving Health* and *Objectives for Improving Health.* 2 vols. Washington, DC: U.S. Government Printing Office.

Welk, G. J. et al. 2000. The utility of the digi-walker step counter to assess daily physical activity patterns. *Medicine and Science in Sports and Exercise* 32(9):5481–5488.

Wilde, B. E., C. L. Sidman, and C. B. Corbin. 2001. A 10,000 step count as a physical activity standard for sedentary women. *Research Quarterly for Exercise and Sport* 72(1):411–414.

 In the News

Bowling and golf are sports considered to be lifestyle physical activities, not because people typically do them as part of their normal daily routine, but because they are of an intensity consistent with activities of this classification. For years, fitness experts discounted the value of these activities. Mark Twain referred to golf as a good way to ruin a long walk. Now we know that, like other lifestyle activities, golf and bowling can be beneficial to your health. One study shows that golf, for those who walk not ride, actually produces heart rates high enough to produce fitness. Both bowling and golf contribute to quality of life associated with social interactions with friends.

Lab 7A Planning and Self-Monitoring (Logging) Your Lifestyle Physical Activity

Name	Section	Date

Purpose: To self-monitor (log) physical activity and use it to plan a lifestyle physical activity program.

Directions: Record the number of 5- or 10-minute activity blocks or steps taken each day (see back for procedures).

Chart 1 ▶ Lifestyle Activity Log

	5-Minute Blocks										10-Minute Blocks						Total Minutes or Steps
Day 1 Date: Activity: Activity: Activity: Activity:	1	2	3	4	5	6	7	8	9	10	1	2	3	4	5	6	Daily Total:
Day 2 Date: Activity: Activity: Activity: Activity:	1	2	3	4	5	6	7	8	9	10	1	2	3	4	5	6	Daily Total:
Day 3 Date: Activity: Activity: Activity: Activity:	1	2	3	4	5	6	7	8	9	10	1	2	3	4	5	6	Daily Total
Day 4 Date: Activity: Activity: Activity: Activity:	1	2	3	4	5	6	7	8	9	10	1	2	3	4	5	6	Daily Total:
Day 5 Date: Activity: Activity: Activity: Activity:	1	2	3	4	5	6	7	8	9	10	1	2	3	4	5	6	Daily Total:
Day 6 Date: Activity: Activity: Activity: Activity:	1	2	3	4	5	6	7	8	9	10	1	2	3	4	5	6	Daily Total:
Day 7 Date: Activity: Activity: Activity: Activity:	1	2	3	4	5	6	7	8	9	10	1	2	3	4	5	6	Daily Total:

Total Steps or Minutes for Week

Procedures:

1. On Chart 1, record the time spent or steps taken per day in the various lifestyle activities.
2. If you record time spent in lifestyle activity list all activities you perform each day. For each activity record the number of minutes you were active using combinations of 5- or 10-minute blocks. For example, if you perform 15 minutes of brisk walking, you would place an X over one 5- and one 10-minute block for that activity. If you cannot keep the log with you during the day, complete it at the end of the day. Total the minutes of activity accumulated during the day and record it in the daily total box.
3. If you wear a pedometer to count daily activity, simply wear the pedometer from the time you get up until the time you go to bed. Record the number of steps taken in the daily total box.
4. Sum the total for each day to determine the total minutes or steps taken for the week.
5. Use the weekly log to help you develop a weekly plan. In Chart 2 record the number of minutes you plan to perform each activity in the coming week, or record the number of steps you plan to take. If you use minutes in your plan, try to reach 30 per day. If you use step counts in your plan, try to achieve 2,000–3,000 steps above your average daily count (if you averaged less than 10,000 steps a day in Chart 1), or at least 10,000 steps per day (if you averaged near or above 10,000 steps in Chart 1). Try to get your steps in blocks of time lasting at least 5 minutes in length.
6. Make a copy of Chart 1 and use it to self-monitor your activity for the week that you institute your plan.
7. Answer the questions in the Results and Conclusions/Interpretations sections.

Chart 2 ▶ Lifestyle Physical Activity Plan

Record the minutes or steps planned for each day. You may mix activities each day.

Activity	Day 1	Day 2	Day 3	Day 4	Day 5	Day 6	Day 7
Brisk walking							
Yard work							
Active house work							
Gardening							
Social dancing							
Occupational activity							
Wheeling self in wheelchair							
Bicycling							
Walking							
Walking up and down stairs							
Other							
Daily Totals							

Results:

Do you think you can consistently do 30 minutes of activity or meet your step goal each day?   Yes   No

Conclusions and Interpretations:

1. Do you feel that you will use lifestyle physical activity as a regular part of your lifetime physical activity plan, either now or in the future? Use several sentences to explain your answer.
2. Did the logging of your activity make you more aware of your daily activity patterns? Explain why or why not.

Cardiovascular Fitness

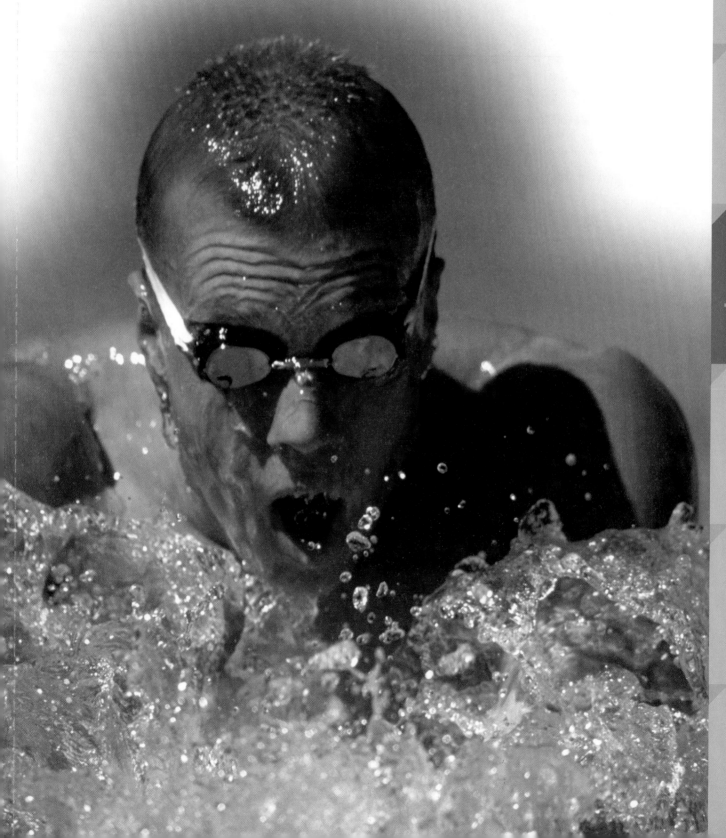

Cardiovascular fitness is probably the most important aspect of physical fitness because of its importance to good health and optimal physical performance.

Health Goals

for the year 2010

- Increase proportion of people who do vigorous physical activity that promotes cardiovascular fitness three or more days a week for 20 minutes per occasion.
- Decrease deaths from heart attack and stroke.
- Decrease incidence of heart attack, high blood pressure, stroke, and high blood lipids.
- Decrease heart disease among females.
- Increase public awareness of symptoms of heart diseases.

Cardiovascular fitness is frequently considered the most important aspect of physical fitness because those who possess it have a decreased risk of heart disease—the number-one killer in our society. This is supported by statements of the American Heart Association, the Surgeon General's office, and the American College of Sports Medicine. Sedentary living is a primary risk factor for heart disease. Physical activity that leads to improved cardiovascular fitness has dramatic health and wellness benefits that extend well beyond heart disease risk reduction. Cardiovascular fitness is important to the effective performance of virtually all types of work and play activities.

Cardiovascular Fitness

Cardiovascular fitness is a term that has several synonyms. Cardiovascular fitness is sometimes referred to as "cardiovascular endurance" because a person who possesses this type of fitness can persist in physical activity for long periods of time without undue fatigue. It has been referred to as "cardiorespiratory fitness" because it requires delivery and utilization of oxygen, which is only possible if the circulatory and respiratory systems are capable of these functions.

The term "aerobic fitness" has also been used as a synonym for cardiovascular fitness because **aerobic capacity** is considered to be the best indicator of cardiovascular fitness, and aerobic physical activity is the preferred method for achieving it. Regardless of the words used to describe it, cardiovascular fitness is complex because it requires fitness of several body systems.

Good cardiovascular fitness requires a fit heart muscle. www.mhhe.com/fit_well/web08 Click 01. The heart is a muscle; to become stronger, it must be exercised like any other muscle in the body. If the heart is exercised regularly, its strength increases; if not, it becomes weaker. Contrary to the belief that strenuous work harms the heart, research has found no evidence that regular, progressive exercise is bad for the normal heart. In fact, the heart muscle will increase in size and power when called upon to extend itself. The increase in size and power allows the heart to pump a greater volume of blood with fewer strokes per minute. For example, the average individual has a resting heart rate between 70 and 80 beats per minute (bpm), whereas a trained athlete's pulse is commonly in the low 50s or even in the 40s.

The healthy heart is efficient in the work that it does. It can convert about half of its fuel into energy. An automobile engine in good running condition converts only one-fourth of its fuel into energy. By comparison, the heart is a more efficient engine. The heart of a normal individual beats reflexively about 40 million times a year. During this time, over 4,000 gallons, or 10 tons, of blood are circulated each day, and every night the heart's workload is equivalent to a person carrying a 30-pound pack to the top of the 102-story Empire State building.

Good cardiovascular fitness requires a fit vascular system. As illustrated in Figure 1, blood containing a high concentration of oxygen is pumped by the left ventricle through the aorta (a major artery), where it is carried to the tissues. Blood flows through a sequence of arteries to capillaries and to veins. Veins carry the blood containing lesser amounts of oxygen back to the right side of the heart, first to the atrium and then to the ventricle. The right ventricle pumps the blood to the lungs. In the lungs, the blood picks up oxygen (O_2), and carbon dioxide (CO_2) is removed. From the lungs, the oxygenated blood travels back to the heart, first to the left atrium and then to the left ventricle. The process then repeats itself.

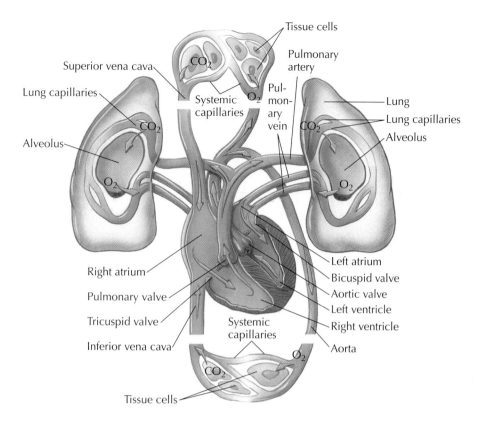

Figure 1 ▶ The cardiovascular system.

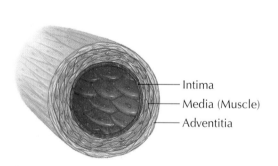

Figure 2 ▶ Healthy, elastic artery.

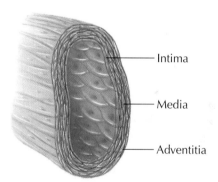

Figure 4 ▶ Healthy, nonelastic vein.

Healthy arteries are elastic, free of obstruction, and expand to permit the flow of blood (see Figure 2). Muscle layers line the arteries and control the size of the arterial opening upon the impulse from nerve fibers. Unfit arteries (see Figure 3) may have a reduced internal diameter (atherosclerosis) because of deposits on the interior of their walls, or they may have hardened, nonelastic walls (arteriosclerosis).

Aerobic Capacity A measure of aerobic or cardiovascular fitness; another term used for maximum oxygen uptake ($\dot{V}O_2$ max).

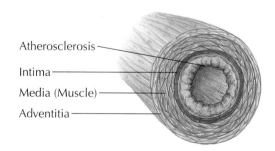

Figure 3 ▶ Unhealthy artery.

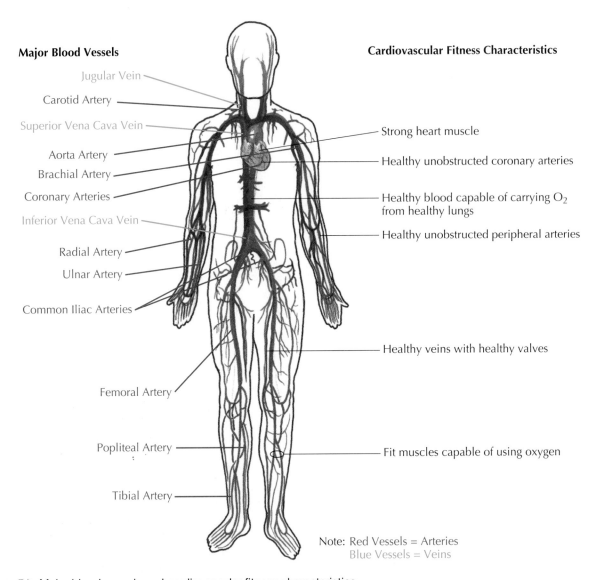

Major Blood Vessels   **Cardiovascular Fitness Characteristics**

Jugular Vein

Carotid Artery

Superior Vena Cava Vein

Aorta Artery

Brachial Artery

Coronary Arteries

Inferior Vena Cava Vein

Radial Artery

Ulnar Artery

Common Iliac Arteries

Femoral Artery

Popliteal Artery

Tibial Artery

Strong heart muscle

Healthy unobstructed coronary arteries

Healthy blood capable of carrying O_2 from healthy lungs

Healthy unobstructed peripheral arteries

Healthy veins with healthy valves

Fit muscles capable of using oxygen

Note: Red Vessels = Arteries
      Blue Vessels = Veins

Figure 5 ▶ Major blood vessels and cardiovascular fitness characteristics.

Fit coronary arteries are especially important to good health. The blood in the four chambers of the heart does not directly nourish the heart. Rather, numerous small arteries within the heart muscle provide for coronary circulation. Poor coronary circulation precipitated by unhealthy arteries can be the cause of a heart attack.

Veins have thinner, less elastic walls than arteries, as shown in Figure 4. Also, veins contain small valves to prevent the backward flow of blood. Skeletal muscles assist the return of blood to the heart. The veins are intertwined in the muscle; therefore, when the muscle is contracted, the vein is squeezed, pushing the blood back to the heart. A malfunction of the valves results in a failure to remove used blood at the proper rate. As a result, venous blood pools, especially in the legs, causing a condition known as varicose veins. Regular physical activity helps reduce pooling of blood in the veins and helps keep the valves of the veins healthy.

Capillaries are the transfer stations where oxygen and fuel are released, and waste products, such as carbon dioxide, are removed from the tissues. The veins receive the blood from the capillaries for the return trip to the heart.

Good cardiovascular fitness requires a fit respiratory system and fit blood. The process of taking in oxygen (through the mouth and nose) and delivering it to the lungs, where it is picked up by the blood, is called external respiration (see Figure 5). External respiration requires fit lungs as well as blood with adequate **hemoglobin** in the red blood cells (erythrocytes). Insufficient oxygen-carrying capacity of the blood is called **anemia,** a condition caused by lack of hemoglobin.

Delivering oxygen to the tissues from the blood is called internal respiration. Internal respiration requires an adequate number of healthy capillaries. In addition to delivering oxygen to the tissues, these systems remove carbon dioxide. Good cardiovascular fitness requires fitness of both the external and internal respiratory systems.

Cardiovascular fitness requires fit muscle tissue capable of using oxygen. Once the oxygen is delivered, the muscle tissues must be able to use oxygen to sustain physical performance. Physical activity that promotes cardiovascular fitness stimulates changes in muscle fibers that make them more effective in using oxygen. Outstanding distance runners have high numbers of well-conditioned muscle fibers that can readily use oxygen to produce energy for sustained running. Training in other activities would elicit similar adaptations in the specific muscles used in those activities.

Cardiovascular Fitness and Health Benefits

Good cardiovascular fitness reduces risk of heart disease, other hypokinetic conditions, and early death. The best evidence indicates that cardiovascular fitness is associated with reduced risk for heart disease. A classic research study at The Cooper Institute for Aerobics Research showed that low-fit people are especially at risk. In addition, it has now been demonstrated that improving your fitness (moving from low fitness to the good fitness zone) can reduce risk of early death and produce the other health benefits described earlier in this text. Among those who are not low in fitness, further fitness increases bring additional health benefits. However, it is generally acknowledged that the principle of diminished returns applies. Figure 6 illustrates that additional fitness yields additional benefits but not equal to

Table 1 ▶ Relative Risk of Major Risk Factors on Heart Disease and Early Death[*]

Risk Factor	Relative Risk of Heart Disease	Relative Risk of Early Death (All Causes)
Low Cardiovascular Fitness	2.69	2.03
Smoking	2.01	1.89
High Systolic Blood Pressure	2.07	1.67
High Cholesterol	1.86	1.45
Obesity (BMI)	1.70	1.33

[*]Statistically adjusted to assure independence of risk factors.
Based on Blair, S. N. et al. (see Suggested Readings).

the benefits received from getting out of the low fitness zone.

Low cardiovascular fitness is associated with greater disease risk, and is independent of other risk factors. Good cardiovascular fitness has been shown to be independent of other risk factors in reducing heart disease risk and of reduction in early death from all causes. Table 1 shows the relative risk of cardiovascular disease in the first column and the relative risk of early death from all causes in the second column. People with virtually no risk factors have a relative risk of 1.0. A person with a relative risk of 2.0 would have two times the risk of a risk-free person. The highest relative risk for heart disease is among people low in cardiovascular fitness (2.69). Those with low cardiovascular fitness also have the highest relative risk of early death (2.03). All of the values in the table were adjusted statistically to exclude the influence of other risk factors. This illustrates that the benefits of good cardiovascular fitness are independent of other primary risk factors for heart disease and early death from all causes.

Good cardiovascular fitness can reduce risk for most people, including those who are overweight. www.mhhe.com/fit_well/web08 Click 02. Some people think that they cannot be fit if they are overweight or overfat. It is now known that appropriate

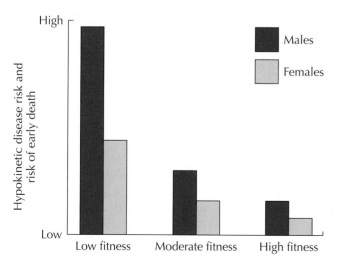

Figure 6 ▶ Risk reduction associated with cardiovascular fitness.

Adapted from Blair et al.

Hemoglobin Oxygen-carrying pigment of the red blood cells.

Anemia A condition in which hemoglobin and the blood's oxygen carrying capacity is below normal.

physical activity can build cardiovascular fitness in all types of people, including those with excess body fat. In fact, having good cardiovascular fitness greatly reduces risk for those who are overweight. Poor cardiovascular fitness on the other hand, increases risk for both lean and overfat people. The greatest risk is among people who are unfit and overfat.

Good cardiovascular fitness enhances the ability to perform various tasks, improves the ability to function, and is associated with a feeling of well-being. Moving out of the low fitness zone is of obvious importance to disease risk reduction. Achieving the good zone on tests further reduces disease and early death risk and promotes optimal wellness benefits and a recent position statement by the American College of Sports Medicine also shows an improved ability to function among older adults. Other wellness benefits include the ability to enjoy leisure activities and meet emergency situations, as well as the health and wellness benefits described earlier in this book. Cardiovascular fitness in the high-performance zone enhances the ability to perform in certain athletic events and in occupations that require high performance level (e.g., firefighters). These benefits are commonly referred to as **performance benefits.**

Heredity influences your cardiovascular fitness. It would be nice if all people who did appropriate physical activity achieved high levels of cardiovascular fitness. Genetic researchers have shown that the type of cardiovascular system you inherit has a good deal to do with your cardiovascular fitness. Further, we do not all respond similarly to physical activity because of our heredity. Figure 7 shows that after fifteen to twenty weeks of training, different people who performed the same amount of physical activity varied greatly in their cardiovascular fitness improvement. This research led the researchers to draw the following conclusion: "Not only is it important to recognize that there are individual differences in the response to regular physical activity, but research indicates that there are non-responders in the population. Heredity may account for fitness differences as large as 3 to 10 fold when comparing low and high responders who have performed the same physical activity program" (Bouchard, see Suggested Readings).

As illustrated in Figure 7, one person showed virtually no gain, while one showed dramatic improvements in cardiovascular fitness even though the activity levels were the same. Those with low fitness in the beginning made more improvements than those who were already fit, but the researchers indicated that heredity was more of a factor than beginning fitness level.

You should not conclude from this information that achieving good cardiovascular fitness is impossible for

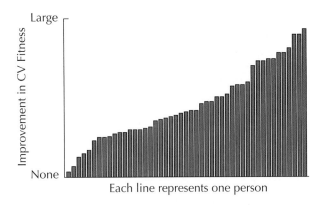

Figure 7 ▶ Difference in cardiovascular fitness improvement in forty-seven different people doing the same activity program for fifteen to twenty weeks.

Adapted from Bouchard.

some people. Rather, you should understand that it is harder for some people to get fit than others. No matter who you are, you can improve your cardiovascular fitness, but it takes longer for some than others. This study also points out the futility of comparing your own performance to others. Comparing yourself to fitness standards associated with good health is more reasonable. The research cited suggests that achieving high-performance levels of cardiovascular fitness will be difficult for some people.

Threshold and Target Zones for Improving Cardiovascular Fitness

Aerobic physical activity that is more vigorous than lifestyle physical activities is necessary to produce optimal gains in cardiovascular fitness. Lifestyle physical activity at the base of the pyramid promotes many health benefits and has positive effects on metabolic fitness. Activities at the second level of the physical activity pyramid, including active aerobics and active sports and recreation, are recommended for promoting good cardiovascular fitness (Figure 8). The word *active* implies that these activities must be relatively vigorous in nature.

Cardiovascular fitness can be developed in three to six days per week. Unlike less-intense lifestyle physical activities, the types of activities that promote cardiovascular fitness may be done as few as three days a week. Additional benefits occur with added days of activity. However, because more vigorous physical activity has been shown to increase risk of orthopedic injury if done too frequently, most experts recommend at least one day a week off.

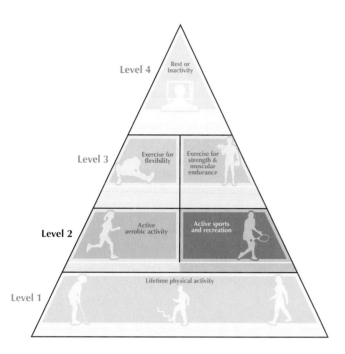

Level 4 — Rest or Inactivity

Level 3 — Exercise for flexibility | Exercise for strength & muscular endurance

Level 2 — Active aerobic activity | Active sports and recreation

Level 1 — Lifetime physical activity

Figure 8 ▶ Select activities from level 2 of the pyramid for optimal cardiovascular fitness.

There are several methods for assessing the intensity of physical activity for building cardiovascular fitness. www.mhhe.com/fit_well/web08 Click 03. The best measure of cardiovascular fitness is **maximum oxygen uptake** ($\dot{V}O_2$ max). This test is usually done on a treadmill. Oxygen use is monitored minute by minute as exercise becomes harder and harder. When the exercise becomes very hard, oxygen use reaches its maximum. The highest amount of oxygen used in one minute of maximum intensity physical activity is your maximum oxygen uptake. Your **resting oxygen uptake** subtracted from your maximum oxygen uptake is your **oxygen uptake reserve** (VO_2R). Calculating a percentage of your VO_2R is the most accurate way to determine if your exercise is intense enough to promote improvements in cardiovascular fitness.

Unfortunately, VO_2R is hard to assess in normal daily activities. For this reason, two different heart rate measures have been developed to help you estimate your VO_2R. The first method is called percentage of **heart rate reserve (HRR),** which is the preferred method because it correlates well with VO_2R. A second method is called percentage of maximal heart rate (max HR). Both of these methods will be described in detail later (see Tables 5 and 6).

Ratings of perceived exertion (RPE) have also been shown to be useful in assessing the intensity of aerobic physical activity. This method will also be described in more detail in a later section (see Table 7).

As noted in a previous concept, calorie counting is useful for assessing the intensity of moderate lifestyle physical activities. The American College of Sports Medicine (ACSM) has cautioned against using this technique for determining intensity of aerobic activity for promoting cardiovascular fitness development; instead, it recommends heart rate monitoring and measures of relative perceived exertion.

The duration of physical activity for building cardiovascular fitness is 20 to 60 minutes. In the past, it was thought that the 20 to 60 minutes of active aerobic activity necessary to promote cardiovascular fitness should be done continuously in one session. Recent ACSM guidelines indicate that activity can be either intermittent or continuous if the total amount of exercise is the same and if the shorter sessions last at least 10 minutes. In other words, three 10-minute exercise sessions appear to give you the same benefit as one 30-minute session if the exercise is at the same intensity level.

There is a FIT formula for building cardiovascular fitness. Table 2 illustrates the threshold of training and target zones for performing physical activity designed to promote cardiovascular fitness and cardiovascular health.

Performance Benefit In this concept, performance benefit refers to an improved score on a cardiovascular fitness test or in performance of activities requiring cardiovascular fitness.

Maximum Oxygen Uptake ($\dot{V}O_2$ max) A laboratory measure held to be the best measure of cardiovascular fitness. Commonly referred to as $\dot{V}O_2$ max or the volume ($\dot{V}$) of oxygen used when a person reaches his or her maximum (max) ability to supply it during exercise.

Resting Oxygen Uptake This is the amount (volume) of oxygen used at rest; also called resting metabolism. One MET is another unit of measure representing resting oxygen uptake.

Oxygen Uptake Reserve (VO_2R) This is the difference between your maximum oxygen uptake and your resting oxygen uptake. A percentage of this value is often used to determine appropriate intensities for physical activities.

Heart Rate Reserve (HRR) The difference between your maximum heart rate (highest heart rate in vigorous activity) and your resting heart rate (lowest heart rate at rest).

Ratings of Perceived Exertion (RPE) The assessment of the intensity of exercise based on how the participant feels; a subjective assessment of effort.

Table 2 ▶ Threshold of Training and Target Zones for Activities Designed to Promote Cardiovascular Fitness*

	Threshold of Training	Target Zone
Frequency	3 days a week	At least 3 days and no more than 6 days a week
Intensity		
Heart rate reserve (HRR)	40%*	40–85%
Maximal heart rate (max HR)	55%*	55–90%
Relative perceived exertion (RPE)	12*	12–16
Time	20 minutes	20 to 60 minutes

*These values are for beginners—the threshold for fit individuals reaches higher into the target zone.

Your current fitness status and activity patterns should influence the type and amount of activity you do to promote cardiovascular fitness. Making proper decisions about how much physical activity you should do is an art that is based on science. It is important that you listen to your body and not do too much too soon. Part of the art of making good decisions about activity is using the principle of progression. The amount of activity performed by a beginner differs from that performed by a person who is more advanced.

Beginners with low fitness may choose to start with lifestyle physical activity of relatively moderate intensity. Performing this type of activity at about 40 percent of HRR or 12 RPE for several weeks will allow the beginner to adapt gradually. Initial bouts of activity may be less than the recommended 20 minutes, but as fitness increases, at least 20 minutes a day should be accumulated. As fitness improves from the low to marginal range, the frequency, intensity, and time of activity can be increased (see Table 3). Cardiovascular fitness improvements for fit and active people are best when activity is at least 50 percent HRR, 65 percent max HR, and 13 RPE. Your current fitness and activity status will affect how quickly you progress. The type of activity you choose should be appropriate for the intensity of activity at each stage of the progression.

Learning to count heart rate at rest and after activity can help you monitor the intensity of your activity to determine if it is adequate to promote cardiovascular fitness. To determine the intensity of physical activity for building cardiovascular fitness, it is important to know how to count your pulse. Each time the heart beats, it pumps blood into the arteries. The surge of blood causes a pulse that can be felt by holding a finger against an artery. Major arteries that are easy to locate and are frequently used for pulse counts include the radial just below the base of the thumb on the wrist (see Figure 9) and the carotid on either side of the Adam's Apple (see Figure 10). In Lab 8A you will have the opportunity to practice counting your resting and postexercise heart rates.

To count the pulse rate, simply place the fingertips (index and middle finger) over the artery at one of the previously mentioned locations. Move the fingers around until a strong pulse can be felt. Press gently so as not to cut off the blood flow through the artery. Counting the pulse with the thumb is *not* recommended because the thumb has a relatively strong pulse of its own, and it could be confusing when counting another person's pulse.

Counting the pulse at the carotid artery is the most popular procedure, probably because the carotid pulse is easy to locate. Some researchers suggest that caution should be used when taking carotid pulse counts because pressing on this artery can cause a reflex that slows the heart rate. This could result in incorrect heart rate counts. More recent research indicates that carotid palpation, when done properly, can be safely used to count

Table 3 ▶ Progression of Activity Frequency, Intensity, and Time Based on Fitness Level

	Low Fitness	Marginal Fitness	Good Fitness
Frequency	3 days a week	3 to 5 days a week	3 to 6 days a week
Intensity			
Heart rate reserve (HRR)	40–50%	50–60%	60–85%
Maximum heart rate (max HR)	55–65%	65–75%	75–90%
Relative perceived exertion (RPE)	12–13	13–14	14–16
Time	10–30	20–40	30–60

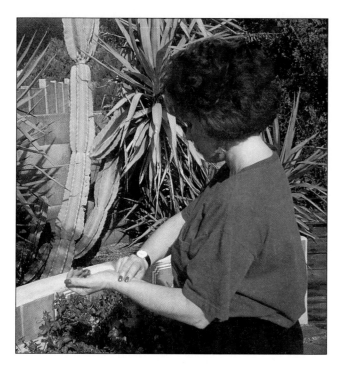

Figure 9 ▶ Counting your radial (wrist) pulse.

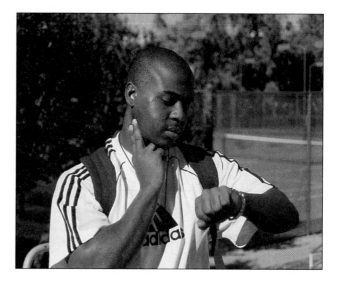

Figure 10 ▶ Counting your carotid (neck) pulse.

heart rate for most people. Some have suggested that if the carotid pulse is taken on the right side of the neck, it should be taken with the right hand to avoid applying too much pressure to the artery. You may choose to use this procedure, though you can learn to be quite effective with either hand. The key is to press gently no matter which hand you use.

The radial pulse is a bit harder to find than the carotid pulse because of the many tendons near the wrist. Moving the fingers around to several locations on the wrist just above the thumb will help you locate this pulse. For older adults or those with known medical problems, the radial pulse is recommended. Though less popular, the pulse can also be counted at the brachial artery. This is located on the inside of the upper arm just below the armpit.

Once the pulse is located, the heart rate can be determined in beats per minute. At rest, this is done simply by counting the number of beats in one minute. To determine exercise heart rate, it is best to count heart beats or pulses during activity; however, during most activities this is difficult. The most practical method is to count the pulse immediately after exercise. During physical activity, the heart rate increases but immediately after exercise, it begins to slow and return to normal. In fact, the heart rate has already slowed considerably within one minute after activity ceases. Therefore, it is important to locate the pulse quickly and to count the rate for a short period of time in order to obtain accurate results. For best results, keep moving while quickly locating the

pulse, then stop and take a 15-second count. Multiply the number of pulses by four to convert heart rate to beats per minute.

You can also count the pulse for ten seconds and multiply by six, or count the pulse for six seconds and multiply by ten to estimate a one-minute heart rate. The latter method allows you to easily calculate heart rates by adding a zero to the six-second count. However, short duration pulse counts increase the chance of error because a miscount of one beat is multiplied by six or ten beats rather than by four beats.

The pulse rate should be counted after regular activity, not after a sudden burst. Some runners sprint the last few yards of their daily run and then count their pulse. Such a burst of exercise will elevate the heart rate considerably. This gives a false picture of the actual exercise heart rate. It would be wise for every person to learn to determine resting heart rate accurately and to estimate exercise heart rate by quickly and accurately making pulse counts after activity.

As noted earlier, two different procedures are commonly used to estimate threshold and target zone heart rates. The first involves calculating a percentage of your HRR, also referred to by some as the working heart rate range or the Karvonen method. The second method, percentage of max HR, is easier to calculate but is less personalized. The heart rate reserve method is considered by many to be the better of the two because it is more personal in that it uses your true resting heart rate in making the calculations. As noted in Table 2, the percentage of heart rate intensity necessary to get you in the target zone differs depending upon which method of heart rate calculation you use. Both methods of determining threshold and target zone heart rates are described in the following paragraphs.

Table 4 ▶ Calculating Maximal Heart Rate (maxHR)		
	208.0	
	−15.4	.7 × 22 (age) = 15.4
	192.6	
maxHR = 193	(rounded up from 192.6)	

Table 5 ▶ Example for Calculating Threshold and Target Heart Rates for Using Percent of Heart Rate Reserve*	
Maximal Heart Rate	193 bpm
Minus Resting Heart Rate	−68 bpm
Equals Heart Rate Reserve (HRR)	125 bpm
Calculating Threshold Heart Rate	
HRR	125 bpm
× 40%	× .40
Equals	50 bpm
Plus Resting Heart Rate	+68 bpm
Equals Threshold Heart Rate	118 bpm
Calculating Upper Limit Heart Rate	
HRR	125 bpm
× 85%	× .85
Equals	106 bpm (106.25)
Plus Resting Heart Rate	+68 bpm
Equals Upper Limit Heart Rate	174 bpm

*Example is for a twenty-two-year-old person with a resting heart rate of 68 bpm. The target zone for this twenty-two-year-old is 118–174 bpm.

Determining Maximal Heart Rate (maxHR)

To calculate your threshold of training and target heart rate, you must first know your maxHR (also referred to as maximum heart rate). Your maxHR is the highest heart rate attained in maximal exercise. It could be determined using an electrocardiogram while exercising to exhaustion; however, for most people it is safer to estimate by using a formula. Until recently a simple formula has been used (220 − age = maxHR). While this formula gives a general estimate, recent research has found that it tends to overpredict for young people (twenty to forty) and underpredict for those over forty. Based on the extensive research involving a review of hundreds of past studies and new laboratory research, a new formula is now recommended. The formula is maxHR = 208 − (.7 × age). The formula has been shown to be useful for both sexes and for people of all activity levels. Table 4 illustrates the calculation of maxHR for a twenty-two-year-old using the new formula. The 193 (rounded up from 192.6) heart rate for the twenty-two-year-old example, is five beats lower than if the old formula had been used.

The new formula is especially beneficial to older adults. Because the previous formula underpredicted maxHR, it also underestimated the true level of physical stress during a treadmill test and underestimated target heart rate values for older adults.

Percentage of Heart Rate Reserve (HRR)

To calculate your HRR, you must know your resting in addition to your maxHR. Resting heart rate is easily determined by counting the pulse for one minute while sitting or lying. Ideally, this should be done early in the morning when you are rested, rather than late in the day when you have been involved in many activities.

HRR is determined by subtracting the resting heart rate from the maximum heart rate. The heart always works in the range between the resting (the lowest) and the maximal (the highest) rate of your pulse. The formula for calculating the working heart rate and an example for the twenty-two-year-old with a resting heart rate of 68 beats per minute are also shown in Table 5.

The threshold of training, or minimum heart rate, for achieving health benefits, is determined by calculating 40 percent of the working heart rate and then adding it to the resting heart rate. The upper limit of the target zone is 85 percent of the working heart rate added to the resting heart rate. The formula for determining threshold and the upper limit of the target heart rate zone, and examples for a hypothetical exerciser, are shown in Table 5. For best results, begin lower in the target zone and gradually increase exercise intensity.

It is important to note that activities that produce heart rates above 85 percent of heart rate reserve are considered to be **anaerobic activities** for most people. Physical activities of this high intensity may be needed for those in training for competition or for special physical tasks; however, it is not necessary for improving cardiovascular fitness associated with good health and wellness. Threshold and target zone values for anaerobic activities will be discussed in later concepts.

Percentage of Maximal Heart Rate

To use this method, first estimate your maximal heart rate just as you did for the previous method, then determine the threshold heart rate by calculating 55 percent of the maximal heart rate. The upper limit of the target zone is determined by calculating 90 percent of the maximal heart rate. Table 6 gives an example for a hypothetical 22-year-old person. This procedure, using a percentage of maximal heart rate, is deemed an acceptable alternative to the procedure using a percentage of heart rate reserve

Table 6 ▶ Examples for Calculating Threshold and Target Heart Rates for Using Percent of Maximal Heart Rate*

Calculating Threshold Heart Rate

Maximal Heart Rate	193 bpm
× 55%	× .55
Equals Threshold Heart Rate	106 bpm (106.15)

Calculating Upper Limit Heart Rate

Maximal Heart Rate	193 bpm
× 85%	× .90
Equals Upper Limit Heart Rate	174 bpm (173.7)

*Example is of a 22-year-old. The target zone for this 22-year old is 106–174.

Technology Update

Heart rate watches are now available that allow you to self-monitor heart rate. A watch (receiver) worn on the wrist, receives a signal from a transmitter attached to a strap worn around the chest. Basic units display heart rates digitally. Medium level units have alarms that indicate when your heart rate is above or below target zone values, display minutes of activity in the target zone, and average heart rate for a workout. The most expensive models have other features such as self-test and BMI calculators. Heart rate watches have the advantage of counting heart rate during, rather than after activity. Consult the "Web Resources" section at the end of this concept for more information.

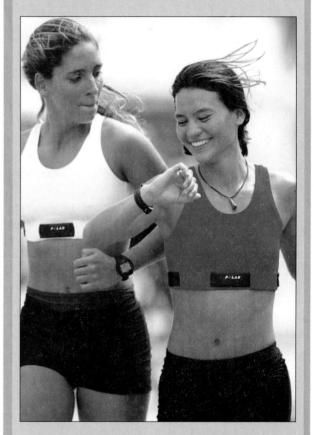

The heart rate watch.

because it provides target heart rates similar to those using 40–85 percent of the HRR method (see Table 6 for a worked example).

The ACSM recently increased the percentage of max HR for calculating threshold heart rates because the percentage formerly used was underestimating these values. As the examples in Tables 5 and 6 indicate, the percent of maximal heart rate formula still underestimates threshold values but provides accurate values for the upper limit of the target zone.

You should learn to calculate your threshold and target heart rate values using one of the two methods. (The first method, percentage of HRR, is a bit more difficult to calculate.) Regardless of which method you use, you should perform activity with enough intensity to bring your heart rate above threshold and into the target zone to get the health benefits of lifestyle physical activity.

It should be noted that several possible sources of error exist in calculating threshold and target heart rates. First, the method of calculating maximal heart rate is an estimate based on typical values for typical people. Second, errors in counting heart rate are possible. Finally, it is possible that the count you make *after* exercise may not actually reflect your heart rate *during* the activity. For this reason, it is important that you make several estimates of your threshold and target heart rates, especially when you are first starting a cardiovascular fitness program.

The recent development of inexpensive watch-sized heart rate monitors has provided a reliable method of heart-rate assessment for those who wish to use them (see Technology Update). They give you a heart-rate count *during* activity, allowing you to easily and quickly determine your heart rate at any time. Though these computerized monitors are helpful to some, they are not a requirement for accurate assessment of physical activity intensity.

Anaerobic Activity Physical activity performed at high intensity followed by rest periods.

Table 7 ▶ Ratings of Perceived Exertion (RPE)	
Rating	**Description**
6	
7	Very, very light
8	
9	Very light
10	
11	Fairly light
12	
13	Somewhat hard
14	
15	Hard
16	
17	Very hard
18	
19	Very, very hard
20	

Data from Borg, G.

Ratings of perceived exertion can be used as a method of monitoring the intensity of physical activity designed to promote cardiovascular fitness. The ACSM suggests that people experienced in physical activity can use RPE to determine if they are exercising in the target zone (see Table 7). Ratings of perceived exertion have been shown to correlate well with VO_2R and HRR. For this reason, RPE can be used to estimate exercise intensity among those who have learned to use the RPE rating categories. This avoids the need to stop and count heart rate during exercise. A rating of 12 (somewhat hard) is equal to threshold, and a rating of 16 (hard) is equal to the upper limit of the target zone. With practice, most people can recognize when they are in the target zone using ratings of perceived exertion.

Strategies for Action

An important step in taking action to develop and maintain cardiovascular fitness is assessing your current status. www.mhhe.com/fit_well/web08 Click 04. For an activity program to be most effective, it should be based on personal needs. Some type of testing is necessary to determine your personal need for cardiovascular fitness. With proper instruction and practice, you can learn to self-assess your cardiovascular fitness.

A person's maximal oxygen uptake ($\dot{V}O_2$ max), commonly referred to as aerobic capacity, is determined in a laboratory by measuring how much oxygen a person can use in maximal exercise. It is a good measure of cardiovascular fitness because you cannot use a great amount of oxygen if you do not have good fitness of all systems, including the heart, blood vessels, blood, respiratory system, and muscles. Great endurance athletes can extract 5 or 6 liters of oxygen per minute from the environment during an all-out treadmill run or bicycle ride. An average person extracts only 2 or 3 liters in a one-minute exercise session. $\dot{V}O_2$ max is often adjusted to account for a person's body size because bigger people may have higher scores due to their larger size. Scores are often reported as milliliters (ml) of oxygen per kilogram (kg) of body weight (ml/O_2/kg). This score is calculated by dividing your $\dot{V}O_2$ max value by your weight in kilograms.

www.mhhe.com/fit_well/web08 Click 05. $\dot{V}O_2$ max is the gold standard for cardiovascular fitness tests, but it is also impractical for regular use by most people because it must be done in a lab with expensive equipment. It is also a maximum test, so it may not be especially appropriate for those with low levels of fitness. Several tests can be done with a minimum of equipment in or near your home. Commonly used tests are the step test, the swim test, the 12-minute run, the Astrand-Ryhming bicycle test, and the walking test. With proper instruction, you can learn to measure your own cardiovascular fitness using one of these methods (see lab resource materials). These tests have been shown to estimate $\dot{V}O_2$ max with reasonable accuracy. Since these tests are not as accurate as laboratory tests of $\dot{V}O_2$ max, using more than one test is recommended to help you get a valid assessment of your cardiovascular fitness.

www.mhhe.com/fit_well/web08 Click 06. The self-assessment you choose depends on your current fitness and activity levels, availability of equipment, and other factors. The walking test is probably best for those at beginning levels because more vigorous forms of activity may cause discomfort and may discourage future participation. The step test is somewhat less vigorous than the running test and takes only a few minutes to complete. The bicycle test is also submaximal or relatively moderate in intensity. It is quite accurate but it does require more equipment than the other tests and requires more expertise. You may need help from a fitness expert to do this test properly. The swim test is especially useful to those with musculoskeletal problems and other disabilities. The running test is the most vigorous and for this reason may not be best for beginners. On the other hand, more advanced exercisers with high levels of motivation may prefer this test.

Results on the walking, running, and swimming tests are greatly influenced by the motivation of the test taker. If the test taker does not try hard, fitness results are underestimated. The bicycle and step tests are influenced less by motivation because one must exercise at a specified workload and at a regular pace. Because heart rate can be influenced by emotional factors, exercise prior to the test, and other factors, tests using heart rate can sometimes give incorrect results. It is important to do your self-assessments when you are relatively free from stress and are rested.

Prior to performing any of these, be sure that you are physically and medically ready. Prepare yourself by doing some regular physical activity for three to six weeks before actually taking the tests. If possible, take more than one test and use the summary of your test results to make a final assessment of your cardiovascular fitness. In Lab 8B, you will have the opportunity to self-assess your cardiovascular fitness using one or more tests.

Web Resources

American College of Sports Medicine **www.acsm.org**
American Heart Association **www.americanheart.org**
The Cooper Institute **www.cooperinst.org**
Good Health Heart Assessment **www.goodhealth.com**
Ordering Information for Heart Rate Watches
    www.polarusa.com

Suggested Readings

 Additional reference materials for concept 8 are available at **www.mhhe.com/fit_well/web08 Click 07.**

Albert, C. M. et al. 2000. Triggering of sudden death from cardiac causes by vigorous exertion. *New England Journal of Medicine* 243(19):1355–1361.

American College of Sports Medicine. 2000. *ACSM's Guidelines for Exercise Testing and Exercise Prescription,* 6th ed. Philadelphia: Lippincott, Williams and Wilkins.

Blair, S. N., and A. S. Jackson. 2001. A guest editorial to accompany physical fitness and activity as separate heart disease risk factors: A meta-analysis. *Medicine and Science in Sports and Exercise* 33(5):762–764.

Booth, F. W., and M. W. Chakravarthy. 2002. Cost and consequences of sedentary living: New battleground for an old enemy. *President's Council on Physical Fitness and Sports* 3(16):1–8.

Bouchard, C. 1999. Heredity and health-related fitness. In Corbin, C. B., and R. P. Pangrazi, *Toward a Better Understanding of Physical Fitness and Activity.* Scottsdale, AZ: Holcomb-Hathaway.

Lee, I., and R. S. Phaffenbarger. 2001. Preventing coronary heart disease: The role of physical activity. *The Physician and Sports Medicine* 29(2):37–52.

Meyers, J. et al. 2002. Exercise capacity and mortality among men referred to for exercise testing. *New England Journal of Medicine* 346(11):793–801.

Schnirring, L. 2001. New formula estimates maximal heart rate. *The Physician and Sports Medicine* 29(7):13–14.

Spain, C. G., and B. D. Franks. 2001. Healthy people 2010: Physical activity and fitness. *President's Council on Physical Fitness and Sports Research Digest* 3(13):1–16.

Tanaka H., K. D. Monahan, and D. R. Seals. 2001. Age-predicted maximal heart rate revisited. *Journal of the American College of Cardiology* 37(1):153–156.

U.S. Department of Health and Human Services. 2000. *Healthy People 2010.* 2nd ed. With *Understanding and Improving Health and Objectives for Improving Health.* 2 vols. Washington, DC: U.S. Government Printing Office.

U.S. Department of Health and Human Services. 1996. *Physical Activity and Health: A Report of the Surgeon General.* Atlanta: U.S. Department of Health and Human Services.

Williams, P. T. 2001. Physical fitness and activity as separate heart disease risk factors: A meta-analysis. *Medicine and Science in Sports and Exercise* 33(5):754–761.

In the News

Is the glass half empty or is it half full? Optimists see the glass as full, not empty. Apparently, optimists also have less risk of heart disease. A recent study followed men for at least ten years and found the higher your optimism the less the risk of having and dying from a heart attack.

Optimistic men were also less likely to have chest pain. Good cardiovascular fitness and regular physical activity help reduce risk of heart disease, but keeping a positive outlook on life can also be important.

Lab 8A: Counting Target Heart Rate and Ratings of Perceived Exertion

Name	Section	Date

Purpose: To learn to count heart rate accurately and to use heart rate and/or ratings of perceived exertion (RPE) to establish the threshold of training and target zones.

Procedure:

1. Practice counting the number of pulses felt for a given period of time at both the carotid and radial locations. Use a clock or watch to count for 15, 30, and 60 seconds. To establish your heart rate in beats per minute, multiply your 15-second pulse by four, and your 30-second pulse by 2.
2. Practice locating your carotid and radial pulses quickly. This is important when trying to count your pulse after exercise.
3. Run a quarter-mile, then count your heart rate at the end of the run. Try to run at a rate you think will keep the rate of the heart above the threshold of training and in the target zone. Use 15-second pulse counts (choose either carotid or radial) and multiply by four to get heart rate in beats per minute (bpm). Record the bpm in the Results section.
4. Rate your perceived exertion (RPE) for the run (see RPE chart below). Record your results.
5. Repeat the run a second time. Try to run at a speed that gets you in the heart rate and RPE target zone. Record your heart rate and RPE results.

Results: Record your **resting** heart rates in the boxes below.

Carotid Pulse		Heart Rate per Minute	Radial Pulse		Heart Rate per Minute
	15 seconds × 4			15 seconds × 4	
	30 seconds × 2			30 seconds × 2	
	60 seconds × 1			60 seconds × 1	

Record your heart rate and rating of perceived exertion for run 1.

Pulse Count		Heart Rate per Minute
	15 seconds × 4	
Rating of Perceived Exertion		

Record your heart rate and rating of perceived exertion for run 2.

Pulse Count		Heart Rate per Minute
	15 seconds × 4	
Rating of Perceived Exertion		

Ratings of Perceived Exertion (RPE)

Rating	Description
6	
7	Very, very light
8	
9	Very light
10	
11	Fairly light
12	
13	Somewhat hard
14	
15	Hard
16	
17	Very hard
18	
19	Very, very hard
20	

Source: Data from Borg, G.

Answer the following questions:

Which pulse-counting technique did you use after the runs?   Carotid ◯   Radial ◯

What is your heart rate target zone (see Chart 8, page 120). _____ bpm

Was your heart rate for run 1 enough to get in the heart rate target zone?   Yes ◯   No ◯

Was your RPE for run 1 enough to get in the target zone (12–16)?   Yes ◯   No ◯

Was your heart rate for run 2 enough to get in the heart rate target zone?   Yes ◯   No ◯

Was your RPE for run 2 enough to get in the target zone (12–16)?   Yes ◯   No ◯

Conclusions and Implications: In several sentences, discuss your results including which method you would use to count heart rate and why. Also discuss heart rate versus RPE for determining the target zone.

Lab Supplement*: You may want to keep track of your exercise heart rate over a week's time or longer to see if you are reaching the target zone in your workouts. Shade your target zone with a highlight pen and plot your exercise heart rate for each day of the week (see sample).

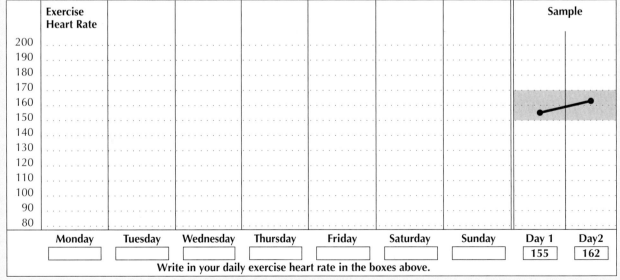

*Thanks to Ginnie Atkins for suggesting this lab supplement.

Lab 8B: Evaluating Cardiovascular Fitness

Name		Section	Date

Purpose: To acquaint you with several methods for evaluating cardiovascular fitness and to help you evaluate and rate your own cardiovascular fitness.

Procedure: Perform one or more of the four cardiovascular fitness tests described in the lab resource materials. Determine your ratings on the test(s) using the rating charts provided.

Results: Record the information obtained from taking the cardiovascular fitness test(s) (one or more) in the space provided.

Walking Test

Time [   ] minutes

Heart rate [   ] bpm

Rating [   ] (see Chart 1, page 117)

The Step Test

Heart rate [   ] bpm

Rating [   ] (see Chart 2, page 117)

The Bicycle Test

Workload [   ] kpm

Heart rate [   ] bpm

Weight [   ] lbs

Weight in kg* [   ]

ml/O$_2$/kg [   ]

Rating [   ] (see Chart 5, page 119)

12-Minute Run

Distance [   ] miles

Rating [   ] (see Chart 6, page 119)

12-Minute Swim Test

Distance [   ] yards

Rating [   ] (see Chart 7, page 120)

*Weight in lbs ÷ 2.2.

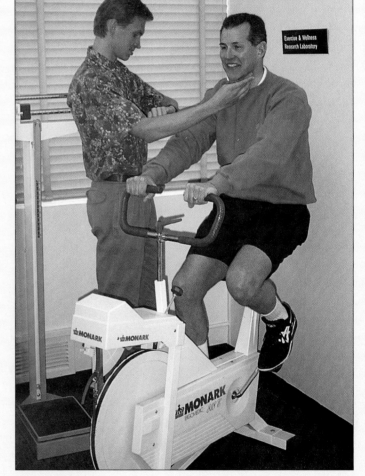

The bicycle test.

Conclusions and Implications:

1. In several sentences, explain why you selected the test or tests you chose. If you only selected one test explain why.

2. In several sentences, explain your results. Discuss your perception of the accuracy of the test results. Also, discuss whether you think you might have gotten different results if you had taken another test, and if so, why.

3. In several sentences, discuss your current level of cardiovascular fitness and steps that you should take in the future to maintain or improve it.

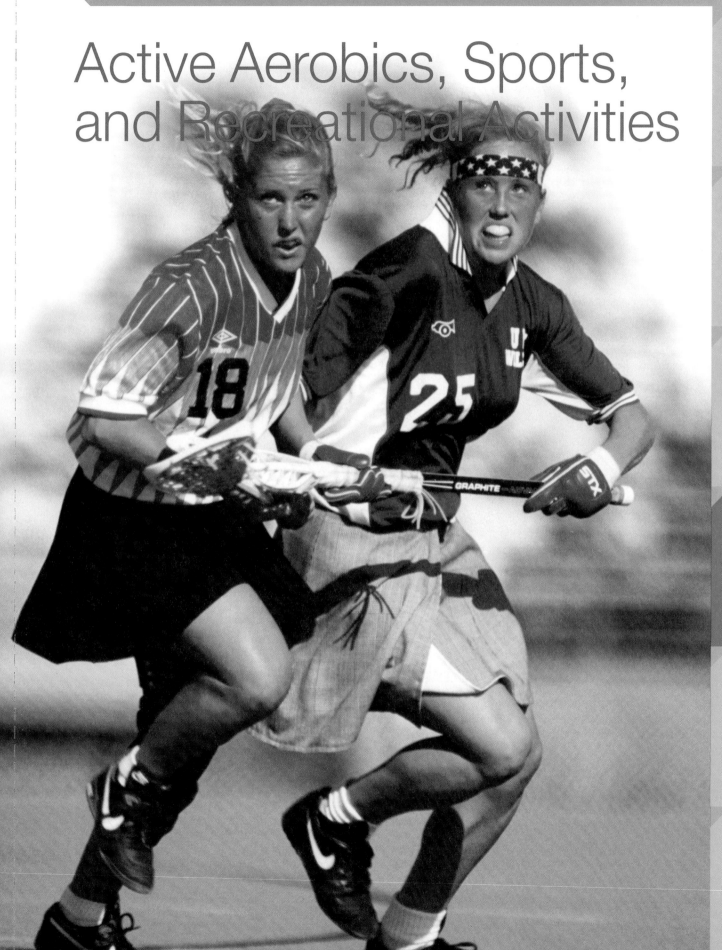

Active Aerobics, Sports, and Recreational Activities

Active aerobics, sports, and recreational activities are effective in promoting health benefits, as well as developing fitness and enhancing performance.

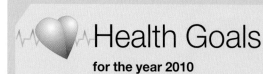

Health Goals

for the year 2010

- Increase proportion of people who do vigorous physical activity that promotes cardiovascular fitness three or more days a week for 20 minutes per occasion.

- Increase the adoption and maintenance of daily physical activity.

- Increase leisure time physical activity.

- Decrease incidence of and deaths from heart diseases.

The two categories of physical activities at the second level of the physical activity pyramid are active aerobics, along with active sports and recreational activities. Some of the more popular activities are described in this concept.

Physical Activity Pyramid: Level 2

Active aerobics are among the most popular physical activities among adults and are included at the second level of the physical activity pyramid. www.mhhe.com/fit_well/web09 Click 01. **Active aerobics** arc placed at the second level of the physical activity pyramid because, next to lifestyle physical activities, they are among the most popular activities among adults (see Figure 1). They are more vigorous than lifestyle physical activities, which are at the base of the pyramid. It is probably because they are more vigorous that active aerobics are not performed as frequently as lifestyle physical activities. Aerobic activities such as swimming, exercising with equipment, cycling, jogging, and aerobic exercise (dance) are among the top fifteen participation activities in the United States (see Table 1). For many of the aerobic activities, the ranks for males and females are quite similar. There are some differences, however. Aerobic exercise (dance) is sixth for females but thirteenth for males and rollerblading is thirteenth for women but not ranked for males.

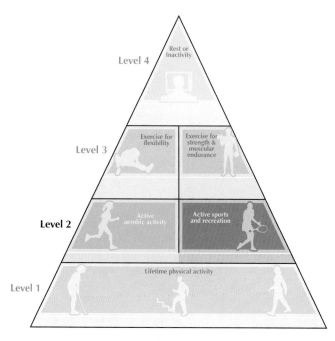

Figure 1 ▶ Active aerobics, sports, and recreational activities are included in the second level of the physical activity pyramid.

As people grow older, they decrease in all types of activity, but decreases in active aerobics are more dramatic than in lifestyle physical activities. Twice as many young people cycle as older people. Young men are three times more likely to jog than men forty-five years of age, and by sixty-five, men are ten times less likely to participate than young men. Young women are three times more likely to participate in aerobic dance than those forty-five years of age, and young women are five times more likely to participate than those sixty-five and older.

Active recreational activities and sports done at moderate to vigorous intensity are included in the second level of the physical activity pyramid. www.mhhe.com/fit_well/web09 Click 02. Experts classify activities such as hiking, boating, fishing, horseback riding, and other outdoor activities as recreational in nature. Recreational activities performed in the target zone for building cardiovascular fitness are considered to be **active recreational activities** and are appropriately included in the second level of the physical activity pyramid. Hiking is an example and is among the top fifteen participation activities (see Table 1). It is equally popular

Table 1 ▶ Most Popular Participation Activities

Activity	Rank	Male	Female
Walking	1	2	1
Swimming	2	3	2
Camping	3	4	4
Fishing	4	1	10
Exercise Equipment	5	8	3
Bowling	6	7	5
Cycling	7	5	7
Billiards/Pool	8	9	8
Basketball	9	10	14
Golf	10	6	*
Hiking	11	13	9
Run/Jog	12	14	11
Aerobics (dance)	13	*	6
Boating	14	15	12
Resistance Training	15	12	15
Hunting	*	11	*
Rollerblading	*	*	13

*not in top 15

Source: National Sporting Goods Association

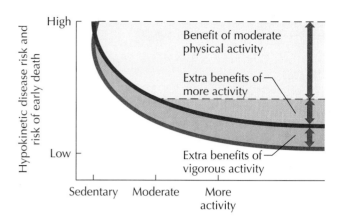

Figure 2 ▶ The extra benefits of vigorous physical activities.

among males and females. Other examples of popular active recreational activities are backpacking, kayaking, and canoeing. Recreational activities such as fishing and boating, also among the most popular activities, are done at less intensity and can be considered as lifestyle physical activities. Fishing and hunting are two activities that are much more popular among men than women.

Active **sports** can also be included in level 2 of the pyramid because they are vigorous in nature. Basketball is the only active sport in the top fifteen activities. It is typically anaerobic and intermittent in nature. It, like racquetball, tennis, and soccer, involves short bursts of vigorous anaerobic activity followed by rest periods. When done consistently with the FIT formula for cardiovascular fitness, these sports can provide benefits similar to active aerobics. Swimming and cycling are popular activities that could be considered sports. However, most people do these activities non-competitively, so they are considered as active aerobics in this book.

Sports such as golf, bowling, and billiards/pool are aerobic in nature but are light to moderate in intensity. For this reason they are classified as lifestyle physical activities. Basketball and golf are much more popular among men than women. Basketball, football, and baseball are most popular among youth and young adults while golf and bowling are much more popular among middle-aged and older adults.

Physical activities at level 2 of the pyramid can produce improvements in cardiovascular fitness and health in addition to those produced by lifestyle physical activities. Lifestyle physical activities are a form of light to moderate aerobic physical activity that promotes significant health benefits. Active aerobics, active sports, and active recreational activities provide similar health benefits and can promote cardiovascular fitness development when performed in the target zone for cardiovascular fitness (see Table 2 in concept 8).

The first curve in Figure 2 illustrates the additional benefits that can result if you do level 2 for the same length of time as less vigorous activity. The more vigorous activity expends more calories, and this produces extra health and fitness benefits. This benefit could occur among those who do less intense activity if they expended 2,000 to 3,500 calories per week. Studies show, however, that most people who do this much run, swim, or do a sport vigorously. One study of runners has shown that running can have significant health benefits over and above those achieved with activity of lesser intensity.

Active Aerobics Active aerobic physical activities are those of enough intensity to produce improvements in cardiovascular fitness. They are more intense than lifestyle physical activities that are also aerobic.

Active Recreational Activities Activities done during leisure time that do not meet the characteristics of sports. Many types of active aerobics are recreational activities.

Sports Typically considered to be competitive physical activities that have an organized set of rules along with winners and losers.

Table 2 ▶ Risk of Injury in Exercise

Activity	Injury per 1,000 Hours of Activity
Skating (including rollerblading)	20
Basketball	18
Average competitive sports	16
Running/jogging	16
Racquetball	14
Average aerobic activity	10
Tennis	8
Cycling	6
High-impact dance aerobics	6
Step aerobics	5
Aerobic exercise machines	3
Walking	2
Low-impact dance aerobics	2

Source: Data from the Center for Sports Medicine at St. Francis Hospital, San Francisco, CA.

The second curve in Figure 2 is based on a long-term study of a large number of people. It illustrates the fact that vigorous aerobic activity and active sports produce added benefits for *the same amount of energy expenditure.* Facts such as those presented in Figure 2 that led the American College of Sports Medicine (ACSM) to emphasize the statement in the Surgeon General's report that "additional benefits can be gained through greater amounts of physical activity."

Activities included in the second level of the activity pyramid can be done less frequently than activities at level 1 of the pyramid. The lower the level in the pyramid, the more frequently an activity should be performed. Lifestyle physical activities need to be performed all, or most, days of the week. Active aerobics, sports, and recreation can be performed as few as three days a week (see FIT formula, Table 3 in Concept 8). They can be done less often because the activities are performed at a more vigorous level. This is important for young people who feel that their time is limited. Performing more vigorous activities provides health and fitness benefits with a relatively small time commitment.

Not all activities at level 2 of the pyramid are equally safe. Sports medicine experts indicate that certain types of physical activities are more likely to result in injury than others. As shown in Table 2, walking and low-impact dance aerobics are among the least risky activities.

Skating, an aerobic activity, is the most risky, followed by basketball and competitive sports. Among the most popular aerobic activities, running has the greatest risk, with cycling, high-impact dance aerobics, and step aerobics having moderate risk of injury. Water activities were not considered in the study on which Table 2 was based. However, swimming and water aerobics are among those least likely to cause injuries because they do not involve impact, falling, or collision. Volume of training is also associated with injury risk. Those who do high volume training have increased risk.

Active Aerobics and Active Recreation

Active aerobics can be done either continuously or intermittently. We generally think of active aerobics as being continuous in nature. Jogging, swimming, and cycling at a steady pace for long periods are classic examples. Experts have shown that aerobic exercise can be done intermittently as well as continuously. Both **continuous** and **intermittent aerobic activities** can build cardiovascular fitness. For example, recent studies have shown that three 10-minute exercise sessions in the target zone were as effective as one 30-minute exercise session. Still, experts recommend bouts of 20 to 60 minutes in length, with several 10 to 15 minute bouts being an acceptable alternative when longer sessions are not possible.

Aerobic interval training and interval dance exercise are examples of intermittent aerobic exercise. The advantages and disadvantages of continuous and intermittent exercise are presented in Table 3.

Table 3 ▶ Continuous versus Intermittent Exercise: Advantages and Disadvantages

Continuous	Intermittent
• Done slowly and continuously, rather than in short, vigorous bursts; considered to be less demanding and more enjoyable.	• When done in the target zone, has the same benefits as continuous.
• Less intense with lower injury risk; may be best for beginners, older people, and those starting after a long layoff.	• If done intensely, can increase risk of soreness and injury.
• Provides health benefits associated with cardiovascular fitness.	• Three 10-minute or two 15-minute sessions easier to schedule than one longer period.
• May not provide optimal performance benefits for competitors.	• May be more interesting to some people.
	• If done at relatively high intensity with alternating rest periods, it can be beneficial in preparing for competition.

There are many popular forms of active aerobics and active recreation. www.mhhe.com/fit_well/web09 Click 03. Some of the most popular forms of aerobic exercise are discussed briefly here. Active recreational activities such as hiking and cross-country skiing are also discussed in this section.

Aerobic Exercise Machines

Many kinds of aerobic exercise machines, including stair-climbers, cross-country ski machines, elliptical trainers, stationary bicycles, and a wide variety of new machines come on the market periodically. The advantages of such machines are that they can be used in the home. Also they do not require excessive amounts of skill. Use of these machines can be fun and interesting initially, but that interest decreases with repeated use. Ski machines would seem to be most useful for people who ski on a regular basis, and stationary bicycles would seem to be most interesting to those who do cycling. Aerobic exercise machines can be useful in developing cardiovascular fitness for people who use them to exercise in the target zone for fitness. The key to the effectiveness of the machines is persistent use over long periods of time.

The type of device you choose should be based on your personal needs and interests. The activity that you personally enjoy is probably the best for you. Beware of claims that certain machines are better because they allow you to expend large numbers of calories in short periods of time. For most people, exercise of such a high intensity would be excessively vigorous and would not foster long-term adherence.

Aerobic Interval Training

Interval training is one of the most common forms of intermittent exercise. Short bursts of energy, commonly referred to as sprints, are alternated with rest periods. Sprints may be in running, swimming, or cycling. For many years, interval training was considered to be exclusively a form of anaerobic training. However, athletes and coaches now feel that aerobic interval training may be important for competitors in a variety of activities. In aerobic interval training, the pace should be slightly beyond a normal aerobic level, and the rest periods should be fairly short (e.g., 400 meter running followed by rest periods of 10 to 15 seconds). Even though this type of activity is aerobic in nature, it is primarily for those interested in competition. For this reason, a more extensive discussion of this type of training is included in the concept on performance.

Bicycling and Spinning

Bicycling, when done in bouts of appropriate length, is a form of aerobic exercise. This activity requires only a

Technology Update

www.mhhe.com/fit_well/web09 Click 04. Global Positioning Systems (GPS) were developed by the federal government primarily for use in national defense but are now used for a variety of other purposes. GPS systems use specially coded satellite signals that can be processed using computers to compute position, velocity, and time. GPS systems are now available for runners and cyclists to determine how far they have traveled and how fast they are going, even over the most rugged terrain. The system includes a GPS receiver and a watch-monitor that are connected by a radio signal. The receiver (typically strapped to the upper arm) gets the signal from a satellite and sends it to the watch for immediate feedback. Because the system uses an atomic clock, data are quite accurate. For more information refer to the "On the Web" site listed above.

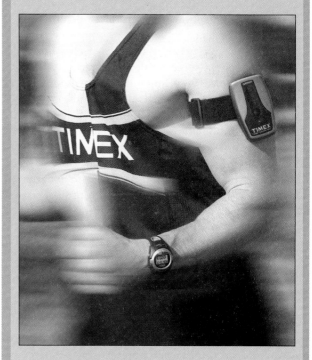
GPS system for runners.

Continuous Aerobic Activity Aerobic activity that is slow enough to be sustained for relatively long periods without frequent rest periods.

Intermittent Aerobic Activity Aerobic activity that is alternated with frequent rest periods; often of relatively high intensity.

bicycle and some safety equipment, such as a helmet, light, and reflectors if done after dark. A tall flag is needed if biking in traffic. To be most effective in building physical fitness, you should pedal continuously, rather than coasting for long periods. Maintaining a steady pace is recommended, though mountain biking often requires hill climbing and faster downhill riding. Periodically, riding a different course can increase enjoyment of the activity. Critical to enjoyable cycling is selecting a bicycle that is of appropriate size. The type of riding you do (touring or off-road) will dictate the type of bicycle you need.

Cycling is more efficient than running and some other aerobic activities because of the mechanical efficiency of the bicycle. Cycling on the level at 5 mph is about three times less intense than running at the same speed. It would take a ride of 13 mph to expend a similar number of calories compared to running at 5 mph. The speed of cycling will give you an indicator of activity intensity, but you should monitor the intensity of the activity using heart rate or perceptions of exertion to determine if it suits your personal needs.

Spinning is a type of stationary cycling that has become popular in some locales. This activity involves alternate bouts of slow cycling followed by faster bouts of low-resistance high-speed pedaling (spinning). Depending on how it is performed, spinning can be either aerobic or anaerobic in nature. It is most likely to be effective for people who like regular cycling. Because it is often relatively high in intensity, it may not be an activity to which large numbers of people are likely to adhere over long periods of time. It may be useful to provide variety for those interested in a change of program.

Circuit Resistance Training (CRT)

Originally, circuit training was a type of physical training involving movement from one exercise station to another. A different type of exercise was performed at each station. In order to complete the circuit, you had to complete all the exercises at all of the stations. The goal was to perform the circuit in progressively shorter periods. Circuit resistance training (CRT) principally promotes muscle fitness development. However, when performed frequently enough and for enough time at the appropriate intensity, CRT can make a significant contribution to cardiovascular fitness. When aerobic exercise, such as riding on stationary bicycles and running on treadmills, is incorporated in the continuous exercise circuit, the contribution of this type of exercise to cardiovascular fitness increases (see concept 11 for additional information).

If cardiovascular fitness is the goal, the best of programs are ineffective if they cannot be performed properly. Some clubs promote exercise circuits as a method of

building both strength and cardiovascular fitness, yet exercise stations are often crowded, and it is next to impossible to perform the circuit without long waiting periods. You may want to add aerobic exercise to your circuit during periods of waiting.

Cooper's Aerobics

www.mhhe.com/fit_well/web09 Click 05. Based on the needs of military personnel, Dr. Kenneth Cooper developed a physical activity program that he called "aerobics." In fact, he popularized the term. His program includes a variety of aerobic activities that have point values for the different types of exercise involved. Examples of activities that earn one point are the following: walking a mile in 14 1/2 to 20 minutes, cycling 2 miles at 10 to 15 mph, and swimming 300 yards in 8 to 10 minutes. To develop fitness (especially cardiovascular fitness) using the aerobics point system, it is necessary to earn thirty aerobic points per week. Aerobic points are part of Cooper's system for helping people know when they are exercising frequently enough, intensely enough, and long enough. Though earning thirty points per week is a good way of achieving fitness, we now know that earning fewer than thirty points can be beneficial to health. For more complete details on the Cooper aerobic points program, the reader is encouraged to read one of Cooper's books (see Suggested Readings).

Continuous Calisthenics

Survey results repeatedly show that calisthenics are among the most frequently performed participant activities. Calisthenics exercises, such as the crunch and push-ups, are designed to build flexibility, strength, or muscular endurance in specific muscle groups. Even though most calisthenics are aerobic, they are usually done intermittently. That is, calisthenic exercises are done a few at a time followed by a rest period. They will do little for cardiovascular fitness or fat control unless they are done continuously.

Continuous calisthenics, or calisthenics that are done without stopping or with walking, jogging, rope jumping, or some other aerobic activity performed during the rest period, can develop almost all health-related aspects of physical fitness. Fitness pioneer Dr. Thomas Cureton long advocated the use of continuous calisthenics, or what he referred to as "continuous rhythmical endurance exercise."

Cross-Country Skiing

In Europe, cross-country skiing is one of the most popular aerobic activities. Of course, this sport requires snow and a certain amount of specialized equipment. For those who can cross-country ski on a regular basis, studies show that it is one of the most effective types of cardiovascular fitness exercise. Cross-country skiing uses both the arms and legs, whereas some aerobic activities primarily use the legs. This is one reason for its effectiveness and why this activity is high in caloric expenditure. Cross-country skiing can be a fun family activity.

Dance

There are many forms of dance that, when done continuously, can contribute significantly to cardiovascular fitness. Among the more popular are ballet, country, disco, folk, hip-hop, Latin (e.g., cha-cha, tango), modern, tap, square, and swing. There are many other forms but to mention them all would take more space than is available. For dance to be considered "active" it should be performed in the target zone for cardiovascular fitness. Less active dance (e.g., slow social dance) is equivalent to a lifestyle activity. Dance and step aerobics are considered next.

Dance and Step Aerobics

This type of activity was first popularized by Jackie Sorensen in the 1970s as "aerobic dance." Since then, other versions of the activity have been promoted as rhythmic aerobics, Jazzercise, and Dancercize, to note just a few of the popular names. Dance aerobics is a choreographed series of dance steps and exercises done to music. Certified instructors may tailor dance routines to individuals, but many dance routines are preplanned (e.g., dance aerobic videos). Most of the early programs were considered to be high-impact because they included jumping, leaping, and hopping dance steps that resulted in stress on the feet and legs.

In an attempt to reduce the risk of injury or soreness, lower-impact dance aerobics were developed. Now dance aerobic activities are commonly divided into three categories: low-impact aerobics, moderate-impact aerobics, and high-impact aerobics. In low-impact dance aerobics, one foot stays on the floor at all times. Low-impact dance aerobics are an especially wise choice for beginners and older exercisers. Moderate-impact dance aerobics alternates between low- and high-impact steps that allow it to be considerably less stressful than high-impact exercise. It is especially useful for people who want more vigorous activity than low-impact but who do not want the intensity of high-impact aerobics. In high-impact aerobics, both feet leave the ground simultaneously for a good part of the routine. It is recommended only for advanced exercisers. Even for these people high-impact aerobics increases injury risk.

Step aerobics, also known as bench stepping and step training, is an adaptation of dance aerobics. In this activity, the performer steps up and down on a bench when performing various dance steps. In most cases, step aerobics is considered to be low-impact but higher in intensity than many forms of dance aerobics. Step training has been used by professional athletic teams to promote cardiovascular fitness. A major benefit is the ability to change the height of the step to meet the needs of individual participants.

Dance and step aerobics, when planned appropriately for individual participants, can be very effective in building cardiovascular fitness for both men and women. One problem with dance aerobics is that it is often a preplanned exercise program; therefore, it requires all participants to do the same activity regardless of their fitness or activity levels. A vigorous routine can cause unfit people to overextend themselves, whereas an easy routine may not result in fitness gains for those who are already quite fit. Also, some dance aerobic routines have been known to include contraindicated exercises. Dance and step aerobics do require skill, so instruction from a qualified instructor and practice are necessary for optimal enjoyment.

Fartlek (Speed Play)

Fartlek is a Swedish word for "speed play." This form of physical activity was developed in Scandinavia where pinewood paths follow curves of lakes and up and down many hills, where the scenery takes your mind off the task at hand. The idea is to get away from the regimen of running or walking on a track and to enjoy the woods, lakes, and mountains. Because of the terrain, the pace is never constant. The uphill path requires a slow pace, while a straight stretch or downhill trail allows for speed. In the speed play, or Fartlek system, you run easily for a time at a steady pace, then sprint for a while, sometimes up or down a hill. Walking typically follows these vigorous bursts.

Hiking and Backpacking

Like walking and jogging, hiking is a recreational activity that can promote cardiovascular fitness. Hiking has the advantage of an outdoors setting, often in a scenic environment. It does require some equipment, such as a rucksack and good hiking shoes, but specialized skills are not needed.

Backpacking is a form of hiking that usually covers longer distances and involves an overnight stay, often in the mountains. Backpacking is excellent for building cardiovascular fitness as well as muscular endurance. Like other aerobic activities, it can be helpful in controlling body fat. In recent years, it has become a popular activity; nearly 11 million American adults report regular involvement in backpacking.

Inline (Rollerblading) and Other Skating

Originally developed for training for skiers in the off season, inline skates (rollerblades) are now used for individual recreation and team activities. The popularity of inline skating has increased in the last decade. Technological

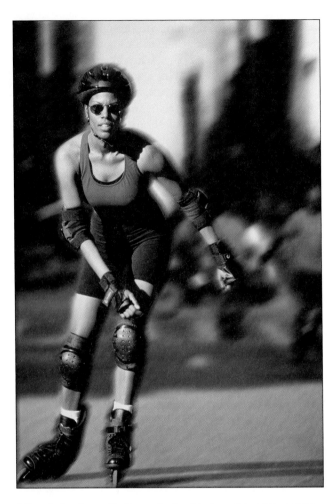

Inline skating is an effective and enjoyable type of aerobic exercise.

advances in equipment have made it much safer, though injury rates are still high compared to other aerobic activities (see Table 2). Inline skating can be done as an individual activity or as part of a team as in roller hockey. Ice skating tends to be regional in its appeal but, like inline skating, can be done as an individual activity or as part of a team as in ice hockey. Roller skating is often limited to those who have access to roller rinks, special recreational, or amusement areas. Because of the injury risk special precautions should be taken for inline and roller skating, especially when performed outdoors. Special equipment is recommended including a helmet, knee and elbow pads, as well as wrist supports and hand protectors. Roller and ice hockey require other protective equipment. Some degree of fitness and skill is necessary to perform skating safely and effectively.

Jogging/Running

A consistently popular form of active aerobics among both adult men and women is jogging or running. Though no official distinction exists between jogging and running, those who run more than a few miles per day, who participate in races, and who are concerned about improving the time in which they run a certain distance often prefer to be called "runners" rather than "joggers." Fifteen to 20 million American adults report that they jog or run on a regular basis.

The major advantage of jogging/running is that it requires only a good pair of running shoes, some inexpensive clothing, and little skill. With effort, almost anyone can benefit from the activity and even improve performance if that is the goal. There are some techniques that every jogger should be familiar with before starting a jogging program.

- *Foot placement.* The heel of the foot hits the ground first in jogging. Your heel should strike before the rest of your foot (but not hard), then you should rock forward and push off with the ball of your foot. Contrary to some opinions, you should *not* jog on your toes. (A flat-foot landing can be all right as long as you push off with the ball of your foot.) Your toes should point straight ahead. Your feet should stay under your knees and *not* swing out to the sides as you jog.
- *Length of stride.* For efficiency, you should have a relatively comfortable stride length. Your stride should be several inches longer than your walking stride. If necessary, you may have to reach to lengthen your stride. Most older people find it more efficient to run with a shorter stride.
- *Arm movement.* While you jog, you should swing your arms as well as your legs. The arms should be bent and should swing freely and alternately from front to back in the direction you are moving, not from side to side. Keep your arms and hands relaxed.
- *Body position.* While jogging, you should hold your upper body in a relatively erect position with your head and chest up. Don't lean forward, as you would with sprinting or fast running.

Martial Arts Exercise

Martial arts exercise, a form of aerobic exercise, has gained popularity in the last decade. Among the more popular forms are aerobic-boxing, cardio-karate, box-fitness, and Tae Bo though there are many other names for this type of activity. This type of activity, as well as traditional martial arts, can be a good form of active aerobics if performed continuously in the target zone for cardiovascular fitness. Because martial arts exercise involves a lot of arm work, people with high blood pressure should have medical clearance before beginning participation. Get basic skill and safety instruction and avoid contraindicated exercises common in some martial arts. If contact is involved it is important to be matched with a person of similar size and ability. Martial arts exercises are often high in intensity so adherence may be difficult for less fit people.

Rope Jumping

Rope jumping is aerobic if done at a slow or moderate pace, but is anaerobic if done vigorously. Even people who are highly trained or who jump at a moderate pace find it difficult to continue this exercise long enough to build cardiovascular fitness because of leg fatigue, high heart rate, or loss of interest in the activity. To be most effective, use a continuous routine involving several different jump steps in combination with other forms of exercise. For example, rope jumping could be a part of a circuit resistance training program or a dance aerobics program. Rope jumping is a relatively high-impact activity, and long-term adherence is likely to result in risk of injury similar to other high-impact activities.

Rowing, Canoeing, and Kayaking

Rowing, canoeing, and kayaking are recreational activities that can be done at a leisurely pace or at a more vigorous pace. When done continuously for periods of ten minutes or longer and with an intensity in the target zone, these activities are classified as a type of active recreation that produces similar benefits to active aerobics. When done at a leisurely pace with more floating than paddling or rowing, the activities are more appropriately considered to be similar to lifestyle physical activity.

Swimming

Public opinion polls typically rank swimming as the first- or second-most popular form of regular physical activity among adults. Data from the *Surgeon General's Report* show that swimming for exercise ranks ninth among participation activities. The discrepancy is probably because many people swim occasionally but fewer people swim as exercise on a regular basis. When done frequently, intensely enough, and for a long enough time, swimming is an excellent form of physical activity to promote cardiovascular fitness. When using heart rate to monitor intensity, it is necessary to adjust the target zone heart rate for swimming. Typically, the heart rate does not increase as rapidly in response to swimming as to other activities. Target zone heart rates are often five to ten beats fewer than for other forms of active aerobics.

Walking

Walking is generally considered as a lifestyle physical activity and is effective in promoting metabolic fitness and health benefits. If cardiovascular fitness is desired, walking must be done intensely enough to elevate the heart rate to target zone levels. As people grow older, walking often provides the intensity necessary for building and maintaining cardiovascular fitness. For younger people, walking would have to be quite brisk to promote cardiovascular fitness.

Water Exercises

Swimming is not the only activity done in the water. Water walking and water exercise are two popular alternatives to swimming. These activities are good for people with arthritis or other musculoskeletal problems and for people relatively high in body fat. The body's buoyancy in water assists the participant and reduces injury risk. The resistance of the water provides an overload that helps the activity promote health and cardiovascular benefits. Exercises done in shallow water are low in impact, and deeper water exercises are considered to be no-impact activities. An advantage of water walking and water exercise is that neither requires the ability to swim. Depending on intensity, they can be classified either as lifestyle activity or active aerobics. Many water exercise programs include activities designed to promote flexibility and muscle fitness development as well as cardiovascular fitness development. Instructors certified by appropriate national organizations, as water exercise instructors and in water safety, are recommended for optimal benefits and water safety.

Active Sports

Some sports are more active than others. Some sports require more activity than others. Activities that involve muscles from different parts of the body are more active than those that involve fewer muscles. Some are of high intensity and others are less intense. When done vigorously, tennis and basketball involve many different muscle groups and are high in intensity. Soccer is an activity that involves many muscle groups and is high in

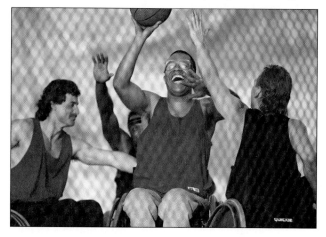

Sports can be effective in promoting fitness and health.

intensity but does not emphasize the use of the arms. Golf, on the other hand, is less intense, and relies more on skill and technique. The action in basketball, tennis, and soccer involves bursts of activity followed by rest but requires persistent vigorous activity over a relatively long period of time. Golf requires little vig-

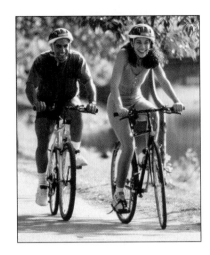

Choose a self-promoting form of physical activity.

orous activity. Sports that have characteristics similar to those of basketball, tennis, and soccer have similar benefits to active aerobic activities. Of course, any given sport can be more or less active depending on how you perform the activity. Shooting baskets or even playing half-court basketball is not as vigorous as a full-court game.

The most popular sports share characteristics that contribute to their popularity. The most popular sports (see Table 1) are often considered to be lifetime sports because they can be done at any age. The characteristics that make these sports appropriate for lifelong participation probably contribute significantly to their popularity. Four of the top five are individual sports that do not require a large group of people to perform them. Often the popular sports are adapted so people without exceptional skill can play them. For example, bowling uses a handicap system to allow people with a wide range of abilities to compete. Slow-pitch softball is much more popular than fast-pitch softball or baseball because it allows people of all abilities to play successfully.

One of the primary reasons sports participation is so popular is that sports provide a challenge. For the greatest enjoyment, the challenge of the activity should be balanced by the person's skill in the sport. If you choose to play against a person with lesser skill, you will not be challenged. On the other hand, if you lack skill or your opponent has considerably more skill, the activity will be frustrating. For optimal challenge and enjoyment, the skills of a given sport should be learned before competing. Likewise, choose an opponent who has a similar skill level.

There are benefits to watching and participating in sports. Active involvement in sports can have many physical, social, and personal benefits. Though watching sports will not build physical fitness, it does have other

benefits. According to recent research, watching sports almost always makes people feel happy when their team wins and gives them a feeling of accomplishment and pride, even though they did not participate. On the downside, when the favorite team loses, feelings of depression and lack of accomplishment may occur. In extreme cases, displays of poor sportsmanship and even violence have occurred. Recent celebrations that have resulted in property destruction and violence after NCAA and NBA championship victories are examples.

Becoming skillful will help you enjoy sports. Improving your performance skill can increase the probability that you will perform sports for a lifetime. The following self-management guidelines can help you improve your sport performance.

- *When learning a new activity, concentrate on the general idea of the skill first; worry about details later.* For example, a diver who concentrates on pointing the toes and keeping the legs straight at the end of a flip may land flat on his/her back. To make it all the way over, the diver should concentrate on merely doing the flip. When the general idea is mastered, then concentrate on details.

- *The beginner should be careful not to emphasize too many details at one time.* After the general idea of the skill is acquired, the learner can begin to focus on the details, one or two at a time. Concentration on too many details at one time may result in **paralysis by analysis.** For example, a golfer who is told to keep the head down, the left arm straight, and the knees bent cannot possibly concentrate on all of these details at once. As a result, neither the details nor the general idea of the golf swing is performed properly.

- *Once the general idea of a skill is learned, a skill analysis of the performance may be helpful.* Be careful not to overanalyze; it may be helpful to have a knowledgeable person help you locate strengths and weaknesses. Movies and videotapes of performances have been known to be of help to learners.

- *In the early stages of learning a lifetime sport or physical activity, it is not wise to engage in competition.* Beginners who compete are likely to concentrate on beating their opponent rather than on learning a skill properly. For example, in bowling, the beginner may abandon the newly learned hook ball in favor of the sure thing straight ball. This may make the person more successful immediately, but is not likely to improve the person's bowling skills for the future.

- *To be performed well, sports skills must be overlearned.* Oftentimes, when you learn a new activity, you begin to play the game immediately. The best way to learn a skill is to overlearn it, or practice it until it becomes habit. Frequently, games do not allow you to overlearn skills. For example, during a tennis match is not a good time to learn how to serve because there may be only a few opportunities to do so. For the beginner, it would be much more productive to hit many serves (overlearn) with a friend until the general idea of the serve is well learned. Further, the beginner *should not* sacrifice speed to concentrate on serving for accuracy. Accuracy will come with practice of a properly performed skill.

- *When unlearning an old (incorrect) skill and learning a new (correct) skill, a person's performance may get worse before it gets better.* For example, a golfer with a baseball swing may want to learn the correct golf swing. It is important for the learner to understand that the score may worsen during the relearning stage. As the new skill is overlearned, skill will improve, as will the golf score.

- *Mental practice may aid skill learning.* Mental practice (imagining the performance of a skill) may benefit performance, especially if the performer has had previous experience in the skill. Mental practice can be especially useful in sports when the performer cannot participate regularly because of weather, business, or lack of time.

- *For beginners, practicing in front of other people may be detrimental to learning a skill.* An audience may inhibit the beginner's learning of a new sports skill. This is especially true if the learner feels that his or her performance is being evaluated by someone in the audience.

- *There is no substitute for good instruction.* Getting good instruction, especially at the beginning level, will help you learn skill faster and better. Instruction will help you apply these rules and to use practice more effectively.

Strategies for Action

You can take steps to become successful in physical activity. You can use several self-management skills to help enjoy activities at the second level of the pyramid.

- *Improve your performance skills.* Consider taking lessons and practice the skills you want to perform using the guidelines listed earlier in this concept.

- *Select self-promoting activities.* **Self-promoting activities** require relatively little skill and can be done in a way that avoids comparison to other people. They allow you to set your own standards of success and can be done individually or in small groups that are suited to your personal needs. Examples include wheelchair distance events, jogging, resistance training, swimming, bicycling, and dance exercise.

- *Change your way of thinking.* You can change your way of thinking so that you feel positively about yourself. Adopting a new way of thinking can help you avoid self-criticism and resist the need to feel bad if you do not perform as well as others. The key is to reward yourself for being active—its what you do that counts.

- *Develop a plan for performing level 2 activities.* All people are not equally good at all activities, but because there are so many activities from which to choose virtually all people can find something in which they can succeed. Lab 9A helps you try jogging, and Lab 9B helps you to plan for any of the different level 2 activities in the pyramid. In Lab 9B you can indicate the activities you plan to do and when you plan to do them. You may do these activities instead of lifestyle physical activities or in addition to them.

- *Self-monitor your activity to help you stick with your plan.* Self-monitoring is a self-management skill that can be valuable in encouraging long-term activity adherence. A self-monitoring chart is provided in Lab 9B to help you log the activities you perform in a one-week period. This is a short-term record sheet. However, charts such as this can be copied to make a log book to allow long-term self-monitoring. You may want to consider using a heart rate monitor to help you determine self-monitor level 2 activities (see concept 8).

Web Resources

American Association for Active Lifestyles and Fitness
   www.aahperd.org/aaalf/aaalf_main.html
American Council on Exercise **www.acefitness.org**
American Running Association **www.americanrunning.org**
Disabled Sports USA **www.dsusa.org**
National Association for Sports and Physical Education
   www.aahperd.org/naspe/naspe_main.html
Ordering Information for GPS system **www.timex.com**

Paralysis by Analysis An overanalysis of skill behavior. This occurs when more information is supplied than a performer can use or when concentration on too many details results in interference with performance.

Self-Promoting Activities Activities that do not require a high level of skill to be successful.

President's Council on Physical Fitness and Sports
www.fitness.gov

Special Olympics International **www.specialolympics.org**

Sport Quest **www.sportQuest.com**

X Sports **www.expn.go.com**

Suggested Readings

 Additional reference materials for concept 9 are available at **www.mhhe.com/fit_well/web09 Click 06.**

Adams, H., C. Norton, and H. Tilden. 2000. *Aquatic Toolbook.* Champaign, IL: Human Kinetics.

Almeida, S. A. et al. 1999. Epidemiological patterns of musculoskeletal injuries and physical training. *Medicine and Science in Sports and Exercise* 31(8):1176–1182.

American College of Sports Medicine. 2000. *ACSM's Guidelines for Exercise Testing and Prescription.* 6th ed. Philadelphia: Lippincott, Williams and Wilkins.

Burke, E. et al. 2000. *Long-Distance Cycling: Build the Strength, Skills and Confidence to Ride as Far as You Want.* Emmaus, PA: Rodale Press.

Cochran, S. 2001. *Complete Conditioning for Martial Arts.* Champaign, IL: Human Kinetics.

Cooper, K. H. 1982. *The Aerobics Program for Total Well-Being.* New York: M. Evans & Co.

Gould, R. H. 2000. *Tennis Anyone?* St. Louis: McGraw-Hill.

Hall, A. 2001. *The Essential Backpacker: A Complete Guide for the Foot Traveler.* St. Louis: McGraw-Hill.

Hannula, D. 2001. *The Swim Coaching Bible.* Champaign, IL: Human Kinetics.

Henderson, J. 2000. *Running 101.* Champaign, IL: Human Kinetics.

Hootman, J. M. et al. 2002. Epidemiology of musculoskeletal injuries among sedentary and physically active adults. *Medicine and Science in Sports and Exercise* 34(5):838–844.

Jaeger, T. M. 1999. *Swimming.* St. Louis: McGraw-Hill.

Kestenbaum, R. 2001. *The Ultralight Backpacker: The Complete Guide to Simplicity and Comfort on the Trail.* St. Louis: McGraw-Hill.

Kluka, D. A., and P. J. Dunn. 2000. *Volleyball.* 3d ed. St. Louis: McGraw-Hill.

Long, J., and M. Hodgson. 2000. *The Complete Hiker.* 2nd ed. St. Louis: McGraw-Hill.

Lovett R. 2001. *The Essential Touring Cyclist: A Complete Guide for the Bicycle Traveler.* 2nd ed. St. Louis: McGraw-Hill.

Lovett, R., and P. Peterson. 2000. *The Essential Cross-Country Skier.* St. Louis: McGraw-Hill.

Magill, R. A. 2001. *Motor Learning: Concepts and Applications.* 6th ed. St. Louis: McGraw-Hill.

Miller, L. 2000. *Advanced Inline Skating.* St. Louis: McGraw-Hill.

Olson, M. S., and H. N. Williford. 1999. Martial arts exercise. *ACSM's Health and Fitness Journal* 3(6):6–14.

Pryor, E. 2000. *Keep Moving: Fitness Through Aerobics and Step.* 4th ed. St. Louis: McGraw-Hill.

Talbot, L. A. et al. 2000. Leisure-time physical activities and their relationship to cardiovascular fitness in healthy men and women. *Medicine and Science in Sports and Exercise* 32(2):412–416.

Townsend, C. 2001. *The Advanced Backpacker: A Handbook of Year Round, Long-Distance Hiking.* St. Louis: McGraw-Hill.

Townsend, C. 2001. *The Backpacker's Pocketguide.* St. Louis: McGraw-Hill.

Winkle, J., and J. Ozmun. 2001. *Teaching Martial Arts for Fitness and Fun.* Champaign, IL: Human Kinetics.

 ## In the News

Because they were associated with X Games created for television, many activities such as snowboarding were considered "extreme sports" prior to the 2002 winter Olympics. Other similar activities are skateboarding, in-line skating, BMX, Moto X, and mountain biking. Many of these activities have now gained popularity as participation rather than spectator activities. Many cities have built, or are now building, municipal skate parks and pay-for-skate parks are becoming popular. Snowboarding, often looked down on by downhill and cross-country skiers, has become accepted since the appearance of medal winners on cereal boxes. Ski resorts have built half-pipe trails and snowboard jumps to accommodate these activities. Special adventure biking trails and facilities have also become popular in recent years. For more information see the "Web Resources" at the end of this concept.

Lab 9A: Jogging/Running

Name	**Section**	**Date**

Purpose: To give you an opportunity to experience one type of jogging program that can be used to develop and maintain cardiovascular fitness and to acquaint you with basic jogging techniques.

Procedure:

1. Work with a partner and evaluate each other on jogging techniques.
   a. Stand 20 yards in front of your partner while he/she jogs toward you; watch his/her arm and leg swing and foot placement.
   b. Jog along 10 yards behind your partner while he/she is jogging and watch for arm and leg swing and foot placement.
   c. Stand 10 yards to one side as your partner jogs past you; watch for body position and foot placement.
   d. Change places with your partner and repeat this procedure.
2. Check the appropriate Correct or Incorrect boxes in Chart 1.
3. Using proper jogging technique, jog for 15 minutes at your own individual cardiovascular threshold of training. You may use a heart rate monitor or count post-exercise heart rate to determine jogging heart rate.

Results:

Record your target zone heart rate here ☐ bpm

Record your heart rate after the jog ☐ bpm

Have your partner evaluate your jogging technique and then record your results in Chart 1.

Chart 1 ▶ Jogging Technique

Body Segment	Check Appropriate Circles Below		Technique
	Correct	**Incorrect**	
Foot placement	◯	◯	Heel hits ground first
	◯	◯	Rock forward, push off ball of foot
	◯	◯	Toes point straight ahead
	◯	◯	Feet under knees, do not swing side to side
Length of stride	◯	◯	Stride is several inches longer than regular step
Arm movement	◯	◯	Elbows bent at 90 degrees
	◯	◯	Arms swing front to back, not side to side
	◯	◯	Arms and legs move in opposition
	◯	◯	Hands and arms are relaxed
Body position	◯	◯	Upper body nearly erect
	◯	◯	Head and chest are up

Conclusions and Implications:

1. In several sentences, give an overall evaluation of your jogging technique.

2. In several sentences, indicate whether jogging is an appropriate activity for you. Indicate your reasons for your answer.

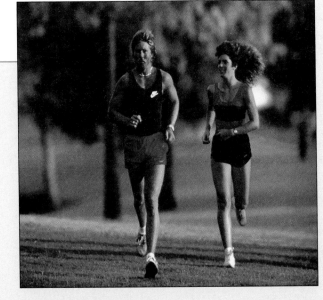

Lab 9B: Planning and Logging Participation in Active Aerobics, Sports, and Recreation

Name		Section	Date

Purpose: To set one-week lifestyle physical activity goals, to prepare a plan, and to self-monitor progress in your one-week active aerobics, active sports, and active recreation plan.

Procedures:

1. Use the planning calendar (Chart 1) to schedule several aerobic exercise sessions for the week. Plan at least three sessions but be realistic in your plan. Schedule activities that you enjoy and that you can conveniently perform. You may mix different activities each day for variety. Indicate the days you expect to do them and the length of time you expect to do the activity.
2. Keep a one-week log of your actual participation using Chart 2. If possible, keep the log with you during the day. Any time you perform an activity for 10 minutes, check one of the boxes. If you perform more than 10 minutes of activity in one session, check additional 10-minute blocks. If you cannot keep the log with you, fill in the log at the end of the day. If you choose to keep a log for more than one week, use the extra log sheet or make copies of the extra log sheet.
3. Log only those activities for which you meet the target zone for cardiovascular fitness. Remember that five to six, rather than seven days a week of more vigorous activity, is recommended. You can create a log book using several log sheets.
4. Sum the total number of minutes for each day by tallying the number of activity blocks.
5. Answer the questions in the Results section.

Chart 1 ▶ Planning Calendar

Write the number of minutes you plan to do each activity each day: You may mix activities each day.	Monday	Tuesday	Wednesday	Thursday	Friday	Saturday	Sunday
Aerobic exercise machines							
Cycling (including stationary)							
Circuit training or calisthenics							
Dance or step aerobics							
Hiking or backpacking							
Jogging or running (or walking)							
Skating/cross-country skiing							
Swimming							
Water activity							
Sport							
Other							
Other							
Daily Totals							

Results:

	Yes	No
Did you do 20 or more minutes at each session?	○	○
Did you do 20 or more minutes of activity on at least three days?	○	○

Conclusions and Interpretations:

1. Do you feel that you will use active aerobics, active sports, or active recreation as a regular part of your lifetime physical activity plan, either now or in the future? Use several sentences to explain your answer.

2. Did the logging of your activity make you more aware of your daily activity patterns? In several sentences, explain why or why not.

Chart 2 ▶ Aerobic Activity Log

Record the type and
length of each activity
you performed.

	10-Minute Blocks						Total Minutes	Comments*
Day 1 Date:	1	2	3	4	5	6		
Activity:								
Activity:								
Activity:								
Daily Total								
Day 2 Date:	1	2	3	4	5	6		
Activity:								
Activity:								
Activity:								
Daily Total								
Day 3 Date:	1	2	3	4	5	6		
Activity:								
Activity:								
Activity:								
Daily Total								
Day 4 Date:	1	2	3	4	5	6		
Activity:								
Activity:								
Activity:								
Daily Total								
Day 5 Date:	1	2	3	4	5	6		
Activity:								
Activity:								
Activity:								
Daily Total								
Day 6 Date:	1	2	3	4	5	6		
Activity:								
Activity:								
Activity:								
Daily Total								

*Optional: Record heart rate, pace, calories, or other details of your session.

141

Chart 3 ▶ Extra Aerobic Activity Log

Record the type and length of each activity you performed.	10-Minute Blocks						Total Minutes	Comments*
Day 1 Date:	1	2	3	4	5	6		
Activity:								
Activity:								
Activity:								
Daily Total								
Day 2 Date:	1	2	3	4	5	6		
Activity:								
Activity:								
Activity:								
Daily Total								
Day 3 Date:	1	2	3	4	5	6		
Activity:								
Activity:								
Activity:								
Daily Total								
Day 4 Date:	1	2	3	4	5	6		
Activity:								
Activity:								
Activity:								
Daily Total								
Day 5 Date:	1	2	3	4	5	6		
Activity:								
Activity:								
Activity:								
Daily Total								
Day 6 Date:	1	2	3	4	5	6		
Activity:								
Activity:								
Activity:								
Daily Total								

*Optional: Record heart rate, pace, calories, or other details of your session.

Flexibility

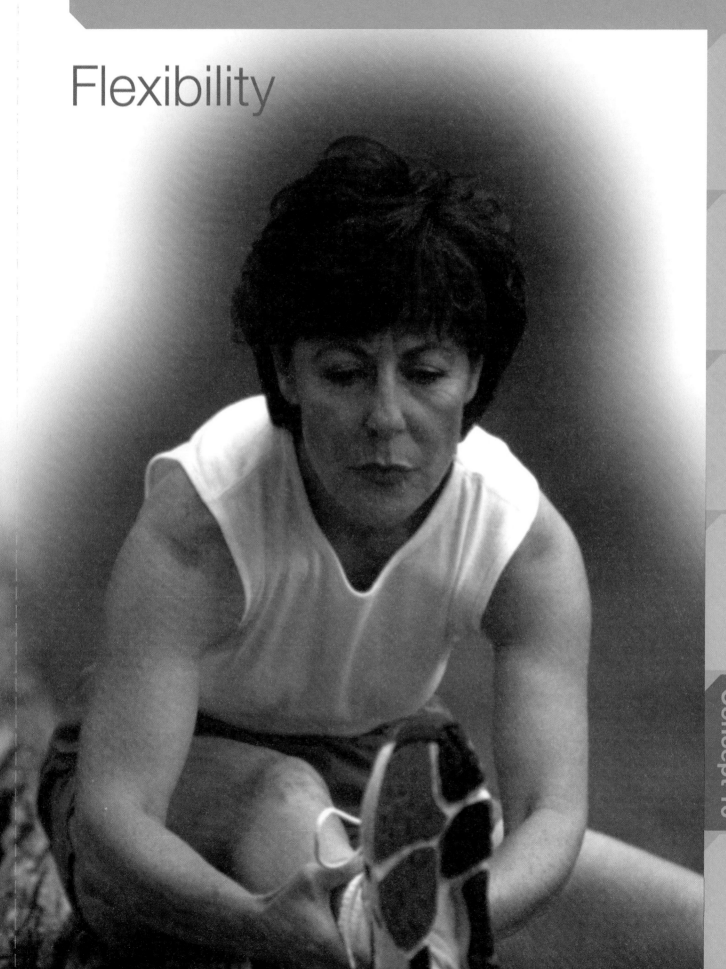

Regular stretching exercises promote flexibility—a component of fitness—that permits freedom of movement, contributes to ease and economy of muscular effort, allows for successful performance in certain activities, and provides less susceptibility to some types of injuries or musculoskeletal problems.

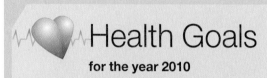

Health Goals

for the year 2010

- Increase proportion of people who regularly perform exercises for flexibility.

Flexibility is a measure of the range of motion available at a joint or group of joints. It is determined by the shape of the bones and cartilage in the joint, and by the length and extensibility of muscles, tendons, ligaments, and fascia that cross the joint. The range of movement at a joint may vary. In some cases, the joint will not bend or straighten and is said to be tight or stiff, or to have contractures. The deformed hand of an arthritic is an example of this extreme. At the other end of the spectrum, a high degree of flexibility is referred to as loose jointedness, hypermobility, or erroneously, as double-jointedness. An example of this extreme is the contortionist seen at the circus. Each person, depending upon his or her individual needs, must have a reasonable amount of flexibility to perform efficiently and effectively in daily life.

Stretching is a type of physical activity done with the intent of improving flexibility. The many types of stretching exercises designed to promote or maintain flexibility are described in this concept.

Factors Influencing Flexibility

Flexibility is not the same thing as stretching. Flexibility is a component of health-related physical fitness. It is a state of being. Stretching is the primary technique used to improve ▶ the state of one's flexibility.

Long muscle-tendon units (MTUs) are important to flexibility. **Range of motion (ROM)** in a joint is an indicator of one's flexibility. Joint ROM is influenced by the extensibility of **ligaments,** the surrounding muscles, and the **tendons** that connect the muscles to the bone. Having long muscles and tendons allows for greater range of motion and better flexibility. Together, the muscles and tendons are referred to as a **muscle-tendon unit (MTU).** Muscle fibers are more extensible and elastic than tendons but both are stretched together. However, for ease of understanding, the phrase "muscle stretching" rather than MTU stretching will be used.

Lack of use, injury, or disease can decrease joint mobility. Arthritis and calcium deposits can damage a joint, and inflammation can cause pain that prevents movement. Failure to move a joint regularly through its full range of motion can lead to a shortening of muscles and ligaments. Static positions held for long periods, such as in poor posture, working postures, and when a body part is immobilized by a cast, lead to shortened tissue and loss of mobility. Improper exercise that overdevelops one muscle group while neglecting the opposing group results in an imbalance that restricts flexibility. For example, body builders who overdevelop their biceps in comparison to the triceps develop a muscle-bound look that is characterized by a restricted range of motion in the elbow joint.

Some people are unusually flexible because of a genetic trait that makes their joints hypermobile. In some families, the trait for loose joints is passed from generation to generation. This **hypermobility** is sometimes referred to as joint looseness. Studies show that people with this trait may be more prone to joint dislocation. There is not much research evidence, but some experts believe that those with hypermobility or **laxity** may also be more susceptible to athletic or dance injuries, especially to the knee, ankle, and shoulder and may be more apt to develop premature osteoarthritis. One recent

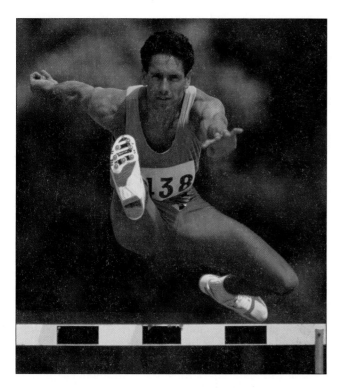

Flexibility aids athletic performance and may help reduce injury risk.

You do not have to sacrifice flexibility in order to develop strength. A person with bulging muscles may become muscle-bound or have a restricted range of motion if strength training is done improperly. In any progressive resistance program, both the muscle being strengthened and the **antagonist muscles** should receive equal training, and all movements should be carried through the full range of motion. Properly conducted strength training does not cause a person to be muscle-bound. A good rule of thumb is: "Stretch what you strengthen and strengthen what you stretch."

Health Benefits of Flexibility and Stretching

No ideal standard for flexibility exists. We do not know how much flexibility any one person should have in a joint. Norms are available that list how hundreds of subjects of various ages, of both sexes, and in many walks of life have performed on different tests. But there is little scientific evidence to indicate that a person who can reach 2 inches past his or her toes on a sit-and-reach test is less fit than a person who can reach 8 inches past the toes. Too much flexibility could be as detrimental as too little. The standards presented in the lab resource materials are based on the best available evidence.

Adequate flexibility may help prevent muscle strain and such orthopedic problems as backache. Back pain is a leading medical complaint in Western culture.

study found that subjects who were loose-jointed used more energy in walking and jogging than those who were medium- or tight-jointed.

In the fifth century, Hippocrates noted the disadvantage of hyperextension of the elbow in archery. The hyperextended position for elbows and knees is not an efficient position from which to move because of a poor angle of muscle pull. For example, it is difficult to perform push-ups when the elbows lock into hyperextension because extra effort is required to unlock the joint. It may be advantageous for loose-jointed people to take extra care to strengthen muscles around the joints most used.

Flexibility is influenced by several factors, including age, sex, and race. Flexibility is generally high in children but declines in early adolescence due to changes with maturation. Girls tend to be more flexible than boys, but the gender difference becomes smaller for adults. The greater flexibility of females may be due to anatomical differences and hormonal influences, as well as to the type and extent of activities that are performed. In adults, there is less difference between the sexes. Some races and ethnic groups have been reported to have specific joints that are hypermobile. For example, the thumb and finger joints of Middle Eastern people and East Indians tend to be more flexible. Older adults frequently have reduced flexibility, principally because of reduced activity. Studies show that regular stretching can help older people maintain good flexibility throughout life.

Range of Motion (ROM) The full motion possible in a joint.

Ligaments Bands of tissue that connect bones. Unlike muscles and tendons, overstretching ligaments is not desirable.

Tendon A fibrous band of collagen tissue that connects muscles to bones and facilitates movement of a joint.

Muscle-Tendon Unit (MTU) The skeletal muscles and the tendons that connect them to bones. Stretching to improve flexibility is associated with increased length of the MTU.

Hypermobility Looseness or slackness in the joint and of the muscles and ligaments (soft tissue) surrounding the joint.

Laxity Motion in a joint outside the normal plane for that joint, due to loose ligaments.

Antagonist Muscles In this concept, antagonist refers to the muscle group on the opposite side of the limb from the muscle group being stretched (e.g., biceps is antagonist of triceps).

One common cause of backache is shortened lower back muscles and hip flexor muscles. Short hamstrings (muscles in the back of the leg) are also associated with lower back problems. Improving flexibility can decrease risk of back problems. For more information concerning the importance of flexibility and muscle fitness to good back health consult concept 13.

Adequate flexibility is necessary for achieving and maintaining optimal posture. When muscles in specific body regions are too short, poor posture can result. Shortness of muscles that can result in back pain is also likely to contribute to a posture problem called swayback. Short shoulder muscles can result in rounded shoulders and forward head.

Adequate flexibility may reduce risk of muscle strain. It has not been conclusively proven that flexibility reduces risk of muscle injuries; however, short, tight muscles are more likely to be involuntarily overstretched than are long ones. Injury to tendons is also thought to be more likely if flexibility is limited.

Flexibility is associated with effective daily functioning, including driving ability, among older adults. Older drivers who perform stretching exercises, to improve their range of motion, are better able to look over their shoulders for blind spots or to parallel park, and back into parking spaces than older drivers with poor flexibility. It is normal for tissue to lose its elasticity with age, but a sedentary lifestyle is clearly the greatest contributor to loss of flexibility with aging. Fortunately, the elderly do respond to training. Spinal mobility is important not only for driving but also for daily activities such as tying one's shoes and reaching and twisting.

Good flexibility can bring about improved athletic performance. Proper stretching can increase muscle length, reduce **stiffness,** and increase **stretch tolerance,** leading most experts to agree that regular stretching and improved flexibility can enhance athletic performance. For example, a diver must have flexibility to perform a pike dive and a hurdler must have good flexibility in the back, hip, and leg to perform well. The most recent evidence, however, suggests that under some circumstances stretching can actually impair performance. For example, one expert suggests that too much stretching during the warm-up can result in short-term decreases in performance. A stretching warm-up is still recommended after a general warm-up, but the warm-up is not the time to conduct an extensive flexibility program, especially for those preparing for a high-level performance. The bulk of stretching is best done toward the end of other training sessions when the muscles are warm and when a performance is not imminent. Other athletes who can benefit from good flexibility are power athletes, such as baseball pitchers and high jumpers, who can apply force through a greater range of motion when they possess good flexibility. Weight lifters may also enhance performances by increasing flexibility.

Performing stretching exercises has benefits in addition to those that result from having good flexibility. As noted earlier in this concept, people who do regular stretching exercises receive benefits in addition to those that come from having good flexibility. However, all people with good flexibility do not do stretching exercises on a regular basis. Of course, one of the benefits of stretching is increased flexibility, so people who are active get both the benefits of good flexibility and regular exercise.

Static muscle stretching is effective in relieving muscle spasms. A muscle spasm or cramp may result for various reasons, including overexertion, dehydration, and heat stress. Stretching a cramped (but not a strained) muscle will help relieve the cramp. Stretching should be done statically and can be done with active or passive assistance, though passive assistance should be applied carefully. For example, a person with a cramp or spasm in the calf muscle can pull the toe toward the shin using the shin muscles, or a partner could push the ball of the foot toward the shin to get the same benefit.

Trigger points may sometimes be prevented or inactivated by static or PNF stretching of the muscles involved. When body parts are held in static positions for long periods, or when muscles are chronically overloaded, fatigued, or chilled, myofascial **trigger points** may cause stiffness and local or referred pain. Often, the trigger point can be deactivated and the pain relieved by gentle but persistent stretching of the muscle, especially if heat or cold packs are applied.

Stretching exercises are useful in preventing and remediating some cases of dysmenorrhea in women. Painful menstruation (dysmenorrhea) of some types can be prevented or reduced by stretching the pelvic and hip joint fascia. Billig's exercise is an example of an effective exercise for this condition.

Static stretching is probably *ineffective* **in preventing muscle soreness.** In the past, it was suggested that stretching during a cool-down will *prevent* muscular soreness. In a controlled study, muscle soreness was deliberately induced in a group of subjects. When half of the group stretched immediately afterward and at intervals for 48 hours, they had no less soreness than the group who did not stretch.

Stretching Methods

To develop flexibility, do exercises from the flexibility exercise section of the physical activity pyramid. The activities in the first two levels of the physical activity pyramid (see Figure 1) do little to develop flexibility. To build this important part of fitness, stretching exercises from the third level of the pyramid are essential. Three commonly used types of stretching exercises are **static stretch, proprioceptive neuromuscular facilitation exercise (PNF),** and **ballistic stretch.**

Static stretching is widely recommended because most experts believe it is less likely to cause injury. Static stretching is done slowly and held for a period of several seconds. With this type of stretch, the probability of tearing the soft tissue is low if performed properly. Static stretches can be performed with **active assistance** or with **passive assistance.**

When active assistance is used, you contract the opposing muscle group to produce a reflex relaxation **(reciprocal inhibition)** in the muscles you are stretching. This enables you to stretch the muscle more easily. For example, when doing a calf stretch exercise (see Figure 2A), the muscles on the front of the shin are contracted to assist in the stretch of the muscles of the calf. For this reason, many experts prefer static stretch with active assistance. However, active assistance to static stretching has one problem. It is almost impossible to produce adequate overload by simply contracting the opposing muscles.

When passive assistance (see Figures 2B, C) is used, an outside force, such as a partner aids you in stretching. For example, in the calf stretch, passive assistance can be provided by another person (Figure 2B), another body part (Figure 2B), or gravity (Figure 2C). This type of stretch does not create the relaxation in the muscle associated with active assisted stretch. An unrelaxed muscle cannot be stretched as far, and injury may happen. Therefore, it is best to combine the active assistance with a passive assistance when performing a static stretch. This gives the advantage of a relaxed muscle and a sufficient force to provide an overload to stretch it.

A good way to begin static stretching exercises is to stretch until you begin to feel tension, back off slightly and hold the position several seconds, then gradually stretch a little farther, back off and hold. Decrease the stretch slowly after the hold.

🌐 **PNF techniques have proven to be most effective at improving flexibility. www.mhhe.com/ fit_well/web10 Click 01.** PNF has been popular for rehabilitation since the 1960s. It consists of dozens of techniques to stimulate muscles to contract more strongly or to relax more fully so that they can be stretched. Several PNF techniques have become popular in fitness programs to improve the flexibility of healthy people. The contract-relax-antagonist-contract (CRAC) technique is the most popular. CRAC PNF involves three steps: (1) move the

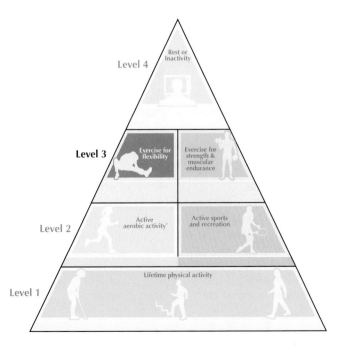

Figure 1 Flexibility or stretching exercises should be selected from level 3 of the physical activity pyramid.

Stiffness Elasticity in the MTU; measured by force needed to stretch.

Stretch Tolerance Greater stretch for the same pain level.

Trigger Point An especially irritable spot, usually a tight band or knot in a muscle or fascia. This often refers pain to another area of the body.

Static Stretch A muscle is slowly stretched, then held in that stretched position for several seconds.

Proprioceptive Neuromuscular Facilitation (PNF) Exercise A type of static stretch most commonly characterized by a precontraction of the muscle to be stretched and a contraction of the antagonist muscle during the stretch.

Ballistic Stretch Muscles are stretched by the force of momentum of a body part that is bounced, swung, or jerked.

Active Assistance An assist to stretch from an active contraction of the opposing (antagonist) muscle.

Passive Assistance Stretch imposed on a muscle with the assistance of a force other than the opposing muscle.

Reciprocal Inhibition Reflex relaxation in stretched muscle during contraction of the antagonist.

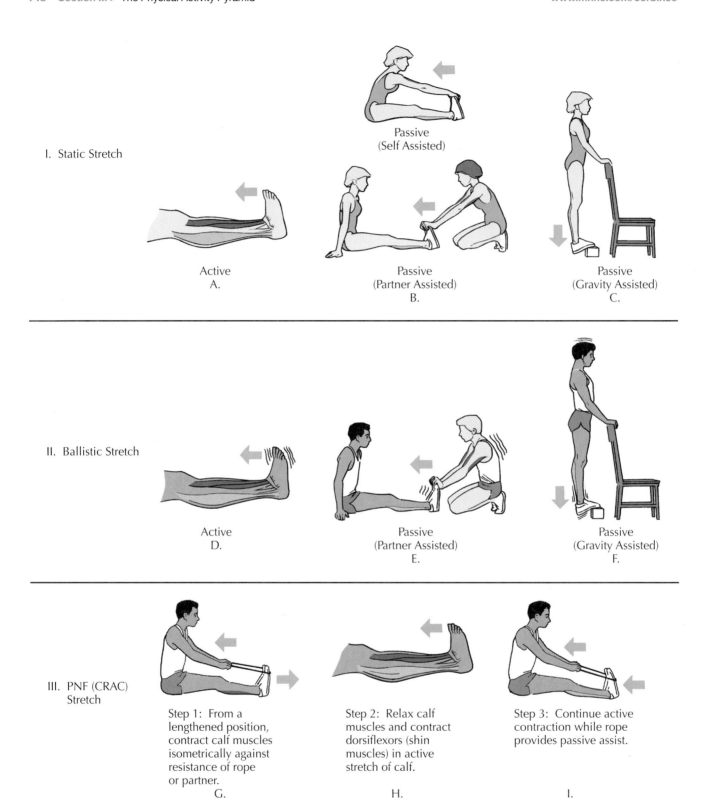

Figure 2 ▶ Examples of static, ballistic, PNF, active, and passive stretches of the calf muscles (gastrocnemius and soleus). Muscles shown in dark pink are the muscles being contracted. Muscles shown in pink are those being stretched.

limb so the muscle to be stretched is elongated initially, then contract it **(agonist muscle)** isometrically for several seconds (against an immovable object or the resistance of a partner); (2) relax the muscle; and (3) immediately statically stretch the muscle with the active assistance of the antagonist muscle and an assist from a partner, gravity, or other body part. Figures 2*G, H,* and *I* provide a detailed illustration of how this technique is applied to the calf stretch. Research shows that this and other types of PNF stretch are more effective than a simple static stretch.

Ballistic stretching may be an important technique for athletes. A ballistic stretch uses momentum to produce the stretch. Momentum is produced by vigorous motion, such as flinging a body part (bobbing) or rocking it back and forth to create a bouncing movement. As with static stretching, the ballistic movement can be provided either actively or passively. For example, in the calf stretch shown in Figures 2*D, E,* and *F,* the foot is actively bounced forward by the antagonist muscle force or passively by an assist from another person or gravity. Some sport-specific examples of ballistic stretch are provided in the concept on performance.

Active lifestyles aid in maintaining range of motion. www.mhhe.com/fit_well/web10 Click 02. Regular stretching is best for optimal flexibility. Merely being active does not overload (stretch) muscles and tendons adequately. However, being active in ways that requires the use of all joints can help you maintain range of motion especially as you grow older.

How Much Stretch Is Enough

A minimum amount of exercise and an optimal amount of exercise (target zone) are necessary for developing flexibility. Threshold and target zones for each type of stretching to improve and maintain flexibility are presented in Table 1. The values in this table illustrate how the principles of overload and progression are best applied to promote and maintain flexibility through regular stretching.

Stretching exercises must be done frequently to improve or maintain flexibility. It is generally agreed that stretching should be done at least three days a week and preferably daily. After a week without stretching, muscle length decreases and stiffness increases, suggesting that stretching one day a week can help maintain muscle length and increase stretch tolerance if more frequent stretching is not possible.

To increase the length of a muscle, you must stretch it more than its normal length (overload) but not overstretch it. There is much that is not known about flexibility, but the best evidence suggests that muscles should be stretched to about 10 percent beyond their normal length to bring about an improvement in flexibility.

> **Agonist Muscles** Refers to the muscle group being stretched.

Table 1 ▶ Flexibility Threshold of Training and Target Zones

	Threshold of Training			Target Zones		
	Static	**Ballistic**	**PNF (CRAC)**	**Static**	**Ballistic**	**PNF (CRAC)**
Frequency	• 3 days per week for all methods			• 3 to 7 days per week for all methods		
Intensity	• Stretch as far as you can go without pain; with slow movement, hold at the end of the range of motion.	• Stretch muscle beyond normal length with gentle bounce or swing, but do not exceed 10 percent of active-static range of motion.	• Same as static except use a maximum isometric contraction of muscle prior to stretch.	• Add assist. • Avoid overstretch and pain for all methods.	• Same as threshold.	• Same as static. • Add assist.
Time	• Hold 15 seconds. • 3 reps. • Rest 30 seconds between reps.	• Continuous reps for 30 seconds (this is 1 set).	• Hold isometric contraction 3 seconds. • Hold stretch 15 seconds. • 3 reps. • Rest 30 seconds between reps.	• Hold 15–60 seconds. • 3–5 reps. • Rest 30 seconds between reps. • Rest 1 minute between sets.	• 1–3 sets. • Rest 1 minute between sets.	• 3–5 reps of 3 second contraction and 15–60 second hold. • Rest 30 seconds between reps. • 1–3 sets. • Rest 1 minute between sets.

More practical indicators of the intensity of stretching are to stretch just to the point of tension or just before discomfort. Exercises that do not cause an overload will not increase flexibility. Excessively intense stretching may actually result in decreased flexibility. Once adequate flexibility has been achieved, **range of motion exercises (ROM)** that do not require stretch greater than normal can be performed to maintain flexibility and joint range of motion.

For flexibility to be increased, you must stretch and hold muscles beyond normal length for an adequate amount of time. When a muscle is stretched (lengthened), sensory receptors (A) in the MTU (muscle-tendon unit) send a signal to sensory neurons (B). They signal the motor neurons (C) that initiates a reflex contraction (shortening) of the muscle (D). This reflex restricts initial efforts at stretching; however, if the stretch is held and maintained over time, the stretch reflex subsides and allows the muscle to lengthen (this phase is called the development phase because it is at this time that improvements occur). This reflex is important to understand because it explains why it is important to hold a stretch for an extended period of time. Attempts to stretch for shorter durations are limited by the opposing action of the stretch reflex (see Figure 3). In the past, stretches of 10 to 30 seconds were recommended. New studies, however, suggest that to get the most benefit for the least effort, stretching for at least 15 seconds and up to 30 to 60 seconds for each repetition is recommended (see Figure 3).

For flexibility to be increased, you must repeat stretching exercises an adequate number of times. Figure 4 provides a graphical representation of the typical responses to a stretched muscle during a series of stretches. Tension in a muscle decreases as the stretch is held. The

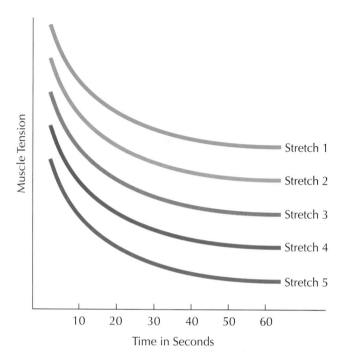

Figure 4 ▶ Typical responses to a stretched muscle during a series of stretches.

majority of the decrease occurs in the first 15 seconds. The tension curves are lower with each successive repetition of stretching, which is why multiple sets of stretching are recommended. The ACSM recommends three to four repetitions because this number seems to give the most benefits for the amount of time spent in exercise. Recent evidence suggests that one or two repetitions are adequate for most healthy people not interested in high-level performance.

Performing warm-up exercises is not the same as doing a stretching workout for flexibility development. The warm-up typically includes stretching exercises to prepare you for the workout and to reduce the risk of injury. Modest static stretching exercises done after a general warm-up are recommended by most experts (see concept on preparing for physical activity). Stretching exercises are typically done later in the workout to promote flexibility.

The best time for stretching is when the muscles are warm. Some studies have shown that increasing the temperature of the muscle through warm-up exercises or applying heat packs has resulted in improved ability to stretch the muscle. Other studies have failed to find a difference between the flexibility of subjects who warmed up and those who did not warm up. Some experts believe that cooling the muscle with ice packs in the final phases of stretching aids in lengthening the muscle, but a recent study has failed to confirm this. Until scientists reach a consensus, it seems wise to perform the stretching phase of your workout when the muscles are warm. This means

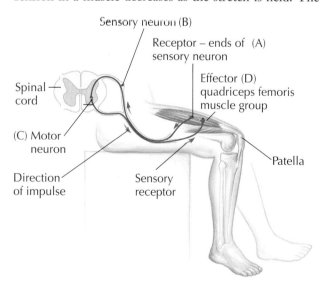

Figure 3 ▶ The stretch reflex.

Source: Shier, D., Butler, J., and Lewis, R.

that stretching can be done in the middle or near the end of the workout. Since some people do not want to interrupt their workout in the middle, they prefer to stretch at the end. Stretching at the end of the workout serves a dual purpose—building flexibility and cooling down. It is, however, appropriate to stretch at any time in the workout after the muscles have been active and are warm.

Guidelines for Safe and Effective Stretching

There is a correct way to perform flexibility exercises. Remember that stretching can *cause* muscle soreness, so "easy does it." Start at your threshold if you are unaccustomed to stretching a given muscle group, then increase within the target zone. The list in Table 2 will help you to gain the most benefit from your exercises.

 Stretching is specific to each muscle or muscle group.   www.mhhe.com/fit_well/web10 Click 03. No single exercise can produce total flexibility. For example, stretching tight hamstrings can increase the length of these muscles but will not lengthen the muscles in other areas of the body. For total flexibility, it is important to stretch each of the major muscle groups of the body and to use the major joints of the body through full range of normal motion.

Overstretching may make a person susceptible to injury or hamper performance. Muscles and tendons have the ability to lengthen (extensibility) and to return to their normal length after stretching (elasticity). Ligaments and the joint capsule are extensible but lack elasticity. When stretched, they remain in the lengthened state. If this occurs, the joint may lack stability and is susceptible to chronic dislocation or movement in an undesirable plane. This is particularly true of weight-bearing joints, such as the hip, knee, and ankle. Loose ligaments may allow the joint to twist abnormally, tearing the cartilage and other soft tissue.

 Technology Update

Technology has provided us with many advancements including computer devices and high tech medicines and procedures. A less sophisticated, but quite effective advancement, is the stretching rope. This type of rope has multiple loops that enable you to change the length of the rope and perform a variety of exercises. The rope allows you to perform static and PNF stretching exercises without the assistance of a partner. There are several different stretching ropes available commercially. For more information consult the Web Resources section at the end of the concept.

Range of Motion (ROM) Exercises   Exercises used to maintain existing joint mobility (to prevent loss of ROM).

Table 2 ► Do and Don't List for Stretching

Do	Don't
Do warm muscles before you attempt to stretch them.	Don't stretch to the point of pain. Remember, you want to stretch muscles, not joints!
Do stretch with care if you have osteoporosis or arthritis.	Don't use ballistic stretches if you have osteoporosis or arthritis.
Do use static or PNF stretching rather than ballistic stretching if you are a beginner.	Don't perform ballistic stretches with passive assistance unless you are under the supervision of an expert.
Do stretch weak or recently injured muscles with care.	Don't ballistically stretch weak or recently injured muscles.
Do use great care in applying passive assistance to a partner; go slowly and ask for feedback.	Don't stretch a muscle after it has been immobilized (such as in a sling or cast) for a long period.
Do perform stretching exercises for each muscle group and at each joint where flexibility is desired.	Don't bounce a muscle through excessive range of motion. Ballistic stretches should be gentle and should not involve excessive range of motion.
Do make certain the body is in good alignment when stretching.	Don't stretch swollen joints without professional supervision.
Do stretch muscles of small joints in the extremities first, then progress toward the trunk with muscles of larger joints.	Don't stretch several muscles all at one time until you have stretched individual muscles. For example, stretch muscles at the ankle, then the knee, then the ankle and knee simultaneously.
Do precede sport-specific ballistic stretch with static or PNF stretching.	

Strategies for Action

An important step in taking action for developing and maintaining flexibility is assessing your current status. www.mhhe.com/fit_well/web10 Click 04. An important early step in taking action to improve fitness is self-assessment. There are dozens of tests of flexibility. Four tests that assess range of motion in the major joints of the body, that require little equipment, and that can be easily administered are presented in the lab resources materials. In Lab 10A you will get an opportunity to try these self-assessments. It is recommended that you perform these assessments before you begin your regular stretching program and use these assessments to reevaluate your flexibility periodically.

Scores on flexibility tests may be influenced by several factors. Your range of motion at any one time may be influenced by your motivation to exert maximum effort, warm-up preparation, muscular soreness, tolerance for pain, room temperature, and ability to relax. Recent studies have found a relationship between leg or trunk length and the scores made on the sit-and-reach test. The sit-and-reach test used in this book is adapted to allow for differences in body build.

Select exercises that promote flexibility in all areas of the body. www.mhhe.com/fit_well/web10 Click 05. The ACSM recommends that adults regularly perform eight to ten stretching exercises for the major muscle groups of the body. Table 3 provides eight exercises referred to as the Basic 8. These exercises are easy to perform and meet the ACSM guidelines. For most people, these will be adequate for building flexibility for health and leisure-time recreational activities.

Additional exercises are provided for people who may want alternatives to the Basic 8 or who want to do more than the basic exercises (see Exercise 2). The exercises presented in Exercise Tables 1 and 2 are static stretching exercises that can also be performed using PNF techniques. Ballistic stretching exercises are discussed in more detail in the concept on performance benefits of physical activity.

Keeping records of progress is important to adhering to a stretching program. An activity logging sheet is provided in Lab 10B to help you keep records of your progress as you regularly perform stretching exercises to build and maintain good flexibility.

Web Resources

Flexibility Exercises www.mhhe.com/fit_well/web10 click 06
Orthopedic Physical Therapy Products (source for stretching ropes) www.optp.com
The Physician and Sports Medicine www.physsportsmed.com

Suggested Readings

Additional reference materials for concept 10 are available at www.mhhe.com/fit_well/web10 Click 07.

Alter, M. J. 1996. *Science of Stretch*. Champaign, IL: Human Kinetics Publishers.

Bracko, M. R. 2002. Can stretching prior to exercise and sports improve performance and prevent injury? *ACSM's Health and Fitness Journal* 6(5):17–22.

Chewning, B., T. M. A. Yu, and J. Johnson. 2000. Tai chi: Effects on health. *ACSM's Health and Fitness Journal* 4(3):17–19.

Fomby, E. W., and M. B. Mellon. 1997. Identifying and treating myofascial pain syndrome. *The Physician and Sports Medicine* 25(2):67.

Gleim, G. W., and M. P. McHugh. 1997. Flexibility and its effect on sports injury and performance. *Sports Medicine* 24:289–299.

Golding, L. A. 1997. Flexibility, stretching, and flexibility testing. *ACSM's Health and Fitness* 1(1):17.

Hootman, J. M. et al. 2002. Epidemiology of musculoskeletal injuries among sedentary and physically active adults. *Medicine and Science in Sports and Exercise* 34(5):838–844.

Knudson, D. 1998. Stretching: From science to practice. *Journal of Physical Education, Recreation and Dance* 69:38–42.

Knudsen, D. V. 2000. Stretching during warm-up: Do we have enough evidence? *Journal of Physical Education, Recreation and Dance* 70(2):271–277.

Knudsen, D. V. et al. 2000. Current issues in flexibility fitness. *President's Council on Physical Fitness and Sports Research Digest* 2(10):1–8.

McAtee, R. 1993. *Facilitated Stretching*. Champaign, IL: Human Kinetics Publishers.

Nieman, D. C. 2000. Exercise soothes arthritis. *ACSM's Health and Fitness Journal* 4(3):20.

Shrier, I., and K. Gossal. 2000. Myths and truths of stretching. *The Physician and Sports Medicine* 28(8):57–63.

In the News

During the past decade, the incidence of injury among major league baseball players has increased dramatically. The average number of injury days has increased by 55 percent compared to ten years ago. Large joint injuries (knee, ankle, elbow, and shoulder) have increased 58 percent. Ligaments and tendons are among the most frequently injured. Many experts suggest that the use of steroids has played a role in the increase in injury rate. Steroids are known to make connective tissue more brittle resulting in less flexibility.

Source: USA Today Research.

Table 3

Table 3 The Basic 8 for Stretching Exercises

1. Calf Stretcher

This exercise stretches the calf muscles and Achilles tendon. Face a wall with your feet two or three feet away. Step forward on your left foot to allow both hands to touch the wall. Keep the heel of your right foot on the ground, toe turned in slightly, knee straight, and buttocks tucked in. Lean forward by bending your front knee and arms and allowing your head to move nearer the wall. Hold. Bend right knee, keeping heel on floor. Stretch and hold. Repeat with other leg.

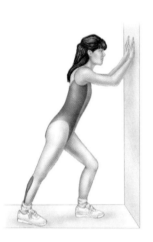

2. Hip and Thigh Stretcher

This exercise stretches the hip (iliopsoas) and thigh muscles (quadriceps) and is useful for people with lordosis and back prob-lems. Place right knee directly above right ankle and stretch left leg backward so knee touches floor. If necessary, place hands on floor for balance.

1. Tilt the pelvis forward by tucking in the abdomen and flattening the back.
2. Then shift the weight forward until a stretch is felt on the front of the thigh; hold. Repeat on opposite side. Caution: Do not bend front knee more than 90 degrees.

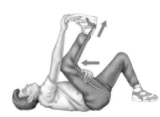

3. Sitting Stretcher

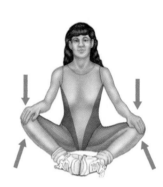

This exercise stretches the muscles on the inside of the thighs. Sit with soles of feet together; place hands on knees or ankles and lean forearms against knees; resist (contract) by attempting to raise knees. Hold. Relax and press the knees toward the floor as far as possible; hold. This exercise is useful for preg-nant women and anyone whose thighs tend to rotate inward causing backache, knock-knees, and flat feet.

4. Hamstring Stretcher

This exercise stretches the muscles on the back of the hip, thigh, knee, and ankle. Lie on your back with your knees bent. Bring right knee to chest and grasp toes with right hand. Place left hand on back of right thigh. Pull knee toward chest and push heel toward ceiling and pull toes toward shin. Attempt to straighten knee. Stretch and hold. Repeat on left side.

Table 3

5. Leg Hug

This exercise stretches the lower back and gluteals. Lie on your back with your knees bent in a hook-lying position. Contract gluteals and lumbar muscles. Lift hips. Hold for 3 seconds. Relax and pull knees to chest with arms as hard as possible; hold. Useful for people with backache and lordosis. Do not place the hands over the knees to apply stretch.

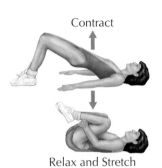

Contract

Relax and Stretch

7. Pectoral Stretch

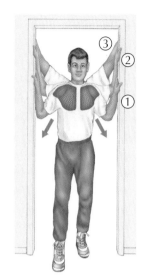

This exercise stretches the chest muscle (pectorals).
1. Stand erect in doorway with arms raised 45 degrees, elbows bent, and hands grasping doorjamb; feet in front-stride position. Press out on door frame, contracting the arms maximally for 3 seconds. Relax and shift weight forward on legs. Lean into doorway so muscles on front of shoulder joint and chest are stretched. Hold.
2. Repeat with arms raised 90 degrees.
3. Repeat with arms raised 135 degrees. Useful to prevent or correct round shoulders and sunken chest.

6. Trunk Twister

This exercise stretches the trunk muscles and muscles on the outside of hip. Sit with right leg extended, left leg bent and crossed over the right knee. Place right arm on the left side of the left leg and push against that leg while turning the trunk as far as possible to the left. Place left hand on floor behind buttocks. Stretch and hold. Reverse position and repeat on opposite side.

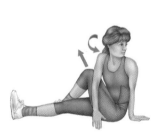

8. Arm Stretcher

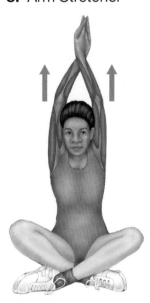

This exercise stretches the arm and chest muscles. Cross arms and turn palms of hands together. Raise arms overhead behind ears. Extend elbows. Stretch as high as possible. Hold.

Table 4

Table 4 Supplemental Stretching Exercises for Flexibility

1. Lower Leg Stretcher

This exercise stretches the calf muscles and Achilles tendon. Stand with the toes on a stair step or thick book. Use hands to balance by holding a rail or wall. Keep toes pointed straight ahead or slightly inward. Rise up on toes (contract) as far as possible and hold for 3 seconds. Relax and lower heels to floor as far as possible; hold. Static stretch may alleviate spasms or cramps in calf muscles.

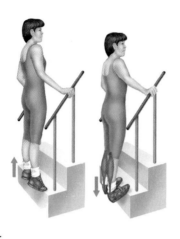

3. Lateral Thigh and Hip Stretch

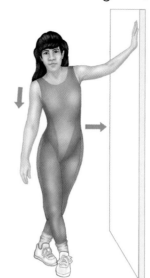

This exercise stretches the muscles and connective tissue on the outside of the legs (iliotibial band and tensor fascia lata). Stand with left side to wall, left arm extended and palm of hand flat on wall for support. Cross the left leg behind right and turn toes of both feet out slightly. Bend left knee slightly and shift pelvis toward wall (left) as trunk bends toward right. Adjust until tension is felt down outside of left hip and thigh. Stretch and hold. Repeat on other side.

2. Standing Thigh Stretcher

This exercise stretches the hip flexor (iliopsoas) and thigh muscles (quadriceps). Stand near a wall so you can use one hand for balance. Place the top of one foot on a flat surface slightly higher than knee height (use a chair or table). Keep the knee of the elevated foot bent. Slide the leg backward until a stretch is felt on the front of the thigh. Keep the top of the pelvis tilted backward so the back does not arch. Repeat with the opposite leg.

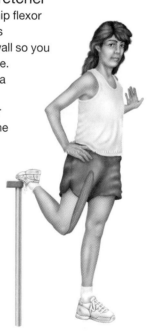

4. Back-Saver Hamstring Stretch

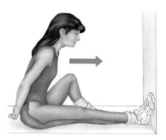

This exercise stretches the hamstrings and calf muscles and helps prevent or correct backache caused in part by short hamstrings. Sit on the floor with the feet against the wall or an immovable object.

Bend left knee and bring foot close to buttocks. Clasp hands behind back. Contract the muscles of the back of the upper leg (hamstrings) by pressing the heel downward toward the floor; hold; relax. Bend forward from hips, keeping lower back as straight as possible. Let bent knee rotate outward so trunk can move forward. Lean forward keeping back flat; hold and repeat on each leg.

5. One-Leg Stretcher

This exercise stretches the lower back and hamstring muscles. Stand with one foot on a bench, keeping both legs straight. Contract the hamstrings and gluteals by pressing down on bench with the heel for 3 seconds, then relax and bend the trunk forward, toward the knee. Hold for 10–15 seconds. Return to starting position and repeat with opposite leg. As flexibility improves, the arms can be used to pull the chest toward the legs. Do not allow either knee to lock. This exercise is useful in relief of backache and correction of lordosis (swayback).

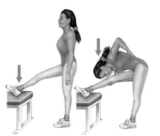

7. Wand Exercise

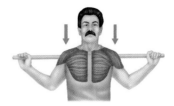

This exercise stretches the front of the shoulders and chest. Sit with wand grasped at ends. Raise wand overhead. Be certain that the head does not slide forward. Keep the chin tucked and neck straight. Bring wand down behind shoulder blades. Keep spine erect. Hold. Press forward on the wand simultaneously by pushing with the hands. Relax, then try to move the hands lower, sliding the wand down the back. Hold again. Hands may be moved closer together to increase stretch on chest muscles. If this is an easy exercise for you, try straightening the elbows and bringing the wand to waist level in back of you.

6. Lateral Trunk Stretcher

This exercise stretches the trunk muscles. Sit on the floor. Stretch the left arm over head to right. Bend to the right at waist, reaching as far to right as possible with left arm and as far as possible to the left with right arm; hold. Do not let trunk rotate. Repeat on opposite side. For less stretch, overhead arm may be bent at elbow. This exercise can be done in the standing position but is less effective.

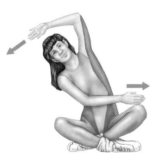

8. Arm Pretzel

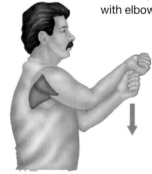

This exercise stretches the shoulder muscles (lateral rotators). Stand or sit with elbows flexed at right angles, palms up. Cross right arm over left; grasp right thumb with left hand and pull gently downward, causing right arm to rotate laterally. Stretch and hold. Reverse arm position and repeat on left arm.

Table 4

Table 4

Table 4 Supplemental Stretching Exercises for Flexibility

9. Shin Stretcher

This exercise relieves shin muscle soreness by stretching muscles on front of shin. Kneel on knees, turn to right, and press down and stretch right ankle with right hand. Move pelvis forward. Hold. Repeat on opposite side. Except when they are sore, most people need to strengthen rather than stretch these muscles.

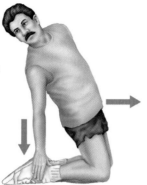

11. Billig's Exercise

This exercise stretches the pelvic fascia, hip flexors, and muscles of the inside thigh. Stand with side to a wall and place the elbow and forearm against the wall at shoulder height. Tilt the pelvis backward, tightening the gluteal and abdominal muscles. Place opposite hand on hip and push the hips toward the wall. Push forward and sideward (45 degrees) with the hips. Do not twist the hips. Hold. Repeat on opposite side. Useful for preventing some cases of dysmenorrhea.

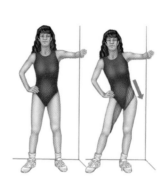

10. Spine Twist

This exercise stretches the trunk rotators and lateral rotators of the thighs. Start in hook-lying position, arms extended at shoulder level. Cross left knee over right; keep arms and shoulders on floor while touching knees to floor on left. Stretch and hold. Reverse leg position and lower knees to right.

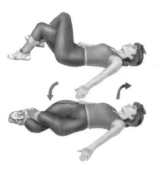

12. Two-Hand Ankle Wrap

This exercise is most useful for athletes or people interested in performance. It should not be done until after individual muscles have been stretched using other exercises. It stretches multiple muscle groups including the back, shoulders, and legs. Stand with heels together. Bend forward and place arms between knees; bend knees and wrap arms around legs, attempting to touch fingers in front of ankles. Hold.

Lab Resource Materials: Flexibility Tests

Directions: To test the flexibility of all joints is impractical. These tests are for joints used frequently. Follow the instructions carefully.

Test

1. *Modified Sit-and-Reach* (Flexibility Test of Hamstrings)
   a. Remove shoes and sit on the floor. Place the sole of the foot of the extended leg flat against a box or bench, and place the head, back, and hips against a wall with a 90-degree angle at the hips.
   b. Place one hand over the other and slowly reach forward as far as you can with arms fully extended. Keep head and back in contact with the wall. A partner will slide the measuring stick on the bench until it touches the fingertips.
   c. With the measuring stick fixed in the new position, reach forward as far as possible, three times, holding the position on the third reach for at least 2 seconds while the partner reads the distance on the ruler. Keep the knee of the extended leg straight (see illustration).
   d. Repeat the test a second time and average the scores of the two trials.

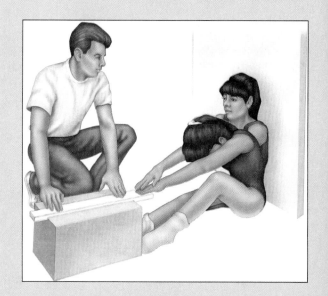

Test

2. *Shoulder Flexibility* ("Zipper" Test)
   a. Raise your arm, bend your elbow, and reach down across your back as far as possible.
   b. At the same time, extend your left arm down and behind your back, bend your elbow up across your back, and try to cross your fingers over those of your right hand as shown in the accompanying illustration.
   c. Measure the distance to the nearest half-inch. If your fingers overlap, score as a plus. If they fail to meet, score as a minus; use a zero if your fingertips just touch.
   d. Repeat with your arms crossed in the opposite direction (left arm up). Most people will find that they are more flexible on one side than the other.

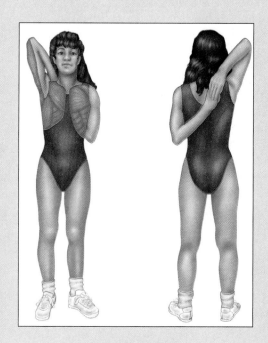

Test

3. *Hamstring and Hip Flexor Flexibility*

   a. Lie on your back on the floor beside a wall.

   b. Slowly lift one leg off the floor. Keep the other leg flat on the floor.

   c. Keep both legs straight.

   d. Continue to lift the leg until either leg begins to bend or the lower leg begins to lift off the floor.

   e. Place a yardstick against the wall and underneath the lifted leg.

   f. Hold the yardstick against the wall after the leg is lowered.

   g. Using a protractor, measure the angle created by the floor and the yardstick. The greater the angle, the better your score.

   h. Repeat with the other leg.*

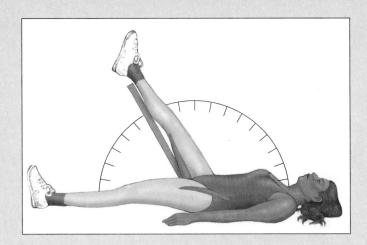

*Note: For ease of testing, you may want to draw angles on a piece of posterboard as illustrated. If you have goniometers, you may be taught to use them instead.

Test

4. *Trunk Rotation*

   a. Tape two yardsticks to the wall at shoulder height, one right side up and the other upside down.

   b. Stand with your left shoulder an arm's length (fist closed) from the wall. Toes should be on the line, which is perpendicular to the wall and even with the 15-inch mark on the yardstick.

   c. Drop the left arm and raise the right arm to the side, palm down, fist closed.

   d. Without moving your feet, rotate the trunk to the right as far as possible, reaching along the yardstick, and hold it 2 seconds. Do not move the feet nor bend the trunk. Your knees may bend slightly.

   e. A partner will read the distance reached to the nearest half-inch. Record your score. Repeat two times and average your two scores.

   f. Next, perform the test facing the opposite direction. Rotate to the left. For this test you will use the second yardstick (upside down) so that the greater the rotation, the higher the score. If you have only one yardstick, turn it right side up for the first test and upside down for the second test.

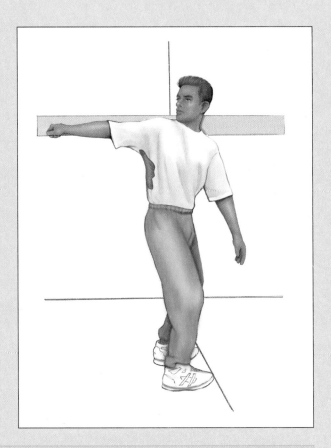

Chart 1 ▶ Flexibility Rating Scale for Tests 1–4

Classification	Men				Women				
	Test 1	Test 2		Test 3	Test 4	Test 1	Test 2		Test 3	Test 4
		Right Up	Left Up				Right Up	Left Up		
High-performance*	16+	5+	4+	111+	20+	17+	6+	5+	111+	20.5 or >
Good fitness zone	13–15	1–4	1–3	80–110	16–19.5	14–16	2–5	2–4	80–110	17–20
Marginal zone	10–12	0	0	60–79	13.5–15.5	11–13	1	1	60–79	14.5–16.5
Low zone	<9	<0	<0	<60	13 or less	<10	<1	<1	<60	14 or <

*Though performers need good flexibility, hypermobility may increase injury risk.

Lab 10A: Evaluating Flexibility

Name	Section	Date

Purpose: To evaluate your flexibility in several joints.

Procedure:

1. Take the flexibility tests outlined in the lab resource materials.
2. Record your scores in the Results section.
3. Use Chart 1 in the lab resource materials to determine your ratings on the self-assessments, then place an X over the circle for the appropriate rating.

Results:

Record Scores:	Record Ratings: High Performance	Good Fitness	Marginal	Poor
Modified sit-and-reach				
Test 1 Left	○	○	○	○
Right	○	○	○	○
Zipper				
Test 2 Left	○	○	○	○
Right	○	○	○	○
Hamstring/hip flexor				
Test 3 Left	○	○	○	○
Right	○	○	○	○
Trunk rotation				
Test 4 Left	○	○	○	○
Right	○	○	○	○

Do any of these muscle groups need stretching? Check one circle for each muscle group.

	Yes	No
Back of the thighs and knees (hamstrings)	◯	◯
Calf muscles	◯	◯
Lower back (lumbar region)	◯	◯
Front of right shoulder	◯	◯
Back of right shoulder	◯	◯
Front of left shoulder	◯	◯
Back of left shoulder	◯	◯
Most of the body	◯	◯
Trunk muscles	◯	◯

Conclusions and Implications: In several sentences, discuss your current flexibility and your flexibility needs for the future. Include comments about your current state of flexibility, need for improvement in specific areas, and special flexibility needs for sports or other special activities.

Lab 10B: Planning and Logging Stretching Exercises

Name	Section	Date

Purpose: To set one-week lifestyle goals for stretching exercises, to prepare a stretching for flexibility plan, and to self-monitor progress in your one-week plan.

Procedures:

1. On Chart 1 check the stretching exercises you plan to perform during the next week. Try to do at least eight exercises three times a week. The Basic 8 are listed. You may substitute other exercises by writing them in the "other" blank. See Exercise 2 for additional exercises.
2. Keep a one-week log of your actual participation using Chart 2. If possible, keep the log with you during the day. Place a check by each of the stretching exercises you perform each day, including ones that you didn't originally have planned. If you cannot keep the log with you, fill in the log at the end of the day. If you choose to keep a log for more than one week, make extra copies of the log before you begin.
3. Answer the questions in the Results section.

Chart 1 ▶ Stretching Exercise Plan

Place a check beside the stretching exercises you plan to do and under the days you plan to do them.	Day 1 Date:	Day 2 Date:	Day 3 Date:	Day 4 Date:	Day 5 Date:	Day 6 Date:	Day 7 Date:
1. Calf stretcher							
2. Hip and thigh stretcher							
3. Sitting stretcher							
4. Hamstring stretcher							
5. Back stretcher (leg hug)							
6. Trunk twister							
7. Pectoral stretcher							
8. Arm stretcher							
Other:							
Other:							
Other:							
Other:							

Results:

	Yes	No
Did you do eight exercises at least three days in the week?	○	○
Did you do eight exercises more than three days in the week?	○	○

Chart 2 ▶ Stretching Exercise Log

Place a check beside the stretching exercises you actually performed and the days on which you performed them.	Day 1 Date:	Day 2 Date:	Day 3 Date:	Day 4 Date:	Day 5 Date:	Day 6 Date:	Day 7 Date:
1. Calf stretcher							
2. Hip and thigh stretcher							
3. Sitting stretcher							
4. Hamstring stretcher							
5. Back stretcher (leg hug)							
6. Trunk twister							
7. Pectoral stretcher							
8. Arm stretcher							
Other:							
Other:							
Other:							
Other:							

Conclusions and Interpretations:

1. Do you feel that you will use stretching exercises as part of your regular lifetime physical activity plan, either now or in the future? Use several sentences to explain your answer.

2. Discuss the exercises you feel benefited you and the ones that did not. What exercises would you continue to do and which ones would you change? Use several sentences to explain your answer.

3. Did the logging of your stretching exercise help you to adhere to your program? In several sentences, explain why or why not.

Muscle Fitness

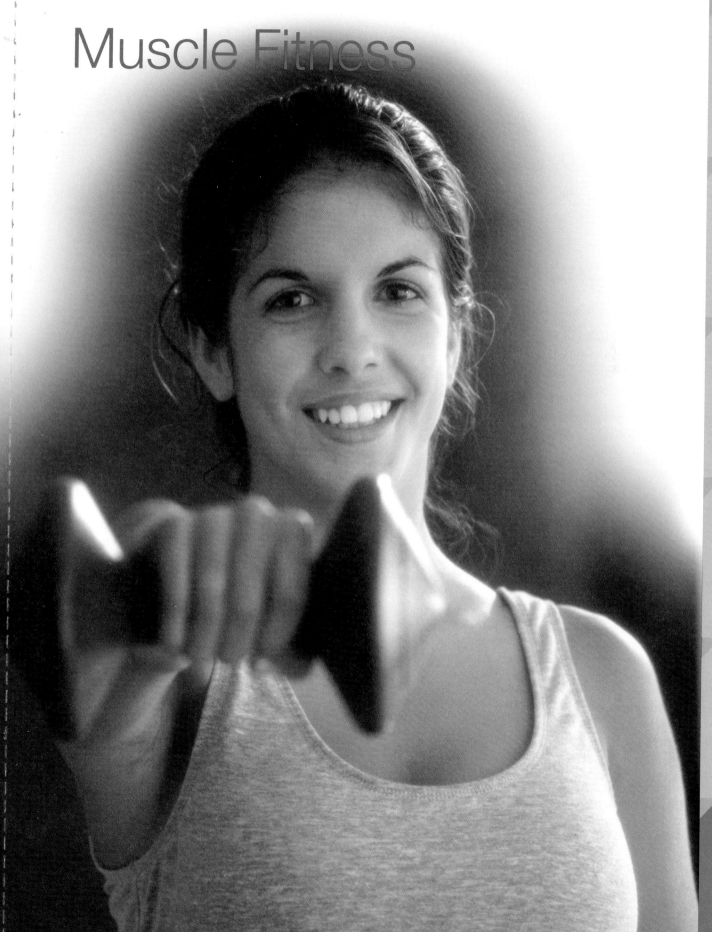

Progressive resistance exercise promotes muscle fitness that permits efficient and effective movement, contributes to ease and economy of muscular effort, promotes successful performance, and lowers susceptibility to some types of injuries, musculoskeletal problems, and some illnesses.

Health Goals

for the year 2010

- Increase proportion of people who regularly perform exercises for strength and muscular endurance.
- Reduce steroid use especially among youth.
- Increase screening and reduce incidence of osteoporosis.
- Reduce activity limitations due to chronic back pain.

There are two components of muscle fitness: strength and muscular endurance. Strength is the amount of force you can produce with a single maximal effort of a muscle group. Muscular endurance is the capacity of the skeletal muscles or group of muscles to continue contracting over a long period of time. You need both strength and muscular endurance to increase work capacity; to decrease the chance of injury; to prevent low back pain, poor posture, and other hypokinetic conditions; to improve athletic performance; and perhaps to save a life or property in an emergency. Muscle fitness training increases the fitness of the bones, tendons, and ligaments, as well as the muscles. It has been found to be therapeutic for patients with chronic pain.

Progressive resistance training is the type of physical activity done with the intent of improving muscle fitness. The many types of progressive resistance exercises designed to promote or maintain muscle fitness are described in this concept.

Factors Influencing Strength and Muscular Endurance

There are three types of muscle tissue. www.mhhe.com/fit_well/web11 Click 01. The three types of muscle tissue—smooth, cardiac, and skeletal—have different structures and functions. Smooth muscle tissue consists of long, spindle-shaped fibers with each fiber containing only one nucleus. The fibers are involuntary and are located in the walls of the esophagus, stomach, and intestines, where they function to move food and waste products through the digestive tract. Cardiac muscle tissue is also involuntary and, as its name implies, it is found only in the heart. These fibers contract in response to demands on the cardiovascular system. The heart muscle contracts at a slow steady rate at rest but contracts more frequently and forcefully during physical activity. Skeletal muscle tissues consist of long, cylindrical, multi-nucleated fibers. They provide the force needed to move the skeletal system and may be controlled voluntarily.

Leverage is an important mechanical principle that influences strength. www.mhhe.com/fit_well/web11 Click 02. The body uses a system of levers to produce movement. Muscles are connected to bones via tendons and some muscles (referred to as "primary movers") cross over a particular joint to produce movement. The movement occurs because when a muscle contracts it physically shortens and pulls the two bones connected by the joint together. Figure 1 shows the two heads of the biceps muscle inserting on the forearm. When the muscle contracts, the forearm is pulled up toward the upper arm (elbow flexion). A person with long arms and legs has a mechanical advantage in most movements since the force that is exerted can act over a longer distance. While it is not possible to change the length of your limbs it is possible to learn to use your muscles more effectively. The ability of Tiger Woods to hit golf balls 350 yards is due to his ability to generate torque and power rather than to his actual strength.

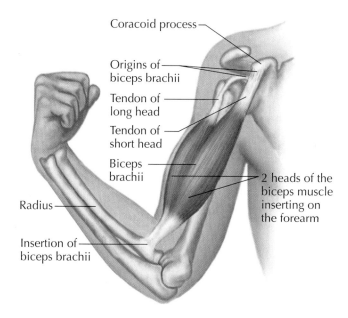

Coracoid process

Origins of
biceps brachii

Tendon of
long head

Tendon of
short head

Biceps
brachii

2 heads of the
biceps muscle
inserting on
the forearm

Radius

Insertion of
biceps brachii

Figure 1 ▶ Muscle action on body levers.

Skeletal muscle tissue consists of different types of fibers that respond and adapt differently to training. There are three distinct types of muscle fibers, slow-twitch (Type I), fast-twitch (Type IIb) and an intermediate fiber type (Type IIa). The slow-twitch fibers are generally red in color and are well-suited to produce energy with aerobic metabolism. Slow-twitch fibers generate less tension but are more resistant to fatigue. Endurance training leads to adaptations in the slow-twitch fibers that allow them to produce energy more efficiently and better resist fatigue. Fast-twitch fibers are generally white in color and are well-suited to produce energy with anaerobic processes. They generate greater tension than slow-twitch fibers, but they fatigue more quickly. These fibers are particularly well-suited to fast, high-force activities such as explosive weight-lifting movements, sprinting, and jumping. Progressive resistance exercise enhances strength primarily by increasing the size (muscle **hypertrophy**) of fast-twitch fibers but cellular adaptations also take place to enhance various metabolic properties. Intermediate fibers have biochemical and physiological properties that are between the slow-twitch and fast-twitch fibers. A distinct property of these intermediate fibers is that they are highly adaptable depending on the type of training that is performed.

An example of fast-twitch muscle fiber in animals is the white meat in the flying muscles of a chicken. The chicken is heavy and must exert a powerful force to fly a few feet up to a perch. A wild duck that flies for hundreds of miles has dark meat (slow-twitch fibers) in the flying muscles for better endurance.

People who want large muscles will use progressive resistance exercises designed to build strength (fast-twitch fibers). People who want to be able to persist in activities for a long period of time without fatigue will want to use progressive resistance training programs designed to build muscular endurance (slow-twitch fibers).

🌐 **Genetics, gender, and age affect muscle fitness performance.** **www.mhhe.com/fit_well/web11 Click 03.** Each person inherits a certain percentage of fast-twitch and slow-twitch muscle fibers. This allocation influences the potential a person has for muscle fitness activities. Individuals with a larger percentage of fast-twitch fibers will generally increase muscle size and strength more readily than individuals endowed with a larger percentage of slow-twitch fibers. People with a larger percentage of slow-twitch fibers have greater potential for muscular endurance performance. Regardless of genetics, all people can improve their strength and muscular endurance with proper training.

Women have smaller amounts of the anabolic hormone testosterone and, therefore, have less muscle mass than men. Because of this, women typically have 60 percent to 85 percent of the **absolute strength** of men. When expressed relative to lean body weight, women have similar **relative strength** as men. For example, a 150-pound female who lifts 150 pounds has equivalent relative strength as a 250-pound male who lifts 250 pounds even though she has less absolute strength. **Absolute muscular endurance** is also greater for males but the difference again is negated if **relative endurance** is considered. Relative strength and endurance are better indicators of muscle fitness since they take into account differences in size and muscle mass, but for some activities, absolute strength and endurance are more important.

Hypertrophy Increase in the size of muscles as the result of strength training; increase in bulk.

Absolute Strength The maximum amount of force one can exert, e.g., maximum number of pounds or kilograms that can be lifted on one attempt.

Relative Strength Amount of force that one can exert in relation to one's body weight or per unit of muscle cross-section.

Absolute Muscular Endurance (Dynamic Type) Endurance measured by the maximum number of repetitions one can perform against a given resistance, e.g., the number of times you can bench press 50 pounds.

Relative Muscular Endurance (Dynamic Type) Endurance measured by the maximum number of repetitions one can perform against a resistance that is a given percentage of one's 1 RM, e.g., the number of times you can lift 50 percent of your 1 RM.

Maximum strength is usually reached in the twenties and typically declines with age. Though muscular endurance declines with age, it is not as dramatic as decreases in absolute strength. As people grow older, regardless of gender, strength and muscular endurance are better among people who train than people who do not. This suggests that progressive resistance training is one antidote to premature aging.

Some endurance tests penalize the weaker person. If you are tested on absolute endurance (the number of times you can move a designated number of pounds), a stronger person has an advantage. However, if you are tested on relative muscular endurance (the number of times you can move a designated percentage of your maximum strength), the stronger person does not have an advantage. For this reason, men and women can compete more evenly in relative muscular endurance activities. In fact, on some endurance tasks women have done as well or better than men. For example, the women at the United States Military Academy do as well as the men on tests of abdominal muscular endurance.

Muscular endurance is related to cardiovascular endurance, but it is not the same thing. Cardiovascular endurance depends upon the efficiency of the heart muscle, circulatory system, and respiratory system. It is developed with activities that stress these systems, such as running, cycling, and swimming. Muscular endurance depends upon the efficiency of the local skeletal muscles and the nerves that control them. Most forms of cardiovascular exercises such as running require good cardiovascular and muscular endurance. For example, if your legs lack the muscular endurance to continue contracting for a sustained period of time, it will be difficult to perform well in running or other aerobic activities.

Health Benefits of Muscle Fitness and Resistance Exercise

Good muscle fitness is associated with reduced risk of injury. www.mhhe.com/fit_well/ web11 Click 04. People with good muscle fitness are less likely to suffer joint injuries (e.g., neck, knee, ankle) than those with poor muscle fitness. Weak muscles are more likely to be involuntarily overstretched than are strong muscles.

Muscle balance is important in reducing the risk of injury. Resistance training should build both agonist and **antagonist muscles.** For example, if you do resistance exercise to build the quadriceps muscles (front of the thigh), you should also exercise the hamstring muscles (back of the thigh). In this instance, the quadriceps are the agonist (muscle being used), and the hamstrings are

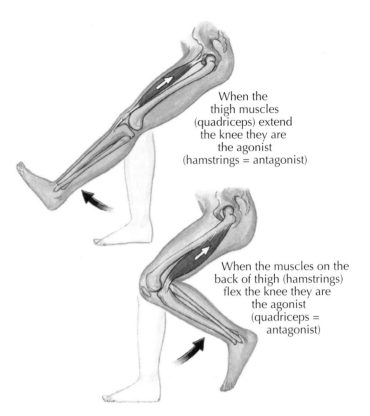

When the thigh muscles (quadriceps) extend the knee they are the agonist (hamstrings = antagonist)

When the muscles on the back of thigh (hamstrings) flex the knee they are the agonist (quadriceps = antagonist)

Figure 2 ▶ Agonist and antagonist muscles.

the antagonist. If the quadriceps become too strong relative to the antagonist hamstring muscles, the risk of injury increases (see Figure 2).

Good muscle fitness is associated with good posture and reduced risk of back problems. www.mhhe.com/fit_well/web11 Click 05. When muscles in specific body regions are weak or overdeveloped, poor posture can result. Lack of fitness of the abdominal and low back muscles is particularly related to poor posture and potential back problems. Excessively strong hip flexor muscles can lead to swayback. Poor balance in muscular development can also result in postural problems. For example, the muscles on the sides of the body must be balanced to maintain an erect posture.

Good muscle fitness can bring about improved athletic performance. Many sports depend on strength and muscular endurance. A football player must have good muscle strength to block and tackle effectively. A swimmer or a wrestler requires good muscular endurance to perform optimally. Also, people in jobs requiring high-level performance such as law enforcement and fire safety are likely to benefit from good muscle fitness.

Good muscular fitness is associated with wellness and quality of life. Wellness is reflected in quality of life and well-being. A person with muscle fitness is able to perform for long periods of time without undue fatigue. As a result, the person has energy to perform daily work efficiently and effectively and has reserve energy to enjoy leisure time. Among older people, maintenance of strength is associated with increased balance, less risk of falling, and greater ability to perform the tasks of daily living independently. Muscle fitness also contributes to looking one's best.

Resistance exercise is associated with reduced risk of osteoporosis. **Progressive resistance exercises (PRE)** provide a positive stress on the bones. Together with good diet, including adequate calcium intake, this stress on the bones reduces the risk of osteoporosis. Evidence suggests that young people who do PRE develop a high bone density. As we grow older, bone mass decreases, so people who have a high bone density when they are young have a "bank account" from which to draw as they grow older. These people have bones that are less likely to fracture or be injured. Injuries to the bones, particularly the hip and back, are common among older adults. Regular PRE can reduce the risk of these conditions. Postmenopausal women are especially at risk for osteoporosis (see concept 6).

PRE contributes to weight control and looking your best. Regular PRE results in muscle mass increases. Muscle or lean body mass takes up less space than fat, contributing to attractive appearance. Further, muscle burns calories at rest so extra muscle built through PRE can contribute to increased resting and basal metabolism. For each pound of muscle gained, a person can burn approximately 35 to 50 calories more per day. A typical strength training program performed at least three times a week can lead to two additional pounds of muscle after eight weeks so this can amount to an additional 100 calories a day or 700 over a week. Conversely, muscle mass tends to decrease with age and this can slow metabolism by a similar amount and contribute to gradual increases in body fatness. PRE can help people retain muscle mass as they grow older.

Types of Progressive Resistance Exercise

The best type of training for muscle fitness is referred to as progressive resistance exercise. The type of training most commonly used to promote muscle fitness is referred to as PRE, or progressive resistance training (PRT). This name is used because the frequency, intensity, and length of time of muscle overload are progressively increased as muscle fitness increases. PREs are typically done in one to three sets of three to twenty-five repetitions (also called reps). A set is a group of reps that are done in succession followed by a rest period.

PRE is not the same thing as weight lifting, powerlifting, or bodybuilding. PRE is a method of training to build muscle fitness that provides health and performance benefits. It should not be confused with the following three competitive activities. Weight lifting is a competitive sport that involves two lifts: the snatch and the clean and jerk. Powerlifting is also a competitive sport that includes three lifts: the bench press, the squat, and the dead lift. Bodybuilding is a competition in which participants are judged on the size and **definition** of their muscles. All three of these competitive events rely on progressive resistance exercise to improve performance. Weight training is a form of PRE and is a method of improving muscle fitness that is different from weight lifting—the competitive event.

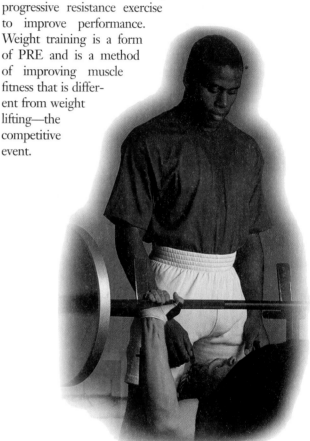

Progressive resistance exercises are methods of training designed to build muscle fitness.

Antagonist Muscles The muscles that have the opposite action from those that are contracting (agonists); normally, antagonists reflexively relax when agonists contract.

Progressive Resistance Exercise (PRE) Exercise done against a resistance; also referred to as progressive resistance training (PRT).

Definition (of Muscle) The detailed external appearance of a muscle.

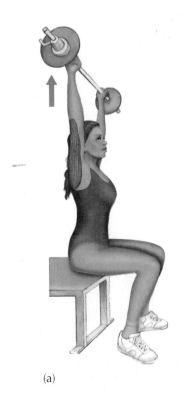
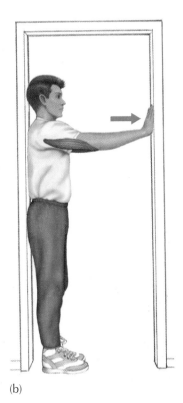
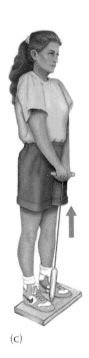

(a)   (b)   (c)

Figure 3 ▶ Examples of three types of muscle fitness exercises (*a*) isotonic, (*b*) isometric, and (*c*) isokinetic.

PRE programs can be performed in a variety of ways and with different equipment. Isotonic exercise refers to activities in which a resistance is raised and then lowered, as in weight training and calisthenics (also called dynamic exercise). When performing isotonic exercise, both **concentric** (shortening) and **eccentric** (lengthening) **contractions** should be used. For example, in an overhead press exercise, the muscles on the back of the arm (triceps) shorten (contract concentrically) to lift the weight overhead (see Figure 3*a*). When the weight is lowered, the muscles lengthen (contract eccentrically) if the weight is lowered slowly. Both concentric and eccentric contractions build the muscle. Eccentric contractions, sometimes called negative contractions, are more likely to cause delayed-onset muscle soreness than concentric contractions. Typically, the stress on the muscle in either concentric or eccentric exercises varies with speed, joint position, and muscle length. Thus, the muscle may work harder at the beginning of a lift than it does near the end of the range of motion.

www.mhhe.com/fit_well/web11 Click 06. **Isometric** exercises are those in which no movement takes place while a force is exerted against an immovable object (see Figure 3*b*). They are effective for developing strength and muscular endurance and require little or no equipment and only minimal space. Isometric exercises build **static strength** and **static muscular endurance** as opposed to **dynamic strength** or **dynamic muscular**

endurance. They work the muscle only at the angle of the joint used in the exercise and promote less hypertrophy and strength than isotonic resistance exercise. Thus, isometric exercises are probably less effective as an overall training method than isotonic exercises. On the other hand, isometrics have been found to be quite useful for some athletes, such as wrestlers and gymnasts, and work especially well for people in the early stages of some rehabilitation programs. Research has shown that strength can be enhanced significantly by using isometric training at the **sticking points** of isotonic lifts.

Isometrics previously have been thought to be dangerous for people with high blood pressure or cardiovascular disease. Recent evidence suggests that may not be the case for all people with these cardiovascular problems. These people should consult a medical expert before using isometric techniques.

www.mhhe.com/fit_well/web11 Click 07. **Isokinetic** exercises are isotonic-concentric muscle contractions performed on machines that keep the velocity of the movement constant through the full range of motion. This rate limiting mechanism prevents the performer from moving faster no matter how much force is exerted. Isokinetic devices essentially match the resistance to the effort of the performer, permitting maximal tension to be exerted throughout the range of motion (see Figure 3*c*). Thus, isokinetic devices overcome the basic weakness of isotonic exercise in which the muscle is only maximally

Table 1 ▶ Advantages and Disadvantages of Isometric, Isotonic, and Isokinetic Exercises		
	Advantages	**Disadvantages**
Isotonic	• Can effectively mimic movements used in sport skills • Enhances dynamic coordination • Promote gains in strength	• Does not challenge muscles through the full range of motion • Requires equipment or machines • May lead to soreness
Isometric	• Can be done anywhere • Low cost/little equipment needed • Can rehabilitate an immobilized joint	• Builds strength at only one position • Less muscle hypertrophy • Poor link or transfer to sport skills
Isokinetic	• Builds strength through a full range of motion • Beneficial for rehabilitation and evaluation • Safe and less likely to promote soreness	• Requires specialized equipment • Cannot replicate natural acceleration found in sports • More complicated to use and cannot work all muscle groups

challenged for a small part of the overall motion. A limitation is that these devices do not permit acceleration, so it is not possible to train specifically for sports skills, such as throwing or kicking, in which the limb is accelerated while applying maximum force. Another limitation is that some of these devices permit only concentric contractions. Isokinetic exercise has the advantage of being safer than most other forms of exercise and may be better for developing power (see concept 14). It is not better for developing pure strength, however. More research is needed to determine the best training regimen for isokinetic exercise.

Some of the advantages and disadvantages of the various forms of progressive resistance exercises, not including plyometrics, are outlined in Table 1.

Plyometrics is a form of isotonic exercise that promotes athletic performance. www.mhhe.com/fit_well/web11 Click 08. **Plyometrics** is a form of isotonic exercise that is especially useful for athletes training for power development. High jumpers, long jumpers, volleyball, and basketball players often use this technique, which includes jumping from boxes, hopping on one foot, and similar types of activities. For most people primarily interested in the health benefits of physical activity, plyometrics are not a preferred type of exercise. In fact, they can increase risk of injury, especially among beginners. For more information on plyometrics, refer to the concept on the performance benefits of physical activity.

Resistance Training Equipment

There are advantages of both free weights and machine weights. Free weights are weights that are not attached to a machine or exercise device. Typically, they come in the form of a barbell or dumbbell that can be adjusted as necessary for different exercises to provide optimal resistance. Weight training with free weights is very popular because it can be done in the home with inexpensive equipment. Because free weights require balance

Isotonic Type of muscle contraction in which the muscle changes length, either shortening (concentrically) or lengthening (eccentrically).

Concentric Contraction An isotonic muscle contraction in which the muscle gets shorter as it contracts, such as when a joint is bent and two body parts move closer together.

Eccentric Contraction An isotonic muscle contraction in which the muscle gets longer as it contracts; that is, when a weight is gradually lowered and the contracting muscle gets longer as it gives up tension. Eccentric contractions are also called negative exercise.

Isometric A type of muscle contraction in which the muscle remains the same length. Also known as static contraction.

Static Strength A muscle's ability to exert a force without changing length. It is also called isometric strength.

Static Muscular Endurance A muscle's ability to remain contracted for a long period. This is usually measured by the length of time you can hold a body position.

Dynamic Strength A muscle's ability to exert force that results in movement. It is typically measured isotonically.

Dynamic Muscular Endurance A muscle's ability to contract and relax repeatedly. This is usually measured by the number of times (repetitions) you can perform a body movement in a given time period. It is also called isotonic endurance.

Sticking Point The point in the range of motion where the weight cannot be lifted any farther without extreme effort or assistance; the weakest point in the movement.

Isokinetic Isotonic concentric exercises done with a machine that regulates movement velocity and resistance.

Plyometrics A training technique used to develop explosive power. It consists of concentric isotonic muscle contractions performed after a prestretch or eccentric contraction of a muscle.

and technique, they may be somewhat difficult for beginners to use. Competitive weight lifters generally prefer them because they can exercise muscle groups in a very specific way.

Resistance training machines can be effective in developing strength and muscular endurance if used properly. They can save time because, unlike free weights, the resistance can be changed easily and quickly. They may be safer because you are less likely to drop weights. A disadvantage is that the kinds of exercises that can be done on these machines are more limited than free weight exercises. They also may not promote optimal balance in muscular development since a stronger muscle can often make up for a weaker muscle in the completion of a lift.

www.mhhe.com/fit_well/web11   Click   09.   Some machines, such as Nautilus and Universal, offer what is called "variable" or "accommodating resistance." The Nautilus, for example, uses a cam to adapt the resistance as the performer moves through the range of motion. The Universal Trainer uses a rolling pivot to do the same thing. These adaptations attempt to compensate for an inherent weakness in isotonic constant-resistance exercises done with free weights and other machines. They are only partially successful, however, in adapting to the shapes, sizes, and torques of individual human bodies. There is no evidence that variable-resistance machines develop more strength or muscular endurance than other devices although they may offer advantages in muscle fitness by allowing movement through an extended range of motion. Table 2 provides a comparison of free weights with weight machines.

Many resistance training exercises can be done with little or no equipment. Calisthenics are among the most popular forms of muscle fitness exercise among adults. Calisthenics, such as curl-ups and push-ups, are suitable for people of different ability levels, and can be used to improve both strength and muscular endurance. One disadvantage is that this type of exercise does little to increase strength unless resistance in addition to your body weight is added. For example, doing a push-up will build strength to a point. However, once you can do several, adding more repetitions will only build muscular endurance but not strength. To develop additional strength, you can add more weights to increase the resistance or change the body position so there is a greater gravitational effect or more torque. For example, you can elevate your feet or wear a weighted vest while doing push-ups.

Other alternatives to expensive resistance training machines or commercially made free weights are homemade weights and elastic exercise bands. Homemade weights can be constructed from pieces of pipe or broom sticks and plastic milk jugs filled with water. Elastic tubes or bands available in varying strengths may be substituted for the weights and for the pulley device used in many resistance training machines to impart resistance.

Muscular endurance can be developed through activities such as running, swimming, circuit training, and aerobic dance if they are designed appropriately. Lifestyle activities such as gardening (e.g., raking, shoveling) or housework (lifting groceries) can also contribute to muscular endurance.

Table 2 ▶ Advantages and Disadvantages of Free Weights and Weight Machines

		Free Weights		Machine Weights
Isolation of Major Muscle Groups	–/+	Movements require balance and coordination; more muscles used for stabilization	+/–	Other body parts are stabilized during lift allowing isolation but muscle imbalances can develop
Applications to Real Life Situations	+	Movements can be developed to be truer to real life	–	Movements are determined by the paths allowed on the machine
Risk of Injury	–	More possibility for injury because weights can fall or drop on toes	+	Safer because weights cannot fall on participants
Needs for Assistance	–	Spotters needed for safety with some lifts	+	No spotters required
Time Requirement	–	More time needed to change weights	+	Easy and quick to change weights or resistance
Number of Available Exercises	+	Unlimited number of exercises possible	–	Exercise options determined by the machine
Cost	+	Less expensive but good (durable) weights are still somewhat expensive	–	Expensive; often have to have access to a club since usually need multiple machines
Space Requirement	+/–	Equipment can be moved but loose weights may clutter areas	–/+	Machines are stationary but take up large spaces

Progressive Resistance Exercise: How Much PRE Is Enough

The overload principle provides the underlying basis for PRE. It was in the area of muscle fitness development that the overload principle was first clearly outlined. Centuries ago, Milo of Crotona was said to have recognized the value of progressive overload. His strength increased as he repeatedly lifted a calf. As the calf grew into a bull, its weight increased, and Milo's strength increased as well. We now know that for most people, PREs are necessary if muscle fitness is to be developed and maintained (see Figure 4). Activities from other levels of the physical activity pyramid rarely promote adequate muscle fitness.

The type of overload for strength is different than for muscular endurance. The stimulus for strength is maximal exertion. Strength training should, therefore, utilize high resistance overload with low repetitions. The stimulus for muscular endurance is repeated contractions with short rests. Muscular endurance exercises should be performed with a relatively high number of repetitions and lower resistance.

The graph in Figure 5 illustrates the relationship between strength and muscular endurance. Training that requires high resistance and low repetitions (top bar) results in the least gain in endurance but the greatest gain in strength. Training with moderate resistance and mod-

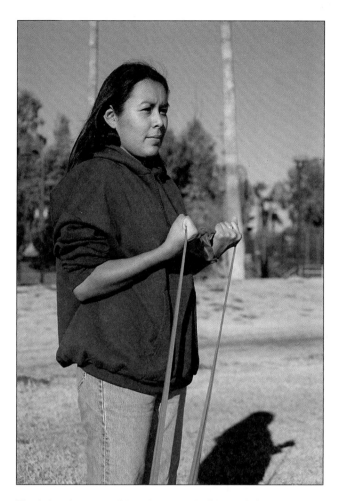

Elastic bands can provide resistance to build muscle fitness.

erate repetitions (second bar) results in moderate gains in both strength and endurance. Training that requires a high number of repetitions and a relatively low resistance (third bar) results in small gains in strength, but large increases in muscular endurance.

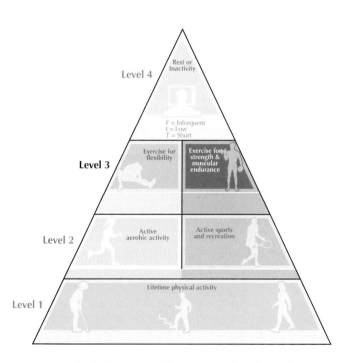

Figure 4 ► To build muscle fitness, activities should be selected from level 3 of the physical activity pyramid.

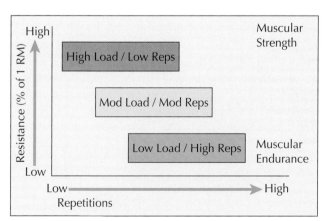

Figure 5 ► Comparison of muscular endurance to muscle strength developed by different repetitions and resistance.

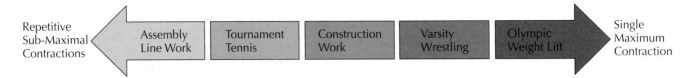

Figure 6 ▶ Muscle strength-endurance continuum.

While strength training promotes strength, studies show that the person who is strength-trained will fatigue as much as four times faster than the person who is endurance-trained. However, there is a modest correlation between strength and endurance. A person who trains for strength will develop some endurance, and a person who trains for endurance will develop some strength.

Muscular endurance and strength are part of the same continuum. Though strength and muscular endurance are developed in different ways, strength and muscular endurance are part of the same continuum (Figure 6). This has led some writers to refer to muscular endurance as strength endurance. "Pure" strength is approached as one nears the end (right) of the continuum, where only one maximum contraction is made. As the number of repetitions increases and the force of the contractions decreases, one nears the other end (left) of the continuum and approaches "pure" endurance. In between the two extremes, varying degrees of strength and endurance are combined. The activities listed along the continuum are examples that might represent points along the scale. Most of the activities of daily living are at the middle of the continuum, indicating that they take a combination of strength and muscular endurance.

The intensity of muscle fitness training is determined using a percentage of the amount of weight you can lift one time (1 RM). The maximum amount of resistance you can move (or weight you can lift) one time is called your one **repetition maximum (RM)**. The amount of resistance you use in a PRE program is based on a percentage of your 1 RM. The percentage of 1 RM used in a program depends on the program goals. For strength, the percentages vary from 60 to 80 percent depending on a person's current strength level. More experienced strength trainers often exercise at a higher percentage of 1 RM than beginners. For muscular endurance, the percentages vary from 20 to 40 percent. People interested in a combination of strength and muscular endurance should use 40 to 60 percent of 1 RM in their training.

🌐 **The muscle fitness workout should be based on the principle of progression. www.mhhe.com/ fit_well/web11 Click 10.** Many beginning resistance trainers experience extreme soreness after the first few days of training. The reason for the soreness is that the principle of progression has been violated. Soreness can occur with even modest amounts of training if the volume of training is considerably more than normal. In the first few days or weeks of training, the primary adaptations in the muscle are due to motor learning factors rather than to muscle growth. Because these adaptations occur no matter how much weight is used, it is prudent to start your program slowly with light weights. After these adaptations occur and the rate of improvement slows down, it would be necessary to follow the appropriate target zone to achieve proper overload.

The most common progression used in resistance training is the double progressive system, so-called because this system periodically adjusts both the resistance and the number of repetitions of the exercise performed. For example, if you are training for strength, you may begin with three repetitions in one set. As the repetitions become easy, additional repetitions are added. When you have progressed to eight repetitions, increase the resistance and decrease the repetitions in each set back to three and begin the progression again.

Other systems can be used within a training session to alter the training effect. Some recommend a "light to heavy" system (Delorme system) in which progressively heavier weights are lifted with each set. Others recommend the "heavy to light" system (Oxford system) in which the heaviest weight is used on the first set when the muscles are most rested. Still others advocate a pre-exhaust routine in which small accessory muscle groups are fatigued before the exercises for major muscle groups are performed.

The principle of specificity applies to PRE. Depending on the specific muscle that you want to develop, you will use different types of resistance training programs. Factors that can be varied in your program are the type of muscle contraction (isometric or isotonic), the speed or cadence of the movement, and the amount of resistance being moved. For example, if you want strength in the elbow extensor muscles (e.g., triceps) so that you could more easily lift heavy boxes onto a shelf, you would train using isotonic contractions, at a relatively slow speed, with a relatively high resistance. If you want muscle fitness of the fingers to grip a heavy bowling ball, much of your training should be done isometrically using the fingers the same way you normally hold the ball. If you are training for a particular skill that requires explosive power, such as in throwing, striking, kicking, or jumping, your strength exercises should be done with less resistance and greater speed. If you are training for a skill that uses both concentric and eccentric contractions or is plyometric, you should perform strength exercises using these characteristics. More information on these techniques is included in the concept on the performance benefits of physical activity.

If you are not training for a specific task, but merely wish to develop muscle fitness for daily living, consider the advantages and disadvantages of isometrics, isotonics, and isokinetics listed in Table 1. You may wish to use a variety of methods.

The principle of diminishing returns applies to resistance training. To get optimal strength gains from progressive resistance training, one or more sets of exercise repetitions is performed. Some high-level performers use as many as five sets of a particular exercise. Research indicates that most of the fitness and health benefits, however, are achieved in one set. As much as 80 to 90 percent of the benefits may result in the first set, with each additional set producing less and less benefit. Because compliance with resistance training programs is less likely as the time needed to complete the program increases, the American College of Sports Medicine (ACSM) recently recommended single-set programs for most adults. They acknowledge that additional benefits are likely with more multiset routines, but they believe that adults are more likely to participate if they can get most of the benefits in a relatively short amount of time. In sports or competition where small performance differences make a big difference, doing multiple sets is important.

The principle of rest and recovery especially applies to strength development. Progressive resistance training for strength development done every day of the week does not allow enough rest and time for recovery. Recent studies have shown that the greatest proportion of strength is accomplished in two days of training per week. Exercise done on a third day does result in additional increases, but the amount of gain is relatively small compared to gains resulting from two days of training per week. For people interested in health benefits rather than performance benefits, two days a week saves time and may result in greater adherence to a strength-training program. For people interested in performance benefits, more frequent training may be warranted. Rotating exercises so that certain muscles are exercised on one day and other muscles are exercised the next allows for more frequent training.

The amount of exercise necessary to maintain strength is less than the amount needed to develop it. Recent evidence suggests that once strength is developed, it may be maintained by performing fewer sets or

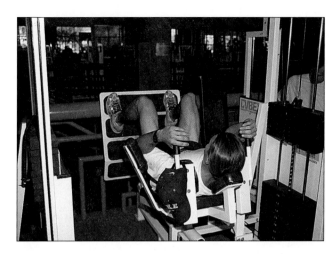

One repetition maximum (1 RM) is a good measure of strength.

exercising fewer days per week. For example, if you have performed three sets of an exercise three days a week to build strength, you may be able to maintain current levels of strength with one set a week. Also you may be able to maintain strength by exercising one or two rather than three days per week. If schedules of fewer sets or days per week result in strength loss, frequency must be increased.

Some muscle groups seem to need training less often to maintain strength levels. For example, evidence suggests that muscle fitness of the back can be maintained using one-day-a-week single-set exercises. Smaller muscles seem to need more frequent exercise.

A threshold of training and a target zone for strength development. The FIT formula for strength defines the threshold and target values for strength development. Table 3 illustrates the FIT formula for isometrics, isotonics, and isokinetic resistance training for typical people. People interested in advanced progressive resistance training, such as body builders or competitive weight lifters, will need special training programs to excel at these activities (refer to the concept on the performance benefits of physical activity).

A threshold of training and a target zone exists for muscular endurance development. There is a frequency, intensity, and time at which a training effect for muscular endurance will begin to take place (threshold). There is also an optimal range, or target zone, where the most effective and efficient improvement will occur (see Table 4). We do not know the exact range, but studies

Repetition Maximum (RM) The maximum amount of resistance one can move a given number of times, for example: 1 RM = maximum weight lifted one time; 6 RM = maximum weight lifted six times.

Table 3 ▶ Strength Threshold of Training and Fitness Target Zones

| | Threshold of Training | | | Target Zone | | |
	Isometrics	Isotonics	Isokinetics	Isometrics	Isotonics	Isokinetics
Frequency	• 2 days a week for each muscle group			• 2 to 3 days per week		
Intensity	• Use 60–65% of maximum contraction (1 RM)	• 60–65% of 1 RM for every rep	• 90% of 1 RM at set speed	• Maximum contractions	• 60–80% 1 RM (for number of reps on every set)	• Maximum effort at set speed
Time	• 1 set • 1 rep held for 2–5 seconds	• 1 set • 3–8 reps	• 2 sets • 3 reps lasting 3–4 seconds (30–60 degrees per second)	• 1 set • 6 reps held 6–8 seconds (or 2 sets of 3 reps each)	• 1–3 sets • 3–8 reps	• 3–5 sets • 3–8 reps lasting 1–2 seconds (70–120 degrees per second)
	• Repeat once a day		• Rest 1 minute between sets	• Rest 30 seconds between reps	• Rest 1 minute between sets	• Rest 1 minute between sets

suggest that it has wide limits. Intensity of effort seems to be important and studies suggest that one set can be nearly as effective as three if done properly.

A combined strength/muscular endurance program provides most of the health benefits associated with PRE. Recent research has shown that for healthy adults most health benefits can be achieved using a combined strength/muscular endurance program. The ACSM's current guidelines suggest the following. For young adults, one set of eight to twelve repetitions performed two days a week provides most of the health benefits of PRE. For older adults (fifty and older), less intense exercises performed ten to fifteen times appears to be most effective. For both age groups, eight to ten basic exercises are recommended so that muscle fitness of the total body is accomplished. Those who want pure strength or high-level muscular endurance for performance will benefit from extra sets and from the specific protocols outlined in Tables 3 and 4. For people interested primarily in health benefits, the FIT formula outlined in Table 5 is recommended.

Circuit resistance training (CRT) is an effective way to build muscular endurance and cardiovascular endurance. CRT consists of the performance of high repetitions of an exercise with low to moderate resistance, progressing from one station to another, performing a different exercise at each station. The stations are usually placed in a circle to facilitate movement. CRT typically employs about twenty to twenty-five reps against a resistance that is 30 to 40 percent of 1 RM for 45 seconds. Fifteen seconds of rest is provided while changing stations. Approximately ten exercise stations are used, and the participant repeats the circuit two to three times (sets). Because of the short rest periods, significant cardiovascular benefits have been reported in addition to muscular endurance gains.

CRT on weight or hydraulic machines has been found to be more effective than standard set weight training for caloric consumption during and after exercise and for improving cardiovascular endurance, although it is not as effective as aerobic exercises, such as cycling or bench stepping.

Programs intended to slim the figure/physique should be of the muscular endurance type. Many men and women are interested in exercises designed to decrease girth measurements. High-repetition, low-resistance exercise is suitable for this because it usually brings about some strengthening and may decrease body fatness, which in turn, changes body contour. Exercises do not spot-reduce fat but they do speed up metabolism so more calories are burned. However, if weight or fat reduction is desired, aerobic (cardiovascular) exercises are best. To increase girth, use strength exercises.

Endurance training may have a negative effect on strength and power. Some studies have shown that for athletes who rely primarily on strength and power in their sports event, too much endurance training can cause a loss of strength and power because of modification of different muscle fibers. Strength and power athletes need some endurance training, but not too much, just as endurance athletes need some strength and power training but not too much.

Table 4 ▶ Muscular Endurance Threshold of Training and Fitness Target Zones

	Threshold of Training	Target Zone
Dynamic Endurance		
Frequency	• 2 days per week	• Every other day
Intensity	• Move 20–30% of the maximum resistance you can lift	• Move 40–60% of the maximum resistance you can lift
Time	• One set of 9 repetitions of each exercise	• 2–5 sets of 9–25 repetitions • Rest 15–60 seconds between sets
Static Endurance		
Frequency	• 3 days per week	• Every other day
Intensity	• Hold a resistance 50–100% of the weight you ultimately will need to hold in your work or leisure activity	• Hold a resistance equal to and up to 50% greater than the amount you will need to hold in your work or leisure activity
Time	• Hold for lengths of time 10%–50% shorter than the time you plan to do the activity. Repeat 10–20 times • Rest 30 seconds between reps	• Hold for lengths of time equal to and up to 20% greater than the time you plan to do the activity. For longer times, use fewer repetitions (5–10) • Rest 30–60 seconds between reps

Table 5 ▶ The FIT Formula for PRE Designed to Achieve Health Benefits

Frequency	Young adults Adults over 50	2–3 days a week 2–3 days a week
Intensity	Young adults Adults over 50	40–60% of 1 RM 30–50% of 1 RM
Time	Young adults Adults over 50	1 set of 8–12 reps 1 set of 10–15 reps

💿 Technology Update

Resistance Training Equipment Over the years, there have been major changes and developments in resistance training machines. Recent developments have allowed machines to overcome some of the well-known limitations. For example, many new machines allow movement to take place in multiple dimensions to allow for converging and diverging movements and independent arm function. Some examples include the Cybex VR2 line, the Paramount ART line and the Arcuate Line by Pacific Fitness. These machines provide additional variety for strength training and a more natural motion. The new Hammer Strength Line (Motion Technology Selectorized or MTS) features independent arm function with dual-weight stacks to avoid one arm dominating the movement. Other companies have developed different "selectorized" technologies using cables and pulleys that allow exercisers to define their own path of motion. These machines allow the user to work multiple muscle groups and to specifically target stabilizer muscles. Examples of this technology can be found in some of the new machines manufactured by Ground Zero, Vortex, Cybex and Life Fitness.

Source: Fitness Management

Is There Strength in a Bottle?

Anabolic steroids are used by some athletes and a significant number of nonathletes to enhance performance and build muscular bodies. Anabolic steroids are a synthetic reproduction of the male hormone testosterone. Physicians prescribe them to treat such conditions as muscle diseases, breast cancer, severe burns, rare types of anemia, and kidney disease. Steroids have also been used to help people with AIDS and muscle-wasting diseases retain muscle mass. Because of their dangerous side effects, doctors prescribe minimal doses. At first, research showed steroids to be ineffective in promoting muscle gain. This was because the doses used in the studies were much smaller than those taken today for performance enhancement. Many athletes and people interested in muscle development have reportedly taken massive doses 20 to 100 times the normal therapeutic dose used for medical conditions. Studies now show that when taken in large doses by people doing regular strength training, gains in muscle mass and strength can be considerable. Steroids act by increasing the rate of protein synthesis and the effects have been shown to occur in a dose-response fashion.

Anabolic Steroid A synthetic hormone similar to the male sex hormone testosterone. It functions androgenically to stimulate male characteristics and anabolically to increase muscle mass, weight, bone maturation, and virility.

Anabolic steroids are typically obtained on the black market or illegally from unethical physicians, coaches, trainers, body builders, athletes, and other entrepreneurs. While athletes use the drugs in an attempt to enhance performance, an increasing number of nonathletes use steroids to enhance their strength or improve their physique or appearance. Two million people are estimated to be using "roids." Steroid use has leveled off among males, but the levels among females has increased dramatically.

Taking anabolic steroids is illegal and a dangerous way to build muscle fitness. A number of significant side effects are associated with steroid use. In women, unlike men, some of these effects are irreversible (Figure 7). As can be seen in the figure, steroids (like all drugs) are dangerous. They can be addictive and produce more than seventy serious side effects, some of which may be fatal. Many deaths have been attributed to their use. Twenty-five athletes from the former Soviet Union who competed in the 1980 Olympics died because of conditions

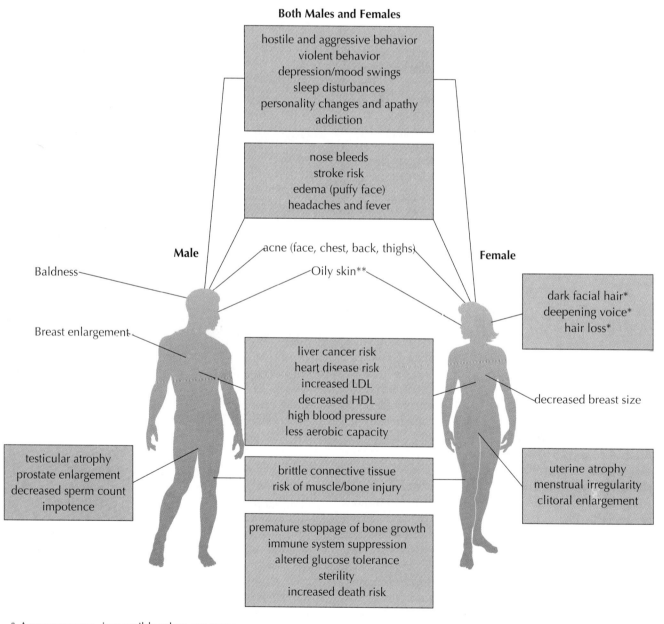

Both Males and Females

hostile and aggressive behavior
violent behavior
depression/mood swings
sleep disturbances
personality changes and apathy
addiction

nose bleeds
stroke risk
edema (puffy face)
headaches and fever

Male

acne (face, chest, back, thighs)
Oily skin**

Baldness

Female

dark facial hair*
deepening voice*
hair loss*

Breast enlargement

liver cancer risk
heart disease risk
increased LDL
decreased HDL
high blood pressure
less aerobic capacity

decreased breast size

testicular atrophy
prostate enlargement
decreased sperm count
impotence

brittle connective tissue
risk of muscle/bone injury

uterine atrophy
menstrual irregularity
clitoral enlargement

premature stoppage of bone growth
immune system suppression
altered glucose tolerance
sterility
increased death risk

* Among women, irreversible when use stops.
** Among women, partially reversible when use stops.

Figure 7 ▶ Adverse effects of anabolic steroids.

attributed to steroid use, and the deaths of several American professional athletes have also been attributed to anabolic steroid use. The death of Lyle Alzado, a former professional football player, was attributed to steroid use. Ken Caminiti, a high-profile former baseball player, indicated in a *Sports Illustrated* magazine article that he used steroids. Jose Conseco made a similar confession in his recent book. Caminiti suggested that a high proportion of active players use steroids. These revelations have resulted in hearings in congress and public polls that show the great majority of fans support mandatory testing of players. Results of studies show that in the last decade muscle injuries among baseball players have increased dramatically. Many consider steroids to be a cause of the increased injuries because of the known effects of steroids on connective tissue (see Figure 7) and because increased muscle size may create forces too great for weakened connective tissue to withstand. Unfortunately, some studies show that many athletes who use anabolic steroids are familiar with the adverse effects, but say, "I don't care and I will use them anyway."

Steroids have also been linked to other dangerous and unhealthy behaviors. Violent behavior, sometimes referred to as "roid rage," has been found to accompany steroid use. Recent research suggests that "roid rage" is most likely to result in people who are mentally unstable prior to use. Evidence indicates that steroid users are at greater risk of hepatitis or HIV/AIDS infections from shared needles.

Steroids taken in pill form are especially dangerous to the kidneys and other organs of the body. This is one reason why many medical experts are especially concerned about "andro," which is sometimes taken in pill form.

Injuries happen more easily and last longer in people who use steroids. Though steroids may make muscles stronger, tendons and ligaments do not proportionately increase in strength. Therefore, a strong muscle contraction can tear a tendon and/or a ligament. This is made more serious because steroids make the injury heal more slowly. When steroids increase muscle size, the extra muscle can grow around the bones and joints, causing them to break more easily.

Androstenedione is a legal supplement, but it is unsafe and banned by many organizations. A popular product in recent years is androstenedione, also called andro. This product causes the body to produce testosterone and has similar effects as taking artificial testosterone. It is controversial because it has been banned by the NCAA and the International Olympic Committee (IOC) but is allowed by other athletic agencies and can be purchased legally. Androstenedione gained instant notoriety when baseball slugger Mark McGuire reported using it during his assault on the season home run record.

Many people assumed that his success was due, at least in part, to the use of the supplement. However, this is unlikely. Studies have shown that andro does not increase testosterone levels unless extremely large doses are used and no performance or strength benefits have been documented even with these doses. The side effects of andro use are similar to those from anabolic steroids. Hormones and lipids are altered and repeated use can increase risk for heart disease, pancreatic cancer, and prostate problems in men.

Human growth hormone (HGH), taken to increase strength, may be even more dangerous than anabolic steroids. HGH is produced by the pituitary gland but is made synthetically. Some athletes are taking it in addition to anabolic steroids or in place of anabolic steroids because it is difficult to detect in urine tests of competitors. The effect of HGH is primarily on increasing bone size and not muscle size. Athletes often use growth hormone in combination with anabolic steroids so they can have gains in muscle mass along with the bone strengthening effects of HGH. Athletes assume that this will protect them from some of the bone injuries that occur among steroid users. However, these athletes are further risking their health as the health risks of steroid use are compounded further with HGH use. Risks of HGH use include irreversible acromegaly (giantism) and gross deformities, cardiovascular disease, goiter, menstrual disorder, excessive sweating, lax muscles and ligaments, premature bone closure, decreased sexual desire, and impotence. In addition, the life span can be shortened by as much as twenty years. Like steroids, there are some medical uses for HGH but they should only be used with physician recommendations and prescriptions.

Another hormone being used by some male athletes is human chorionic gonadotropin (HCG), a substance found in the urine of pregnant women. It is being used to stimulate testosterone production before competition. The IOC has banned its use, but no test has been developed to detect it.

Creatine use is becoming increasingly popular among people training for strength development. www.mhhe.com/fit_well/web11 Click 11. Creatine is produced naturally by your body from foods containing protein such as meat and fish. It is stored in the muscles and helps supply energy for muscle contraction. Because it is classified as a food supplement and not a drug, it is legal for people in competition. Users typically consume creatine as a powder that is dissolved in a liquid. Creatine supplements increase the creatine level in the muscle above the amount possible from normal food intake. The theory is that extra creatine in the muscle will allow quicker recovery from intense exercise such as vigorous strength training and sprinting. Further theory suggests that creatine supplements can keep muscle creatine levels higher than normal, resulting in faster recovery from vigorous short-duration exercise bouts. This, in turn, may allow more intense workouts. An important point is that if strength gains result they are the result of the increased training stimulus and not from the supplement itself. There are some studies that support the theory described earlier. However, a recent study that statistically analyzed all of the recent research on creatine suggests that "creatine supplementation does not improve anaerobic performance." The authors further state that ". . . the ergogenic effect of creatine, although widely publicized and believed, is not supported by the available data . . ." (see Misic and Kelley, suggested readings).

Even those who believe in the benefits of creatine supplementation for anaerobic performance concede that the benefits do not extend to performance in swimming, distance running events, and other performances involving muscular endurance. Studies show that creatine supplementation causes relatively immediate increases in body weight, but it is mostly a result of water retention. The extra weight resulting from water retention may actually impair endurance performance and may also negatively affect sports such as high jumping because the body has to lift the extra weight over the bar.

Recently, the deaths of three college wrestlers led the Food and Drug Administration (FDA) to study creatine to determine if it was in some way associated with these deaths. No evidence of creatine involvement was found, though the various organizations have warned that creatine supplementation may precipitate dehydration. This could be a problem among athletes who want to lose weight by losing body water. The long-term effects of creatine supplementation are unknown, and public health officials are concerned. Short-term side effects include stomach distress and cramping. Many people using the supplement take doses far in excess of those recommended for optimal saturation in the muscles. A recent position statement by the ACSM suggests that doses of 20 to 25 grams per day for five days followed by much smaller doses of 3 to 5 grams per day will result in maximal muscle saturation. Though not recommended for most people, if you are going to take creatine, it should not be taken in doses greater than those listed above. Further, changes in the law in 1994 leave quality control issues up to the manufacturer rather than the government. For this reason, the quality of any food supplement (which creatine is considered) is only as good as the integrity of the supplier.

Some people have turned to other dietary supplements and glandular extracts, which have been promoted as substitutes for anabolic steroids. In an effort to avoid the undesirable side effects of anabolic steroids or the detection of its use by sports-governing bodies who have banned it, some athletes or body builders are taking chemicals and supplements such as boron, chromium picolinate, gamma oryzanol, and L-carnitine (see concept on quackery). There is also a considerable market for "glandulars" such as ground-up bull testes, hypothalamus and pituitary glands, hearts, livers, spleens, and brains. These products have been advertised as steroid alternatives. Dietitians, the FDA, and the National Council for Reliable Health Information are alarmed and consider these products potentially dangerous because they have not been tested on humans or animals for safety and effectiveness. Little is known about some of them. No published scientific evidence substantiates claims for improved human performance. An article in the *Journal of the American Medical Association* has cautioned people concerning the use of such "body-building" supplements.

Table 6 ▶ How to Prevent Injury (for the Beginner)
• Warm up 10 minutes before the workout and stay warm during the workout.
• Do not hold your breath while lifting. This may cause blackout or hernia.
• Avoid hyperventilation before lifting a weight.
• Avoid dangerous or high-risk exercises.
• Progress slowly.
• Use good shoes with good traction.
• Avoid arching your back. Keep the pelvis in normal alignment.
• Keep the weight close to the body.
• Do not lift from a stoop (bent over with back rounded).
• When lifting from the floor, do not let the hips come up before your upper body.
• For bent-over rowing, lay your head on a table and bend the knees, or use one-arm rowing and support the trunk with the free hand.
• Stay in a squat as short a time as possible and do not do a full squat.
• Be sure collars on free weights are tight.
• Use a moderately slow, continuous, controlled movement and hold the final position a few seconds.
• Overload but don't overwhelm! A program that is too intense can cause injuries.
• Do not pause between repetitions.
• Keep a steady rhythm.
• Do not allow the weights to drop or bang.
• Do not train without medical supervision if you have a hernia, high blood pressure, fever, infection, recent surgery, heart disease, or back problems.
• Use chalk or a towel to keep hands dry when handling weights.

Guidelines for Safe and Effective Resistance Training

There is a proper way to perform resistance training. While resistance training offers considerable health benefits, there are also some risks if the exercises are not performed correctly or if safety procedures are not followed. A recent survey published in the *Physician and Sports Medicine* estimated that there were over 1 million emergency room visits in the United States attributed to weight training during the twenty-year period from 1978 to 1998. The leading predictor of injury identified in this survey was improper use of equipment. If you are unfamiliar with how to operate resistance training equipment, be sure to follow printed guidelines on the equipment and/or ask for general instruction. See Table 6 for specific safety tips.

Beginners should emphasize lighter weights and progress their program gradually. When beginning a resistance training program, start with weights that are too light so that you can learn proper technique and avoid soreness and injury. As mentioned, most of the adaptations that occur in the first few months after beginning a program are due to improvements in the body's ability to recruit muscle fibers to contract effectively and efficiently. These neural adaptations occur in response to the movement itself and

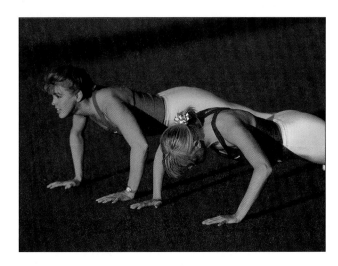

Well-planned resistance training helps you look your best.

are not due to how much weight is used. After training for several months, you may wish to increase the resistance to provide a greater stimulus for strength or to experiment with other types of more advanced training methods.

There are many fallacies, myths, and superstitions associated with resistance training. Some common misconceptions about resistance training are described in Table 7.

Table 7 ▶ Facts and Fallacies about Resistance Training

Myths and Fallacies	Facts
"Resistance training will make you muscle bound and cause you to lose flexibility."	Normal resistance training will not reduce flexibility if exercises are done through the full range of motion and with proper technique. Powerlifters who do highly specific movements have been shown to have poorer flexibility than other weight lifters.
"Women will become masculine looking if they gain strength."	Women will not become masculine looking from resistance exercise. Women have less testosterone and do not bulk up from resistance training to the same extent as men. Women and men can make similar relative gains in strength and hypertrophy from a resistance training program however. The greater percentage of fat in most women prevents the muscle definition possible in men and camouflages the increase in bulk.
"Strength training makes you move more slowly and look uncoordinated."	Strength training, if done properly, can enhance sport specific strength and increase power. There are no effects on coordination from having high levels of muscular fitness.
"No pain—no gain."	It is not true that you have to get to the point of soreness to benefit from resistance exercise. It may be helpful to strive until you can't do a final repetition but you should definitely stop before it is painful. Slight tightness in the muscles is common one to two days following exercise but is not necessary for adaptations.
"Soreness occurs because lactic acid builds up in the muscles."	Lactic acid is produced during muscular work but is converted back into other substrates within 30 minutes after exercising. Soreness is due to microscopic tears or damage in the muscle fibers but this damage is repaired as the body builds the muscle. Excessive soreness occurs if you violate the law of progression and do too much too soon.
"Strength training can build cardiovascular fitness and flexibility."	Resistance exercise can increase heart rate but this is due primarily to a pressure overload rather than a volume overload on the heart that occurs from endurance (aerobic) exercise. Gains in muscle mass do cause an increase in resting metabolism that can aid in controlling body fatness.
"Strength training is only beneficial for young adults."	Studies have shown that people in their 80s and 90s can benefit from resistance exercise and improve their strength and endurance. Most experts would agree that resistance exercise increases in importance with age rather than decreases.

Use good technique to enhance the safety and effectiveness of the lifts. Be sure to complete all lifts through the full range of motion using only the intended muscle group. If you have to jerk the weight or use momentum to lift it then the weight is too heavy. Lifting at a slow cadence will also provide a greater stimulus to the muscles. A common recommendation is to take two seconds on the lifting (concentric) phase and four seconds on the lowering (eccentric) phase.

Provide sufficient time to rest during and between workouts. The body needs time to rest in order to allow beneficial adaptations to occur. Choose an exercise sequence that alternates muscle groups so muscles have a chance to rest before another set. Lifting every other day or alternating muscle groups (if lifting more than three to four days per week) is also important in providing rest for the muscles.

Include all body parts and balance the strength of antagonistic muscle groups. A common mistake made by many beginning lifters is to perform only a few different exercises or to emphasize a few body parts. Training the biceps without working the triceps, for example, can lead to muscle imbalances that can compromise flexibility and increase risks of injury. In some cases, training must be increased in certain areas to compensate for stronger antagonist muscle groups. Many sprinters, for example, pull their hamstrings because the quadriceps are so over-developed that they overpower the hamstrings. The recommended ratio of quadriceps to hamstring strength should be 60:40.

Customize your training program to fit your specific needs. Athletes should train muscles the way that they will be used in their skill, employing similar patterns, range of motion, and speed (the principle of specificity). If you wish to develop a particular group of muscles, remember that the muscle group can be worked harder when isolated than when worked in combination with other muscle groups.

Strategies for Action

An important step in taking action for developing and maintaining muscle fitness is assessing your current status. www.mhhe.com/fit_well/web11 Click 12. An important early step in taking action to improve fitness is self-assessment. A 1 RM test of isotonic strength is described in the lab resource materials. This test allows you to determine absolute and relative strength for the arms and legs. In addition, the 1 RM values can be used to help you select the appropriate resistance for your muscle fitness training program. A grip strength test of isometric strength is also provided in the resource materials for Lab 11A. In addition to descriptions of the 1 RM test, a body weight test for isotonic strength is provided in the Web Resources for people who do not have the equipment to perform the 1 RM assessment.

www.mhhe.com/fit_well/web11 Click 13. Three tests of muscular endurance are described in the Lab Resource Materials for Lab 11B. It is recommended that you perform the assessments for both strength and muscular endurance before you begin your progressive resistance training program. Periodically reevaluate your muscle fitness using these assessments.

Many factors other than your own basic abilities affect muscle fitness test scores. If muscles are warmed up before lifting, more force can be exerted and heavier loads can be lifted. Muscle endurance performance may also be enhanced by a warm-up. Do not perform your self-assessments after vigorous exercise because that exercise can cause fatigue and result in suboptimal test results. It is appropriate to practice the techniques involved in the various tests on days preceding the actual testing. People who have good technique achieve better scores and are less likely to be injured when performing tests than those without good technique. It is best to perform the strength and muscular endurance tests on different days.

Choose exercises that build muscle fitness in the major muscle groups of the body. www.mhhe.com/fit_well/web11 Click 14. The ACSM recommends eight to ten basic exercises for muscle fitness. Eight basic exercises, the Basic 8, for free weights (Table 8), resistance machines (Table 9), isometric exercises (Table 10), and calisthenics (Table 11) are presented to help you meet your muscle fitness needs. For most people performing the Basic 8 exercises using any of the four types of exercise, the majority of the benefits associated with muscle fitness will result. The Basic 8 for free weight and resistance machines would need to be supplemented with one or both of the abdominal exercises included in Table 12.

People interested in additional exercises that serve as alternates or that focus on improving fitness in other muscle groups are referred to the supplemental exercises in Web Resources. Web Resources also includes eight basic exercises using elastic bands.

Keeping records of progress is important to adhering to a PRE program. An activity logging sheet is provided in Lab 11C to help you keep records of your progress as you regularly perform PRE to build and maintain good muscle fitness. A guide to the different muscles of the body is presented in Figure 8.

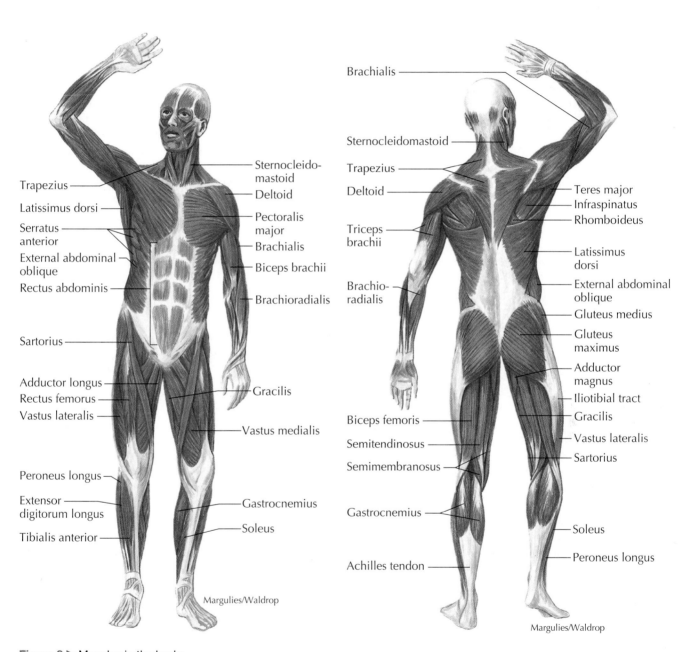

Figure 8 ▶ Muscles in the body.

Table 8

Table 8 The Basic 8 for Free Weights

1. Bench Press

This exercise develops the chest (pectoral) and triceps muscles. Lie supine on bench with knees bent and feet flat on bench or flat on floor in stride position. Grasp bar at shoulder level. Push bar up until arms are straight. Return and repeat. Do not arch lower back. Note: Feet may be placed on floor if lower back can be kept flattened. Do not put feet on the bench if it is unstable.

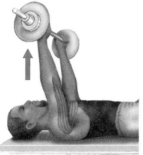

3. Biceps Curl

This exercise develops the muscles of the upper front part of the arms (biceps). Stand erect with back against a wall, palms forward, bar touching thighs. Spread feet in comfortable position. Tighten abdominals and back muscles. Do not lock knees. Move bar to chin, keeping body straight and elbows near the sides. Lower bar to original position. Do not allow back to arch. Repeat. Spotters are usually not needed. Variations: Use dumbbell and sit on end of bench with feet in stride position, work one arm at a time; or use dumbbell with the palm down or thumb up to emphasize other muscles.

2. Overhead (Military Press)

This exercise develops the muscles of the shoulders and arms. Sit erect, bend elbows, palms facing forward at chest level with hands spread (slightly more than shoulder width). Have bar touching chest, spread feet (comfortable distance). Tighten your abdominal and back muscles. Move bar to overhead position (arms straight). Lower bar to chest position. Repeat. Caution: Keep arms perpendicular and do not allow weight to move backward or wrists to bend backward. Spotters are needed.

4. Triceps Curl

This exercise develops the muscles on the back of the upper arms (triceps). Sit erect, elbows and palms facing up, bar resting behind neck on shoulders, hands near center of bar, feet spread. Tighten abdominal and back muscles. Keep upper arms stationary. Raise weight overhead, return bar to original position. Repeat. Spotters are needed. Variation: Substitute dumbbells (one in each hand, or one held in both hands, or one in one hand at a time).

5. Wrist Curl

This exercise develops the muscles of the fingers, wrist, and forearms. Sit astride a bench with the back of one forearm on the bench, wrist and hand hanging over the edge. Hold a dumbbell in the fingers of that hand with the palm facing forward. To develop the flexors, lift the weight by curling the fingers then the wrist through a full range of motion. Slowly lower and repeat. To strengthen the extensors, start with the palm down. Lift the weight by extending the wrist through a full range of motion. Slowly lower and repeat. Note: Both wrists may be exercised at the same time by substituting a barbell in place of the dumbbell.

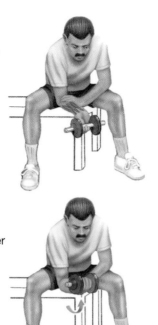

7. Lunge

This exercise develops the thigh and gluteal muscles. Place a barbell (with or without weight) behind your head and support with hands placed slightly wider than shoulder-width apart. In a slow and controlled motion, take a step forward and allow the leading leg to drop so that it is nearly parallel with the ground. The lower part of the leg should be near vertical and the back should be maintained in an upright posture. Take stride with opposite leg to return to standing posture. Repeat with other leg, remaining stationary or moving slowly in a straight line with alternating steps.

6. Half-Squat

This exercise develops the muscles of the thighs and buttocks. Stand erect, feet turned out 45 degrees. Rest bar behind neck on shoulders. Spread hands in a comfortable position. Squat slowly, keeping back straight, eyes ahead. Bend knees to approximately 90 degrees, and keep knees over feet. Pause, then stand. Repeat. Spotters are needed. Variations: Substitute dumbbell in each hand at sides.

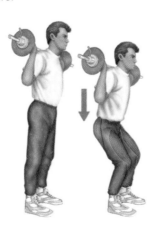

8. Heel Raise

This exercise develops the muscles of the legs (calf). Stand erect with palms facing forward, hands wider than shoulder-width apart, bar resting behind neck on shoulders. Rest balls of feet on two-inch block with heels on floor. Toes together, heels apart. Rise on toes quickly, hold for one second. Lower heels to floor. Repeat. Keep toes turned in slightly. Spotters are needed. Note: Some people do this with toes straight ahead or turned out; however, this tends to weaken the foot muscles.

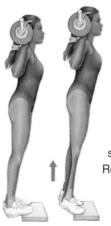

Table 9

Table 9 The Basic 8 for Resistance Machine Exercises

1. Chest Press

This exercise develops the chest (pectoral) and tricep muscles. Position seat height so that arm handles are directly in front of chest. Position backrest so that hands are at a comfortable distance away from the chest. Push handles forward to full extension and return to starting position in a slow and controlled manner. Repeat. Note: Machine may have a foot lever to help position, raise, and lower the weight.

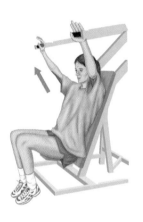

3. Bicep Curl

This exercise develops the elbow flexor muscles on the front of the arm, primarily the biceps. Adjust seat height so that arms are fully supported by pad when extended. Grasp handles palms up. While keeping the back straight, flex the elbow through the full range of motion.

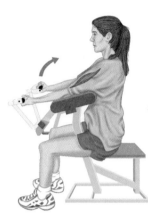

2. Seated Press

This exercise develops the muscles of the shoulders and arms. Position seat so that arm handles are slightly above shoulder height. Grasp handles with palms facing away and push lever up until arms are fully extended. Return to starting position and repeat. Note: Some machines may have an incline press.

4. Tricep Press

This exercise develops the extensor muscles on the back of arm, primarily the triceps. Adjust seat height so that arm handles are slightly above shoulder height. Grasp handles with thumbs toward body. While keeping the back straight, extend arms fully until wrist contacts the support pad (arms straight). Return to starting position and repeat.

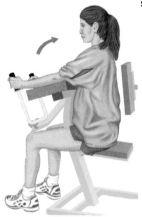

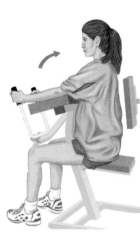

Table 9

5. Lat Pull Down

This exercise primarily develops the latissmus dorsi, but the biceps, chest, and other back muscles may also be developed. Sit on the floor. Adjust seat height so that hands can just grasp bar when arms are fully extended. Grasp bar with palms facing away from you and hands shoulder-width (or wider) apart. Pull bar down to chest and return. Repeat.

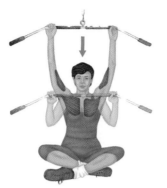

7. Knee Extension

This exercise develops the thigh (quadriceps) muscles. Sit on end of bench with ankles hooked under padded bar. Grasp edge of table. Extend knees. Return and repeat. Alternative: Leg press (similar to half-squat). Note: The knee extension exercise isolates the quadriceps but places greater stress on the structures of the knee than the leg press or half-squat.

6. Seated Rowing

This exercise develops the muscles of the back and shoulder. Adjust the machine so that arms are almost fully extended and parallel to the ground. Grasp handgrip with palms turned down and hands shoulder-width apart. While keeping the back straight, pull levers straight back to chest. Slowly return to starting position and repeat.

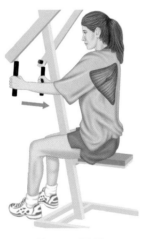

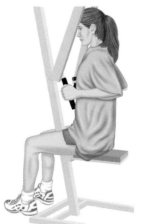

8. Hamstring Curl

This exercise develops the hamstrings (muscles on back of thigh) and other knee flexors. Lie prone on bench with ankles hooked under padded bar. Rest chin on hands or grasp bench. Flex knees as far as possible without allowing hips to raise. Return and repeat. Caution: Do not hyperextend the knees while assuming the starting position. If necessary, ask a partner to raise the pads while you place the heels under the bar.

Table 10

Table 10 The Basic 8 for Isometric Exercises

1. Arm Press in Doorway

This exercise develops the tricep and pectoral muscles. Stand in doorway, back flat on one side of doorway, hands placed on other side. Push with maximum force.

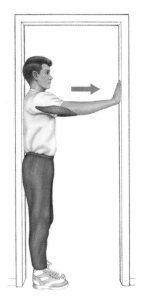

3. Curls

This exercise develops the muscles on the front of the arms. Place rope or towel loop behind thighs while standing in a half-squat position. Grasp loop, palms up, shoulder-width apart. Lift upward with maximum effort. Variation: Repeat, gripping with palms down.

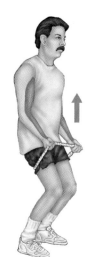

2. Overhead Press in Doorway

This exercise develops the muscles of the arms and shoulders. Stand in doorway, face straight ahead, hands shoulder-width apart, elbows bent. Tighten leg, hip, and back muscles. Push upward as hard as possible.

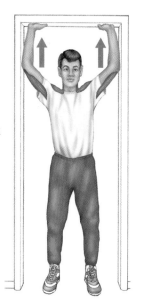

4. Triceps Press

This exercise develops the muscles on the back of the upper arm (triceps). Grasp towel or rope at both ends. Hold left hand at small of back, right hand over shoulder. Pull hands apart with maximum force. Repeat exercise, reversing position of hands.

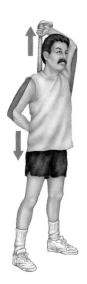

5. Pelvic Tilt

This exercise develops the muscles of the abdomen and buttocks. Assume a supine position with the knees bent and slightly apart. Press the spine down on the floor and hold for several seconds. Keep abdominal and gluteal muscles tightened.

7. Wall Seat

This exercise develops the muscles of the legs and hips. Assume a half-sit position, back flat against wall, knees bent to 90 degrees. Push back against wall with maximum force and hold for several seconds.

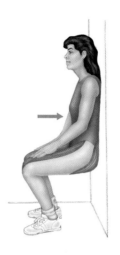

6. Leg Press in Doorway

This exercise develops the muscles of the legs and hips. Sit in doorway facing side of door frame. Grasp molding behind head. Keep back flat on side of doorway, feet against other side. Push legs with maximum force and hold for several seconds.

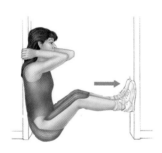

8. Hamstring Curl

This exercise develops the muscles on back of legs. Stand on rope or towel loop with left foot. Place loop around right ankle. Flex knee until taut. Apply maximum force upward.

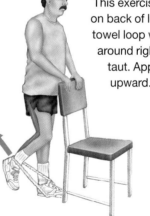

Table 11

Table 11 The Basic 8 for Calisthenics

1. Bent Knee Push-Ups and Let-Down

This exercise develops the muscles of the arms, shoulders, and chest. Lie on the floor face down with the hands under your shoulders. Keep your body straight from the knees to the top of the head. Push up until the arms are straight. Slowly lower chest (let-down) to floor. Repeat. Variation: full push-up and let-down performed the same way except body is straight from the toes to the top of head. Variation: Start from the up position and lower until the arm is bent at 90 degrees; then push up until arms are extended. Caution: Do not arch back.

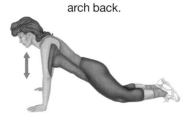

2. Modified Pull-Ups

This exercise develops the muscles of the arms and shoulders. Hang (palms forward and shoulder-width apart) from a low bar (may be placed across two chairs), heels on floor, with the body straight from feet to head. Bracing the feet against a partner or fixed object is helpful. Pull up, keeping the body straight, touch the chest to the bar, then lower to the starting position. Repeat. Note: This exercise becomes more difficult as the angle of the body approaches horizontal and easier as it approaches the vertical. Variation: Perform so that the feet do not touch the floor (full pull-up). Variation: Perform with palms turned up. When palms are turned away from the face, pull-ups tend to use all the elbow flexors. With palms facing the body, the biceps are emphasized more.

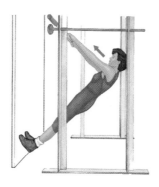

3. Dips

This exercise will develop the latissimus dorsi (on the back) and also the tricep. Start in a fully extended position with hands grasping the bar (palms facing in). Slowly drop down until the upper part of the arm is horizontal or parallel with the floor. Extend the arms back up to the starting position and repeat. Note: Many gyms have a dip/pull-up machine with accommodating resistance that provides a variable amount of assistance to help you complete the exercise.

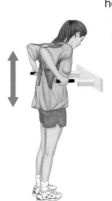

4. Crunch (Curl-Up)

This exercise develops the upper abdominal muscles. Lie on the floor with the knees bent and the arms extended or crossed with hands on shoulders or palms on ears. If desired, legs may rest on bench to increase difficulty. For less resistance, place hands at side of body (do not put hands behind head or neck). For more resistance, move hands higher. Curl up until shoulder blades leave floor, then roll down to the starting position. Repeat. Note: Twisting the trunk on the curl-up develops the oblique abdominals.

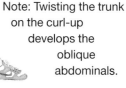

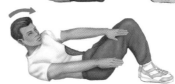

Table 11

5. (Trunk) Lift

This exercise develops the muscles of the upper back and corrects round shoulders. Lie face down with hands clasped behind the neck. Pull the shoulder blades together, raising the elbows off the floor. Slowly raise the head and chest off the floor by arching the upper back. Return to the starting position; repeat. For less resistance, hands may be placed under thighs. Caution: Do not arch the lower back. Lift only until the sternum (breastbone) clears the floor. Variations: arms down at sides (easiest), hands by head, arms extended (hardest).

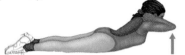

7. Lower Leg Lift

This exercise develops the muscles on the inside of thighs. Lie on the side with the upper leg (foot) supported on a bench. Note: If no bench is available, bend top leg and cross it in front of bottom leg for support. Raise the lower leg toward the ceiling. Repeat. Roll to opposite side and repeat. Keep knees pointed forward.
Variation: An ankle weight may be added for greater resistance.

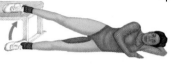
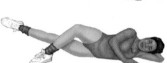

6. Side Leg Raises

This exercise develops the muscles on the outside of thighs. Lie on your side. Point knees forward. Raise the top leg 45 degrees, then return. Do the same number of repetitions with each leg. Caution: Keep knee and toes pointing forward. Variation: Ankle weights may be added for greater resistance.

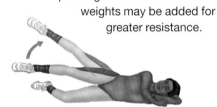

8. Alternate Leg Kneel

This exercise develops the muscles of the legs and hips. Stand tall, feet together. Take a step forward with the right foot, touching the left knee to the floor. The knees should be bent only to a 90-degree angle. Return to the starting position and step out with the other foot. Repeat, alternating right and left. Variation: Dumbbells may be held in the hands for greater resistance.

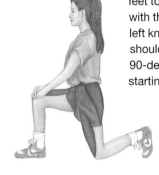

Table 12

Table 12 Exercises for the Abdominals

1. Crunch (Curl-Up)

This exercise develops the upper abdominal muscles. Lie on the floor with the knees bent and the arms extended or crossed with hands on shoulders or palms on ears. If desired, legs may rest on bench to increase difficulty. For less resistance, place hands at side of body (do not put hands behind neck). For more resistance, move hands higher. Curl up until shoulder blades leave floor, then roll down to the starting position. Repeat. Note: Twisting the trunk on the curl-up develops the oblique abdominals.

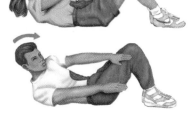

2. Reverse Curl

This exercise develops the lower abdominal muscles. Lie on the floor. Bend the knees, place the feet flat on the floor, and place arms at sides. Lift the knees to the chest, raising the hips off the floor. Do not let the knees go past the shoulders. Return to the starting position. Repeat.

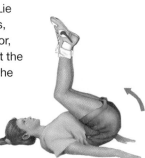

1. Seated Press (Chest Press)

This test can be performed using a seated press (see below) or using a bench press machine. When using the seated press position the seat height so that arm handles are directly in front of the chest. Position backrest so that hands are at comfortable distance away from the chest. Push handles forward to full extension and return to starting position in a slow and controlled manner. Repeat. Note: machine may have a foot lever to help position, raise, and lower the weight.

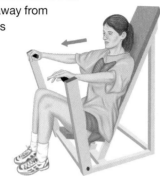

2. Leg Press

To perform this test use a leg press machine. Typically, the beginning position is with the knees bent at right angles with the feet placed on the press machine pedals or a foot platform. Extend the legs and return to beginning position. Do not lock the knees when the legs are straightened. Typically handles are provided. Grasp the handles with the hands when performing this test.

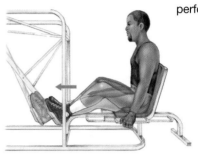

Web Resources

American College of Sports Medicine **www.acsm.org**

Muscle Fitness Exercises **www.mhhe.com/phys_fit/web11 click 15**

National Athletic Trainers Association www.nata.org

National Strength and Conditioning Association **www.nsca-cc.org**

The Physician and Sports Medicine Online **www.physsportsmed.com**

Suggested Readings

 Additional reference materials for concept 11 are available at **www.mhhe.com/fit_well/web11 Click 16**.

American College of Sports Medicine. 2000. *ACSM's Guidelines for Exercise Testing and Prescription*. 6th ed. Philadelphia: Lippincott, Williams and Wilkins.

American College of Sports Medicine. "Creatine Supplementation: Current Content." (www.acsm.org).

Baechle, T. R., and R. W. Earle. (eds.). 2000. *Essentials of Strength Training and Conditioning*. 2nd ed. Champaign, IL: Human Kinetics.

Earnest, C. P. 2001. Dietary androgen supplements. *The Physician and Sports Medicine* 29(5):63–79.

Francis, P. R. et al. 2001. An electromyographical approach to the evaluation of abdominal exercises. *ACSM's Health and Fitness Journal* 5(4):8+.

Hartgens, F. et al. 2001. Androgenic-anabolic steroid-induced body changes in strength athletes. *The Physician and Sports Medicine* 29(1):49–66.

Holt, S. July 2001. Mechanics of machines: Selecting the right piece of equipment. *Fitness Management* 56+.

Jones, C. S., C. Christenson, and M. Young. 2000. Weight training injury trends: A 20-year survey. *The Physician and Sports Medicine* 28(7):61–72.

Katzmarzyk, P. T. and L. C. Cora. 2002. Musculoskeletal fitness and risk of mortality. *Medicine and Science in Sports and Exercise* 34(5):740–744.

King, J. M. July 2001. The evolution of equipment. *Fitness Management* 46–51.

Misic, M., and G. A. Kelley. 2002. The impact of creatine supplementation on anaerobic performance: A meta-analysis. *American Journal of Sports Medicine* 4:116–124.

Schilling, B. K. et al. 2001. Creatine supplementation and health variables. *Medicine and Science in Sports and Exercise* 33(2):183–188.

Verducci, T. et al. Totally juiced. *Sports Illustrated*. 96(23) 34A.

Volek, J. S. 1999. Update: What we know about creatine. *ACSM's Health and Fitness Journal* 3(3):27–33.

Westcott, W. L., and T. R. Baechle. 1999. *Strength Training for Seniors*. Champaign, IL: Human Kinetics.

Yesalis, C. E., and Cowart, V. S. 1998. *The Steroids Game*. Champaign, IL: Human Kinetics.

 ## In the News

Research on PRE has proven challenging due to the large number of variables that can be manipulated (load, repetitions, sets) as well as the variability in individuals in regard to strength, endurance, nutrition status, etc. A number of recent studies have used well-controlled research designs to answer important questions about PRE.

Speed of Lifting

One study reported that slower lifting produced greater gains in strength than regular speed lifting. Individuals in the study were novice exercisers who completed 8 to 10 weeks of training (2–3 times per week) using a Nautilus circuit. The participants performed one set of each exercise in the circuit using either a standard cadence for the lift or a "Super Slow" training. Gains in 10 RM and 5 RM lifts were significantly greater for the Super Slow group than for the normal pace group although both groups improved.

Frequency of Lifting

Another study compared different frequencies of exercise when the total volume of work was held constant between the groups. One group lifted one day per week and did three sets and another group lifted 3 days per week and did one set of each exercise. The intensity (percent of 1 RM) was varied throughout the study in both groups by using a periodized repetition range of 3 to 10 and participants were instructed to do as many repetitions as possible. The group lifting one day a week had significant gains in strength but they were less than those for the group lifting 3 days per week. This study suggests that a higher frequency of resistance training produces larger gains in strength (and muscle mass) even when the overall amount of lifting is the same.

Varying Resistance Levels

Another study compared the effect of doing 3 days of lifting at 80 percent of 1 RM versus three different intensities (80 percent, 65 percent, and 50 percent). The gains were similar but the group performing the varied intensities had lower ratings of exertion of an assessment of "daily activity tasks" indicating better gains in endurance.

Lab Resource Materials: Muscle Fitness Tests

Evaluating Isotonic Strength: 1 RM

1. Use a weight machine for the leg press and seated arm press (or bench press) for the evaluation.
2. Estimate how much weight you can lift two or three times. Be conservative; it is better to start with too little weight than too much. If you lift the weight more than ten times, the procedure should be done again on another day when you are rested.
3. Using correct form, perform a leg press with the weight you have chosen. Perform as many times as you can up to ten.
4. Use Chart 1 to determine your 1 RM for the leg press. Find the weight used in the left-hand column and then find the number of repetitions you performed across the top of the chart.
5. Your 1 RM score is the value where the weight row and the repetitions column intersect.
6. Repeat this procedure for the seated arm press.
7. Record your 1 RM scores for the leg press and seated arm press in the Results section.
8. Next, divide your 1 RM scores by your body weight in pounds to get a "strength per pound of body weight" (str/lb/body wt.) score for each of the two exercises.
9. Finally, determine your strength rating for your upper body strength (arm press) and lower body (leg press) using Chart 2.

Chart 1 ▶ Predicted 1 RM Based on Reps-to-Fatigue

Wt	Repetitions										Wt	Repetitions									
	1	2	3	4	5	6	7	8	9	10		1	2	3	4	5	6	7	8	9	10
30	30	31	32	33	34	35	36	37	38	39	170	170	175	180	185	191	197	204	211	219	227
35	35	37	38	39	40	41	42	43	44	45	175	175	180	185	191	197	203	210	217	225	233
40	40	41	42	44	46	47	49	50	51	53	180	180	185	191	196	202	209	216	223	231	240
45	45	46	48	49	51	52	54	56	58	60	185	185	190	196	202	208	215	222	230	238	247
50	50	51	53	55	56	58	60	62	64	67	190	190	195	201	207	214	221	228	236	244	253
55	55	57	58	60	62	64	66	68	71	73	195	195	201	206	213	219	226	234	242	251	260
60	60	62	64	65	67	70	72	74	77	80	200	200	206	212	218	225	232	240	248	257	267
65	65	67	69	71	73	75	78	81	84	87	205	205	211	217	224	231	238	246	254	264	273
70	70	72	74	76	79	81	84	87	90	93	210	210	216	222	229	236	244	252	261	270	280
75	75	77	79	82	84	87	90	93	96	100	215	215	221	228	235	242	250	258	267	276	287
80	80	82	85	87	90	93	96	99	103	107	220	220	226	233	240	247	255	264	273	283	293
85	85	87	90	93	96	99	102	106	109	113	225	225	231	238	245	253	261	270	279	289	300
90	90	93	95	98	101	105	108	112	116	120	230	230	237	244	251	259	267	276	286	296	307
95	95	98	101	104	107	110	114	118	122	127	235	235	242	249	256	264	273	282	292	302	313
100	100	103	106	109	112	116	120	124	129	133	240	240	247	254	262	270	279	288	298	309	320
105	105	108	111	115	118	122	126	130	135	140	245	245	252	259	267	276	285	294	304	315	327
110	110	113	116	120	124	128	132	137	141	147	250	250	257	265	273	281	290	300	310	321	333
115	115	118	122	125	129	134	138	143	148	153	255	256	262	270	278	287	296	306	317	328	340
120	120	123	127	131	135	139	144	149	154	160	260	260	267	275	284	292	302	312	323	334	347
125	125	129	132	136	141	145	150	155	161	167	265	265	273	281	289	298	308	318	329	341	353
130	130	134	138	142	146	151	156	161	167	173	270	270	278	286	295	304	314	324	335	347	360
135	135	139	143	147	152	157	162	168	174	180	275	275	283	291	300	309	319	330	341	354	367
140	140	144	148	153	157	163	168	174	180	187	280	280	288	296	305	315	325	336	348	360	373
145	145	149	154	158	163	168	174	180	186	193	285	285	293	302	311	321	331	342	354	366	380
150	150	154	159	164	169	174	180	186	193	200	290	290	298	307	316	326	337	348	360	373	387
155	155	159	164	169	174	180	186	192	199	207	295	295	303	312	322	332	343	354	366	379	393
160	160	165	169	175	180	186	192	199	206	213	300	300	309	318	327	337	348	360	372	386	400
165	165	170	175	180	186	192	198	205	212	220	305	305	314	323	333	343	354	366	379	392	407

This chart is reprinted with permission from the *Journal of Physical Education, Recreation & Dance*, January 1993, p. 89. *JOPERD* is a publication of the American Alliance for Health, Physical Education, Recreation and Dance, 1900 Association Drive, Reston, VA 22091.

Evaluating Isometric Strength

Test: Grip Strength

Adjust a hand dynamometer to fit your hand size. Squeeze it as hard as possible. You may bend or straighten the arm, but do not touch the body with your hand, elbow, or arm. Perform with both right and left hands. *Note:* When not being tested, perform the Basic 8 isometric strength exercises, or squeeze and indent a new tennis ball (*after* completing the dynamometer test).

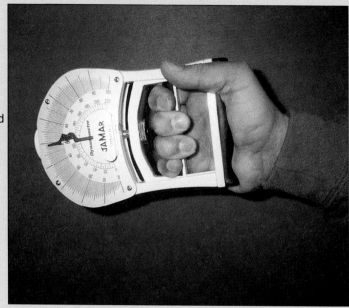

Evaluating Muscular Endurance

1. Curl-Up (Dynamic)

Sit on a mat or carpet with your legs bent more than 90 degrees so your feet remain flat on the floor (about halfway between 90 degrees and straight). Make two tape marks 4$\frac{1}{2}$ inches apart or lay a 4$\frac{1}{2}$ inch strip of paper or cardboard on the floor. Lie with your arms extended at your sides, palms down and the fingers extended so that your fingertips touch one tape mark (or one side of the paper or cardboard strip). Keeping your heels in contact with the floor, curl the head and shoulders forward until your fingers reach 4$\frac{1}{2}$ inches (second piece of tape or other side of strip). Lower slowly to beginning position. Repeat one curl-up every three seconds. Continue until you are unable to keep the pace of one curl-up every three seconds.

Two partners may be helpful. One stands on the cardboard strip (to prevent movement) if one is used. The second assures that the head returns to the floor after each repetition.

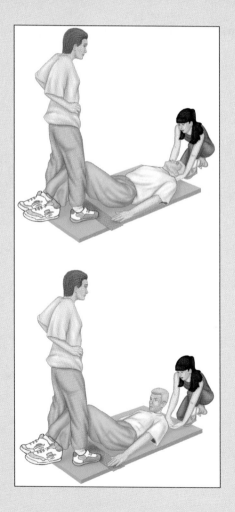

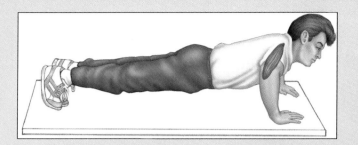

2. Ninety-Degree Push-Up (Dynamic)
Support the body in a push-up position from the toes. The hands should be just outside the shoulders, the back and legs straight, and the toes tucked under. Lower the body until the upper arm is parallel to the floor or the elbow is bent at 90 degrees. The rhythm should be approximately one push-up every three seconds. Repeat as many times as possible up to 35.

3. Flexed-Arm Support (Static)
Women: Support the body in a push-up position from the knees. The hands should be outside the shoulders, and the back and legs straight. Lower the body until the upper arm is parallel to the floor or the elbow is flexed at 90 degrees.
Men: Use the same procedure as for women except support the push-up position from the toes instead of the knees. (Same position as for 90-degree push-up, see previous page.) Hold the 90-degree position as long as possible, up to 35 seconds.

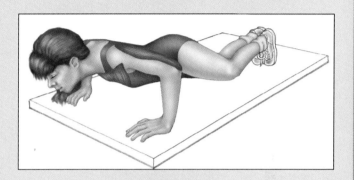

Chart 2 ▶ Strength Per Pound of Body Weight Ratings

Rating: Age:	Leg Press			Arm Press		
	30 or Less	31–50	51+	30 or Less	31–50	51+
Men						
High-performance zone	2.06+	1.81+	1.61+	1.26+	1.01+	.86+
Good fitness	1.96–2.05	1.66–1.80	1.51–1.60	1.11–1.25	.91–1.00	.76–0.85
Marginal	1.76–1.95	1.51–1.65	1.41–1.50	.96–1.10	.86–0.90	.66–0.75
Low fitness	1.75 or less	1.50 or less	1.40 or less	.96 or less	.80 or less	.65 or less
Women						
High-performance zone	1.61+	1.36+	1.16+	.75+	.61+	.51+
Good fitness	1.46\–1.60	1.21\–1.35	1.06–1.15	.65–0.75	.56–0.60	.46–0.50
Marginal	1.31–1.45	1.11–1.20	.96–1.05	.56–0.65	.51–0.55	.41–0.45
Low fitness	1.30 or less	1.10 or less	.95 or less	.55 or less	.50 or less	.40 or less

Chart 3 ▶ Isometric Strength Rating Scale (Pounds)

Classification Men	Left Grip	Right Grip	Total Score
High-performance zone	125+	135+	260+
Good fitness zone	100–124	110–134	210–259
Marginal zone	90–99	95–109	185–209
Low zone	less than 90	less than 95	less than 185
Women			
High-performance zone	75+	85+	160+
Good fitness zone	60–74	70–84	130–159
Marginal zone	45–59	50–69	95–129
Low zone	less than 45	less than 50	less than 95

Suitable for use by young adults between 18 and 30 years of age. After 30, an adjustment of 0.5 of 1 percent per year is appropriate because some loss of muscle tissue typically occurs as you grow older.

Chart 4 ▶ Rating Scale for Dynamic Muscular Endurance

Age: Classification Men	17–26 Curl-Up	17–26 Push-Ups	27–39 Curl-Up	27–39 Push-Ups	40–49 Curl-Up	40–49 Push-Ups	50–59 Curl-Up	50–59 Push-Ups	60+ Curl-Up	60+ Push-Ups
High-performance zone	35+	29+	34+	27+	33+	26+	32+	24+	31+	22+
Good fitness zone	24–34	20–28	23–33	18–26	22–32	17–25	21–31	15–23	20–30	13–21
Marginal zone	15–23	16–19	14–22	15–17	13–21	14–16	12–20	12–14	11–19	10–12
Low zone	<15	<16	<14	<15	<13	<14	<12	<12	<11	<10
Women										
High-performance zone	25+	17+	24+	16+	23+	15+	22+	14+	21+	13+
Good fitness zone	18–24	12–16	17–23	11–15	16–22	10–14	15–21	9–13	14–20	8–12
Marginal zone	10–17	8–11	9–16	7–10	8–15	6–9	7–14	5–8	6–13	4–7
Low zone	<10	<8	<9	<7	<8	<6	<7	<5	<6	<4

Chart 5 ▶ Rating Scale for Static Endurance (Flexed-Arm Support)

Classification	Score in Seconds
High-performance zone	30+
Good fitness zone	20–29
Marginal zone	10–19
Low zone	10

Lab 11A Evaluating Muscle Strength: 1 RM and Grip Strength

Name	**Section**	**Date**

Purpose: To evaluate your muscle strength using 1 RM and to determine the best amount of resistance to use for various strength exercises.

Procedure: 1 RM refers to the maximum amount of resistance you can lift for a specific exercise. Testing yourself to determine how much you can lift only one time using traditional methods can be fatiguing and even dangerous. The procedure you will perform here allows you to estimate 1 RM based on the number of times you can lift a weight that is less than 1 RM.

Evaluating Strength Using Estimated 1 RM

1. Use a resistance machine for the leg press and arm or bench press for the evaluation part of this lab.
2. Estimate how much weight you can lift two or three times. Be conservative; it is better to start with too little weight than too much. If you lift a weight more than ten times, the procedure should be done again on another day when you are rested.
3. Using correct form, perform a leg press with the weight you have chosen. Perform as many times as you can up to 10.
4. Use Chart 1 to determine your 1 RM for the leg press. Find the weight used in the left-hand column and then find the number of repetitions you performed across the top of the chart.
5. Your 1 RM score is the value where the weight row and the repetitions column intersect.
6. Repeat this procedure for the arm or bench press using the same technique.
7. Record your 1 RM scores for the leg press and bench press in the Results section.
8. Next divide your 1 RM scores by your body weight in pounds to get a "strength per pound of body weight" (str/lb/body wt.) score for each of the two exercises.
9. Determine your strength rating for your upper body strength (arm press) and lower body (leg press) using Chart 2 in the lab resource materials. Record in the Results section. If time allows, assess 1 RM for other exercises you choose to perform (see Lab 11C).
10. If a grip dynamometer is available, determine your right-hand and left-hand grip strength using the procedures in the lab resource materials. Use Chart 3 to rate your grip (isometric) strength.

Results:

Arm press
(or bench press):

Wt. selected [　　] Reps [　　] Estimated 1 RM [　　]
(Chart 1, lab resource materials)

Strength per lb. body weight [　　] Rating [　　]
(1 RM ÷ body weight) (Chart 2, lab resource materials)

Leg press:

Wt. selected [　　] Reps [　　] Estimated 1 RM [　　]
(Chart 1, lab resource materials)

Strength per lb. body weight [　　] Rating [　　]
(1 RM ÷ body weight) (Chart 2, lab resource materials)

Grip strength:

Right grip score [　　] Right grip rating [　　]

Left grip score [　　] Left grip rating [　　]

Total score [　　] Total rating [　　]

Conclusions and Implications: In several sentences, discuss your current strength, whether you believe it is adequate for good health, and whether you think that your "strength per pound of body weight" scores are really representative of your true strength.

Lab 11B Evaluating Muscular Endurance

Name		Section	Date

Purpose: To evaluate the dynamic muscular endurance of two muscle groups and the static endurance of the arms and trunk muscles.

Procedure:

1. Perform the curl-up, push-up, and flexed-arm support tests described in the Lab Resource Materials.
2. Record your test scores in the Results section. Determine and record your rating from Charts 4 and 5 in the lab resource materials.

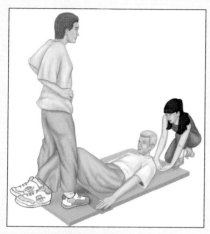

1. Curl-up (dynamic)

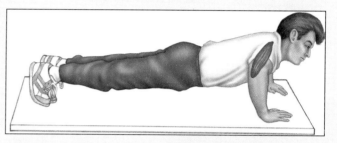

2. Ninety-degree push-up (dynamic)

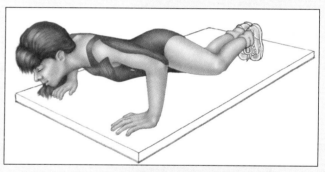

3. Flexed-arm support (static): women in knee position and men in full support position

Results:

Record your scores below.

Curl-up [ ]   Push-up [ ]   Flexed-arm support (seconds) [ ]

Check your ratings below.

Chart 1 ▶ Rating Scale for Static Endurance (Flexed-Arm Support)

	High Performance	Good Fitness	Marginal	Poor
Curl-up	◯	◯	◯	◯
Push-up	◯	◯	◯	◯
Flexed-arm support	◯	◯	◯	◯

On which of the tests of muscular endurance did you score the lowest? ◯ Curl-up ◯ Push-up ◯ Flexed-arm support

On which of the tests of muscular endurance did you score the best? ◯ Curl-up ◯ Push-up ◯ Flexed-arm support

Conclusions and Implications: In several sentences, discuss your current level of muscular endurance and whether this level is enough to meet your health, work, and leisure-time needs in the future.

Lab 11C Planning and Logging Muscle Fitness Exercises: Free Weights or Resistance Machines

Name		Section	Date

Purpose: To set lifestyle goals for muscle fitness exercise, to prepare a muscle fitness exercise plan, and to self-monitor progress for the one-week plan.

Procedures:

1. The Basic 8 exercises are listed for free weights and resistance machines. Use Chart 1 to select eight exercises to represent your Basic 8 exercises. If you would like to add other exercises to your program, then list them on the lines at the bottom of the chart. Descriptions of the exercises are provided in Exercise Tables 9 and 10.

2. In Chart 1, also indicate the days of the week that you plan on performing the exercises and the number of reps and the number of sets. Be sure to base your program on your goals (strength/endurance). If you are just starting out it is best to start with one set of twelve to fifteen repetitions. Use the 1 RM procedure described in Lab 11A, to help you determine the amount of weight or resistance to use. Plan to do at least eight exercises, two or three times a week. Note: All exercises do not have to be performed on the same day, but many people find this more convenient.

3. Though abdominal exercises are not typically done using free weights or resistance machines, an abdominal exercise is recommended as part of a resistance exercise program. Two abdominal exercises are provided in the "other" category for you to consider (see Table 8).

4. In Chart 2, keep a one-week log of your actual participation. For best results, keep the log with you during your workout session. Indicate the exercises you performed, including any that you didn't plan on performing when you developed your schedule. If you would like to keep a log for more than one week, make extra copies of the log before you begin.

5. Answer the questions in the Results section.

Chart 1 ▶ Muscle Fitness Exercise Plan

What is your goal? Check one or more: Strength ☐   Endurance ☐   General Fitness ☐
Check boxes beside at least 8 exercises, note days, reps, sets, and resistance to be used.

Primary Body Parts to Be Exercised	Free Weight Exercises (Basic 8)	Machine Weight Exercises (Basic 8)	Day 1 Date	Day 2 Date	Day 3 Date	How Many Reps?	How Many Sets?	Weight or Setting
Chest	Bench press	Chest press						
Shoulder	Overhead press	Seated press						
Arm (bicep)	Bicep curl	Bicep curl						
Arm (tricep)	Tricep curl	Tricep press						
Arm (wrist)	Wrist curl	(No equivalent*)						
Back	(No equivalent*)	Lat pull down						
Back (lower)	(No equivalent*)	Seated rowing						
Hip/leg (thigh)	Lunge	(No equivalent*)						
Leg (thigh)	Half squat	Knee extension						
Leg (hamstring)	(No equivalent*)	Hamstring curl						
Leg (calf)	Heel raise	(No equivalent*)						
Other exercises								
Abdominal	Crunch	Reverse curl						

*Note: Some free weight and machine exercises do not have equivalents.

203

Chart 2 ▶ Muscle Fitness Exercise Log

Check the exercises you performed and the days you performed them.

Primary Body Parts to Be Exercised	Free Weight Exercises (Basic 8)	Machine Weight Exercises (Basic 8)	Day 1 Date	Day 2 Date	Day 3 Date
Chest	Bench press	Chest press			
Shoulder	Overhead press	Seated press			
Arm (bicep)	Bicep curl	Bicep curl			
Arm (tricep)	Tricep curl	Tricep press			
Arm (wrist)	Wrist curl	(No equivalent*)			
Back	(No equivalent*)	Lat pull down			
Back (lower)	(No equivalent*)	Seated rowing			
Hip/leg (thigh)	Lunge	(No equivalent*)			
Leg (thigh)	Half squat	Knee extension			
Leg (hamstring)	(No equivalent*)	Hamstring curl			
Leg (calf)	Heel raise	(No equivalent*)			
Other exercises					
Abdominal	Crunch	Reverse curl			

*Note: Some free weight and machine exercises do not have equivalents.

Results:

Were you able to do your Basic 8 exercises at least two days in the week?　　◯ Yes　◯ No

Conclusions and Implications:

1. Do you feel that you will use muscle fitness exercises as part of your regular lifetime physical activity plan, either now or in the future? Use several sentences to answer.

2. Discuss the exercises you feel benefited you and the ones that did not. What modifications would you make in your program for it to work better for you? Use several sentences to answer.

Lab 11D Planning and Logging Muscle Fitness Exercises: Calisthenics or Isometric Exercises

Name	**Section**	**Date**

Purpose: To set lifestyle goals for muscle fitness exercises that can easily be performed at home, to prepare a muscle fitness exercise plan, and to self-monitor progress for a one-week plan.

Procedures:

1. The Basic 8 exercises are listed for calisthenics and isometric exercises. Use Chart 1 to select eight exercises to represent your Basic 8. If you would like to add other exercises to your program, then list them on the lines at the bottom of the chart. Descriptions of the exercises are provided in Tables 11 and 12.
2. In Chart 1, indicate the days of the week that you plan to perform the exercises and the number of reps and the number of sets. Plan to do at least eight exercises, two or three times a week. Note: All exercises do not have to be performed on the same day, but many people find this more convenient. Do what is best for your schedule.
3. In Chart 2, keep a one-week log of your actual participation. For best results, keep the log with you during your workout session. Indicate the exercises you performed, including any that you did not plan on. If you would like to keep a log for more than one week, make extra copies of the log before you begin.
4. Answer the questions in the Results section.

Chart 1 ▶ Muscle Fitness Exercise Log

What is your goal? Check one or more: Strength ☐   Endurance ☐   General Fitness ☐
Check boxes beside at least 8 exercises, note days, reps, sets, and resistance to be used.

Primary Body Parts to Be Exercised	Calisthenic Exercises (Basic 8)	Isometric Exercises (Basic 8)	Day 1 Date	Day 2 Date	Day 3 Date	How Many Reps?	How Many Sets?
Chest	Knee push-up	Arm press in door					
Shoulder	(No equivalent*)	Overhead press in door					
Arm (bicep)	Modified pull-up	Bicep curl					
Arm (tricep)	Dips	Tricep press					
Trunk/back	Trunk lift	(No equivalent*)					
Abdominals	Crunch	Pelvic tilt					
Leg (outer)	Side leg raise	(No equivalent*)					
Leg (inner)	Lower leg lift	(No equivalent*)					
Leg (thigh)	Leg kneel	Leg press					
Leg (thigh)	(No equivalent*)	Wall seat					
Leg (hamstring)	(No equivalent*)	Hamstring exercise					
Other							

*Note: Calisthenics and isometric exercises may not have exact equivalents.

Chart 2 ▶ Muscle Fitness Exercise Log

Check the exercises you performed and the days you performed them.

Primary Body Parts to Be Exercised	Calisthenic Exercises (Basic 8)	Isometric Exercises (Basic 8)	Day 1 Date	Day 2 Date	Day 3 Date
Chest	Knee push-up	Arm press in door			
Shoulder	(No equivalent*)	Overhead press in door			
Arm (bicep)	Modified pull-up	Bicep curl			
Arm (tricep)	Dips	Tricep press			
Trunk/back	Trunk lift	(No equivalent*)			
Abdominals	Crunch	Pelvic tilt			
Leg (outer)	Side leg raise	(No equivalent*)			
Leg (inner)	Lower leg lift	(No equivalent*)			
Leg (thigh)	Leg kneel	Leg press			
Leg (thigh)	(No equivalent*)	Wall seat			
Leg (hamstring)	(No equivalent*)	Hamstring exercise			
Other					

*Note: Calisthenics and isometric exercises may not have exact equivalents.

Results:

Were you able to do your Basic 8 exercises at least two days in the week? ◯ Yes ◯ No

Conclusions and Implications:

1. Do you feel that you will use these muscle fitness exercises as part of your regular lifetime physical activity plan, either now or in the future? Would the convenience of being able to do these exercises anywhere make it easier for you to stick with your program? Use several sentences to answer.

2. Discuss the exercises you feel benefited you and the ones that did not. What modifications would you make in your program for it to work better for you? Use several sentences to answer.

Safe Physical Activity and Exercises

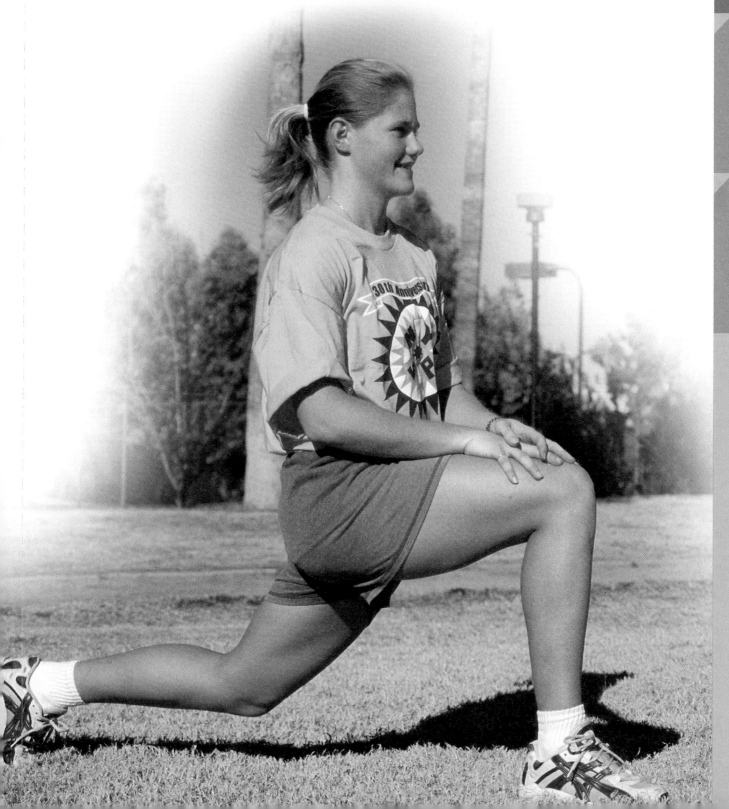

There are safe exercises that can be used as alternatives to questionable exercises that may cause more harm than good.

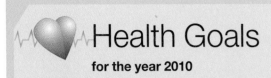

Health Goals

for the year 2010

- Increase incidence of people reporting "healthy days."
- Increase "active days" without pain.
- Reduce activity limitations.

One can choose from thousands of exercises, but they must be chosen carefully because not all exercises are good for all people. Some exercises should be avoided because there is some risk of injury. We term these exercises "questionable" or "hazardous." Some of these exercises so drastically violate the mechanics of the human frame that they are dangerous and should never be used by anyone.

Studies indicate that many fitness centers and health clubs do not employ properly trained instructors. Those most likely to be qualified to advise you about exercise have college degrees and four to eight years of study in such courses as anatomy, physiology, kinesiology, preventive and therapeutic exercise, and physiology of exercise. These qualified individuals are most likely to be athletic trainers, biomechanists, kinesiotherapists, physical educators, physical therapists, or strength and conditioning specialists. On-the-job training, good physique or figure, or good athletic or dancing ability are not sufficient qualifications for teaching or advising about exercise. People with appropriate training will have the appropriate college degree and additional certifications to document their knowledge of the topic.

If you have had knowledgeable instructors, you may recognize some questionable exercises, but others listed here may set off a protest such as: "I've been doing that all my life and it never has hurt me!"

This concept explains the difference between individually prescribed exercise and mass prescription; what is good for one person may not be good for another. The difference between microtrauma and acute injury, and the significance of the number of repetitions, will also be discussed. Potentially hazardous exercises for most people are presented with the reasons for classifying them as such. Safer alternative exercises are suggested. The old saying

"when in doubt, don't do it" is a good philosophy when choosing exercises because you can always find safe, effective alternative exercises for any specific muscle group.

Harmful Effects of Questionable Exercises

Exercises that are good when prescribed for a particular individual differ from those that are good for everyone (mass prescription).

Individual Prescription

In the clinical setting, a therapist works with one patient. A case history is taken and tests made to determine which muscles are weak or strong, short or long. Exercises are then prescribed for that specific person. The patient is supervised in the correct execution of the exercises.

For example, in a back care program for an individual with lumbar lordosis, back hyperextension exercises might be **contraindicated.** However, another client might have a flat lumbar spine with limited range of motion, in which case, a set of back hyperextension exercises would be indicated. Thus, the classification of exercises in this concept does not necessarily apply to the setting where individual prescription is done by a qualified professional.

Mass Prescription

When a physical educator, aerobics instructor, or coach leads a group of people in exercises, or a book or magazine describes a great exercise to "slim and trim," and all participants in the group or all readers perform the same exercise, this is a mass prescription. There is little if any consideration for individual differences except perhaps some allowance made in the number of repetitions or in the amount of weight (resistance) used.

Some of the exercises that would be appropriate for an individual would not be appropriate for all individuals in the group. Since it is not practical to prescribe individually for everyone, it is necessary to consider what the needs of the majority may be and choose the least harmful (but most effective) exercises for the group.

Some exercises can produce microtrauma, and some may cause acute injuries. **www.mhhe.com/fit_well/web12 Click 01. Microtrauma** refers to "a silent injury"; that is, an injury that results from repetitive motions such as those used in calisthenics or sports. These

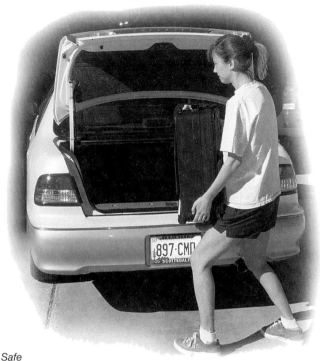

Safe exercise includes performing activities of daily living properly.

Technology Update

Ergonomics, also known as Human Factors Engineering, is a discipline that helps to develop tools and workplace settings that put the least amount of strain on the body. Biomechanical principles are used to help identify movements and positions that may put individuals at greater risk for specific injuries or microtrauma. Many worksites take an active interest in ergonomic principles since repetitive motion injuries and other musculoskeletal conditions are the leading cause of work-related ill health.

One application of ergonomics is the design of effective workstations for computer users. Proper fitting desks and chairs and effective positioning of the computer on the desk have been shown to minimize problems such as carpal tunnel syndrome (CTS), a painful and debilitating injury of the median nerve at the wrist. Risk of CTS increases if the fingers are forced to be above the wrists while typing so care should be used to ensure proper desk and chair height. Wrist rests can also be used to provide support for the wrist. The Human Factors and Ergonomics Society has recently released a guidebook called "Human Factors Engineering of Computer Workstations" (for more information check On the Web **www.mhhe.com/fit_well/web12 Click 02**).

injuries also occur in occupations. Other terms that frequently appear in the scientific literature include repetitive motion syndrome, repetitive strain injury (RSI), cumulative trauma disorder (CTD), and overuse syndrome. They all refer to injury caused by repetitive movement. We may violate the integrity of our joints by performing, for example, forty backward arm circles with the palms down three days per week for ten or twenty years. The wear and tear is not usually noticed by the participant until the friction over time wears down the tendon, ligament, and/or bone, resulting in tendonitis, faciitis, bursitis, arthritis, and nerve compression. The injury may not become apparent until later in life. Chances are, when the injury reaches an acute stage in later life, the cause of the injury is never really identified and will be attributed to old age. Because the injury is unseen and unfelt, the participant views the exercise as harmless. Note: Many of the changes in the musculoskeletal system normally attributed to aging are found in young athletes. Degenerated disks are a common finding.

The term *acute injury* as used here refers to the stress, strain, or sprain that produces pain at the time it occurs or within a few hours of performing the exercise. For example, violating the integrity of the knee joint by placing torque on it during a toe touch or knee bend can tear the ligament and cartilage on the inside of the knee so the participant knows immediately that an injury occurred during that exercise. Some of the exercises considered questionable in this concept are capable of producing this kind of injury, whereas others in the list are more apt to produce the "silent" microtrauma. Some exercises can produce both types of injury.

Some exercises may be reasonably safe for most people when performed only once but may become hazardous when done repetitively. An acute exercise injury in any hazardous activity may occur the first time you place yourself at risk, or it may never happen. Microtrauma, on the other hand, occurs with each repetition of an exercise that violates physiologic movements or normal joint mechanics. We cannot avoid all wear and tear on the body, and it is true that we must "use it or lose it," but we can reduce wear and tear by eliminating hazardous activities, because if we do not use it correctly, then we will also lose it! Some of the exercises considered questionable because of microtrauma can probably be performed safely when the number of repetitions is small and they are rarely used. For example, if hyperextending the back in the prone press-up feels comfortable, then it is probably safe when done once as a static stretch after a series of abdominal strengthening exercises, but repetitive hyperextension exercises, even if comfortable, are hazardous.

Contraindicated A term used to describe treatments or exercises that are not recommended because of the potential for harm.

Microtrauma Injury so small it is not detected at the time it occurs.

Some Guidelines for Avoiding Hazardous Exercises

Most hazardous exercises occur at the extreme ranges of motion. The human body is made to move. Nevertheless, there are certain movements that put the joints and musculoskeletal system at risk and should therefore be avoided. Most of the contraindicated exercises involve positions at the extreme ranges of motion. General guidelines for safer exercises are presented at the end of this concept. With respect to back health, many contraindicated movements involve hyperflexion or hyperextension movements. Hyperflexion causes the disk to bulge outward where it can impinge on the spinal cord. Hyperextension causes scraping and "wear and tear" on the facet joints that join each vertebral segment (see Figure 1). Hyperflexion and extension of the knee also puts excessive stress on the ligaments and joint capsule. Care should be used to avoid these movements during normal daily activity and to avoid exercises that involve these positions.

Other Important Facts

If sports or special jobs require dangerous movements or exercises, developing and maintaining high levels of physical fitness is especially important. In baseball, the catcher has to assume and maintain a deep squat position for long periods of time. This causes microtrauma to the knee. Gymnasts frequently perform double-leg raises and movements resulting in hyperextension of the back. These movements cause microtrauma to the spine. Some workers (e.g., postal workers and construction workers) may also perform movements that produce microtrauma even when adhering to guidelines for efficient and safe exercise. It is especially important that these people develop muscle fitness and flexibility in the regions of the body that are exposed to the dangerous movements. Baseball catchers should be sure to strengthen the muscles around the knee and stretch the hamstring and quadriceps muscles. Gymnasts should exercise to build strong abdominal and back muscles as well as stretch to lengthen the back, hamstring, and hip flexor muscles. Workers should similarly strengthen and lengthen the muscles associated with the movements commonly used in their jobs.

Some exercises performed in training for sports can predispose a person to injury. Many young athletes perform certain exercises because their coaches recommend them or their friends and teammates perform them in practice. Ballistic stretching or passive forms of resistance are often used in training programs but these can lead to injury or instability in certain joints. Competitive swimmers, for example, often perform a variety of

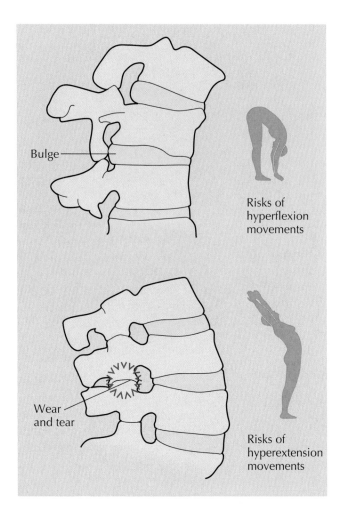

Figure 1 ▶ Risks of hyperflexion and hyperextension.

ballistic stretches or use passive forms of resistance to loosen up their shoulder muscles prior to swimming. One common exercise involves pulling the arms backward at shoulder level until they cross each other behind the back or pulling the bent elbows together making them touch while the hands are on the back of the head. Competitive swimmers sometimes begin such practices while they are in children's swimming programs and continue them through their competitive years. Such overstretching has resulted in painful shoulders and disability.

Tiptoeing exercises such as those performed in dance class will develop the calf muscles, but they will overstretch the muscles and ligaments supporting the long arch of the foot. Heel walking may have the same effect; that is, it may develop strong shin muscles while further weakening the arch. The harm is lessened if these exercises are performed with the toes turned in slightly.

Jogging and aerobic dance exercise may not be appropriate activities for all people. www.mhhe.com/fit_well/web12 Click 03. Jogging and aerobic dance exercises are excellent for cardiovascular conditioning, weight control, and improvement of a variety of conditions; however, reasonable caution should be observed. Jogging has been used successfully in rehabilitating cardiac patients and a variety of other health problems. Like many other exercises, jogging should not be done without a physician's approval for people with arthritis, osteoporosis, and heart and circulatory diseases. The pounding from repeated strides can lead to shin splints, blisters, and a variety of foot, ankle, knee, and hip problems. Wearing the proper footwear and learning how to jog correctly will minimize these hazards. If you have poor leg or foot alignment, you would be wise to jog only three or four days per week because studies show that the risk of injury is greatest for those who jog every day. Or you should choose another activity such as cycling or swimming. The same fitness levels will result with less risk of injury.

Aerobic dance exercise has some of the same hazards as jogging; these include the overstress syndromes from too many hours of high-impact landings on the floor. The most common problems are shin splints, Achilles tendon injuries, arch strains, and pain under the knee cap. Most of these problems can be prevented by warming up and stretching properly before exercising, by using low-impact movements, and by avoiding hazardous exercises such as those described in this concept. More recently, there have been increasing reports of dizziness, hearing loss, and impaired balance in pupils and in teachers. Loud music can cause hearing loss, and high-impact landings may cause inner ear damage, but the causes are not yet understood. Some women may need to wear a special bra as a comfort measure for either jogging or dance exercise.

Movements and postures during daily activities can also put the body at risk. Most people are aware that standing toe touches put a lot of strain on the low back. The reason is that it causes hyperflexion in the low back which increases the pressure on the vertebral disks. Slouching in a chair can also put the back at risk (see Figure 2). Because we spend a large amount of time sitting it is important to adopt good sitting postures to reduce damage to the low back. More on back care can be found in concept 13.

The valsalva maneuver should be avoided when exerting great force in weight lifting, calisthenics, and isometrics. Many people mistakenly hold their breath when lifting weights or exerting force. This action, known as a **valsalva maneuver** is potentially dangerous and should be avoided. A sharp increase occurs in thoracic pressure and arterial blood pressure when force is exerted in this way. The pressure decreases rapidly when the breath is released and can lead to a lag in blood flow to the heart. This can lead to dizziness,

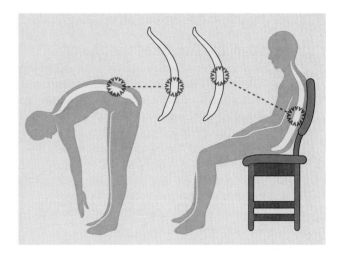

Figure 2 ► Poor sitting posture puts the back at risk.

blackouts, and inguinal hernias. Do not hold your breath during exercises. **Hyperventilation** should also be avoided.

Strategies for Action

Common exercises when misused or abused are potentially harmful. www.mhhe.com/fit_well/ web12 Click 04. A number of commonly used exercises are considered by experts to be contraindicated or not recommended for most individuals. These exercises typically put the body in a position that compromises the integrity of the joint or put extra strain on the muscles and ligaments that support the body. No harm may be associated with doing the exercise once but repeated use over time can lead to instability or more significant problems. In most cases, safer exercises target the same muscles or areas more effectively. Table 1 on the following pages shows a number of questionable exercises and safer alternatives.

Valsalva Maneuver Exerting force with the epiglottis closed. This action increases pressure in the thorax and raises arterial blood pressure. When released, arterial pressure drops rapidly, blood vessels expand and are then filled, causing a lag in blood flow to the left ventricle. When this occurs, the subject may become dizzy or feel faint. May be caused by holding the breath while exerting force.

Hyperventilation Overbreathing; forced, rapid, or deep breathing.

Table 1

Table 1 Questionable Exercises and Safe Alternatives

Questionable Exercise: The Swan

This exercise hyperextends the lower back and stretches the abdominals. These muscles are too long and weak in most people and should not be lengthened further. It can be harmful to the back, potentially causing an impingement on the nerve, compression, and even herniation of the disc, and myofascial trigger points. Other exercises in which this occurs include: cobras, backbends, straight-leg lifts, straight-leg sit-ups, prone-back lifts, donkey kicks, fire hydrants, prone swans, backward trunk circling, weight lifting with the back arched, and landing from a jump with the back arched.

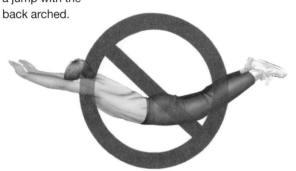

Questionable Exercise: Back-Arching Abdominal Stretch

This exercise can stretch the hip flexors, quadriceps, and shoulder flexors (such as the pectorals), but it also stretches the abdominals, which is not desired. Because of the armpull, it can potentially hyperflex the knee joint.

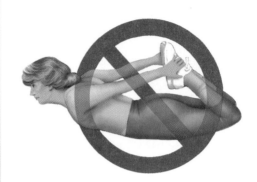

Safer Alternative Exercise: Back Extension

Lie prone over a roll of blankets or pillows and extend the back to a neutral or horizontal position.

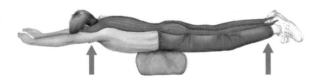

Safer Alternative Exercise: PNF Pectoral Stretch

Stand erect in the doorway with arms raised 45 degrees, elbows bent, and hands grasping door jambs, and feet in front stride position. Press forward on door frame, contracting the arms maximally for several seconds. Relax and shift weight on legs so muscles on front of shoulder joint and chest are stretched. Hold. Repeat with arms at 90 and 135 degrees. If your goal is stretching the hip flexors and quadriceps, substitute the hip and thigh stretcher.

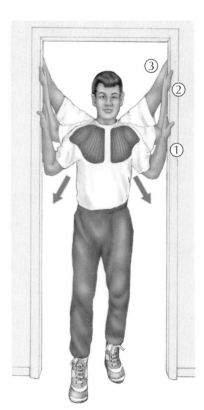

Table 1

Questionable Exercise: Donkey Kick

This exercise may involve touching the nose with the knee followed by a ballistic backward kick, hyperextending the neck and the lower back when the leg is lifted above the horizontal.

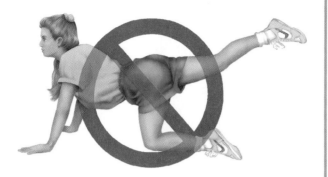

Questionable Exercise: Double-Leg Lift

This exercise is usually used with the intent of strengthening the lower abdominals, when in fact it is primarily a hip flexor (iliopsoas) strengthening exercise. Most people have overdeveloped the hip flexors and do not need to further strengthen those muscles because this may cause forward pelvic tilt. Even if the abdominals are strong enough to contract isometrically to prevent hyperextension of the lower back, the exercise produces excess compression on the discs.

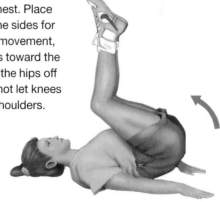

Safer Alternative Exercise: Knee-to-Nose

Kneel on all fours. While looking forward, pull the knee up under the chest, then extend the leg backward, being sure not to raise the leg higher than the horizontal. Change legs.

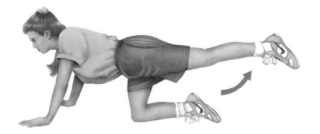

Safer Alternative Exercise: Reverse Curl

This exercise strengthens the lower abdominals. Lie on your back on the floor and bring your knees in toward the chest. Place the arms at the sides for support. For movement, pull the knees toward the head, raising the hips off the floor. Do not let knees go past the shoulders. Return to starting position and repeat.

Table 1

Table 1 Questionable Exercises and Safe Alternatives

Questionable Exercise: The Windmill

This exercise involves simultaneous rotation and flexion (or extension) of the lower back, which is contraindicated. Because of the shape of the facet joints in the lumbar spine, these movements violate normal joint mechanics, placing tremendous torsional stress on the joint capsule.

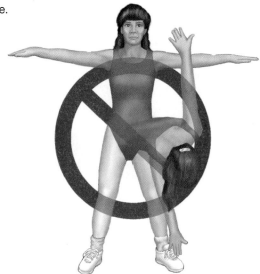

Questionable Exercise: Neck Circling

This exercise and other exercises that require neck hyperextension (e.g., neck bridging) can pinch arteries and nerves in the neck and at the base of the skull, grind down the discs, and produce dizziness or myofascial trigger points. In people with degenerated discs, it can cause dizziness, numbness, or even precipitate strokes. It also aggravates arthritis and degenerated discs.

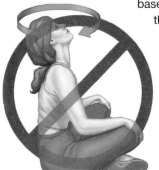

Safer Alternative Exercise: Back-Saver Hamstring Stretch

This exercise stretches the hamstring and lower back muscles. Sit with one leg extended and one knee bent, foot turned outward and close to the buttocks. Clasp hands behind back. Bend forward from the hips, keeping the low back as straight as possible. Allow bent knee to move laterally so trunk can move forward. Stretch and hold. Repeat with the other leg.

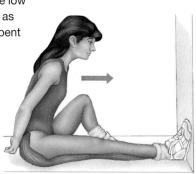

Safer Alternative Exercise: Head Clock

This exercise relaxes the muscle of the neck. Assume a good posture (seated with legs crossed or in a chair), and imagine that your neck is a clock face with the chin at the center. Flex the neck and point the chin at 6:00, hold, lift the chin; repeat pointing chin to 4:00, to 8:00, to 3:00 and finally to 9:00. Return to center position with chin up after each movement.

214

Questionable Exercise: Shoulder Stand Bicycle

This exercise and the yoga positions called the plough and the plough shear (not shown) force the neck and upper back to hyperflex. It has been estimated that 80 percent of the population has forward head and kyphosis (humpback) with accompanying weak muscles. This exercise is especially dangerous for these people. Neck hyperflexion results in excessive stretch on the ligaments and nerves. It can also aggravate preexisting thin discs and arthritic conditions. If the purpose for these exercises is to reduce gravitational effects on the circulatory system or internal organs, lie on a tilt board with the feet elevated. If the purpose is to warm up the muscles in the legs, slow jog in place. If the purpose is to stretch the lower back, try the leg hug exercise.

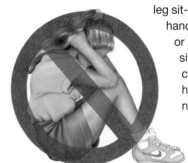

Questionable Exercise: Straight-Leg and Bent-Knee Sit-Ups

There are several valid criticisms of the sit-up exercise. Straight-leg sit-ups can displace the fifth lumbar vertebra causing back problems. A bent-knee sit-up creates less shearing force on the spine, but some recent studies have shown it produces greater compression on the lumbar discs than the straight-leg sit-up. Placing the hands behind the neck or head during the sit-up or during a crunch results in hyperflexion of the neck.

Safer Alternative Exercise: Leg Hug

Lie on your back with the knees bent at about 90 degrees. Bring your knees to the chest and wrap the arms around the back of the thighs. Pull knees to chest and hold.

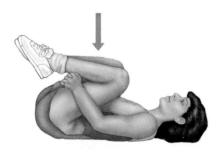

Safer Alternative Exercise: Crunch

Lie on your back with the knees bent more than 90 degrees. Curl up until the shoulder blades lift off the floor, then roll down to starting position and repeat. There are several safe arm positions. The easiest is with the arms extended straight in front of the body. Alternatives are with the arms crossed over the chest or the palms or fist held beside the ears.

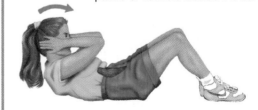

Table 1 Questionable Exercises and Safe Alternatives

Table 1

Questionable Exercise: Standing Toe Touches or Double-Leg Toe Touches

These exercises—especially when done ballistically—can produce degenerative changes at the lumbosacral joint. They also stretch the ligaments and joint capsule of the knee. Bending the back while the legs are straight may cause back strain, particularly if the movement is done ballistically. If performed only on rare occasions as a test, the chance of injury is less than if incorporated into a regular exercise program. Safer stretches of the lower back include the leg hug, the single knee-to-chest, the hamstring stretcher, and the back-saver toe touch.

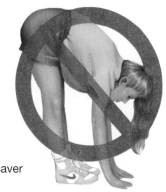

Questionable Exercise: Bar Stretch

This type of stretch may be harmful. Some experts have found that when the extended leg is raised 90 degrees or more and the trunk is bent over the leg, it may lead to **sciatica** and **pyriformis syndrome,** especially in the person who has limited flexibility.

Safer Alternative Exercise: Back-Saver Toe Touch

Sit on the floor. Extend leg and bend the other knee, placing the foot flat on the floor. Bend at the hip and reach forward with both hands. Grasp one foot, ankle, or calf depending upon the distance you can reach. Pull forward with your arms trying to touch your head to your knee. Slight bend in the knee is acceptable. Hold. Repeat with the opposite leg.

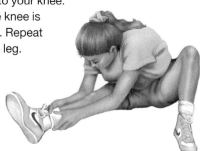

Safer Alternative Exercise: Hamstring Stretcher

Lie on your back with the knees bent at about 90 degrees. Draw one knee to the chest by pulling on the thigh with the hands, then extend the knee and point the foot toward the ceiling. Hold. Pull to chest again and return to the starting position. Repeat with the other leg.

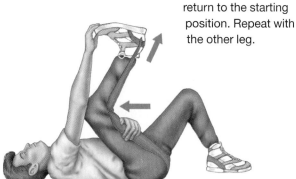

Questionable Exercise: Shin and Quadriceps Stretcher

This exercise causes hyperflexion of the knee. When the knee is hyperflexed to 120 degrees or more, the ligaments and joint capsule are stretched and the cartilage may be damaged. In many cases, people who do this exercise place the knee in a rotated position with **torque** on the flexed knee, which stretches the ligaments and capsule, and may damage the cartilage. Note: One of the quadriceps, the rectus femoris, is not stretched by these exercises because it crosses the hip as well as the knee joint. If the exercise is used to stretch the quadriceps, substitute the hip and thigh stretcher. For most people it is not necessary to stretch the shin muscles, since they are often elongated and weak; however, if you need to stretch the shin muscles to relieve muscle soreness, try the shin stretcher.

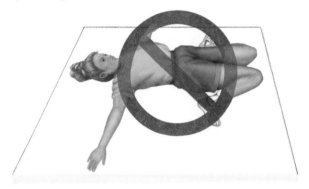

Questionable Exercise: The Hero

Like the shin and quadriceps stretcher this exercise causes hyperflexion of the knee. It also causes torque on the hyperflexed knee. For these reasons the ligaments and joint capsule are stretched and the cartilage may be damaged. This exercise does not stretch the rectus femoris, one of the quadriceps muscles. For most people it is not necessary to stretch the shin muscles since they are often elongated and weak; however, if you need to stretch the shin muscles use the shin stretcher. If this exercise is used to stretch the quadricps substitute the hip and thigh stretcher.

Safer Alternative Exercise: Hip and Thigh Stretcher

Kneel so that the front leg is bent at 90 degrees (front knee directly above the front ankle). The knee of the back leg should touch the floor well behind the front foot. Press the pelvis forward and downward. Hold. Repeat with the opposite leg forward. Do not bend the front knee more than 90 degrees.

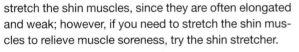

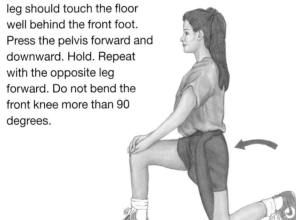

Safer Alternative Exercise: Shin Stretcher

Kneel on your knees, turn to right and press down on right ankle with right hand. Hold. Keep hips thrust forward to avoid hyperflexing the knees. Do not sit on the heels. Repeat on the left side.

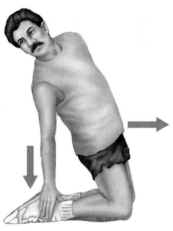

Sciatica Pain along the sciatic nerve in the buttock and leg.

Pyriformis Syndrome Muscle spasm and nerve entrapment in the pyriformis muscle of the buttocks region causing pain in the buttock and referred pain down the leg (sciatica).

Torque A twisting or rotating force.

Table 1 Questionable Exercises and Safe Alternatives

Questionable Exercise: Deep Squatting Exercises

This exercise, with or without weights, places the knee joint in hyperflexion, tends to "wedge it open," stretching the ligaments, irritating the synovial membrane, and possibly damaging the cartilage. The joint has even greater stress when the lower leg and foot are not in straight alignment with the knee. If you are performing squats to strengthen the knee and hip extensors, then try substituting the alternate leg kneel or half-squat with free weight or leg presses on a resistance machine.

Questionable Exercise: Knee Pull-Down

This exercise can result in hyperflexion of the knee. The arms or hands placed on top of the shin places undue stress on the knee joint.

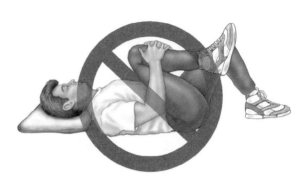

Safer Alternative Exercise: Alternate Leg Kneel

From a standing position, with or without a free weight, take a step forward with right foot, touching left knee to floor. The front knee should be bent only to a 90-degree angle. Return to start and lunge forward with other foot. Repeat, alternating right and left.

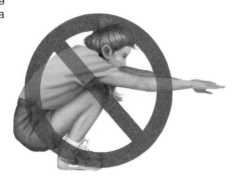

Safer Alternative Exercise: Single Knee-to-Chest

From the hook-lying position, draw one knee to the chest by pulling on the thigh with the hands, then extend the knee and point the foot toward the ceiling. Hold. Pull to chest again and return to starting position. Repeat with other leg.

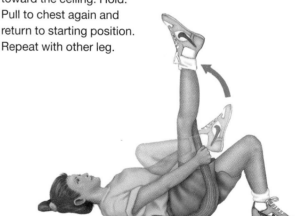

Table 1

Questionable Exercise: Seated Forward Arm Circles with Palms Down

This exercise (arms straight out to the sides) may cause the bony knob in the shoulder to squeeze the muscles and the **bursa** in the shoulder every time the arm is lifted. In addition, the tendency is to emphasize the use of the stronger chest muscles (pectorals) rather than to stretch those muscles and emphasize the weaker upper back muscles.

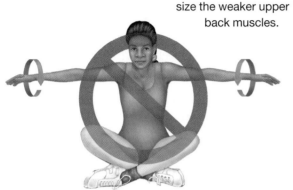

Safer Alternative Exercise: Seated Backward Arm Circles with Palms Up

Sit, turn palms up, pull in chin, and contract abdominals. Circle arms backward.

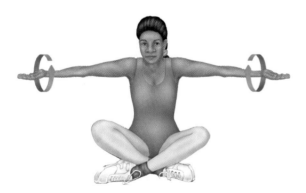

Bursa Small sac filled with fluid and situated between muscles, or between muscles and bones, to prevent friction.

Web Resources

American Academy of Orthopaedic Surgeons **www.aaos.org**
Human Factors and Ergonomics Society **www.hfes.org**
Safe Exercises **www.mhhe.com/phys_fit/web12 Click 05.**

Suggested Readings

Additional reference materials for concept 12 are available at **www.mhhe.com/fit_well/web12 Click 06.**

Almeida, S. A. et al. 1999. Epidemiological patterns of musculoskeletal injuries and physical training. *Medicine and Science in Sports and Exercise* 31(8):1182.

Hootman, J. M. et al. 2002. Epidemiology of musculoskeletal injuries among sedentary and physically active adults. *Medicine and Science in Sports and Exercise* 34(5):838–844.

Jones, C. S., C. Christenson, and M. Young. 2000. Weight-training injury trends: A 20-year survey. *The Physician and Sports Medicine* 28(7):61–72.

Liemohn, W., T. Haydu, and D. Phillips. 1999. Questionable exercises. *President's Council on Physical Fitness and Sports Research Digest* 3(8):1–8.

McGill, S. M. 2001. Low back stability: From formal description to issues for performance and rehabilitation. *Exercise and Sports Science Reviews* 29(1):26–31.

Neiman, D. C. 2000. Exercise soothes arthritis: Joint effects. *ACSM's Health and Fitness Journal* 4(3):20–27.

Pope, R. P., R. D. Herbert, and J. D. Kirwan. 2000. A randomized study of preexercise stretching for prevention of lower-limb injury. *Medicine and Science in Sports and Exercise* 31(2):271–277.

Wallman, H. 1998. Low back pain: Is it really all behind you? An excellent 7-step abdominal strengthening program. *ACSM's Health and Fitness* 2(5):30.

 In the News

Do Glucosamine and Chondroitin Work to Treat Osteoarthritis and Improve Joint Health?

Osteoarthritis is a degenerative condition in which the joints and surrounding tissue become impaired over time. The incidence of osteoarthritis increases with age and may be indirectly caused or influenced by microtrauma that occurred earlier in life. Recently, there has been considerable interest in the potential of two related neutraceuticals (glucosamine and chondroitin) for treating osteoarthritis problems. Glucosamine is a substance that is produced naturally in the synovial fluid of joints to help promote cartilage formation. Chondroitin is a molecule found in connective tissue that makes cartilage more pliable, and

therefore, better for shock absorption. Because these substances are produced in only small quantities and are not found naturally in foods, some experts have recommended that patients take these "chondroprotective" supplements. Some evidence has indicated that glucosamine can help to rebuild damaged cartilage. Results from a large, well-controlled study reported better outcomes over a three-year period for participants taking the supplement than those taking the placebo. Other experts have not yet been convinced and point out that substances have not been fully tested for long-term use. Because a consensus has not been reached, users should remain cautious about using these substances.

Lab 12A: Safe Exercises

Name		Section	Date

Purpose: To perform safe exercises that are good alternatives to commonly performed questionable exercises and to self-monitor progress in your one-week plan.

Procedures:

1. On Chart 1 check the questionable exercises you have performed.
2. Perform the safe exercises listed in the chart. Use the descriptions in this concept to help you perform them properly.
3. Place a check by the exercises you think you might consider using as part of your regular program.
4. Answer the questions in the Results section.

Chart 1 ▶ Questionable Exercises and Safe Alternatives

Place a check beside the questionable exercises you have performed in the past.	Place a check beside the safe exercises you think you might include in your exercise program.
○ 1. The swan	○ 1. Back extension
○ 2. Back-arching abdominal stretch	○ 2. Pectoral stretch
○ 3. Donkey kick	○ 3. Knee-to-nose
○ 4. Double-leg lift	○ 4. Reverse curl
○ 5. The windmill	○ 5. Back-saver hamstring stretch
○ 6. Neck circling	○ 6. Head clock
○ 7. Shoulder stand bicycling, plough, or plough shear	○ 7. Leg hug
○ 8. Straight-leg or bent-knee sit-ups	○ 8. Crunch
○ 9. Standing toe touches	○ 9. Back-saver toe touch
○ 10. Bar stretch	○ 10. Hamstring stretcher
○ 11. Shin and quadriceps stretcher	○ 11. Shin stretcher
○ 12. Hero	○ 12. Hip and thigh stretcher
○ 13. Deep squatting exercise	○ 13. Alternate leg kneel
○ 14. Knee pull-down	○ 14. Single knee-to-chest
○ 15. Forward arm circles (palms down)	○ 15. Backward seated arm circles (palms up)

Results: How many of the questionable exercises listed above have you performed? ☐

Conclusions and Interpretations:

1. In most cases, it takes a considerable amount of time for a questionable exercise and the microtrauma it causes to result in noticeable damage to the body. To what extent do you think that you might be affected by questionable exercises you have done in the past? Use several sentences to explain.

2. Will you change your way of exercising as a result of learning about questionable exercises and safe alternatives? Use several sentences to explain your answer.

Body Mechanics: Posture and Care of the Back and Neck

Proper body mechanics should be employed for both static and dynamic postures to ensure the health, integrity, and function of the back and the neck.

Health Goals

for the year 2010

- Increase healthy and active days.
- Reduce days with pain and activity limitations.
- Increase assistance to those with pain and activity limitations.
- Increase proportion of people who regularly perform exercises for strength and muscular endurance.
- Increase proportion of people who regularly perform exercises for flexibility.

Body mechanics is the application of physical laws to the human body. The bones of the body act as levers or simple machines, with the muscles supplying the force to move them. The discipline of biomechanics applies mechanical laws and principles to study how the body can perform more and better work with less energy. Biomechanical principles are often used to enhance sports technique, but they are also applied to understand factors that can lead to strain or injury.

This concept focuses on four aspects of body mechanics. The first part of the concept discusses the mechanics of body alignment while sitting or standing (static postures). The second part of the concept emphasizes the prevention of low back and neck pain through proper body mechanics. The third section of the concept stresses dynamic postures for activities of daily living. The fourth section includes exercises that are effective in correcting postural problems and removing the cause of neck and back pain.

Elements and Benefits of Good Posture

Good posture has aesthetic benefits. **Posture** is an important part of nonverbal communication. The first impression a person makes is usually a visual one and good posture can help convey an impression of alertness, confidence, and attractiveness.

Proper posture allows the body segments to be balanced. www.mhhe.com/fit_well/web13 Click 01. The body is made in segments that are balanced in a vertical column by muscles and ligaments. Proper posture helps to maintain this balance. In the standing position, the head should be centered over the trunk, the shoulders should be down and back, but relaxed, with the chest high and the abdomen flat. The spine should have gentle curves when viewed from the side (**lordotic curve**), but should be straight as seen from the back. When the pelvis is tilted properly, the pubis falls directly underneath the lower tip of the sternum. The knees should be relaxed, with the kneecaps pointed straight ahead. The feet should point straight ahead, and the weight should be borne over the heel, on the outside border of the sole, and across the ball of the foot and toes (see Figure 1).

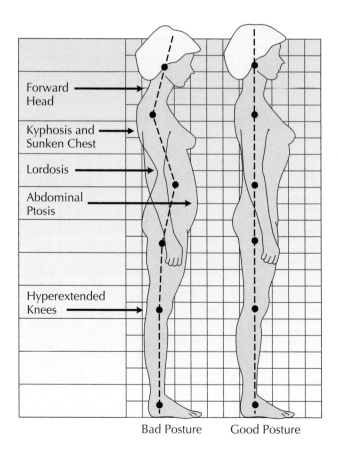

Forward Head

Kyphosis and Sunken Chest

Lordosis

Abdominal Ptosis

Hyperextended Knees

Bad Posture   Good Posture

Figure 1 ▶ Comparison of bad and good posture.

Table 1 ▶ Health Problems Associated with Poor Posture

Posture Problem	Definition	Health Problem
Forward head	The head is aligned in front of the center of gravity; also called poke neck.	Headache, dizziness, and pain in the neck, shoulders, or arms.
Kyphosis	Excessive curvature (flexion) in the upper back; also called hump back.	Impaired respiration as a result of sunken chest and pain in the neck, shoulders, and arms.
Lumbar lordosis	Excessive curvature (hyperextension) in the lower back (lumbar region), with a forward pelvic tilt; commonly known as swayback.	Back pain and/or injury, protruding abdomen, low back syndrome, and painful menstruation.
Abdominal ptosis	Excessive protrusion of abdomen, also called protruding abdomen.	Back pain and/or injury, lordosis, low back syndrome, and painful menstruation.
Hyperextended knees	The knees bend backward excessively.	Greater risk of knee injury and excessive pelvic tilt (lordosis).

If one part of the body is out of line, other parts must compensate to balance it, thus increasing the strain on muscles, ligaments, and joints. If gravity or a short muscle pulls one segment out of line, other portions of the body will move out of alignment to compensate (see Figure 1). For example, if the abdomen sticks out over the belt line, the pelvis can tip forward, increasing strain on the low back. Chronic strain from poor alignment can lead to other postural deviations, producing worse posture, more stress and strain, and possible deformity of the musculoskeletal system.

Chronic postural problems can lead to a variety of health problems. With proper posture, the lower spine (lordotic curve) should have a slight inward curvature. This curve helps support the body weight and promote balance about the trunk. If the lower back curve is too great (lumbar lordosis), the muscles of the low back are more easily fatigued, more likely to suffer muscle spasms, and more prone to injury. If the lower back curve is absent, problems associated with "flat back" posture (lumbar kyphosis) can occur. Some examples of specific health problems that result from these or other postural problems are described in Table 1.

Maintaining proper alignment requires a balance of flexibility and strength in muscles supporting the trunk. Muscles of the legs, trunk, and neck work in combination to maintain body alignment and posture (Figure 2). The abdominal muscles pull the bottom of the pelvis upward and keep the top of the pelvis tipped backward, eliminating excessive back curve. Strong hamstring muscles also help keep the pelvis tipped backward. If the hip flexor muscles are too strong, or not long enough, they have the opposite effect of strong abdominal muscles; that is, they tip the top of the pelvis forward, causing excessive low back curve (lordosis). (See Figure 3.) This is why it is important to have long, but not too strong, hip flexor

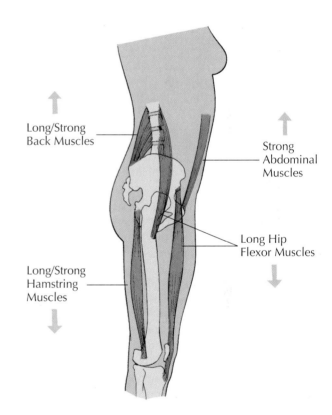

Long/Strong Back Muscles

Strong Abdominal Muscles

Long Hip Flexor Muscles

Long/Strong Hamstring Muscles

Figure 2 ▶ Balanced muscle strength and length permit good postural alignment.

Posture The relationship of body parts, whether standing, lying, sitting, or moving. Good posture is the relationship of body parts that allows you to function most effectively, with the least expenditure of energy and with a minimum amount of strain on muscles, tendons, ligaments, and joints.

Lordotic Curve Normal curvature of the spine that is necessary for good posture and body mechanics.

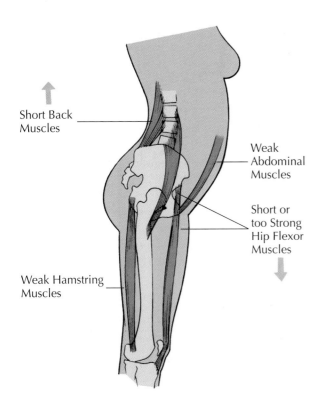

Figure 3 ▶ Unbalanced muscular development may cause poor posture or back problems.

Short Back Muscles

Weak Abdominal Muscles

Short or too Strong Hip Flexor Muscles

Weak Hamstring Muscles

muscles. As a general rule, flexibility exercises are needed to lengthen the hip flexor muscles, and strength and endurance exercises are recommended for the abdominal muscles. Sample exercises are provided later in this concept. Exercises to increase the strength of the hip flexor muscles are not recommended for people with back pain.

In addition to body alignment problems, hereditary, congenital, and disease conditions, as well as certain environmental factors, can cause poor posture. Some environmental factors that may contribute to poor posture include ill-fitting clothing and shoes, chronic fatigue, improperly fitting furniture (including poor chairs, beds, and mattresses), emotional and personality problems, poor work habits, poor physical fitness due to inactivity, and lack of knowledge relating to good posture. Some posture problems, such as **scoliosis**, may be congenital, hereditary, or acquired, but may be corrected with exercise, braces, and/or other medical procedures. Early detection is critical in treating scoliosis.

Backaches and Neck Aches

Most people (more than half) will see a physician about a backache during their lifetime. Backaches are second only to headaches as a common medical complaint. An estimated 30 to 70 percent of Americans have recurring back problems, and 2 million of these people cannot hold jobs as a result. It is also the most common

reason for workers' compensation claims and for lost workdays among employed individuals. Because of this, improving back health and minimizing back problems is a high priority for many worksite wellness programs.

Back problems most often affect people between the ages of twenty-five and sixty but one study indicated that up to 26 percent of teenagers reported backaches. Athletes also have back problems, but the condition is more common in people who are not highly fit. Unfortunately, studies also indicate that back pain is the leading cause of inactivity among individuals under the age of forty-five. Therefore, taking preventive measures to reduce risk of back pain is important.

The cause of backache is rarely a dramatic event such as trauma in a diving or an automobile accident. Incorrect posture when standing, sitting, lying, or working is responsible for many back problems. Compounding this are weak muscles and muscular imbalance. Other causes of low back pain include improper exercises; incorrect techniques in lifting and in sports; repetitive, forced hyperextension of the back; and other preventable causes (see Table 1). This list excludes some uncontrollable causes such as trauma, tumors, and congenital abnormalities. You will have the opportunity to assess your back and neck risk factors in the questionnaire in Lab 13A. You may be familiar with many of the causes listed in Table 1, but what you may not know is that in 80 percent of the cases, physicians are unable to pinpoint the exact cause of back and neck problems.

The overwhelming majority of backaches and neck aches are avoidable. A common cause of backache is muscular strain, frequently precipitated by poor body mechanics in daily activities or during exercise. When lifting improperly, you exert great pressure on the lumbar discs and severe stress on the lumbar muscles and ligaments. Many popular exercises place great strain on the back (see concept on safe physical activity). Sleeping flat on the back or abdomen on a soft mattress can also cause lower back strain.

Poor posture can lead to back strain and pain. www.mhhe.com/fit_well/web13 Click 02. Lumbar lordosis (excessive curvature in the low back) causes the pelvis to tip forward and puts the spine in an unsupported and vulnerable position. In this position, the lumbar vertebrae can press on nerve roots and contribute to low back pain or **sciatica**. To avoid this position, some experts recommend that individuals with lordosis and weak abdominals should eliminate all exercises that hyperextend the spine.

Individuals who sit for long periods of time with the back flat and pelvis tilted backward can have the opposite postural problem of lumbar kyphosis ("flat back"). These individuals probably need to regain a normal lordotic curve and probably need to perform relaxed static stretches with the back in the hyperextended position, such as the press-up exercise. They may also benefit from the use of lumbar support (rolls or pillows) placed behind the back during sitting.

There is no such thing as a slipped disc. Disc problems are frequently misunderstood. **Intervertebral discs** may herniate or rupture, but they do not slip (Figure 4). Material from the pulpy center part of the disc (the nucleus pulposus) may bulge outward and press on spinal nerves, causing pain, and a protective reflex muscle spasm may occur to protect it. This causes a lack of circulation to the muscle and more pain, and more muscles tense up to prevent movement. Stiffness results and the muscles become weaker; chronic back pain may set in unless this vicious pain cycle can be stopped. If it persists, bones may develop spurs, discs may degenerate, the patient may go to bed and worry and tense up, and the cycle may go on indefinitely.

The discs in the lumbar area are subjected to greater compression and torque because they are at the bottom of the spine. They are, therefore, more susceptible to damage. Sudden twisting and flexion or extension movements, such as suddenly reaching for a ball in tennis or racquetball, may precipitate a **herniated disc.** It is more apt to happen when the disc is degenerated from overuse (Figure 5). It is more common in men than women and in people who do heavy manual labor. Degenerated discs are normal with aging, and common in athletes. One study showed that gymnasts' discs were comparable to the discs of sixty-five-year-old men. However, in spite of what popular literature and certain unethical "back doctors" may tell you, studies show that a herniated disc is rarely the cause of back pain, which occurs in only 5 to 10 percent of the cases.

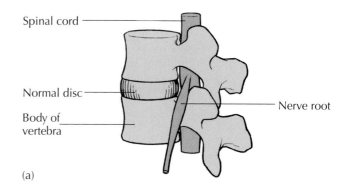

(a)

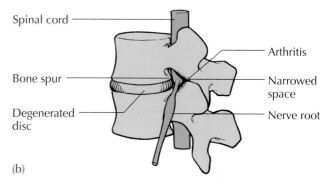

(b)

Figure 5 ▶ Normal disc (*a*) and degenerated disc with nerve impingement and arthritic changes (*b*).

The neck is probably strained more frequently than the lower back. The neck is constructed with the same curve and has the same mechanical problems as the lower back. The postural fault of forward head places a chronic strain on the posterior neck muscles. Tension in these muscles can lead to **myofascial trigger points,** causing headache or **referred pain** in the face, scalp, shoulder, arm, and chest.

Scoliosis A lateral curvature with some rotation of the spine; the most serious and deforming of all postural deviations.

Sciatica Pain radiating along the course of the sciatic nerve in the back of the hip and leg.

Intervertebral Disc Spinal disc; a cushion of cartilage between the bodies of the vertebrae. Each disc consists of a fibrous outer ring (annulus fibrosus) and a pulpy center (nucleus pulposus).

Herniated Disc The soft nucleus of the spinal disc that protrudes through a small tear in the surrounding tissue; also called prolapse.

Myofascial Trigger Points A sensitive spot in the muscle and muscle fascia caused by muscle spasms.

Referred Pain Pain that appears to be located in one area though it actually originates in another area.

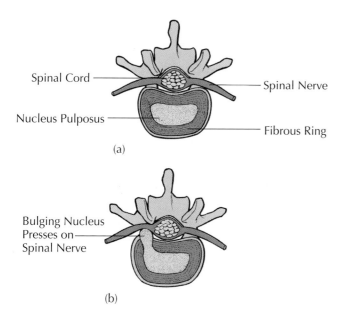

Figure 4 ▶ Normal disc (*a*) and herniated disc (*b*).

Kyphosis is a contributing factor in neck pain. The more the upper back is flexed, the greater the compensating curve (**cervical lordosis**) in the neck. The sharpest angle is between the fourth and sixth cervical vertebrae, creating wear and tear (microtrauma) that accelerates disc degeneration and arthritic changes, which can ultimately result in nerve and artery impingement.

Because the exact causes of chronic neck pain are many and they vary from individual to individual, diagnosis is difficult. Some of the causes of chronic neck pain (and the often accompanying shoulder pain) include workplace design, poor posture, work habits, and physical fitness, and too much stress. Some examples of good body mechanics to prevent problems are shown in Figure 6.

Table 2 ▶ Body Mechanics Guidelines for Posture and Back/Neck Care	
Sitting	• Use a hard chair with a straight back and armrests, placing the spine against the back of the chair. A foot rest reduces fatigue (see Figure 6). • Keep one or both knees lower than the hips and feet supported on the floor. • If your back flattens when you sit, place a lumbar roll behind your lower back. • When sitting at a table, keep the back and neck in good alignment. • Do not sit in front-row theater seats, which forces you to tip your head back. • When driving a car, pull the seat forward so the legs are bent when operating the pedals. If your back flattens when you drive, use a lumbar support pillow. • Whenever possible, sit while working but stand occasionally.
Standing	• When standing for long periods of time, keep the lower back flat by propping a foot on a stool; alternate feet. • Avoid tilting the head backward (when shaving or washing your hair).
Lying	• Avoid lying on the abdomen. • When lying on the back, a pillow or lift should be placed under the knees. Do not use a thick head pillow. • When lying on your side, keep your knees and hips bent; place a pillow between the knees.
Lifting and Carrying	• When lifting, avoid bending at the hips. Keep the back straight, bend the knees, and lift with the legs. Assume a side-stride position with the object between the feet to allow you to get low and near the object (see Figure 6). • Perform one-hand lifting the same way as two-hand lifting; use the nonlifting hand (see Figure 6) for support. • When lifting, do not twist the spine. This can be more damaging from a sitting position than from a standing position. • When lifting, keep the object close to the body; do not reach to lift. Tighten the back muscles before lifting. • If possible, avoid carrying objects above waist level. • When objects must be carried above the waist, carry them in the midline of the body, preferably on the back (use a backpack). Keep backpack weight low and use both straps for support. • Push or pull heavy objects, rather than lifting them. It takes thirty-four times more force to lift than to slide an object across the floor. Pushing is preferred over pulling. • Do not lift or carry loads too heavy for you. The most economical load for the average adult is about 35 percent of the body weight. Obviously, with strength training, you can lift a greater load, but heavy loads are a backache risk factor. • Divide the load if possible, carrying half in each hand/arm. If the load cannot be divided, alternate it from one side of the body to the other (see Figure 6). • When lifting and lowering an object from overhead, avoid hyperextending the neck and the back. Any lift above waist level is inefficient. • When objects must be carried in front of the body above the level of the waist, lean backward to balance the load, and avoid arching the back.
Working	• When working above head level, get on a stool or ladder to avoid tipping the head backward. • Work at eye level; for example, computer monitors should not be too high or low. • To avoid back and neck strain, climb a ladder or stand on a stool so you don't have to raise your arms over your head. • When working with the hands, the workbench or kitchen cabinet should be about 2 to 4 inches below the waist. The office desk should be about 29 to 30 inches high for the average man and about 27 to 29 inches high for the average woman. • Tools most often used should be the closest to reach. • Avoid constant arm extension, whether forward or sideward. • The arms should move either together or in opposite directions. When the conditions allow, use both hands in opposite and symmetrical motions while working. • Organize work to save energy. Vary the working position by changing from one task to another before feeling fatigued. When working at a desk, get up and stretch occasionally to relieve tension. • Use proper tools and equipment to reduce neck strain; for example, use a paint roller with an extension to reach overhead, thus reducing the need to hold the arms overhead and to hyperextend the neck. • Avoid stooping or unnatural positions that cause strain.

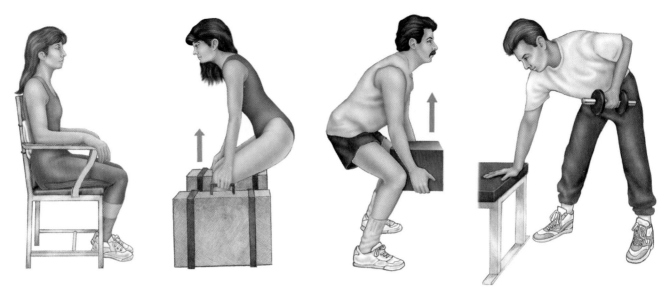

Figure 6 ▶ Good body mechanics can help prevent back and neck ache.

Prevention and Intervention

Practicing good body mechanics and posture can help prevent back problems. Several practical suggestions for modifying everyday activities to improve posture and reduce the risk of back and neck problems are illustrated and described in Table 2.

Some additional general guidelines will help in preventing posture, back, and neck problems. In addition to the suggestions for improving body mechanics noted in the previous sections, these guidelines should be helpful.

- Do exercises to strengthen abdominal and hip extensors and to stretch the hip flexors and lumbar muscles if they are tight (see Tables 3–9).
- Avoid hazardous exercises (see concept on safe physical activity).
- Do regular physical activity for the entire body, such as walking, jogging, swimming, and bicycling.
- Warm up before engaging in strenuous activity.
- Sleep on a firm mattress or place a 3/4-inch-thick plywood board under the mattress.
- Avoid sudden, jerky back movements, especially twisting.
- Avoid obesity. The smaller the waistline, the lesser the strain on the lower back.
- Use appropriate back and seat supports when sitting for long periods.
- Maintain good posture when carrying heavy loads; do not lean forward, sideways, or backward.
- Adjust sports equipment to permit good posture; for example, adjust bicycle seat and handle bars to permit good body alignment.

- Avoid long periods of sitting at a desk or driving; take frequent breaks and adjust the seat and headrest for maximum support.

Exercises for Posture and Back/Neck Care

 Exercise is one of the most frequently prescribed treatments for back or neck pain. www.mhhe.com/fit_well/web13 Click 03. Treatments range from surgical removal of a disc or fusion, to more conservative measures such as injections, electrical stimulation, muscle relaxants, anti-inflammatory drugs, vapo-coolant spray, bracing, traction, bed rest, heat, cryotherapy, massage, and therapeutic exercise. Regardless of the treatment used, 70 to 85 percent of back patients recover spontaneously. Of those, 70 percent will have no symptoms by the end of three weeks, and 90 percent will recover in two months. The various treatment modalities may simply make patients more comfortable or they may hasten the recovery.

Exercise has been found to be helpful in treating all kinds of chronic pain. (Resistance exercises and aerobic exercises have been particularly helpful in pain clinics.) Aerobic exercise is also known to help nourish the spinal discs.

Cervical Lordosis Excessive hyperextension in the neck region (swayback of the neck).

Technology Update

Therapeutic Exercise Machines for Back Health
While general resistance training may help to improve the strength and endurance of the back muscles the exercises may not be specific enough to target the specific problems contributing to back pain. For years, physical therapists have used various rehabilitation devices to study muscle function in the back. Many of the equipment innovations used in clinical settings are becoming available to consumers in some fitness clubs. The inclusion of these new machines in many clubs reflects the growing interest and awareness in the population (and fitness professionals) about the importance of back care. One line of machines is made by a company called MedX. Similar to some clinical devices, these machines use a strain gauge and computer to evaluate isometric contractions at specific angular positions to determine the resistance profile supplied by the machine (this is similar to what clinical machines do). The machines include low minimal resistance levels and small increments in resistance to allow the machines to be used for individuals with different levels of back strength (see Web Resources for information).
www.mhhe.com/ fit_well/web13 Click 04.

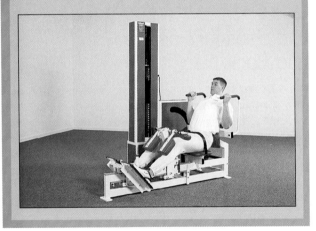

Exercise can prevent or correct some of the underlying causes of back and neck pain by strengthening weak muscles and stretching short ones. In the process of creating muscle balance, exercise improves postural alignment and body mechanics and relaxes muscle spasms.

Exercise can often correct muscle imbalance, the underlying cause of many postural and back problems. www.mhhe.com/fit_well/web13 Click 05. If the muscles on one side of a joint are stronger than the muscles on the opposite side, the body part is pulled in the direction of the stronger muscles. Corrective exercises are usually designed to strengthen the long, weak muscles and to stretch the short, strong ones in order to have equal pull in both directions. For example, people with lumbar lordosis may need to strengthen the abdominals and hamstrings, and stretch the lower back and hip flexor muscles (see Figures 2 and 3).

Some people are unable to lift loads safely because tight and/or weak muscles may prevent them from using proper body mechanics. Some people have backaches because they lift improperly. In many instances, the poor technique is caused by muscle imbalance. Examples include: hamstrings or gluteals that are too tight to permit the lower back to retain its normal curve during lifting; calf muscles that are too tight to allow the heels to remain on the floor during squatting; abdominal muscles that are too weak to support the back; or quadriceps and gluteals that are too weak to lift. Proper exercise can correct these problems.

Strategies for Action

 An important step in taking action to assure good posture and good back and neck care is assessing your current status. www.mhhe.com/fit_well/web13 Click 06. An important early step in taking action is self-assessment. The Healthy Back Test consists of eight pass or fail items that will give you an idea of the areas in which you might need improvement. The Healthy Back Test is described in the lab resource materials. You will have the opportunity to take this test in Lab 13A.

A posture test is included in Lab 13B to help you determine if you have any of the posture problems described in Table 1. Rating charts for both the back and posture tests are included in the lab resource materials.

Experts have identified behaviors associated with potential future back and neck problems. In addition to the back and posture tests, it may be useful to assess your risk factors. A questionnaire is provided in Lab 13A for assessing these risk factors.

Specific exercises are sometimes needed to prevent or help rehabilitate posture, neck, and back problems. www.mhhe.com/fit_well/web13 Click 07. Exercises included in previous concepts were presented with health-related fitness in mind. The exercises included in this concept are not really so different. They are either flexibility or strength/muscle endurance exercises for specific muscle groups; however, each is selected specifically to help correct a postural problem or to remove the cause of neck and back pain. To that extent, these exercises may be classified as therapeutic. These same exercises may be called preventive because they can be used to prevent postural or spine problems. Whether therapeutic or preventive, the exercises will not be effective unless they are done faithfully and with the FIT formula applied. People who have back and neck pain should seek the advice of a physician to make certain that it is safe for them to perform the exercises.

The exercises in Tables 3–9 are not necessarily intended for all people. Rather you should choose exercises based on your own individual circumstances. Use your results on the Healthy Back Test and the posture test to determine the exercises that are most appropriate for you.

To facilitate the use of these exercises for back or postural problems, the most effective exercises for various maladies are organized in Tables 3 through 9. Lab 13C is designed to help you choose specific exercises related to test items in Lab 13A.

Keeping records of progress is important to adhering to a back care program. An activity logging sheet is provided in Lab 13C to help you keep records of your progress as you regularly perform exercises to build and maintain good back and neck fitness.

Table 3

Table 3 Stretching Exercises for the Hip Flexors and Hamstrings, and for Pelvic Stabilization

These exercises are designed to address the root problems associated with lumbar lordosis and to train the muscles that provide postural stability. Stretching the hip flexors and training the pelvic stabilization muscles will make it easier to maintain a **neutral pelvis.** Exercises for the hamstrings are provided because they can effectively combat low back pain caused by lordosis. These exercises are good for most people because long hip flexors and hamstrings and fit postural stabilization muscles are beneficial to those who do not have lordosis. Once the muscles have been developed, be aware of your posture and use your muscles to maintain it.

1. Back-Saver Hamstring Stretch

This exercise stretches the hamstrings and calf muscles and helps prevent or correct backache caused in part by short hamstrings. Sit on the floor with the feet against the wall or an immovable object. Bend left knee and bring foot close to buttocks. Clasp hands behind back. Bend forward from hips, keeping lower back as straight as possible. Let bent knee rotate outward so trunk can move forward keeping back flat. Hold and repeat on each leg.

3. Low Back Stretcher

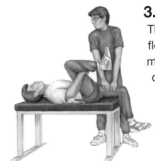

This exercise stretches the hip flexors, gluteals, and lumbar muscles and helps prevent or correct lumbar lordosis and backache. Lie on your back. Draw one knee up to the chest and pull thigh down tightly with the hands, then slowly return to the original position. Repeat with other knee. Do not grasp knee—grasp thigh. If a partner or a weight stabilizes the extended leg, the hip flexor muscles on that leg will be stretched.

2. Single Knee-to-Chest

This exercise stretches the lower back, gluteals, and hamstring muscles and helps prevent or correct lordosis and backache. Lie on your back with knees bent. Use hands on back of thigh to draw one knee to the chest, then extend the knee and point the foot toward the ceiling. Hold. Return to the starting position by drawing the knee back to the chest before sliding the foot to the floor. Repeat with other leg.

4. Hip and Thigh Stretcher

This exercise stretches the hip flexor muscles and helps prevent or correct forward pelvic tilt, lumbar lordosis, and backache. Place right knee directly above right ankle and stretch left leg backward so knee touches floor. If necessary, place hands on floor for balance. Press pelvis forward and downward. Hold. Repeat on opposite side. Caution: Do not bend front knee more than 90 degrees.

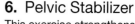

Table 3 & 4

Stretching Exercises for the Hip Flexors and **Table 3** Hamstrings, and for Pelvic Stabilization

5. Bridging

This exercise strengthens the hip extensors, especially the gluteal muscles, and helps prevent and correct lordosis and forward pelvic tilt. Lie on your back with knees bent and feet close to buttocks. Contract gluteals, lifting buttocks, and lower back off floor. Hold, relax, and repeat. Do not allow the lower back to arch.

6. Pelvic Stabilizer

This exercise strengthens the postural muscles needed to maintain a pelvic tilt. Lie on your back. Bend both knees up to chest. Place arms on floor for support. Perform pelvic tilt by flattening the back against the floor. Slowly extend one leg as far as possible without arching the back. Return knee to chest.

Exercises for Muscle Fitness of the Abdominals **Table 4**

These exercises are designed to increase the strength of the abdominal muscles. Strong abdominal muscles are important for maintaining a neutral pelvis, maintaining good posture, and preventing backache associated with lordosis.

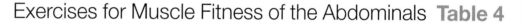

1. Reverse Curl

This exercise develops the lower abdominal muscles, corrects abdominal ptosis, and helps prevent backache. Lie on your back. Bend the knees and bring knees in toward the chest. Place arms at sides for balance and support. Pull the knees toward the chest, raising the hips off the floor. Do not let the knees go past the shoulders. Return to the starting position. Repeat.

2. Crunch (Curl-Up)

This exercise develops the upper abdominal muscles, corrects abdominal ptosis and lordosis, and aids in backache prevention. Lie on your back with your knees bent and the arms extended or crossed with hands on shoulders or palms on ears. If desired, legs may rest on bench to increase difficulty. For less resistance, place hands at side of body. For more resistance, move hands higher. Curl up until shoulder blades leave floor, then roll down to the starting position. Repeat.

Neutral Pelvis Proper position of the pelvis to maintain a normal lordotic curve. The pelvis is neither tipped forward nor backward but is in stable, neutral position.

Table 4

Table 4 Exercises for Muscle Fitness of the Abdominals

3. Crunch with Twist (on Bench)

This exercise strengthens the oblique abdominals and helps prevent or correct lumbar lordosis, abdominal ptosis, and backache. Lie on your back with your feet on a bench, knees bent at 90 degrees. Arms may be extended or on shoulders or hands on ears (the most difficult). Same as crunch except twist the upper trunk so the right shoulder is higher than the left. Reach toward the left knee with the right elbow. Hold. Return and repeat to the opposite side.

5. Pelvic Tilt

This exercise strengthens the abdominals and helps prevent or correct lumbar lordosis, abdominal ptosis, and backache. Lie on your back with knees bent. Tighten the abdominal muscles and tilt the pelvis backward. Try to flatten the lower back against the floor. At the same time, tighten the hip and thigh muscles. Do not push with the legs. Hold, then relax. Breathe normally during the contraction; do not hold your breath.

4. Sitting Tucks

This exercise strengthens the lower abdominals, increases their endurance, improves posture, and prevents backache. (This is an advanced exercise and is not recommended for people who have back pain.) Sit on floor with feet raised, arms extended for balance. Alternately bend and extend legs without letting back or feet touch floor.

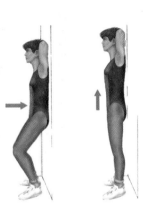

6. Wall Slide

This exercise helps prevent or correct poor spinal alignment by teaching the feel of flattening the neck and back, and tilting the pelvis. Stand with heels 4 to 6 inches from wall, arms at sides. Flatten neck and lumbar region to wall by flexing knees and sliding down wall until spine can be forced against it. Slide up wall, maintaining flat spine. Walk away from wall, keeping curves flat. Return to wall and check alignment. Repeat with hands behind neck and elbows touching wall. Repeat with arms at sides and sandbag on head. Repeated flexion and extension of the knees can develop strength in the quadriceps muscles on the front of the thigh.

Table 5

Stretching and Strengthening Exercises **Table 5**
for the Muscles of the Neck

These exercises are designed to increase strength in the neck muscles and to improve neck range of motion. They are helpful in preventing and resolving symptoms of neck pain and for relieving trigger points.

1. Neck Rotation Exercise

This PNF exercise strengthens and stretches the neck rotators. It should always be done with the head and neck in axial extension (good alignment). It is particularly useful for relieving **trigger point** pain and stiffness. Place palm of left hand against left cheek. Point fingers toward ear and point elbow forward. Turn head and neck to the left while gently resisting with left hand. Hold six seconds. Relax and turn head to right as far as possible; hold ten seconds. Repeat four times; repeat on opposite side.

3. Chin Tuck

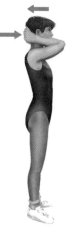

This exercise stretches the muscles at the base of the skull and reduces headache symptoms. Place hands together at the base of the head. Tuck in the chin and gently press head backward into your hands, while looking straight ahead. Hold.

2. Isometric Neck Exercises

This exercise strengthens the neck muscles and prevents or corrects forward head and cervical lordosis, as well as upper back and neck trigger points and pain. Sit and place one or both hands on the head as shown. Assume good head and neck posture by tucking the chin, flattening the neck, and pushing the crown of the head up (axial extension). Apply resistance (a) sideward, (b) backward, and (c) forward. Contract the neck muscles to prevent the head and neck from moving. Hold for six seconds. Repeat each exercise up to six times. Note: For neck muscles, it is probably best to use a little less than a maximal contraction, especially in the presence of arthritis, degenerated discs, or injury.

4. Upper Trapezius Stretch

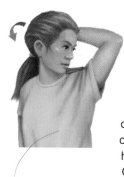

This exercise stretches the upper trapezius muscle and relieves neck ache and headache. Place right hand behind back and place left hand on back of head. Gently move chin toward your chest, turning head toward the left underarm. Gently press head forward with left hand for more stretch. Hold. Repeat to the opposite side.

Trigger Point An especially irritable spot, usually a tight band or knot in a muscle or fascia. It often refers pain to another area of the body. For example, a trigger point in the shoulder might cause a headache. This condition is referred to as myofascial pain syndrome and is often caused by muscle tension, fatigue, or strain.

235

Table 6

Table 6 Exercises for the Trunk and Mobility

These exercises are designed to increase strength and mobility of muscles that move the trunk. They are especially helpful for people with chronic back pain.

1. Upper Trunk Lift

This exercise develops upper back strength. Lie on a table, bench, or a special-purpose bench designed for trunk lifts with the upper half of the body hanging over the edge. Have a partner stabilize the feet and legs while the trunk is raised parallel to the floor, then lower the trunk to the starting position. Place hands behind neck or on ears. Do not raise past the horizontal or arch the back or neck.

3. Side Bender

This exercise stretches the trunk lateral flexors and helps prevent and correct backaches by maintaining flexibility in the spine. Stand with feet shoulder-width apart. Stretch left arm overhead to right. Bend to right at waist reaching as far to right as possible with left arm; reach as far as possible to the left with right arm. Hold. Do not let trunk rotate or lower back arch. Repeat on opposite side. Note: This exercise is made more effective if a weight is held down at the side in the hand opposite the side being stretched. More stretch will occur if the hip on the stretched side is dropped and most of the weight is borne by the opposite foot.

2. Trunk Lift

This exercise develops the muscles of the upper back and corrects round shoulders. Lie face down with hands clasped behind the neck. Pull the shoulder blades together, raising the elbows off the floor. Slowly raise the head and chest off the floor by arching the upper back. Return to the starting position. Repeat. For less resistance, hands may be placed under thighs. Caution: Do not arch the lower back or neck. Lift only until the sternum (breastbone) clears the floor. Variations: arms down at sides (easiest), hands by head, hands extended (hardest).

4. Supine Trunk Twist

This exercise increases the flexibility of the spine and stretches the rotator muscles. Lie on your back with your arms extended at shoulder level. Place left foot on right knee cap. Twist the lower body by lowering left knee to touch floor on right. Turn head to left. Keep shoulders and arms on floor. Hold for several seconds.

These exercises are designed to strengthen and restore normal curve to the back. They are *not* recommended for people with lordosis.

1. Lower Trunk Lift

This exercise develops low back and hip strength. Lie on your stomach on bench or table with legs hanging over the edge. Have a partner stabilize the upper back or grasp the edges of the table with hands. Raise the legs parallel to the floor and lower them. Do not raise past the horizontal or arch the back. Suggested progression: (1) begin by alternating legs; (2) when you can do 25 reps, add ankle weights; (3) when you can do 25 reps, lift both legs simultaneously (no weights).

2. Press-Up (McKenzie Extension Exercise)

This exercise increases flexibility of the lumbar spine, reduces tension on posterior discs and longitudinal ligaments, and restores normal lordotic curve, especially for people with a flat lumbar spine. Lie on your stomach with hands under the face. Slowly press up to a rest position on forearms. Keep pelvis on floor. Relax and hold ten seconds. Repeat once. Do several times a day. Progress to gradually straightening the elbows while keeping the pubic bone on the floor. Caution: Do not perform if you have lordosis or if you feel any pain or discomfort in the back or legs. Note: A prone press-up will feel good as a stretch after doing abdominal strength or endurance exercises. This relaxed lordotic position can be performed while standing. Place the hands in the small of the back and gently arch the back and hold. This should feel good after sitting for a long period with the back flat.

Table 8

Table 8 Stretching and Strengthening Exercises for Round Shoulders

These exercises are designed to stretch the muscles of the chest and strengthen the muscles that keep the shoulders pulled back in good alignment (scapular adduction).

1. Arm Lift

This exercise strengthens the scapular adductors and helps prevent or correct round shoulders and kyphosis. Lie on stomach with arms in reverse-T. Rest forehead on floor. Maintain the arm position and contract the muscles between the shoulder blades, lifting the arms as high as possible without raising head and trunk. Hold. Relax and repeat. Note: If the arms are first pressed against the floor before lifting, this becomes a PNF exercise and range of motion may be greater. Variation: This more advanced exercise is performed in the same way except the arms are extended overhead.

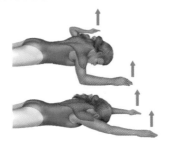

2. Seated Rowing

This exercise strengthens the scapular adductors (rhomboid and trapezius) and prevents or corrects kyphosis, round shoulders, head forward or cervical lordosis, and neck pain. Sit facing pulley, feet braced and knees slightly bent. Grasp bar, palms down with hands shoulder-width apart. Pull bar to chest, keeping elbows high, and return.

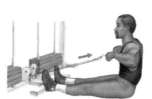

3. Wand Exercise

This exercise helps prevent and correct round shoulders and kyphosis by stretching the muscles on the anterior side of the shoulder joint. Sit with wand grasped at ends. Raise wand overhead. Be certain that the head does not slide forward into a "poke neck" position. Keep the chin tucked and neck straight. Bring wand down behind shoulder blades. Keep spine erect; hold. Hands may be moved closer together to increase stretch on chest muscles.

4. Pectoral Stretch

This exercise stretches the chest muscle (pectorals) and prevents or corrects round shoulders and sunken chest.

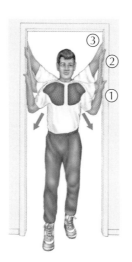

1. Stand erect in doorway with arms raised 45 degrees, elbows bent, and hands grasping door jambs; feet in front stride position. Press out on door frame, contracting the arms maximally for three seconds. Relax and shift weight forward on legs. Lean into doorway so muscles on front of shoulder joint and chest are stretched. Hold.
2. Repeat with arms raised 90 degrees.
3. Repeat with arms raised 135 degrees.

Lumbar Stabilization Exercises with Physioballs (Swiss Balls) Table 9

These exercises are designed to help improve the ability of the back to stabilize and support the trunk. The physioballs provide a useful way to learn to balance the body in these positions. Physioballs are available at many commercial fitness centers.

Table 9

1. Balancing

Contract abdominal muscles. Straighten one knee and raise opposite arm over head. Alternate sides. Then slowly walk the ball forward and backward with legs. To increase difficulty, position ball farther from your body.

Varriation: Slowly walk ball forward or backward with legs. Be careful not to arch back.

3. Wall Support

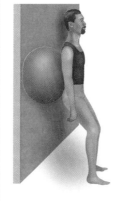

Stand against a wall with ball supporting low back. Contract abdominal muscles. Slowly bend knees 45 to 90 degrees and hold five seconds. Straighten knees and repeat. Raise both arms over head to increase difficulty.

2. Marching

Sit up straight with hips and knees bent 90 degrees. Contract abdominal muscles. Slowly raise one heel and opposite arm over head. Alternate sides. To increase difficulty, slowly raise one foot 2 inches from floor, alternating sides.

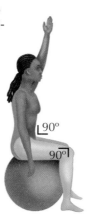

90°
90°

4. Stomach Roll

Lie on your stomach with the ball supporting your lower abdomen. Contract abdominal muscles. Straighten one knee and raise legs 2 to 4 inches off the floor. Alternate legs. To increase difficulty, raise the opposite arm and leg. Be careful not to arch your back.

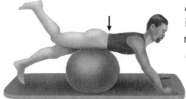

Web Resources

American Back Care Company **www.americanback.com**

Body and Back Care **www.backandbodycare.com**

MedX Machine **www.medxonline.com**

National Safety Council: back care **www.nsc.org**

Suggested Readings

Web review materials for concept 13 are available at **www.mhhe.com/fit_well/web13 Click 08.**

Drezner, J. A., and S. A. Herring. 2001. Managing low back pain. *Physician and Sports Medicine* 29(8):37–43.

Katzmarzyk, P. T., and L. C. Cora. 2002. Musculoskeletal fitness and risk of mortality. *Medicine and Science in Sports and Exercise* 34(5):740–744.

Kuritzky, L., and J. White. 1998. Low back pain. *The Physician and Sports Medicine* 25(1):56.

McGill, S. M. 2001. Low back stability. *Exercise and Sport Science Reviews* 29(1):26–31.

Plowman, S. A. 1999. Physical fitness and healthy low back function. In Corbin, C. B., and R. P. Pangrazi, (eds.), *Towards a Better Understanding of Physical Fitness and Activity.* Scottsdale, AZ: Holcomb-Hathaway.

Pollock, M. L., and K. R. Vincent. 1999. Resistance training for health. In Corbin, C. B., and R. P. Pangrazi, (eds.), *Towards a Better Understanding of Physical Fitness and Activity.* Scottsdale, AZ: Holcomb-Hathaway.

U.S. Department of Health and Human Services. Nov. 2000. *Healthy People 2010.* 2nd ed. *With Understanding and Improving Health and Objectives for Improving Health.* 2 vols. Washington, DC: U.S. Government Printing Office.

Walters, P. H. 2000. Back to the basics: Strengthening the neglected lower back. *ACSM's Health and Fitness Journal* 4(4):19–25.

In the News

The prevention of back problems is an important goal in many worksite health promotion programs. Back pain is one of the top reasons that employees seek medical care and it is also one of the primary causes of long-term disability as well as absenteeism. Most employers today cover the majority of health-care costs for their employees. Employers also lose productivity if their staff of employees are absent or on disability. By reducing medical claims/disability related to back problems and absenteeism related to back pain, companies save money. Therefore, there are major economic incentives for companies to work to promote back health among employees.

Back care programs in worksites can include structured exercise programs, the use of ergonomic chairs and equipment, as well as educational programs and awareness messages about proper lifting and carrying in the workplace. A recent study identified a number of predictive factors that contributed to employees requiring sick leave of eight days or more due to low back pain. The main predictors were a past history of low back pain, a low employment grade, heavy smoking, existing pain, required bending backward or forward at work every day, overall social integration, and low social support at work. This study revealed that biomechanical exposure and the psychosocial work environment influence risk for significant back pain. Studies such as this help worksite health promotion professionals to develop appropriate prevention programs for the employees in their company.

Lab Resource Materials: Healthy Back Tests

Chart 1 ▶ Healthy Back Tests

Physicians and therapists use these tests, among others, to make differential diagnoses of back problems. You and your partner can use them to determine if you have muscle tightness that may put you at risk for back problems. Discontinue any of these tests if they produce pain, numbness, or tingling sensations in the back, hips, or legs. Experiencing any of these sensations may be an indication that you have a low back problem that requires diagnosis by your physician. Partners should use *great caution* in applying force. Be gentle and listen to your partner's feedback.

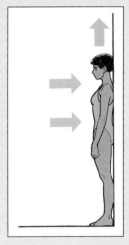

Test 1-Back to Wall

Stand with your back against a wall with head, heels, shoulders, and calves of legs touching the wall as shown in the diagram. Flatten your neck and the hollow of your back by pressing your buttocks down against the wall. Your partner should just be able to place a hand in the space between the wall and the small of your back.

- If this space is greater than the thickness of his/her hand, you probably have lordosis with shortened lumbar and hip flexor muscles.

Test 2-Straight-Leg Lift

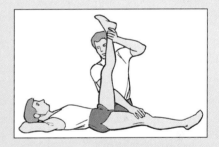

Lie on your back with hands behind your neck. The partner on your left should stabilize your right leg by placing his/her right hand on the knee. With the left hand, your partner should grasp the left ankle and raise your left leg as near to a right angle as possible. In this position (as shown in the diagram), your lower back should be in contact with the floor. Your right leg should remain straight and on the floor throughout the test.

- If your left leg bends at the knee, short hamstring muscles are indicated. If your back arches and/or your right leg does not remain flat on the floor, short lumbar muscles or hip flexor muscles (or both) are indicated. Repeat the test on the opposite side. (Both sides must pass in order to pass the test.)

Test 3-Thomas Test

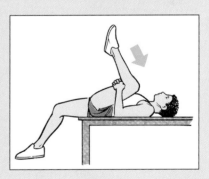

Lie on your back on a table or bench with your right leg extended beyond the edge of the table (approximately one-third of the thigh off the table). Bring your left knee to your chest and pull the thigh down tightly with your hands. Lower your right leg to the table. Your lower back should remain flat against the table as shown in the diagram. Your right thigh should remain on the table.

- If your right thigh lifts off the table while the left knee is hugged to the chest, a tight hip flexor (iliopsoas) on that side is indicated. Repeat on the opposite side. (Both sides must pass in order to pass the test.)

Test 4-Ely's Test

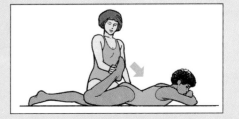

Lie prone: flex right knee. Partner *gently* pushes right heel toward the buttocks. Stop when resistance is felt or when partner expresses discomfort.

- If pelvis leaves the floor or hip flexes or knee fails to bend freely (135 degrees) or heel fails to touch buttocks, there is tightness in the quadriceps muscles. Repeat with left leg. (Both sides must pass in order to pass the test.)

Chart 1 ▶ Healthy Back Tests *(Continued)*

Test 5-Ober's Test

Lie on left side with left leg flexed 90 degrees at the hip and 90 degrees at the knee. Partner places right hip in neutral position (no flexion) and right knee in 90-degree flexion. Partner then allows the weight of the leg to lower it toward the floor.

- If there is no tightness in the iliotibial band (fascia and muscles on lateral side of leg), the knee touches the floor without pain and the test is passed. Repeat on the other side. (Both sides must pass in order to pass the test.)

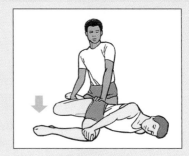

Test 6-Press-Up (Straight Arm)

Perform the press-up.

- If you can press to a straight-arm position, keeping your pubis in contact with the floor, and if your partner determines that the arch in your back is a continuous curve (not just a sharp angle at the lumbosacral joint), then there is adequate flexibility in spinal extension.

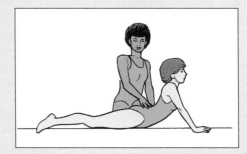

Test 7-Knee Roll

Lie supine with your knees and hips flexed 90 degrees, arms extended to the sides at shoulder level. Keep the knees and hips in that position and lower them to the floor on the right and then on the left.

- If you can accomplish this and still keep your shoulders in contact with the floor, then you have adequate rotation in the spine, especially at the lumbar and thoracic junction. (Both sides must pass in order to pass the test.)

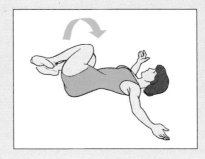

Test 8-Leg Drop Test*

Lie on your back on a table or on the floor with both legs extended overhead. Flatten the low back against the table or floor. Slowly lower legs while keeping the back flat.

- If your back arches before you reach a 45-degree angle, the abdominal muscles are too weak. A partner should be ready to support your legs if needed to prevent lower back arching or strain to the back muscles.

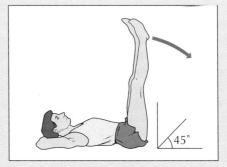

*The double leg-drop is suitable as a diagnostic test when performed one time. It is not a good exercise to be performed regularly by most people. If it causes pain, stop the test.

Chart 2 ▶ Healthy Back Test Ratings

Classification	Number of Tests Passed
Excellent	7–8
Very good	6
Good	5
Fair	4
Poor	1–3

Lab 13A: The Healthy Back Test and Back/Neck Questionnaire

Name	**Section**	**Date**

Purpose: To self-assess your potential for back problems using the Healthy Back Test and the Back/Neck Questionnaire.

Procedures:

1. Answer the questions in the Back/Neck Questionnaire below. Count your points for nonmodifiable factors, modifiable factors, and total score and record these scores in the Results section. Use Chart 1 to determine your rating for all three scores and record them in the Results section.
2. With a partner, administer the Healthy Back Test to each other (see lab resource materials). Determine your rating using Chart 2. Record your score and rating in the Results section. If you did not pass a test, list the muscles you should develop to improve on that test.
3. Answer the questions in the Conclusions and Implications section.

Risk Factor Questionnaire for Back and Neck Problems

Directions: Place an X in the appropriate circle after each question. Add the scores for each of the circles you checked to determine your modifiable risk, nonmodifiable risk, and total risk scores.

Nonmodifiable:

1. Do you have a family history of osteoporosis, arthritis, rheumatism, or other joint disease?   (0) No   (1) Yes

2. What is your age?   (0) < 40   (1) 40–50   (2) 51–60   (3) 61+

3. Did you participate extensively in these sports when you were young (gymnastics, football, weight lifting, skiing, ballet, javelin, or shot put)?   (0) No   (1) Some   (3) Extensive

4. How many previous back or neck problems have you had?   (0) None   (1) 1   (2) 2   (5) 3+

Modifiable:

5. Does your daily routine involve heavy lifting?   (0) No   (1) Some   (3) A lot

6. Does your daily routine require you to stand for long periods?   (0) No   (1) Some   (3) A lot

7. Do you have a high level of job-related stress?   (0) No   (1) Some   (3) A lot

8. Do you sit for long periods of time (computer operator, typist, or similar job)?   (0) No   (1) Some   (3) A lot

9. Does your daily routine require repetitive movements or holding objects for long periods of time (e.g., baby, briefcase, sales suitcase)?   (0) No   (1) Some   (3) A lot

10. Does your daily routine require you to stand or sit with poor posture (e.g., poor chair, reaching required while standing)?   (0) No   (1) Some   (3) A lot

11. What is your score on the Healthy Back Test?   (0) 6–7   (1) 5   (3) 4   (5) 0–3

12. What is your score on the Posture Test in Lab 13B?   (0) 0–2   (1) 3–4   (3) 5–7   (4) 8+

Results:

Test	Pass	Fail	If you failed, what exercise should you do?
1. Back to wall	○	○	
2. Straight-leg lift	○	○	
3. Thomas test	○	○	
4. Ely's test	○	○	
5. Ober's test	○	○	
6. Press-up	○	○	
7. Knee roll	○	○	
8. Leg drop	○	○	

Total

Chart 1 ▶ Back/Neck Questionnaire Ratings

Rating	Alterable Score	Unalterable Score	Total Score
Very high risk	7+	12+	19+
High risk	5–6	6–11	11–18
Average risk	3–4	4–6	7–10
Low risk	0–2	0–3	0–6

Chart 2 ▶ Healthy Back Test Ratings

Classification	Number of Tests Passed
Excellent	7–8
Very good	6
Good	5
Fair	4
Poor	1–3

Back/Neck Questionnaire

Score _____ Rating _____

Back Test

Score _____ Rating _____

Conclusions and Implications: In several sentences, discuss your need to do exercises for care of the back and neck. Include in your discussion whether you think your muscles are fit enough to prevent problems, the areas in which you are most likely to experience problems, and steps you might take to prevent future problems. Use your test results to answer.

Lab 13B: Evaluating Posture

Name	Section	Date

Purpose: To learn to recognize postural deviations and thus become more posture conscious and to determine your posture limitations in order to institute a preventive or corrective program.

Procedures:

1. Wear as little clothing as possible (bathing suits are recommended) and remove shoes and socks.
2. Work in groups of two or three, with one person acting as the subject while partners serve as examiners, then alternate roles.
   a. Stand by a vertical plumb line.
   b. Using Chart 1 and Figure 1, check any deviations and indicate their severity (see points scale below).
   c. Total the score and determine your posture rating from the Posture Rating Scale (Chart 2).
3. If time permits, perform back and posture exercises (see Lab 13C).

Results:

Record your posture score ☐

Record your posture rating from the Posture Rating Scale below ☐

Chart 1 ▶ Posture Evaluation

Side View	Points	Back View	Points
Head forward	_____	Tilted head	_____
Sunken chest	_____	Protruding scapulae	_____
Round shoulders	_____	Symptoms of scoliosis Shoulders uneven	_____
Kyphosis	_____	Hips uneven	_____
Lordosis	_____	Lateral curvature of spine (Adam's position)	_____
Abdominal ptosis	_____	One side of back high (Adam's position)	_____
Hyperextended knees	_____		
Body lean	_____	Total score	☐

Rate each using this point system:

- 0 = none
- 1 = slight
- 2 = moderate
- 3 = severe

Chart 2 ▶ Posture Rating Scale

Classification	Total Score
Excellent	0–2
Very good	3–4
Good	5–7
Fair	8–11
Poor	12 or more

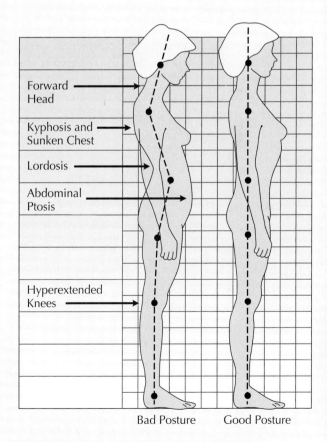

Forward Head

Kyphosis and Sunken Chest

Lordosis

Abdominal Ptosis

Hyperextended Knees

Bad Posture   Good Posture

Figure 1 ▶ Comparison of bad and good posture.

Conclusions and Implications:

Were you aware of the deviations that were found?   Yes ◯   No ◯

1. List the deviations that were moderate or severe.

2. In several sentences, describe your current posture status. Include in this discussion your overall assessment of your current posture, whether you think you will need special exercises in the future, and the reasons why your posture rating is good or not so good.

Lab 13C: Planning and Logging Exercises: Care of the Back and Neck

Name		Section	Date

Purpose: To select several exercises for the back and neck that meet your personal needs and to self-monitor progress for one of these.

Procedures:

1. On Chart 1 check the tests from the Healthy Back Test that you did *not* pass. Select at least one exercise from the group associated with those items. In addition, select several more exercises (a total of eight to ten) that you think will best meet your personal needs. If you passed all of the items, select eight to ten exercises that you think will best prevent future back and neck problems. Check the exercises you plan to perform in Chart 1.
2. Perform each of the exercises you select three days in one week.
3. Keep a one-week log of your actual participation using the last three columns in Chart 1. If possible, keep the log with you during the day. Place a check by each of the exercises you perform for each day, including ones that you didn't originally have planned. If you cannot keep the log with you, fill in the log at the end of the day. If you choose to keep a log for more than one week, make extra copies of the log before you begin.
4. Answer the questions in the Results section.

Chart 1 ▶ Back and Neck Exercise Plan

Check the tests you failed:	√	Place a check beside the exercises you plan to do. In the last 3 columns, check the exercises done and the days done.	√	Day 1 Date:	Day 2 Date:	Day 3 Date:
1. Back to wall		Pelvic tilt				
		Bridging				
		Wall slide				
		Pelvic stabilizer				
2. Straight-leg lift		Back-saver hamstring stretch				
		Calf stretcher				
3. Thomas test		Hip and thigh stretcher				
4. Ely's test		Single knee-to-chest				
5. Ober's test		Lateral hip and thigh stretcher				
6. Press-up		Upper trunk lift				
		Trunk lift				
7. Knee roll		Side bender				
		Supine trunk twist				
8. Leg drop		Reverse curl				
		Crunch				
Choose other exercises for the neck and shoulders		Chin tuck				
		Neck rotation				
		Arm lift				
		Pectoral stretch				

Results:

Did you do eight to ten exercises at least three days in the week?

Yes   No

○   ○

Conclusions and Interpretations:

1. Do you feel that you will use back and neck exercises as part of your regular lifetime physical activity plan, either now or in the future? Use several sentences to explain your answer.

2. Discuss the exercises you did. What exercises would you continue to do and which ones would you change? Use several sentences to explain your answer.

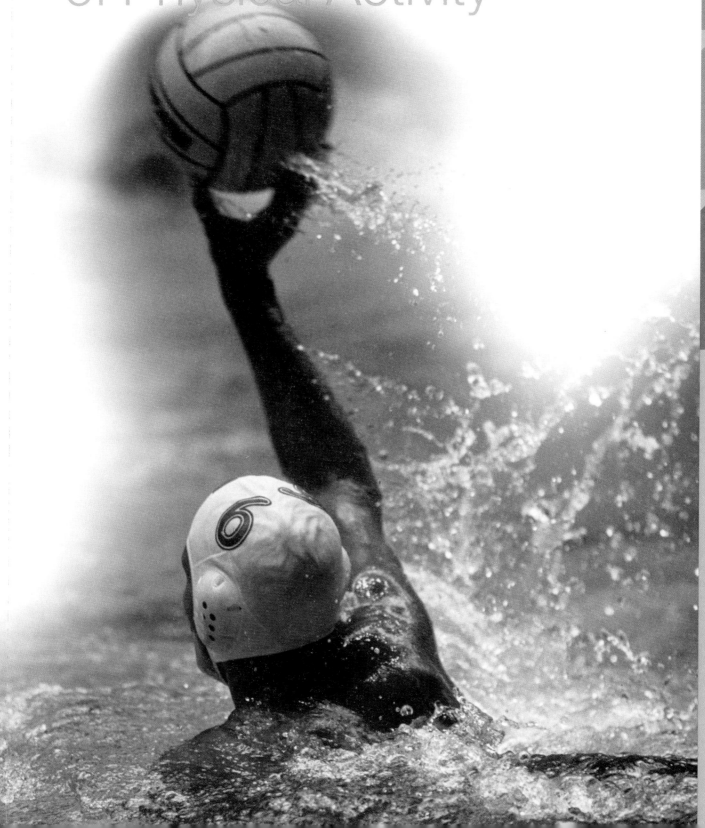

Performance Benefits
of Physical Activity

Physical activity provides performance benefits above and beyond the benefits to health. These performance benefits can promote quality of life for the typical person and enhance the abilities of athletes and people in jobs requiring high levels of performance.

Health Goals

for the year 2010

- Increase leisure time physical activity.

- Increase adoption and maintenance of regular daily physical activity.

- Increase proportion of people who participate in employee sponsored activity programs.

- Reduce steroid use especially among young people.

Sports and competitive athletics are compelling challenges to many individuals. Participation in physical activity provides opportunities for individuals to explore the limits of their ability and to challenge themselves in competition. Some individuals enjoy challenges associated with competitive aerobic activities such as running, cycling, swimming, and triathlons. Others enjoy the challenges associated with competitive resistance training activities, such as powerlifting or bodybuilding. Competitive opportunities are also available in various sport activities. While competitive activities provide health benefits and recreation opportunities, many individuals are more interested in improving their performance. High-level performance is also a requirement for some types of work. Examples are fire safety, military service, and police work. The heroic efforts of fire fighters, law enforcement and Port Authority officials following the events of September 11, 2001 are a clear example of how important high-level performance is in these careers.

In this concept, specific attention is devoted to the methods used to train for high-level performance. Several types of training will be discussed including aerobic training, anaerobic training, special forms of resistance training (including plyometrics), and advanced techniques for flexibility. Methods for maximizing skill-related fitness and skill will also be presented.

High-Level Performance and Training Characteristics

Improving performance requires more specific training than the type needed to improve health. High levels of performance require good genetics, high levels of motivation, and a commitment to regular training. The effort and training required to excel in sports, competitive athletics, or work requiring high-level performance are greater than the amount required for good health and wellness. Because adaptations to exercise are specific to the type of activity that is performed, training should be matched to the specific needs of a given activity.

High-level performance requires health-related, skill-related fitness and specific motor skills necessary for the performance. People who possess good fitness levels for each of the five health-related fitness components have enhanced health and wellness, as well as reduced risk of disease. To succeed in sports and certain jobs, high performance levels of health-related physical fitness are necessary, over and above what the normal person needs to enhance health. This is illustrated in Figure 1. **Training** (regular physical activity) builds health-related fitness to enhance health and high-level performance. This is why arrows in Figure 1 extend from health-related fitness to both health and high-level performance. To some extent, it can be said that high-level health-related fitness is much like skill-related fitness. High performance levels are not necessary for all people, only those who need exceptional performances. A distance runner needs exceptional cardiovascular fitness and muscular endurance, a lineman in football needs exceptional strength, a volleyball player needs power for jumping, and a gymnast needs exceptional flexibility.

Exceptional performance also requires high-level skill-related physical fitness. Skill-related physical fitness

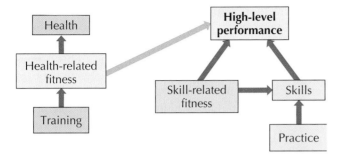

Figure 1 ▶ Factors influencing high-level performance.

is especially affected by heredity. For example, speed is influenced greatly by the number of fast-twitch fibers you inherit, and reaction time is associated with the innate characteristics of your nervous system. With specific training, you can make modest modifications in your skill-related fitness, but most experts believe that it is more important to do regular practice to enhance performance skills associated with the specific tasks of your sport or job. It is important to understand that skill-related fitness and skills are not the same thing!

Skill-related fitness components are abilities that help you learn skills faster and better, thus the arrow in Figure 1 from skill-related fitness to skills. Skills, on the other hand, are things like throwing, kicking, catching, and hitting a ball. Practice enhances skills (see arrow from practice to skills). Therefore, practicing the specific skills of a sport or a job is more productive to performance enhancement than more general drills associated with changing skill-related fitness. The most successful performers will be those who inherit good potential for health and skill-related fitness, who train

High-level performers need high-performance levels of fitness.

to improve their health-related fitness, and who do extensive practice to improve the skills associated with the specific activity in which they hope to excel.

Periodization of training may help prevent overtraining. www.mhhe.com/fit_well/web14 Click01. When a person trains for a single performance or perhaps several competitive events such as games or matches during a sport season, it requires careful planning to reach peak performance at the right time and to avoid overtraining and injuries. Periodization is a modern concept of manipulating repetition, resistance, and exercise selection so there are periodic peaks and valleys during the training program. The peaks are needed to challenge the body, and the valleys are needed to allow the body to recover and adapt fully. Over the course of the season, there should be a gradual progression that allows the person to peak at just the right time. To accomplish this, training begins with an emphasis on base training in which the volume of training is gradually increased (increasing reps or performing large numbers of sets). As the season progresses, the focus shifts to an emphasis on the intensity of training (going faster or lifting heavier weights). Because higher intensity exercise requires more time for recovery, the volume of training should be reduced at these times. A key concept in periodization is to provide opportunities for the body to fully adapt and recover prior to competition. Thus, the phase immediately prior to competition (**tapering**) is characterized by a reduced volume and intensity of training. By applying periodization to their training, athletes are able to optimize performance and minimize the risk of overtraining (see Figure 2).

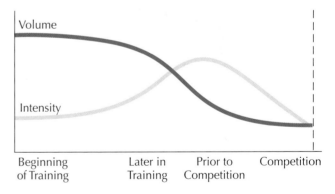

Figure 2 ▶ Volume and intensity of training during periodization.

Tapering A reduction in training volume and intensity that is used prior to competition to elicit peak performance.

Training A term typically used to describe the type of physical activity performed by people interested in high-level performance, e.g., athletes, people in specialized jobs.

Training for Speed and Endurance

Many types of high-level performance require aerobic capacity. Regardless of the type of activity you perform, you derive energy from high-energy fuel that must be available to the muscle fibers. The breakdown of this high-energy fuel in the muscle cells allows you to perform all types of exercise. To continue exercising, the body must replenish these energy stores on a continual basis.

For some performers, success depends on the ability to sustain activity for long periods of time without stopping. Distance runners and swimmers are good examples. These types of performers are in special need of high levels of cardiovascular fitness or aerobic capacity. In aerobic exercise, adequate oxygen is available to use the carbohydrates and fats available in the body to rebuild the high-energy fuel the muscles need to sustain performance. Aerobic exercise increases aerobic capacity (cardiovascular fitness) by enhancing the body's ability to supply oxygen to the muscles as well as their ability to use it. Slow-twitch muscle fibers appear to benefit most from aerobic exercise. Any performance that involves long sustained performance places special demands on the slow-twitch fibers and requires a high level of aerobic capacity (cardiovascular fitness). The best measure of cardiovascular fitness is $\dot{V}O_2$ max (see cardiovascular fitness concept).

Many types of high-level performance require anaerobic capacity. www.mhhe.com/fit_well/web14 **Click 02.** If adequate oxygen is supplied, activity can be sustained for long periods. Unfortunately, the energy resulting from the breakdown of the body's high-energy fuel is used in a matter of seconds if adequate oxygen is not supplied. Carbohydrates stored in the cells can be broken down to replenish the high-energy fuel supply to allow performance to continue for an additional time (30 to 40 seconds for most people). Short-term, vigorous exercise performed in the absence of an adequate oxygen supply is called **anaerobic exercise.** Anaerobic exercise results in **lactic acid** build-up in the process of energy production. Muscle fatigue occurs when anaerobic energy supplies are depleted, and lactic acid build-up occurs. Regular anaerobic exercise seems to allow the muscle to tolerate higher lactic acid levels before fatigue occurs. Also, anaerobic exercise improves anaerobic energy production capabilities, primarily in the fast-twitch fibers. These fibers appear to benefit most from anaerobic exercise.

Anaerobic capacity, or the ability to perform vigorous, short-term bouts of exercise and repeat them after relatively short rest periods, is necessary for success in many sports and jobs that require high-level performance. Anaerobic capacity is often measured in the laboratory using the Wingate test, an all-out, 30-second stationary bicycle ride at high resistance.

Interval training is effective in building anaerobic capacity. www.mhhe.com/fit_well/web14 **Click 03.** In anaerobic **interval training,** the goal is to challenge the anaerobic energy systems. This is typically accomplished with repeated high-intensity bouts of activity. In response to this training, the body improves its ability to produce energy anaerobically and also improves its ability to tolerate and remove lactic acid from the blood.

Anaerobic interval training can be performed with either short or long intervals. Short-interval workouts should use maximum speed with rest intervals lasting from ten seconds to two minutes. These should be repeated eight to thirty times. Long-interval training should use 90 to 100 percent speed with rest intervals lasting from 3 to 15 minutes. These should be repeated four to fifteen times. A sample short anaerobic interval program and a sample long interval running program are presented in Table 1. These plans could be modified for use with other types of activities.

Principles of interval training can be modified for different activities. The principles of interval training can be applied to specific sports or specific jobs that require high levels of anaerobic performance. Basketball, for example, requires anaerobic sprints up and down the court. Simulated games that require repeated sprints with appropriate rest periods between intervals are a form of interval training specific to the needs of basketball performers. Similar specific types of interval training can be developed for virtually any activity.

Recently, interval training has also been adapted to different forms of exercise such as dance exercise. A recent increase in interest in high-level performance in this area has resulted in the development of dance interval training. This involves vigorous dance exercise alternated with frequent rest periods. In some cases, other forms of exercise, such as running, are alternated with dance exercise bouts.

Table 1 ▶ Sample Anaerobic Interval Training Program (Moderate Intensity)

Short Intervals	Long Intervals
1. Do a flexibility and cardiovascular warm-up.	1. Do a flexibility and cardiovascular warm-up.
2. Run at 100% speed for 10 seconds (approximately 70–100 yards).	2. Run at 90% speed for one minute (approximately 300–500 yards).
3. Rest for ten seconds by walking slowly.	3. Rest for four minutes by walking slowly.
4. Alternately repeat steps 2 and 3 until twenty runs have been completed.	4. Alternately repeat steps 2 and 3 until five runs have been completed.

Fartlek training is a modified form of interval training. As noted in an earlier concept, *Fartlek* is a Swedish word for speed play. This exercise was developed in Scandinavia where pinewood paths follow curves of lakes and up and down many hills. The idea is to get away from the regimen of running on a track and to enjoy the woods, lakes, and mountains. Because of the terrain, the pace is never constant. The uphill path requires a slow pace, while a straight stretch or downhill trail allows for speed. In the speed play, or Fartlek, system, you run easily for a time at a steady, hard speed, walk rapidly following that, alternate short sprints with walking, go full speed uphill, and perhaps at a fast pace for a while. You can plan your own speed-play program using your own course, which may include uphill and downhill running with other variations.

Training for activities requiring high levels of aerobic capacity can be achieved using a variety of techniques. www.mhhe.com/fit_well/web14 **Click 04.** The ability to perform sustained aerobic performance can be enhanced using a variety of techniques. The most common procedure is to perform the activity in which you plan to participate. For example, people who plan to run a marathon or a 10K race will commonly perform regular distance running at speeds similar to those required for their specific event. This type of training is also supplemented with aerobic interval training and long-slow distance training. Some training to enhance anaerobic capacity is also performed by most people interested in aerobic activities. Performers in other activities such as swimming and cycling will use similar schedules of training.

Interval training can be done aerobically. Many people think only of interval training as an anaerobic method of training. In fact, aerobic interval training can be very effective in performance enhancement. In aerobic interval training, the goal is to challenge the aerobic system to work near maximal levels for extended periods of time. Research suggests that a period of four to six minutes of activity is needed to cause the aerobic system to elicit maximal adaptations that will improve aerobic capacity ($\dot{V}O_2$ max). The use of repeated mile runs at a faster-than-normal training pace would provide this type of challenge to the aerobic system. Alternately, shorter exercise bouts can be performed with brief rest periods to achieve the same goal. For example, a series of quarter-mile repeats with short rests would be suitable as long as the total time at a high intensity was similar. In this case, the rest intervals must be short enough to only allow partial recovery between intervals.

Aerobic intervals are typically conducted at paces slower than the pace an individual would use in a race. An example of a schedule of aerobic interval training for a 10-km runner is illustrated in Table 2. To use the schedule, locate your typical 10-km time in the left-hand column. Perform 400-meter runs at the time specified in the "pace" column. Repeat twenty times with intervals of 10 to 15 seconds between runs. Similar schedules can be developed with other activities such as swimming and cycling. This activity, however, is not recommended for those just beginning exercise. If your heart rate exceeds your target zone, you will need to modify the running time for each interval.

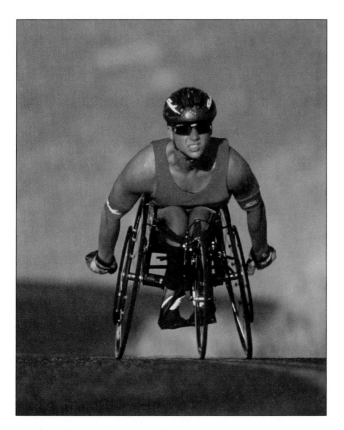

Interval training can be adapted for performers in a variety of activities.

Anaerobic Exercise Anaerobic means "in the absence of oxygen." Anaerobic exercise is performed at an intensity that is greater than the body's ability to provide energy through the aerobic system.

Lactic Acid Substance that results from the process of supplying energy during anaerobic exercise; a cause of muscle fatigue.

Interval Training A training technique often used for high-level aerobic and anaerobic training; uses repeated bouts of activity followed by rest to maximize the quality of the workout.

Table 2 ▶ Aerobic Interval Training Schedules for a 10-Kilometer Runner				
Best 10-km Times (Min:Sec)	Reps	Distance (Meters)	Rest (Sec)	Pace (Min:Sec)
46:00	20	400	10–15	2:00
43:00	20	400	10–15	1:52
40:00	20	400	10–15	1:45
37:00	20	400	10–15	1:37
34:00	20	400	10–15	1:30

Source: Wilmore J. H. and Costill D. L.

Long-slow distance training is important for enhancing performances requiring aerobic capacity. The training techniques described in previous sections are necessary to achieve high-level aerobic performance. However, there is evidence that **long-slow distance training (LSD)** is also needed to promote high-level aerobic performances (such as long-distance running, cycling, or swimming). The reason for this is that there are specific adaptations that take place within the muscles when used for long periods of time. These adaptations improve the muscles' ability to take up and use the oxygen in the bloodstream. Adaptations within the muscle cell also improve the body's ability to produce energy from fat stores. Long slow-distance training involves performances longer than the event for which you are performing but at a slower pace. For example, a mile runner will regularly perform 6 to 7 mile runs (at 50 to 60 percent of racing pace) to improve aerobic conditioning even though the event is much shorter. A marathoner may perform runs of 20 miles or more to achieve even higher levels of endurance. While this 20-mile distance is shorter than the marathon race distance, research suggests that ample adaptations occur from this volume of exercise. Excess mileage in this case may just wear the body down. Long-slow distance training should be performed once every one to two weeks, and a rest day is recommended on the subsequent day to allow the body to recover fully.

Improved anaerobic capacity can contribute to performance in activities considered to be aerobic. Many physical activities commonly considered to be aerobic—such as tennis, basketball, and racquetball—have an anaerobic component. These activities require periodic vigorous bursts of exercise. Regular anaerobic training will help you resist fatigue in these activities. Even participants in activities such as long-distance running can benefit from anaerobic training, especially if performance times or winning races is important. A fast start may be anaerobic, a sprint past an opponent may be anaerobic, and a kick at the end will no doubt be anaerobic. Anaerobic training can help prepare a person for these circumstances.

Some training methods can interfere with performance. Some research studies have shown that certain techniques may cause a decrease in performance. For example, when distance runners were trained with weighted wristlets, anklets, and belts, they performed worse than runners who did not wear weights in training. In another study, people who were running and bicycling for aerobic endurance six days per week combined those exercises with a strength training program five days per week. The results suggest that doing intense training for aerobic capacity and muscle fitness simultaneously had somewhat limited muscle fitness benefits.

Training for Strength and Power

The amount of progressive resistance training for high-level performance differs from techniques used to build strength for health. In the concept on muscle fitness, basic training techniques were described. The focus was on health enhancement. Training techniques for people interested in health differ from those who want high-level performance. The American College of Sports Medicine (ACSM) recently released a Position Stand on "Progression Models in Resistance Training for Healthy Adults." Progression in this document was described as the "act of moving forward or advancing toward a specific goal." Individuals performing high-level resistance training may have different goals even though

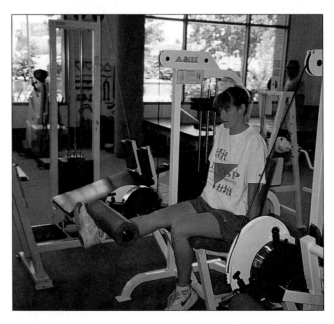

Strength training for high-level performance differs from strength training for health.

they use the same basic equipment and lifts. Olympic weight lifting competitors use free weights and compete in two exercises: the snatch, and the clean and jerk. Powerlifting competitors use free weights and compete in three lifts: the bench press, squat, and dead lift. Bodybuilding competitors use several forms of resistance training and are judged on muscular hypertrophy and **definition of muscle.** Performers in these activities as well as those in a variety of other activities use advanced resistance training techniques, some of which are described in the sections that follow.

Performers training for high-level strength should use multiple sets with heavier weights. www.mhhe.com/fit_well/web14 Click 05. While a single set of exercises for each muscle group is sufficient for novice lifters, or for general health goals, guidelines for advanced lifters call for multiple sets of exercises ranging from one to twelve repetitions. The additional sets are needed to overload more effectively muscles that have already been trained to some extent. For continued progress and improvement, systematically vary the training volume and intensity of efforts (periodization). Multiple joint exercises such as the bench press have been found to be more effective in strength enhancement since they allow a greater load to be lifted.

The sequencing of exercises within a workout is also an important consideration for strength development. When training all major muscle groups in a workout, large muscle groups should be done before small muscle groups, and multiple-joint exercises should be done before single-joint ones.

Performers training for bulk and definition often use extra reps and/or sets. www.mhhe.com/fit_well/web14 Click 06. Bodybuilders are more interested in definition and hypertrophy (large muscles) than in absolute strength. Gaining both size and definition requires a balance between strength and muscle endurance training. Most bodybuilders use three to seven sets of ten to fifteen repetitions, rather than the three sets of three to eight repetitions recommended for most weight lifters. Sometimes definition is difficult to obtain because it is obscured by fat. It should be noted that people with the largest-looking muscles are not always the strongest.

"Negative" exercise has no advantage over other types of exercise for muscle fitness development. Contrary to the claims of some enthusiasts, eccentric (negative) and concentric (positive) exercises show no difference in terms of their effectiveness in developing strength or muscular endurance. Weight can be handled more comfortably with eccentric exercise, but this type of exercise has a tendency to cause more muscle soreness. This type of exercise also requires the assistance of another person or

the use of special machines such as the Kin Com Biodex or Keiser dynamometers. The most common application of eccentric exercise has been in rehabilitation settings where it has been found to be useful in promoting muscle function and recovery from injury.

Eccentric contractions are combined with concentric contractions in most sports. For example, if you lift something, you also lower it. Thus, to apply the law of specificity, progressive resistance exercises should generally include both types of contractions. This can be accomplished with a slow, steady concentric lifting phase and a slower, eccentric lowering phase (see discussion of technique later in the concept).

Training for cardiovascular fitness at the same time as strength training may prevent maximum results in both. Studies have shown that training simultaneously for strength and cardiovascular fitness may not produce the same result as one could obtain while training for either one separately. Some people have interpreted this to mean that they interfere with each other. The cause of this is not clear. It may be that the time spent on each one is less or that overtraining occurs rather than one inhibiting the other. Whatever the cause, the differences are relatively minor and should not prevent an individual from doing both concurrently.

Muscular endurance is important to high-level performance. Muscular endurance training (see concept 11) is necessary for performers in various activities. For people training for distance events, muscular endurance training can complement cardiovascular fitness training and enhance performance. Resistance training for this type of performance would focus on high repetitions rather than high resistance. For performers in activities requiring strength, the amount of muscular endurance training depends on the specific nature of the activity. For example, if the activity requires a short duration and has a high strength requirement, muscular endurance training involving high repetitions may actually impair performance. The sport of weight lifting would be an example. On the other hand, activities such as blocking in football require repeated strength performance. For performers doing this type of activity, the ability to persist (muscular endurance) is important so training should use a relatively high number of repetitions.

LSD Training A training technique that emphasizes long, slow distance. It is used by marathon runners and other endurance performers.

Definition (of Muscle) The detailed external appearance of a muscle.

Advanced Muscle Endurance Training should include multple sets of ten to twenty-five repetitions. Rest periods of one to two minutes are recommended for high repetition sets and periods of less than one minute should be used for lower repetition sets. This challenges the muscles to perform over time. Variation in the order in which exercises are performed is also recommended. Intermediate lifters should aim for two to four times per week but advanced lifters may perform up to six sessions a week if appropriate variation in muscle groups is used between workouts.

Power is a combination of strength and speed, and is both health-related and skill-related. Most experts classify power as a skill-related component of fitness because it is partially dependent on speed. On the other hand, power is also dependent on strength and can be classified as a health-related component to the extent that strength is involved. Thus, power falls somewhere in between the two distinct groups of fitness attributes. Certainly its use is not limited to sports and dance. We use power extensively in our daily activities every time we apply a force to move something quickly. Power is important in protective movements, such as a pedestrian jumping to dodge a car or a driver jerking the steering wheel to avoid a collision or slamming on the brakes to stop in an emergency. A worker heaves a heavy load from a truck to a dock, and a carpenter uses force to hammer a nail.

Power is usually neglected in fitness literature. Some experts consider power to be the most functional mode in which all human motion occurs. Still, if the typical person builds adequate muscle fitness using the guidelines described earlier in this text, adequate power for daily living will occur. Power is exceptionally important in activities such as hitting a baseball, blocking in football, putting the shot, or throwing the discus. Power is also essential for good vertical jumping—a movement critical for basketball and many other sports. Clearly people interested in high-level performances should consider appropriate exercises that develop power.

The stronger person is not necessarily the more powerful. Power is the amount of work per unit of time. To increase power, you must do more work in the same time or the same work in less time. If you extend your knee and move a 100-pound weight through a 90-degree arc in one second, you have twice as much power as a person who needs two seconds to complete the same movement. Power requires both strength and speed. Increasing one without the other limits power. Some power athletes (for example, football players) might benefit more by achieving less strength and more speed.

The principle of specificity applies to power development. If you need power for an activity in which you are required to move heavy weights, then you need to develop *strength-related power* by working against heavy resistance at slower speeds. If you need to move light objects at great speed, such as in throwing a ball, you need to develop *speed-related power* by training at high speeds with relatively low resistance. There must be trade-offs between speed and power because the heavier the resistance, the slower the movement. Training adaptations are also specific to the type of training performed. Power exercises done at high speeds will help to enhance muscular endurance while power exercises that use heavy resistance at lower speeds will increase strength.

Performers who need explosive power to perform their events should use training that closely resembles the event. Jumpers, for example, should jump as a part of their training programs in order to learn correct timing at the same time they are developing power. This also applies to Olympic weight lifters, shot putters, jumpers, ballet dancers, and others. These athletes need both strength and endurance; however, studies show that too much of either can have a negative effect on performance. If they use machines, it is better to use the leg press than a knee extension machine because the press more nearly resembles the leg action of the jump.

The performer's program should use similar speed, force, angle, and range of motion, as the activity. However, if a performer is unable to do the specific skill because of weather or injury or is seeking variety, then plyometrics, isokinetics, and weight training (especially with free weights or pulleys if simulating a sport skill) are effective means of developing power.

Power training can be done with weight equipment but care is needed to ensure safety and efficacy. Resistance training can be performed to optimize power development but these movements are not recommended for beginning lifters. Studies have shown that heavy resistance training can actually decrease power unless training also includes some explosive movements. Current guidelines from the ACSM recommend heavy loading (85 percent to 100 percent of 1 RM) to increase the force component of the power equation and light to moderate loading (30 percent to 60 percent of 1 RM) performed at an explosive velocity to enhance the speed component of power. The guidelines recommend that a multiple set power program (three to six sets) be integrated within an overall strength training program. Exercises for power are most effectively done with free weights or pulleys to simulate sport-related movements more effectively. Isokinetic devices, such as isokinetic swim benches, may also be useful for enhancing sport specific power.

Plyometrics may be useful in training for tasks or events requiring power. www.mhhe.com/fit_well/web14 Click 07. A quick prestretch, or eccentric contraction of a muscle, immediately followed by an isometric

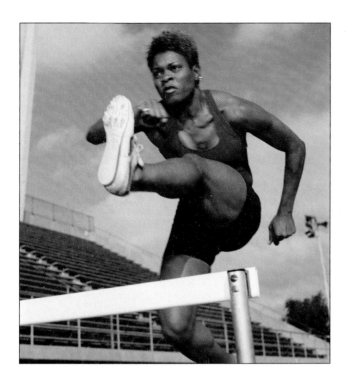

Plyometric enhances power.

Table 3 ▶ Safety Guidelines for Plyometrics

- Plyometrics for growing teens should begin moderately and progress slowly compared to adults.
- Progression should be gradual to avoid extreme muscle soreness.
- Adequate strength should be developed prior to plyometric training. (As a general rule, you should be able to do a half-squat with one-and-a-half times your body weight.)
- Get a physician's approval prior to doing plyometrics if you have a history of injuries or if you are recovering from injury to the body part being trained.
- The landing surface should be semiresilient, dry, and unobstructed.
- Shoes should have good lateral stability, be cushioned with an arch support, and have a nonslip sole.
- Obstacles used for jumping-over should be padded.
- The training should be preceded by a general and specific warm-up.
- The training sequence should:
  - precede all other workouts (while you are fresh);
  - include at least one spotter;
  - be done no more than twice per week, with 48 hours rest between bouts;
  - last no more than 30 minutes;
  - (for beginners) include 3 or 4 drills, with 2 or 3 sets per drill, 10–15 reps per set and 1–2 minutes rest between sets.

Source: G. Brittenham.

or concentric contraction, produces power. This has been called "pre-exertion countermovement," "wind up," or **plyometrics.** Former Soviet Olympic coaches pioneered this technique, developing drills for their athletes. Track and field athletes may do a hopping drill for 30 to 100 meters or alternate jumping from a box to the floor and back to the box (called depth jumping, drop jumping, or bounce loading). As the body lands, some of the major leg muscles lengthen in an eccentric contraction, then follow immediately with a strong concentric contraction as the legs push off for the next jump or stride. The prestretch of the muscle during landing adds an elastic recoil that provides extra force to the push-off.

Plyometrics are used to apply the specificity principle to training for certain skills. Because eccentric exercise tends to result in more muscular soreness, it would be wise to proceed slowly with this type of training. It would also be important to have good flexibility before beginning a plyometrics program. Some guidelines are listed in Table 3.

Training for High-Level Performance: Flexibility

Stretching for performance may differ from stretching for good health. Guidelines for building flexibility using a variety of stretching exercises are presented in the concept on flexibility. It was noted in that concept that static stretching techniques are recommended for the warm-up, even for high-level performers. Ballistic stretching is appropriate for high-level performers because many of the motions of the activities in which they perform require ballistic movements. Nevertheless, it is recommended that ballistic stretch used as a training technique should be performed after initiating the workout with static or PNF stretch.

After the static stretching phase of the workout, the ballistic stretching phase should use stretches that closely approximate the performance activity. Examples of ballistic stretching exercises for specific performances are presented in Table 4.

Plyometrics A training technique used to develop explosive power. Referred to as "speed-strength training" in Eastern Europe and the former Soviet Union, where it originated, it consists of concentric isotonic contractions performed after a prestretch or eccentric contraction of a muscle.

Table 4

Table 4 Examples of Ballistic Stretch to Enhance Performance

Ballistic Stretch for Throwing and Striking

This exercise is to improve flexibility to aid one-handed throwing and striking skills (for example, racket sports forehand, backhand, and serve; baseball throw, or discus and shot put); and/or two-handed throwing or striking skills (for example, batting a softball or executing a golf drive or hammer throw). Assume a position at the end of the backswing for any skill listed above. Partner grasps hand(s) and resists movement while the performer turns the trunk away from the partner, making a series of gentle bouncing movements, attempting to rotate the trunk as if performing the skill. Alternate roles with the partner. Note: Avoid overstretching by too vigorous bouncing. If no partner is available, use a door frame for resistance, or these sports actions can be practiced using elastic bands or inner tubes (attached to fixed objects) as resistance.

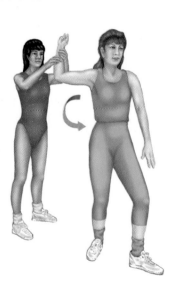

Ballistic Stretch for Golf Swing

This exercise is to improve flexibility for the golf swing. A similar exercise can be performed using one-handed throwing and striking skills (for example, racket sports forehand, backhand, and serve; baseball throw, or discus and shot put); and/or two-handed throwing or striking skills (for example, batting a softball or hammer throw). Stand and swing the club with or without a weight on the implement or on the wrist. Start by swinging backward and forward rhythmically and continuously. Gradually increase the speed and vigor of the swing to finally resemble the actual skill.

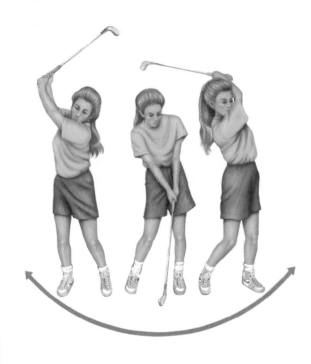

Training for High-Level Performance: Skill-Related Fitness and Skill

Many factors contribute to high-level performance. Possessing high levels of the six primary components of skill-related physical fitness (agility, coordination, balance, reaction time, speed, and power) make it easier to learn the skills important to high-level performance. However, other abilities also contribute to performing skills. For example, many experts consider various perceptual abilities such as depth and distance perception (ability to judge depth and distances accurately) and visual tracking (ability to visually follow a moving object) to be skill-related parts of physical fitness. Skill-related physical fitness is also called **motor fitness** or **sports fitness.**

 Technology Update

Advances in equipment technology can make the difference between winning and losing for highly elite athletes. Speed skaters in the recent 2002 winter Olympics in Salt Lake City used a new type of skate called klap skates (named for the sound it makes). The skates have a spring-loaded front hinge that allows the skater to raise their heel off of the blade while skating. Speed skaters also wear special skin-tight racing suits to reduce wind resistance. These recent advances in technology led to a number of record setting performances at the games. Advances in clothing were also evident among swimmers in the 2000 summer Olympic games. At these games, most swimmers were wearing "skinsuits" that have less resistance than skin when gliding through the water. Some suits are made of knitted lycra but the latest suits are made with woven lycra and are called paper suits because of the texture. Information about the latest in equipment technology can be found at the U.S. Olympic Center website **http://www.usoc.org/** or through various trade magazines that cover specific sports.

   Mechanical ergogenic aids such as those discussed here are likely to only be beneficial for highly trained competitive athletes. Other innovations in clothing and equipment, however, can make exercise safer and more enjoyable. "Wickable" fabrics (e.g., CoolMax) and waterproof fabrics (e.g., Gore-Tex) can help to keep you more comfortable while exercising in hard conditions. Therefore, stay abreast of these innovations.

There are sub-components of each component of skill-related physical fitness. Most of the six parts of skill-related physical fitness have sub-components. For example, coordination includes foot-eye coordination

and hand-eye coordination, which are measured quite differently. The tests in this concept measure some of the skill-related fitness aspects most important to sports performance.

   An individual might possess ability in one area and not in another. For this reason, general motor ability probably does not really exist, and individuals do not have one general capacity for performing. Rather, the ability to play games or sports is determined by combined abilities in each of the separate skill-related components. However, some performers will probably be above average in many areas.

Exceptional performers tend to be outstanding in more than one component of skill-related fitness. Though people possess skill-related fitness in varying degrees, great athletes are likely to be above average in most, if not all, aspects. Indeed, exceptional athletes must be exceptional in many areas of skill-related fitness. Different sports require different skills, each of which requires varying degrees of the six components of skill-related fitness.

Excellence in one skill-related fitness component may compensate for a lack in another. Each individual possesses a specific level of each skill-related fitness aspect. The performer should learn his or her other strengths and weaknesses in order to produce optimal performances. For example, a tennis player may use good coordination to compensate for lack of speed.

Excellence in skill-related fitness may compensate for a lack of health-related fitness when playing sports and games. As you grow older, health-related fitness potential declines more rapidly than many components of skill-related fitness. You may use superior skill-related fitness to compensate. For example, a baseball pitcher who lacks the strength and power to dominate hitters may rely on a pitch such as a knuckle ball, which is more dependent on coordination than on power.

Practice can help skill-related fitness but is probably not as effective as practice to improve the specific skills of the activity you expect to perform. As noted in a previous section, power is the component of fitness especially likely to be changed with training. Drills for enhancing other aspects of skill-related physical fitness can

Motor Fitness A term commonly used for skill-related physical fitness.

Sports Fitness A term commonly used for skill-related fitness.

help improve these abilities. For example, agility drills can improve scores on the specific agility drill that is practiced. Speed in running can be improved by increasing strength. However, experts generally agree that heredity highly influences skill-related fitness.

As illustrated in Figure 1, learning specific skills (not skill-related fitness) through regular practice is the preferred method of improving performance. To achieve high-level performance, lengthy practice of the appropriate kind is essential.

Hyperkinetic Conditions

Just as too little physical activity can result in health problems, too much can also contribute to illness and injury. Hypokinetic means too little physical activity. Conversely, hyperkinetic means too much. Just as reasonable amounts of physical activity can help reduce the risk of hypokinetic health problems, excessive exercise can lead to **hyperkinetic conditions** that have negative effects on health and wellness. High-level performance requires high-level training.

Many athletes push themselves too hard in their pursuit of high-level performance, not allowing adequate time for rest. This overtraining results in "overload" syndrome characterized by fatigue, irritability, and sleep problems, as well as one or more hyperkinetic conditions. Some types of common hyperkinetic conditions are presented in the sections that follow.

One type of hyperkinetic condition is musculoskeletal overuse injuries. Periodic rest is necessary to allow the body to recover from the stress of continuous and vigorous training. For example, runners who train seven days a week have more muscle and joint injuries than runners who take off at least one day a week or reduce training levels several days a week. The most common overuse injuries are joint injuries to the foot, ankle, and knee; stress fractures in the lower extremities; and muscle/connective tissue injuries such as shin splints, strained hamstring muscles, and calf pain. These injuries are apparent among exercisers who overdo it. For example, dance aerobics instructors are particularly likely to have overuse injuries. Tennis and baseball players often have similar problems, but their problems occur in different parts of the body (the arm and shoulder). The best way to prevent this type of hyperkinetic condition is periodic rest. Pain, the body's warning signal, is a good clue that the body needs rest.

Overtraining is a common hyperkinetic condition among serious athletes. Overtraining syndrome refers to "untreated overreaching that results in chronic decreases in performance and impaired ability to train."

Other health problems may be associated with the syndrome and may require medical attention. Those interested in training for high-level performance should be aware of the symptoms, causes, and treatments for the syndrome, as well as the methods of prevention. The key seems to be a well-conceived training program that does not "overreach." If you plan to begin training for high-level performance, you should seek more information about the overtraining syndrome (see suggested readings). Lab 14B will help you identify some of the symptoms of overtraining.

Compulsive physical activity is referred to as activity neurosis. People with activity neurosis become irrationally concerned about their exercise regimen. They may exercise more than one time a day, rarely take a day off, or feel the need to exercise even when ill or injured. Musculoskeletal overuse injuries are especially common among activity neurotics. The excessive desire to be active can also be the source of poor performance in other aspects of life, as well as a source of stress. Competitive athletes with this condition may have reduced performance, and among females, amenorrhea (no menstrual flow).

Anorexia nervosa can be considered as a hyperkinetic condition. Anorexia nervosa is an eating disorder associated with an obsessive desire to be lean. Evidence exists that many anorexics use compulsive exercise, as well as undereating, to keep body fat at low levels. For this reason, anorexia nervosa can often be considered a hyperkinetic condition. Recent data suggest that at least 25 percent of people with anorexia do compulsive exercise (see concept 15 for more information).

A recently defined type of hyperkinetic condition is body neurosis. Body neurosis is an obsessive concern for having an attractive body. Among females, it is associated with an extreme desire to be lean. In some cases, it can lead to anorexia. Among males, this condition is associated with an extreme desire to be muscular. Recent research indicates that increasing numbers of males are interested in leanness, and a number of females are now compulsive about muscle mass gains. People with body neurosis are often compulsive exercisers.

Ergogenic Aids

Many athletes look to ergogenic aids as an additional way to improve performance. Athletes are always looking for a competitive edge. In addition to pursuing rigorous training programs, many athletes look for alternative ways to improve their performance. Substances, strategies, or treatments that are designed to improve physical performance beyond the effects of normal training are collectively referred to as **ergogenic aids.** People interested in improving their appearance (including those with body neurosis) also abuse products they think will enhance their appearance. The types of ergogenic aids can be classified as mechanical, psychological, and physiological. Each category will be discussed in the subsequent sections.

Mechanical ergogenics (technology or equipment) may improve efficiency and performance. Most competitive activities require equipment or special clothing. New technology has produced better designs that improve mechanical efficiency. An example of mechanical ergogenics is the improved aerodynamics resulting from advances in bicycling clothing and equipment. Another example is the improved performance resulting from oversized, composite tennis racquets. These aids can help you enjoy an activity and may provide an advantage in competition.

Psychological ergogenics improve concentration and focus during competitive activities. Many competitive activities require extreme levels of concentration and focus. Athletes who are able to maintain this mental edge during an event are at a clear advantage over athletes who cannot. Psychological ergogenics are strategies such as mental imagery and hypnosis, which have been shown to help athletes achieve peak performance. Athletes are encouraged to use these psychological aids but to be wary of untested or unproven techniques since quackery is prominent in this area.

Physiological ergogenics are designed to improve performance by enhancing biochemical and physiological processes in the body. Physiological ergogenics refer primarily to nutritional supplements that are thought to have a positive effect on various metabolic processes. An example is fluid replacement drinks that athletes consume during endurance exercise. Consumption of these drinks has been shown to maintain blood sugar levels and delay fatigue in exercise lasting over one hour. While the ergogenic benefit of fluid replacement beverages is clearly established, the safety and effectiveness of most other supplements are questionable. Because the supplement industry is largely unregulated, many products are developed and marketed with little or no research to document their effects. These products prey on an athlete's lack of knowledge and concern over performance. Products with little or no evidence of benefits also have questionable safety so consumers should be cautious. Table 5 summarizes the potential effectiveness and safety issues of many commercially available supplements.

Strategies for Action

You can maximize your chances for success by selecting activities that match your abilities. Whether your goal is high-level performance or finding an activity that you can enjoy during your leisure time, your choice of activity is important. To give yourself the best chance of being successful, you should consider choosing an activity that matches your abilities. Assessing your skill-related physical fitness abilities can help you determine your areas of strength. In Lab 14A, you have the opportunity to assess your skill-related fitness and build a fitness profile. Using Table 6, you can determine the sports and activities that best match your individual abilities.

It should be noted that the assessments provided in Lab 14A are but a few of the many tests that can be done for each of the skill-related fitness parts. You may want to try other tests if you want more information about your abilities. If you have a personal desire to train for a specific sport or activity, but do not have a fitness profile that predicts success, you should not be deterred. Lab 14A will help you find an activity that you will enjoy and in which you have a good chance of success. People with good motivation, who persist in training, can often excel over others with greater ability. Lab 14B will provide an assessment of overtraining for individuals who may be pursuing some type of high-level training or competitive sport.

Hyperkinetic Conditions   Condition caused by too much physical activity and/or insufficient rest.

Ergogenic Aids   Substances, strategies, or treatments that are theoretically designed to improve performance in sports or competitive athletics.

Table 5 ▶ Effectiveness and Safety of Various Physiological Ergogenic Aids

Name of Supplement	Ergogenic Aids with Strong Evidence for a Performance Benefit	
	Proposed Effect (Claims)	Safe?
Alkaline salts (e.g., sodium bicarbonate, sodium citrate)	Buffer metabolic acidosis produced from lactic acid buildup	Yes
Caffeine	Increases rate of fat metabolism and sparing glycogen depletion	Yes, in moderation, can dehydrate
Carbohydrates (e.g., glucose, fructose)	Maintain blood glucose levels and delay glycogen depletion	Yes
Creatine	Muscular strength	Side effects include dehydration and cramps; long-term safety unknown
Water	Minimizes dehydration during endurance exercise in the heat	Yes

Name of Supplement	Ergogenic Aids with Some Evidence for a Performance Benefit	
	Proposed Effect (Claims)	Safe?
Aspartate salts (e.g., potassium, magnesium aspartate)	Mitigate the accumulation of ammonia during exercise	Probably safe
Carbohydrate metabolites (e.g., DHAP, pyruvate)	Maintain blood glucose levels and delay glycogen depletion	Probably safe
Glycerol	Promotes hyperhydration and improves thermoregulation during exercise in the heat	Probably safe
Phosphates	Phosphates are a component of 2,3-DPG, which is essential for the release of oxygen from hemoglobin	Not clear

Name of Supplement	Ergogenic Aids with Little or No Evidence for a Performance Benefit	
	Proposed Effect (Claims)	Safe?
Amino acids (general)	Alleged increase in muscle mass, prevents protein catabolism	Probably, unless consumed in extremely high doses
Amino acids (e.g., arginine, ornithine)	Alleged increase in strength by increasing levels of human growth hormone and insulin	Probably safe; however, extreme protein consumption is harmful
Androstenedione	Alleged hormone precursor to testosterone	Not established
L-carnitine	Allegedly facilitates the transport of fatty acids, and oxidation of amino acids and pyruvate, which delays glycogen depletion	Not established
Choline	Allegedly maintains acetylcholine levels during exercise; acetylcholine is thought to be related to onset of fatigue	Not established
Chysin	Allegedly prevents conversion of excess testosterone to estrogen, which would allow higher testosterone levels	Not established
Coenzyme Q10 (Ubiquinone)	Allegedly improves oxygen uptake in the mitochondria	Not established
Dehydroepiandrosterone	Alleged hormone precursor to testosterone	Not established
Hydroxy beta-methylbutyrate (HMB)	Allegedly a metabolite of leucine, thought to improve cellular repair of muscle	Not established
Inosine	A nucleic acid in DNA purported to increase energy production	Not established
Lipid metabolites (medium chain triglycerides)	Allegedly increases fat metabolism by increasing the availability of dietary fats in the circulation	Yes, if consumed as a part of diet
Protein metabolites (e.g., tryptophan and branched chain amino acids [BCA])	Alter the formation of serotonin, a neurotransmitter alleged to influence central nervous system fatigue	Yes, if consumed as a part of diet

Source: Williams, M. H.

Table 6 ▶ Skill-Related Requirements of Sports and Other Activities

Activity	Balance	Coordination	Reaction Time	Agility	Power	Speed
Archery	***	****	*	*	*	*
Backpacking	**	**	*	**	**	*
Badminton	**	****	***	***	**	***
Baseball/softball	***	****	****	***	****	***
Basketball	***	****	****	****	****	***
Bicycling	****	**	**	*	**	**
Bowling	***	****	*	**	**	**
Canoeing	***	***	**	*	***	*
Circuit training	**	**	*	**	***	**
Dance, aerobic	**	****	**	***	*	*
Dance, ballet	****	****	**	****	***	*
Dance, disco	**	***	**	****	*	**
Dance, modern	****	****	**	****	***	*
Dance, social	**	***	**	***	*	**
Fencing	***	****	****	***	***	****
Fitness calisthenics	**	**	*	***	***	*
Football	***	***	****	****	****	****
Golf (walking)	**	****	*	**	***	*
Gymnastics	****	****	***	****	****	**
Handball	**	****	***	****	***	***
Hiking	**	**	*	**	**	*
Horseback riding	***	***	**	***	*	*
Interval training	**	**	*	*	*	**
Jogging	**	**	*	*	*	*
Judo	***	****	****	****	****	****
Karate	***	****	****	****	****	****
Mountain climbing	****	****	**	***	***	*
Pool; billiards	**	***	*	**	**	*
Racquetball	**	****	***	****	**	***
Rope jumping	**	***	**	***	**	*
Rowing, crew	**	****	*	***	****	**
Sailing	***	***	***	***	***	*
Skating	****	***	**	***	**	***
Skiing, cross-country	**	****	*	***	****	**
Skiing, downhill	****	****	***	****	***	*
Soccer	**	****	***	****	***	***
Surfing	****	****	***	****	***	*
Swimming (laps)	**	***	*	***	**	*
Table tennis	**	***	***	**	**	**
Tennis	**	****	***	***	***	***
Volleyball	**	****	***	***	**	**
Walking	**	**	*	*	*	*
Waterskiing	***	***	*	***	**	*
Weight training	**	**	*	*	**	*

* = minimal needed; **** = a lot needed.

Web Resources

Gatorade Sports Science Institute **www.gssiweb.com**
National Athletic Trainers Association **www.nata.org**
National Collegiate Athletic Association **www.ncaa.org**
National Strength and Conditioning Association
  www.nsca-cc.org
Special Olympics International **www.specialolympics.org**
United States Olympic Committee **www.usoc.org**
Women's Sports Foundation
  www.womenssportsfoundation.org

Suggested Readings

 Additional reference materals for concept 14 are available at **www.mhhe.com/fit_well/web14 Click 08.**

ACSM. 1997. Position stand on the female athlete triad. *Medicine and Science in Sports and Exercise* 29(5):i.

Albert, C. M. et al. 2000. Triggering of sudden death from cardiac causes by vigorous exertion. *New England Journal of Medicine* 243(19):1355–1361.

Baechle, T. R., and R. W. Earle, (eds.). 2000. *Essentials of Strength Training and Conditioning.* 2nd ed. Champaign, IL: Human Kinetics.

Chu, D. A. 1998. *Jumping Into Plyometrics.* Champaign, IL: Human Kinetics.

Dufek, J. S. 2002. Exercise variability: A prescription for overuse injury prevention. *ACSM's Health and Fitness Journal* 6(4):18–23.

Hill, K. L. 2000. *Frameworks for Sports Psychologists: Enhancing Sports Performance.* Champaign, IL: Human Kinetics.

Kraus, D. 2000. *Mastering Your Inner Game.* Champaign, IL: Human Kinetics.

Manore, M., and J. Thompson. 2000. *Sport Nutrition for Health and Performance.* Champaign, IL: Human Kinetics.

Morgan, J. F. 2000. From Charles Atlas to Adonis Complex: Fat is more than a feminist issue. *Lancet* 356:1372–1373.

Nelson, T. F., and H. Wechsler. 2001. Alcohol and college athletes. *Medicine and Sciences in Sports and Exercise* 33(1):43–47.

Raglin, J., and A. Barzdukas. 1999. Overtraining in athletes: The challenge of prevention—A consensus statement. *ACSM's Health and Fitness Journal* 3(2):27–31.

USA Today. 15 April 2002. Dietary supplement use: Troubling side effects. *USA Today.*

Uusitalo, A. L. 2001. Overtraining. *The Physician and Sports Medicine* 29(5):35–50.

Williams, M. H. 1998. Nutritional ergogenics and sports performance. *PCPFS Research Digest* (10):1.

In the News

Sudden Death in Elite Athletes

Athletes are often held up as pillars of strength and fitness yet each year there are surprising accounts of elite athletes dying. The deaths of St. Louis Cardinal baseball player Daryl Kyle and the apparent heat-related death of Minnesota Vikings football lineman Corey Stringer are recent examples but other publicized cases include Hank Gathers, Len Bias, and Reggie Lewis. The majority of nontraumatic sports deaths are primarily cardiovascular in nature; however, 20 to 25 percent of these deaths are thought to be due to noncardiovascular causes, including heat-related illness, rhabdomyolysis in individuals with sickle cell trait, and drug-related deaths.

Data from the National Center for Catastrophic Sports Injury Research indicate that approximately sixteen nontraumatic sports deaths per year occur in organized high school and college athletics in the United States. When the participation rates were factored in, the estimated annual death rates were 7.5 and 1.3 deaths per million male and female athletes, respectively (death rates among pro athletes are probably similar but due to smaller numbers the events appear to be less common). Over the years, sudden death has occurred more among football and basketball players, but this has been attributed to the greater number of participants in these sports rather than an increased risk.

Athletes in competitive sports often undergo preparticipation physicals to screen for potential cardiac arrhythmias or conditions that may increase risk of sudden death. Unfortunately, recreational athletes may not take the same precaution. The best advice is to get a physical prior to beginning serious training. This is especially critical if there is a family history of heart problems. Also, refrain from using supplements containing ephedra or other stimulants as this has been implicated in some cases of sudden death.

Lab Resource Materials: Skill-Related Physical Fitness

Important Note: Because skill-related physical fitness does not relate to good health, the rating charts used in this section differ from those used for health-related fitness. The rating charts that follow can be used to compare your scores to those of other people. You *do not* need exceptional scores on skill-related fitness to be able to enjoy sports and other types of physical activity; however, it is necessary for high-level performance. After the age of thirty, you should adjust ratings by 1 percent per year.

Evaluating Skill-Related Physical Fitness

I. Evaluating agility: The Illinois agility run

An agility course using four chairs 10 feet apart, and a 30-foot running area will be set up as depicted in this illustration. The test is performed as follows:

1. Lie prone with your hands by your shoulders and your head at the starting line. On the signal to begin, get on your feet and run the course as fast as possible.
2. Your score is the time required to complete the course.

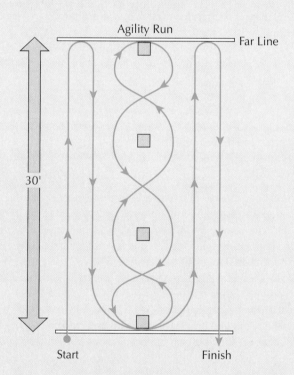

II. Evaluating balance: The Bass test of dynamic balance

Eleven circles (9 1/2 inch) are drawn on the floor as shown in the illustration. The test is performed as follows:

1. Stand on the right foot in circle X. *Leap* forward to circle 1, then circle 2 through 10, alternating feet with each leap.
2. The feet must leave the floor on each leap and the heel may not touch. Only the ball of the foot and toes may land on the floor.
3. Remain in each circle for five seconds before leaping to the next circle. (A count of five will be made for you aloud.)
4. Practice trials are allowed.
5. The score is 50, plus the number of seconds taken to complete the test, minus the number of errors.
6. For every error, deduct three points each. Errors include touching the heel, moving the supporting foot, touching outside a circle, or touching any body part to the floor other than the supporting foot.

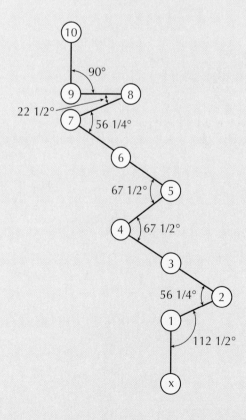

Chart 1 ► Agility Rating Scale

Classification	Men	Women
Excellent	15.8 or faster	17.4 or faster
Very good	16.7–15.9	18.6–17.5
Good	18.6–16.8	22.3–18.7
Fair	18.8–18.7	23.4–22.4
Poor	18.9 or slower	23.5 or slower

Source: Adams et al.

Chart 2 ▶ Balance Test Rating Scale

Rating	Score
Excellent	90–100
Very good	80–89
Good	60–79
Fair	30–59
Poor	0–29

III. Evaluating coordination: The stick test of coordination

The stick test of coordination requires you to juggle three wooden sticks. The sticks are used to perform a one-half flip and a full flip as shown in the illustrations.

1. *One-half flip*—Hold two 24-inch (one-half inch in diameter) dowel rods, one in each hand. Support a third rod of the same size across the other two. Toss the supported rod in the air so that it makes a half turn. Catch the thrown rod with the two held rods.
2. *Full flip*—Perform the preceding task, letting the supported rod turn a full flip.

The test is performed as follows:
1. Practice the half-flip and full flip several times before taking the test.
2. When you are ready, attempt a half-flip five times. Score one point for each successful attempt.
3. When you are ready, attempt the full flip five times. Score two points for each successful attempt.

Chart 3 ▶ Coordination Rating Scale

Classification	Men	Women
Excellent	14–15	13–15
Very good	11–13	10–12
Good	5–10	4–9
Fair	3–4	2–3
Poor	0–2	0–1

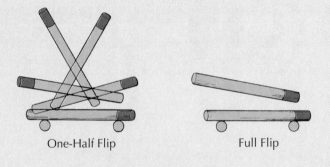

One-Half Flip   Full Flip

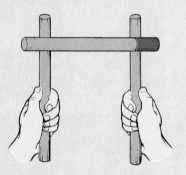

Hand Position

IV. Evaluating power: The vertical jump test

The test is performed as follows:

1. Hold a piece of chalk so its end is even with your fingertips.
2. Stand with both feet on the floor and your side to the wall and reach and mark as high as possible.
3. Jump upward with both feet as high as possible. Swing arms upward and make a chalk mark on a 5′ × 1′ wall chart marked off in half-inch horizontal lines placed 6 feet from the floor.
4. Measure the distance between the reaching height and the jumping height.
5. Your score is the best of three jumps.

Chart 4 ▶ Power Rating Scale		
Classification	**Men**	**Women**
Excellent	25 1/2″ or more	23 1/2″ or more
Very good	21″–25″	19″–23″
Good	16 1/2″–20 1/2″	14 1/2″–18 1/2″
Fair	12 1/2″–16″	10 1/2″–14″
Poor	12″ or less	10″ or less

Metric conversions for this chart appear in Appendix B.

V. Evaluating reaction time: The stick drop test

To perform the stick drop test of reaction time, you will need a yardstick, a table, a chair, and a partner to help with the test. To perform the test, follow these procedures:

1. Sit in the chair next to the table so that your elbow and lower arm rest on the table comfortably. The heel of your hand should rest on the table so that only your fingers and thumb extend beyond the edge of the table.
2. Your partner holds a yardstick at the top, allowing it to dangle between your thumb and fingers.
3. The yardstick should be held so that the 24-inch-mark is even with your thumb and index finger. No part of your hand should touch the yardstick.
4. Without warning, your partner will drop the stick, and you will catch it with your thumb and index finger.
5. Your score is the number of inches read on the yardstick just above the thumb and index finger after you catch the yardstick.
6. Try the test three times. Your partner should be careful not to drop the stick at predictable time intervals so that you cannot guess when it will be dropped. It is important that you react only to the dropping of the stick.
7. Use the middle of your three scores (for example: if your scores are 21, 18, and 19, your middle score is 19). The higher your score, the faster your reaction time.

Chart 5 ▶ Reaction Time Rating Scale	
Classification	**Score**
Excellent	More than 21″
Very good	19″–21″
Good	16″–18 3/4″
Fair	13″–15 3/4″
Poor	Below 13″

Metric conversions for this chart appear in Appendix B.

VI. Evaluating speed: Running test of speed

To perform the running test of speed, it will be necessary to have a specially marked running course, a stopwatch, a whistle, and a partner to help you with the test. To perform the test, follow this procedure:

1. Mark a running course on a hard surface so that there is a starting line and a series of nine additional lines, each 2 yards apart, the first marked at a distance 10 yards from the starting line.

2. From a distance 1 or 2 yards behind the starting line, begin to run as fast as you can. As you cross the starting line, your partner starts a stopwatch.

3. Run as fast as you can until you hear the whistle that your partner will blow exactly three seconds after the stopwatch is started. Your partner marks your location at the time when the whistle was blown.

4. Your score is the distance you were able to cover in three seconds. You may practice the test and take more than one trial if time allows. Use the better of your distances on the last two trials as your score.

Chart 6 ▶ Speed Rating Scale

Classification	Men	Women
Excellent	24–26 yards	22–26 yards
Very good	22–23 yards	20–21 yards
Good	18–21 yards	16–19 yards
Fair	16–17 yards	14–15 yards
Poor	Less than 16 yards	Less than 14 yards

Metric conversions for this chart appear in Appendix B.

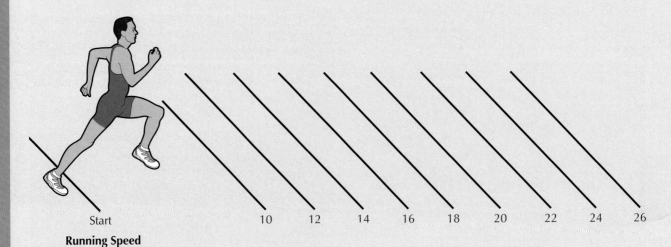

Start 10 12 14 16 18 20 22 24 26

Running Speed

Lab 14A: Evaluating Skill-Related Physical Fitness

Name	**Section**	**Date**

Purpose: To help you evaluate your own skill-related fitness, including agility, balance, coordination, power, speed, and reaction time. This information may be of value in helping decide which sports match your skill-related fitness abilities.

Procedure:

1. Read the direction for each of the skill-related fitness tests presented in the Lab Resource Materials.
2. Take as many of the tests as possible, given the time and equipment available.
3. Be sure to warm up before and to cool down after the tests.
4. It is all right to practice the tests before trying them. However, you should decide ahead of time which trial you will use to test your skill-related fitness.
5. After completing the tests, write your scores in the appropriate places in the Results section.
6. Determine your rating for each of the tests from the rating charts in the Lab Resource Materials.

Results:

Place a check in the circle for each of the tests you completed.

Agility (Illinois run)   ◯

Balance (Bass test)   ◯

Coordination (stick test)   ◯

Power (vertical jump)   ◯

Reaction time (stick drop test)   ◯

Speed (three-second run)   ◯

Record your score and rating in the following spaces.

	Score	Rating	
Agility			(Chart 1)
Balance			(Chart 2)
Coordination			(Chart 3)
Power			(Chart 4)
Reaction time			(Chart 5)
Speed			(Chart 6)

Conclusions and Implications: In two or three paragraphs, discuss the results of your skill-related fitness tests. Comment on the areas in which you did well or did not do well, the meaning of these findings, and the implications of the results with specific reference to the activities you will perform in the future.

Lab 14B: Identifying Symptoms of Overtraining

Name	Section	Date

Purpose: To help you identify symptoms associated with overtraining.

Procedures:

1. Answer the questions concerning overtraining syndrome in the Results section. If you are in training, rate yourself; if not, evaluate a person you know who is in training. As an alternative you may evaluate a person you know who was formerly in training (and who experienced symptoms) or evaluate yourself when you were in training (if you trained for performance in the past).
2. Use Chart 1 to rate the person (yourself or another person) who is (or was) in training.
3. Use Chart 2 to identify some steps that you might take to treat or prevent overtraining syndrome.
4. Answer the questions in the conclusions section.

Results:

Place a check in the circle by any of the overtraining symptoms you (or the person you are evaluating) experienced.

○ 1. Has performance decreased dramatically in the last week or two?

○ 2. Is there evidence of depression?

○ 3. Is there evidence of atypical anger?

○ 4. Is there evidence of atypical anxiety?

○ 5. Is there evidence of general fatigue that is not typical?

○ 6. Is there general lack of vigor or loss of energy?

○ 7. Have sleeping patterns changed (inability to sleep well)?

○ 8. Is there evidence of heaviness of the arms and/or legs?

○ 9. Is there evidence of loss of appetite?

○ 10. Is there a lack of interest in training?

Chart 1 ▶ Ratings for Overtraining Syndrome

Number of Yes Answers	Rating
9–10	Overtraining syndrome is very likely present. Seek help.
6–8	Person is at risk of overtraining syndrome if it is not already present. Seek help to prevent additional symptoms.
3–5	Some signs of overtraining syndrome are present. Consider methods of preventing further symptoms.
0–2	Overtraining syndrome is not present, but attention should be paid to the few symptoms that do exist.

Conclusions and Implications:

Chart 2 lists some of the steps that may be taken to help eliminate or prevent overtraining syndrome. Check the steps that you think would be (or would have been) most useful to the person you evaluated.

Chart 2 ▶ Steps for Treating or Preventing Overtraining Syndrome
◯ 1. Consider a break from training.
◯ 2. Taper the program to help reduce symptoms.
◯ 3. Seek help to redesign the training program.
◯ 4. Alter your diet.
◯ 5. Evaluate other stressors that may be producing symptoms.
◯ 6. Reset performance goals.
◯ 7. Talk to someone about problems.
◯ 8. Have a medical check-up to be sure there is no medical problem.
◯ 9. If you have a coach, consider a talk with him/her.
◯ 10. Add fluids to help prevent performance problems from dehydration.

Discuss overtraining syndrome in general. Elaborate on one or two of the steps in Chart 2 that you think would be (or would have been) most effective in treating or preventing overtraining syndrome for the person you evaluated.

Body Composition

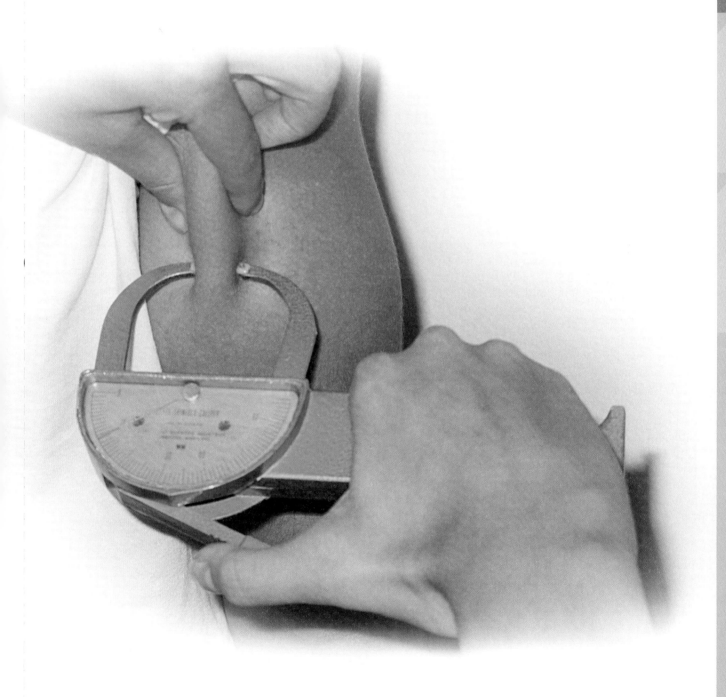

Possessing an optimal amount of body fat contributes to health and wellness.

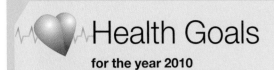

Health Goals

for the year 2010

- Increase the proportion of adults who are at a healthy weight.

- Reduce the proportion of adults who are obese.

- Reduce the proportion of children and adolescents who are overweight or obese.

B ody composition refers to the relative percentage of muscle, fat, bone, and other tissue of the body. Of primary concern, because of its association with various health problems, is body fatness. Being overfat or underfat can result in health concerns.

Despite general public awareness and concerns about weight control, the prevalence of obesity has continued to rise. Current estimates suggest that more than 60 percent of Americans are overweight and about 20 to 25 percent of these individuals also meet the criterion for obesity. A highly publicized article in *Journal of the American Medical Association (JAMA)* documented that the prevalence of obesity has increased by over 50 percent in the last decade, indicating that this is a relatively recent trend. Increases in obesity were evident for both sexes and the trends were also consistent across all ages, across different socioeconomic classes, and across all regions of the country. The fact that similar trends are occurring in nearly all industrialized countries in the world suggests that the "epidemic of obesity" should really be considered pandemic. The World Health Organization (WHO) recently concluded that "obesity's impact is so diverse and extreme that it should now be regarded as one of the greatest neglected public health problems of our time with an impact on health which may well prove to be as great as that of smoking." Since eating disorders such as anorexia nervosa and bulimia are also a significant health concern, especially among teens, the national goal is to keep the percentage of overfat teens from increasing while at the same time reducing the incidence of those who have too little fat associated with eating disorders.

Understanding and Interpreting Body Composition Measures

There are standards that have been established to determine how much body fat an individual should possess. www.com/fit_well/web15 Click 01. Every person should possess at least a minimal amount of fat **(percent body fat)** for good health. This fat is called **essential fat** and is necessary for temperature regulation, shock absorption, and regulation of essential body nutrients, including vitamins A, D, E, and K. The exact amount of fat considered essential to normal body functioning has been debated, but most experts agree that males should possess no less than 5 percent and females no less than 10 percent. For females, an exceptionally low body fat percentage **(underfat)** is especially of concern. **Amenorrhea** may occur among women at fat levels of higher than 10 percent and sometimes at 11 to 16 percent. (11 to 16 percent for many women). Some people feel that amenorrhea, when associated with low body fat levels, is a reversible condition that is merely the body's method of preventing pregnancy. However, low body fat levels, accompanied by amenorrhea, places a woman at risk of bone loss (osteoporosis). A body fat level below 10 percent is one of the criteria often used by clinicians for diagnosing eating disorders such as anorexia nervosa.

Close inspection of Table 1 reveals an overlap between essential fat, borderline, and high-performance classifications for body fatness. As noted previously, essential fat levels are those necessary for normal body functioning. Because individuals differ in their response to low fatness, a borderline range is provided. No particular health benefits appear to be associated with being in the borderline range, and for some people there are health risks. Even

Table 1 ▶ Standards for Body Fatness (Percent Body Fat)

Classification	Males	Females
Essential fat	No less than 5%	No less than 10%
Borderline	5%–9%	10%–16%
High performance	5%–15%	10%–23%
Good fitness (healthy)	10%–20%	17%–28%
Marginal	21%–25%	29%–35%
Overfat	25%+	35%+

though low body fat levels (borderline range) are not generally recommended, some individuals are interested in high-level performance and seek low body fatness in an attempt to enhance performance. Standards for high-level performers are typically lower than for normally active people primarily interested in good health. Performance levels considered to be in the borderline area for nonperformers can be acceptable if the performer eats well, avoids overtraining, and practices a healthy lifestyle. If symptoms such as amenorrhea, bone loss, and frequent injury occur, then levels of body fatness should be reconsidered, as should training techniques and eating patterns. For many people in training, maintaining performance levels of body fatness is temporary, thus the risk of long-term health problems is diminished.

Nonessential fat is fat above essential fat levels that accumulates when you take in more calories than you expend. When nonessential fat accumulates in excessive amounts, **overfatness** or even **obesity** can occur. Just as the percent of body fat should not drop too low, it should not get too high either. A desirable range of fatness is associated with good metabolic fitness, good health, and wellness. It is referred to as the good fitness or healthy fatness range. People with more than healthy fat levels but who are not considered obese have scores in the marginal zone. While reaching the healthy fitness zone is desirable, it will be harder to reach for some people. Most experts agree that fat levels in the marginal zone are healthier than those in the overfatness zone.

The location of body fat can influence the health risks associated with obesity. Studies have shown that upper body fat poses a greater health risk than lower body fatness. For this reason, it is important to keep both your total and abdominal fat levels low, especially as you grow older. A useful indicator of fat distribution is the waist-to-hip circumference ratio. A high ratio between the waist and hip has been shown to be correlated with a high incidence of heart attack, stroke, chest pain, breast cancer, and death. Recent evidence indicates that people who exercise regularly accumulate less fat in the upper central regions of the body as they get older. This suggests that regular physical activity throughout life will result in a smaller waist-to-hip ratio and a reduced risk of various lifestyle diseases.

Body composition is considered a component of health-related fitness but can also be considered a component of metabolic fitness. Body composition is generally considered to be a health-related component of physical fitness. Most national fitness tests include either a skinfold test or the **body mass index (BMI)** as an indicator of this component. Like the other parts of health-related physical fitness, body composition is related to good health. However, body composition is unlike the other parts of health-related physical fitness in that it is not a performance measure. Cardiovascular fitness,

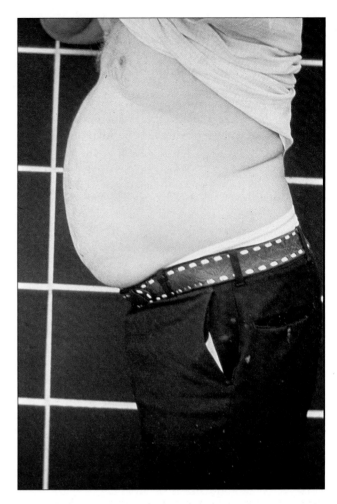

Abdominal fat is associated with increased disease risk.

Percent Body Fat The percentage of total body weight that is composed of fat.

Essential Fat The minimum amount of fat in the body necessary to maintain healthful living.

Underfat Too little of the body weight composed of fat (see Table 1).

Amenorrhea Absence of, or infrequent, menstruation.

Nonessential Fat Extra fat or fat reserves stored in the body.

Overfat Too much of the body weight composed of fat (see Table 1).

Obesity Extreme overfatness.

Body Mass Index (BMI) A measure of body composition using a height-weight formula. High BMI values have been related to increased disease risk.

strength, muscular endurance, and flexibility can be assessed using some type of movement or performance such as running, lifting, or stretching. Body composition requires no movement or performance. This is one reason why some experts prefer to consider body composition as a component of metabolic fitness.

Metabolic fitness includes other nonperformance measures associated with increased risk of health problems, such as high blood fat, high blood pressure, and high blood sugar levels. Some experts have hypothesized that metabolic fitness is really one syndrome characterized by body composition (body fat) and the other highly related nonperformance measures described earlier. Whether you consider body composition to be a part of health-related or metabolic fitness, it is an important health-related factor.

Assessing body weight too frequently can result in making false assumptions about body composition changes. Taking body weight measurements too frequently can provide incorrect information and lead to false assumptions. For example, people vary in body weight from day to day and even hour to hour based solely on their level of hydration. Short-term changes in weight are often due to water loss or gain, yet many people attribute the weight changes to their diet, a pill they have taken, or the exercise they are doing. In fact, short-term weight changes are more likely water changes than real body composition changes. We know this to be true because it takes a relatively long period of time for diet or exercise to affect weight changes. Monitoring your weight less frequently, once a week for example, is more useful than daily or multiple daily measures because it is more likely to represent real changes in body composition. Weighing at the same time of day, preferably early in the morning, is best because it reduces the chances that your weight variation will be a result of body water changes. Of course, it is best to use body composition assessments in addition to those based on body weight if accurate evaluations are expected.

Decisions about body composition should be based on more than one measurement. In Lab 15A, you will have the opportunity to do several different measurements of body composition. Using only one of the methods may result in misinformation and unrealistic goals, which is why it is wise to use several techniques when making decisions about personal body composition goals. As you read about the various ways to assess body composition, consider the strengths and weaknesses of each technique and learn to use the techniques that provide the most information to you personally.

Being overfat is more important than overweight in making decisions about health and wellness. Many of the measures described in the following

sections of this concept are indicators of the amount of body fat a person possesses. Others focus primarily on body weight. People who do regular physical activity and possess a large muscle mass can be high in body weight without being too fat. This is one of the limitations of measures based primarily on weight. Also, weight measures vary greatly based on your state of hydration or dehydration. You can lose weight merely by losing body water (becoming dehydrated) or gain weight by gaining body water (becoming hydrated). For this reason, measures that use weight as the primary indicator of body composition should be viewed with caution.

Methods Used to Assess Body Composition

Methods of body composition vary by accuracy and practicality. www.mhhe.com/fit_well/web15 Click 02. Underwater weighing, also referred to as hydrostatic weighing, is a laboratory procedure for assessing body composition. In this procedure, a person is weighed underwater and out of the water. Corrections are made for the amount of air in the lungs when the underwater weight is measured. Using Archimedes' principle, the body's density can be determined. Because the density of various body tissues is known, the amount of the total body fat can be determined. Body fatness is usually expressed in terms of a percentage of the total body weight. Underwater weighing was considered the best method, but dual-energy X-ray absorptiometry (DXA) has now become the accepted "gold standard" for body composition measurements. This technique is only available in research laboratories or medical centers but it may lead to changes in the accuracy with which other measures can estimate body fatness. (See Technology Update.)

Other more commonly used methods for measuring body fatness include skinfold measurements, bioelectric impedance, body circumferences, near-infrared interactance, and BMI. Table 2 provides a summary of the effectiveness of these methods. The procedures vary in terms of practicality and accuracy so it is important to understand the limitations of each method.

A variety of other technologies have been developed to assess body composition. Different types of X-rays and magnetic resonance machines (including DXA) have been used to assess body fatness in specific regions of the body for clinical research. Another relatively new device called the Bod Pod, uses air displacement (rather than water displacement as in underwater weighing) to assess body composition. Evidence suggests that it provides an acceptable alternative to underwater weighing and is particularly useful for special populations (obese, older people, and the physically challenged).

Table 2 ► Ratings of the Validity and Objectivity of Body Composition Methods

Method	Precise	Objective	Accurate	Valid Equations	Overall Rating
Skinfold measurement	4.0	3.5	3.5	3.5	3.5
Bioelectric impedance	4.0	4.0	3.5	3.5	3.5
Circumferences	4.0	4.0	3.0	3.0	3.0
Near-infrared interactance	5.0	4.5	2.0	2.0	2.5
Body mass index (BMI)	5.0	5.0	1.5	1.5	2.0

Precise: Can the same person get the same results time after time?

Accurate: Do values compare favorably to underwater weighing?

5 = excellent; 4 = very good; 3 = good; 2 = fair; 1 = unacceptable.

Adapted from Lohman, T. G., Houtkooper, L. H., and Going, S. B.

Objective: Can two different people get the same results consistently?

Valid: Is the formula accurate for predicting fat from measurements?

Technology Update

Dual-energy X-ray absorptiometry (DXA) has emerged in recent years as the most accepted criterion measure of body composition. The technique utilizes the attenuation of two energy sources in order to estimate the density of the body. A specific advantage of DXA is that it can provide whole body measurements of body fatness as well as amounts stored in different parts of the body. For the procedure, the person lies on a table and the machine scans up along the body. While some radiation exposure is necessary with the procedure, it is quite minimal compared with X-ray and other diagnostic scans. Because the machine is quite expensive, this procedure is only found in medical centers and well-equipped research laboratories. Still, the use of this procedure as a gold standard can indirectly improve the accuracy of other measures such as skinfold or bioelectric impedence since these measures rely on comparisons with a criterion measure in order to provide estimates of body fatness.

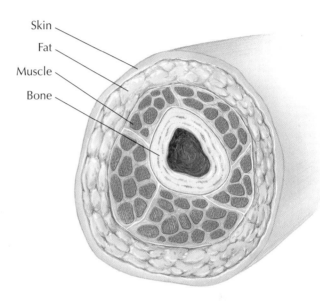

Figure 1 ► Location of body fat.

 Skinfold measurements are a preferred, practical method of assessing body fatness. www.mhhe.com/fit_well/web15 Click 03. Body fat is distributed throughout the body. About one-half of the body's fat is located around the various body organs and in the muscles. The other half of the body's fat is located just under the skin, or in skinfolds (Figure 1). A skinfold is two thicknesses of skin and the amount of fat that lies just under the skin. By measuring skinfold thicknesses of various sites around the body it is possible to estimate total body fatness (Figure 2). Skinfold measurements are often used because they are relatively easy to do. They are not nearly as costly as underwater weighing and other methods that require

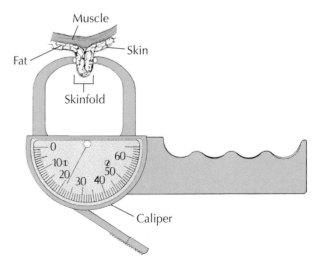

Figure 2 ► Measuring skinfold thickness.

expensive equipment. A set of calipers is used to make the measurements. The better, more accurate calipers cost several hundred dollars. However, considerably less expensive calipers are now available.

In general, the more skinfolds measured, the more accurate the body fatness estimate. However, measurements with two or three skinfolds have been shown to be reasonably accurate and can be done in a relatively short period. Two skinfold techniques are used in Lab 15A. You are encouraged to try both. With adequate training, most anyone can learn to use calipers to get a good estimate of fatness. When performed by a trained person, skinfold techniques are rated favorably by experts (see Table 2), but it is a skill that takes practice. Measurements made by an untrained person can be inaccurate.

Body circumference measures can be used to assess body fatness. Body circumference, or girth measurements, can be used to estimate body fatness using various weight, height, waist, thigh, hip, and other girth measurements. They are not rated as favorably as skinfold measurements (see Table 2), but they are easy to do. One weakness of circumference measures is they may misclassify people who have a large muscle mass. For this reason, they are not as useful as skinfold measures for active people who have a relatively large muscle mass compared to inactive people. As the sole measure of fatness, they should be used with caution. They can provide a useful second or third source of information about body fatness, however. Another technique that uses body circumferences—the waist-to-hip ratio—will be discussed in a later section.

Bioelectric impedance analysis has become a practical alternative for body fatness assessment. www.mhhe.com/fit_well/web15 **Click 04.** Bioelectric impedance analysis ranks quite favorably for accuracy and has similar overall

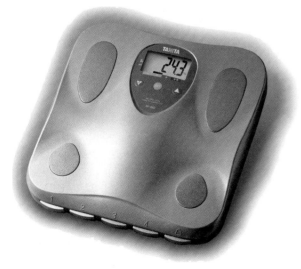

Bioelectric Impedance Scale.

rankings to skinfold measurement techniques. The test can be performed quickly and is more effective for people high in body fatness (a limitation of skinfolds). The technique is based on measuring resistance to current flow. Electrodes are placed on the body and low doses of current are passed through the skin. Because muscle has greater water content than fat, it is a better conductor and has less resistance to current. The overall amount of resistance and body size are used to predict body fatness. Dehydration can bias the result and it is also critical to not have measures taken within three to four hours after a meal. Accurate measures require the use of high quality equipment but some commercially available "scales" now provide estimates of body fatness that are based on the same principles. Instead of electrodes, you simply stand on metal plates that measure the current flow.

Infrared sensors are sometimes used to assess body fatness. Near-infrared interactance machines use the absorption of light to estimate body fatness. The technique was originally developed to measure the fat content of meats. Commercially available units for humans have not been shown to be effective for estimating body fat.

The BMI is considered to be a better measure than height and weight charts, but it has its limitations. www.mhhe.com/fit_well/web15 **Click 05.** Individuals who are interested in controlling their weight often consult height and weight tables to determine their "desirable" weight. Being 20 percent or more above the recommended table weight is one commonly used indicator of obesity. New tables adopted by the federal government are based on relative risk of health problems rather than normative comparisons to other people. A limitation of height and weight tables is that they do not take into account a person's degree of body fatness. A person who has a large muscle mass as a result of regular physical activity could appear to be **overweight** using a height and weight table and still not be too fat. A more accurate way to use height and weight is with the body mass index. BMI is calculated using a special formula and has a higher correlation with true body fatness than weights determined from height-weight tables. Nevertheless, the BMI may misclassify active people who have a large muscle mass. You can calculate your BMI using the procedures described in the Lab Resource Materials. After much debate, there has been some consensus regarding standards of overweight and obesity based on BMI values. The accepted international standards used by the United States and the WHO is a BMI > 25 for overweight and a BMI > 30 for obesity.

Consensus regarding the definition of these body composition categories now makes it easier to examine trends within the United States or to compare body composition levels and research results across countries. For example, BMI is the measure that public health officials have used to determine that over half of the U.S. population is either overweight or obese and to document increases in the past 10 years. Nearly all other developed countries are observing similar trends in the prevalence of obesity.

While the BMI is a useful indicator for large-scale research applications or to examine differences in groups, it is less valuable for making measurements for one specific individual at one particular point in time. Because the BMI is widely cited in news reports, it is important for all people to know how to calculate it and how to use it properly. Plotting changes in BMI over time can be useful in tracking personal changes. Together with other techniques, the BMI can provide useful information, but the risk of misclassification is high among active people with a high amount of muscle if the BMI is used by itself.

Health Risks Associated with Overfatness

Obesity has recently been elevated from a secondary to a primary risk factor for heart disease. Prior to 1998, obesity was considered to be a secondary risk factor for heart disease. The reason for this was that the effects of obesity were thought to be mediated by other risk factors such as blood pressure and blood lipids. Because of the mounting evidence of the relationship of obesity to health risk, especially risk of heart disease, the American Heart Association classifies obesity as a primary risk factor along with high blood lipids, high blood pressure, tobacco use, and sedentary living.

Physical fitness provides protection from health risks of obesity. www.mhhe.com/fit_well/ **web15 Click 06.** Recent research suggests that people who are above normal standards for BMI are not especially at risk if they participate in regular physical activity and possess relatively high levels of cardiovascular fitness (see Figure 3). In fact, active people who have a high BMI are at less risk than inactive people with normal BMI levels. Even high levels of body fatness may not be especially likely to increase disease risk if a person has good metabolic fitness as indicated by healthy blood fat levels, normal blood pressure, and normal blood sugar levels. It is when several of these factors are present at the same time that risk levels increase dramatically. For this reason, it is important to consider your cardiovascular and metabolic fitness levels before drawing conclusions about the effects of high body weight or high body fat levels on health and wellness. This information also points out the importance of periodically assessing your cardiovascular and metabolic fitness levels.

Overfatness or obesity can contribute to degenerative diseases, health problems, and even shortened life. Some diseases and health problems are

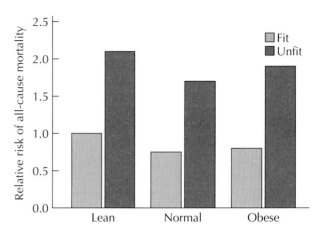

Figure 3 ▶ Risks of fatness vs. fitness.
Source: Wei M. et al.

associated with overfatness and obesity. In addition to the higher incidence of certain diseases and health problems, evidence shows people who are moderately overfat have a 40 percent higher than normal risk of shortening their lifespan. More severe obesity results in a 70 percent higher than normal death rate. This is evidenced by the exorbitant life insurance premiums paid by obese individuals.

Heart disease is not the only disease that is associated with obesity. Diabetes is another leading killer that is associated with all components of metabolic fitness including obesity. The incidence of diagnosis of this disease has increased sixfold in the last 40 years. Recent studies also indicate a significant increase in risk of breast cancer among the obese. High blood pressure and asthma are examples of other conditions associated with obesity.

Statistics indicate that underweight people also have a higher than normal risk of premature death. Though adequate evidence shows extreme leanness can be life threatening (e.g., anorexia nervosa), many underweight people included in these studies have lost weight because of a medical condition such as cancer. It appears that the medical problems are often the reason for low body weight rather than low body weight being the source of the medical problem. Most experts agree that people who are free from disease and who have lower than average amounts of body fat have a lower than average risk of premature death.

Excessive abdominal fat and excessive fatness of the upper body can increase the risk of various diseases. As noted earlier, research studies have shown that a relationship exists between the amount of abdominal fat and various health problems. Fat in the upper part of the body is sometimes called "Northern hemisphere"

Overweight Weight in excess of normal; not harmful unless it is accompanied by overfatness.

fat and is considered more risky than "Southern hemisphere" fat, such as in the hips and upper legs. People who have abdominal fatness are sometimes considered to have the "apple" fat pattern, while people with lower body fatness levels are considered to have the "pear" fat pattern. Regardless of the name used, it is clear that people who distribute fat around their middle as opposed to in the limbs are at greater risk of various health problems. The waist-to-hip ratio described in the previous section provides a means of assessing central body fatness. In general, men have higher waist-to-hip ratio than women and postmenopausal women have higher ratios than premenopausal women. As you grow older, you must monitor your waist-to-hip ratio.

Health Risks Associated with Excessively Low Body Fatness

Excessive desire to be thin or low in body weight can result in health problems. In Western society, the near obsession with thinness has been, at least in part, responsible for health conditions referred to as eating disorders. Eating disorders, or altered eating habits, involve extreme restriction of food intake and/or regurgitation of food to avoid digestion. The most common disorders are anorexia nervosa, bulimia, and anorexia athletica. All of these disorders are most common among highly achievement-oriented girls and young women, although they affect virtually all segments of the population.

Anorexia nervosa is the most severe eating disorder. If untreated, it is life-threatening. Anorexics restrict food intake so severely that their bodies become emaciated. Among the many characteristics of *anorexia nervosa* are fear of maturity and inaccurate body image. The anorexic starves herself/himself and may exercise compulsively or use laxatives to prevent the digestion of food in an attempt to attain excessive leanness. The anorexic's self-image is one of being too fat even when the person is too lean for good health. Assessing body fatness using procedures such as skinfolds and observation of the eating habits may help identify people with anorexia. Among anorexic girls and women, development of an adult figure is often feared. People with this disorder must obtain medical and psychological help immediately, as the consequences are severe. People with anorexia may also have some of the characteristics of the person with bulimia. About 25 percent of those with anorexia do compulsive exercise in attempt to stay lean.

Bulimia is a common eating disorder characterized by bingeing and purging. Disordered eating patterns become habitual for many people with *bulimia*. They alternate between bingeing and purging. Bingeing means the periodic eating of large amounts of food at one time. A binge might occur after a relatively long period of dieting and often consists of junk foods containing empty calories. After a binge, the bulimic purges the body of the food by forced regurgitation or the use of laxatives. Another form of bulimia is bingeing on one day and starving on the next. The consequences of bulimia are not as severe as anorexia, but can result in serious mental, gastrointestinal, and dental problems. Bulimics may or may not be anorexic. It may not be possible to use measures of body fatness to identify bulimia, as the bulimic may be lean, normal, or excessively fat.

Anorexia athletica is a recently identified eating disorder that appears to be related to participation in sports and activities that emphasize body leanness. *Anorexia athletica* is a recently identified eating disorder that appears to be related to participation in sports and activities, such as ballet, that emphasize excessive body leanness. Studies show that participants in sports such as gymnastics, wrestling, body building, and activities such as ballet and cheerleading are most likely to develop anorexia athletica. This disorder has many of the symptoms of anorexia nervosa, but not of the same severity. In some cases, anorexia athletica can lead to anorexia nervosa.

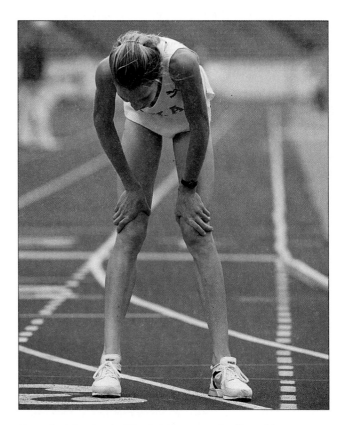

Excessively low levels of body fatness pose health problems.

Female athlete triad is an increasingly common condition among female athletes. *Female athlete triad* is an increasingly common condition among female athletes. The three health concerns (the triad) that characterize the condition are eating disorders, amenorrhea, and osteoporosis. The disordered eating patterns may be extreme as in anorexia or bulimia, or less severe as evidenced by poor eating habits. Because they are athletes, females with this condition are very active. Together, the poor eating habits and high levels of activity typically result in low body fat levels. The triad of symptoms is often accompanied by considerable pressure to perform well, resulting in high stress levels. In addition to the triad of symptoms, the combination of poor eating, overexercise, and competitive stress can result in other problems, such as depression and anxiety, and even risk of suicide. Many female athletes train extensively and have relatively low body fat levels but experience none of the symptoms of the triad. Eating well, training properly, using stress-management techniques, and monitoring health symptoms are the keys to their success. (See In the News.)

Fear of obesity is a less severe condition but it can still have negative health consequences. *Fear of obesity* is a less severe condition, but it can still have negative health consequences. This condition is most common among achievement-oriented teenagers who impose a self-restriction on caloric intake because they fear obesity. Consequences include stunting of growth, delayed puberty, delayed sexual development, and decreased physical attractiveness. It is important to avoid excessive eating and inactivity to prevent the problems associated with overfatness and obesity; however, an excessive concern for leanness can also result in serious health problems.

Society can help reduce the incidence of the problems associated with disordered eating and desire to be thin by changing its image of attractiveness, especially among young women. Many of the models and movie stars who convey the "ideal" image are anorexic or are exceptionally thin. Teachers and athletic coaches can help by educating people about these disorders, by not placing too much emphasis on leanness, and by screening students for extreme leanness using procedures such as skinfolds and body mass index. Parents and friends can help by looking for excessive changes in body weight and lack of eating. Once an eating disorder is identified, it is important to help the individual obtain treatment for the problem. While regular physical activity is good, excessive activity can be harmful. It is important to help athletes learn not to overdo it and to keep competition in perspective so that it does not become excessively stressful.

Conflicting news reports should not deter efforts to maintain a healthy body fat level. One recent headline said "Excess pounds deadly." One week later the headline read "It may be better to be a little fat." Adding to the confusion is that BMI standards have been lowered in recent years so that more people are now classified as overweight using this measurement technique. At the same time, some of the standards for body fatness are now more lenient than they were in the past. In both cases, the changes are made based on new scientific evidence.

Sometimes people read conflicting headlines and adopt a defeatist attitude. Do not let one headline influence your overall plan of fat control. The debate will continue in the years ahead as to just how much you should weigh or how much fat you should have for your good health and wellness. In the meantime, the message is clear. If possible, make several different assessments and consider all of the results before making decisions (see charts in Lab Resource Materials). For some people, meeting the standards described in this book may be difficult. It is far better to be close to the standard than to say "I can't meet the standard, so I won't even try." Some experts feel that many people are overfat because they have repeatedly failed to meet unrealistic body fatness or weight goals. Adopting a realistic personal standard of fatness is very important. Using many different self-assessments and adopting realistic goals based on personal information rather than comparisons to others can help you make informed decisions about your body composition.

The Origin of Fatness

Heredity plays a role in fatness. Some people have suggested that every individual is born with a predetermined weight (sometimes called your set-point). This implies that you have little control over your weight or body fat levels. In fact, you do have considerable control over your weight and level of fatness as evidenced by the fact that calories taken in (diet) and calories expended (activity) are the two most important factors associated with fat control. Nevertheless, research suggests that people are born with a predisposition toward fatness or leanness. For years, some scholars have suggested that your body type, or **somatotype,** is inherited. Clearly, some people will have more difficulty than others controlling fatness because of their body types and because they come from families with a history of obesity. In fact, recent research by a well-respected team of scholars indicates the body has a "natural" fatness range, which is influenced by heredity. If you deviate more than 10 to 15 percent from this range, your body may actually alter its metabolism in an attempt to maintain

Somatotype Inherent body build: ectomorph (thin), mesomorph (muscular), and endomorph (fat).

your "natural" fatness level. But even these changes are temporary. If you continue the behavior that caused the weight gain (eating more or exercising less), after a period of time your body accepts your new weight as your "natural" level. Scientists caution people not to overgeneralize the importance of heredity to body fatness. Such overgeneralizations could lead to incorrect conclusions about regulation of body fat levels.

Recently the "ob-gene" (or gene responsible for obesity) was discovered. It is true that this is an important scientific discovery, but it is unlikely that it will result in a cure for overfatness in the near future. In the meantime, more conventional methods of fat control must be used. Even if you come from a family with a history of obesity, you should not conclude that nothing can be done to prevent obesity. Virtually all people have a natural fatness level below obese levels. Those with a predisposition to high fatness will have a harder time having a low body fat level, but with healthy lifestyles, even these people can maintain body fat levels within normal ranges. Research shows that regular physical activity is especially effective in the control of genetically determined predispositions to fatness.

Glandular disorders are not a cause of overfatness for most people. Glandular disorders can cause or contribute to overfatness. For example, thyroid problems can cause a low metabolic rate that results in fat gain. However, most experts suggest that only 1 to 2 percent of all

overfatness is directly caused by problems of this type. Medical treatment is necessary for people suffering from these problems.

Fatness early in life leads to adult fatness. Research studies have documented that body composition levels tend to track through the life span. While there are exceptions, individuals that are overweight or obese as children are more likely to be overweight or obese as adults. One explanation for this is that overfatness in children causes the body to produce more fat cells. Since adults can only increase or decrease the size of existing fat cells, the number of fat cells becomes an important factor influencing body fat levels.

Maintaining healthy levels of body fat is an important objective for children and adults. It was previously thought that only adult obesity was related to health problems but it is now apparent that teens who are overfat are at a greater risk of heart problems and cancer than leaner peers. Obese children have been found to have symptoms of "adult-onset diabetes" indicating that the effects of obesity can impair health even for young people.

Changes in basal metabolic rate can be the cause of obesity. The amount of energy you expend each day must be balanced by your energy intake if you are to maintain your body fat and body weight over time (see Figure 4). Your energy intake is determined by the calories you eat. Expenditure is determined by a combination

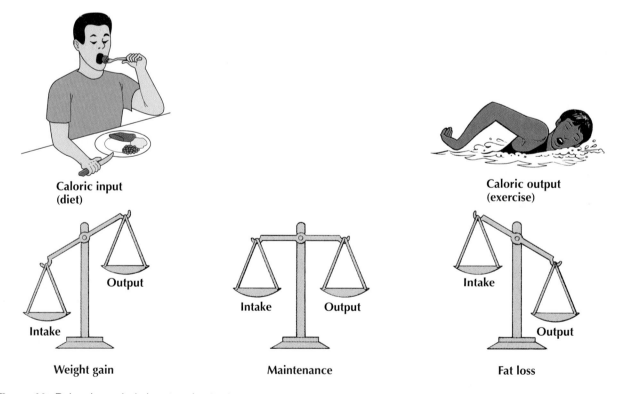

Figure 4 ▶ Balancing caloric input and output.

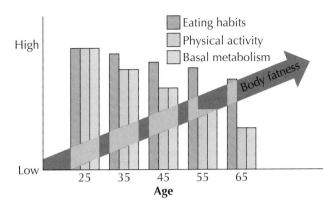

Figure 5 ▶ The creeping obesity.

of several factors. You expend calories just to exist even when you are inactive. Your **basal metabolic rate (BMR)** is the indicator or your energy expenditure when your are totally inactive. You also expend calories digesting food and, of course, in the activities of daily living.

BMR is highest during the growing years. The amount of food eaten increases to support this increased energy expenditure. When growing ceases, if eating does not decrease or activity level increase, fatness can result. Basal metabolism also decreases gradually as you grow older. One major reason for this is the loss of muscle mass associated with inactivity. Regular physical activity throughout life helps keep the muscle mass higher, resulting in a higher BMR. Recent evidence suggests that regular exercise can contribute in other ways to increased BMR. The higher BMR of active people helps them prevent overfatness, particularly in later life.

"Creeping obesity" is a problem as you grow older. People become less active and their BMR gradually decreases with age. Caloric intake does seem to decrease somewhat with age, but the decrease does not adequately compensate for the decreases in BMR and activity levels. For this reason, body fat increases gradually for the typical person with age (see Figure 5). This increase in fatness over time is commonly referred to as "creeping obesity" because the increase in fatness is gradual. For a typical person, creeping obesity could result in a gain of one-half to one pound per year. People who stay active can keep muscle mass high and delay changes in BMR. For those who are not active, it is suggested that caloric intake should decrease by 3 percent each decade after twenty-five so that by age sixty-five, caloric intake is at least 10 percent less than it was at age twenty-five. The decrease in caloric intake for active people need not be as great.

Excess caloric intake results in an increase in fat cell size. Overfatness can result in an increase in the number of fat cells among children. For adults, overfatness

is a result of the increase in size of fat cells (hypertrophy). When fat cells become excessively large, they can cause dimples or lumps under the skin. Some people refer to these large fat cells as cellulite. Quacks say that this type of fat is different from other types of fat and is removed from the body in different ways than regular fat. This is not true. All fatness among adults is a result of enlarged fat cells. All fat is lost as a result of reduction in fat cell size.

The Relationship Among Diet, Physical Activity, and Fatness

A combination of regular physical activity and dietary restriction is the most effective means of losing body fat. Studies indicate that regular physical activity combined with dietary restriction is the most effective method of losing fat. One study of adult women indicated that diet alone resulted in loss of weight, but much of this loss was lean body tissue. Those who were dieting as well as exercising experienced similar weight losses, but this loss included more body fat. For optimal results, all weight loss programs should combine a lower caloric intake with a good physical exercise program (see Figure 5). Thresholds of training and target zones for body fat reduction, including information for both physical activity and **diet** are presented in Table 3.

Good physical activity and diet habits can be useful in maintaining desirable body composition. Table 3 illustrates how fat can be lost through regular physical activity and proper dieting. However, not all people want to lose fat. For those who wish to maintain their current body composition, a **caloric balance** between intake and output is effective. For people who want to increase their lean body weight, increased caloric intake with increased exercise can result in the desired changes.

🌐 **Physical activity is one effective means of controlling body fat.** www.mhhe.com/fit_well/web15 **Click 07.** Though physical activity or exercise will not result in immediate and large decreases in body fat levels, there is

---

Basal Metabolic Rate (BMR) Your energy expenditure in a basic or rested state.

Diet The usual food and drink for a person or animal.

Caloric Balance Consuming calories in amounts equal to the number of calories expended.

| Table 3 ▶ Threshold of Training and Target Zones for Body Fat Reduction | | | | |

| | Threshold of Training* | | Target Zones* | |
	Physical Activity	Diet	Physical Activity	Diet
Frequency	• To be effective, activity must be regular, preferably daily, though fat can be lost over the long term with almost any frequency that results in increased caloric expenditure.	• It is best to reduce caloric intake consistently and daily. To restrict calories only on certain days is not best, though fat can be lost over a period of time by reducing caloric intake at any time.	• Daily moderate activity is recommended. For people who do regular vigorous activity, three to six days per week may be best.	• It is best to diet consistently and daily.
Intensity	• To lose 1 pound of fat, you must expend 3,500 calories more than you normally expend.	• To lose 1 pound of fat, you must eat 3,500 calories fewer than you normally eat.	• Slow, low-intensity aerobic exercise that results in no more than 1 to 2 pounds of fat loss per week is best.	• Modest caloric restriction resulting in no more than 1 to 2 pounds of fat loss per week is best.
Time	• To be effective, exercise must be sustained long enough to expend a considerable number of calories. At least 15 minutes per exercise bout are necessary to result in consistent fat loss.	• Eating moderate meals is best. Do not skip meals.	• Exercise durations similar to those for achieving aerobic cardiovascular fitness seem best. An exercise duration of 30 to 60 minutes is recommended.	• Eating moderate meals is best. Skipping meals or fasting is not most effective.

*Note: It is best to combine exercise and diet to achieve the 3,500 caloric imbalance necessary to lose a pound of fat. Using both exercise and diet in the target zone is most effective.

increasing evidence that fat loss resulting from physical activity may be more lasting than fat loss from dieting. Vigorous exercise can increase the resting energy expenditure up to thirteen times (13 **METs**).

Physical activity that can be sustained for relatively long periods is considered the most effective for losing body fat. Physical activities from virtually any level of the physical activity pyramid can be effective in controlling body fatness because all physical activities expend calories. Among the most effective activities are those in the aerobic activity section of the pyramid because they can be done for relatively long periods of time. Lifestyle activities are also effective, if performed regularly for extended periods of time. Table 4 shows the caloric expenditures for one hour of involvement in various physical activities. Heavier people expend more **calories** than lighter people because more work is required to move larger bodies.

Popular books have recently claimed that vigorous activities are not effective in helping with body fat loss because they say vigorous activities burn less fat than less intense activities. While this is true in theory, it has little practical meaning for most people. It is the total calories expended in your activity that counts. If you run for the same period of time that you walk, you will expend more calories in running.

Even though vigorous activity can be effective, it will not work if you do not do it regularly. For this reason, more vigorous activity may not be as effective as some less vigorous activities for certain people. For example, running at 10 miles per hour (a 6-minute mile) will cause a 150-pound person to expend 900 calories in one hour. Jogging about half as fast, or at 5 1/2 miles per hour (approximately an 11-minute mile), will result in an expenditure of about 650 calories in the same amount of time. At first glance, the more vigorous exercise seems to be a better choice. But how many people can continue to run at a 10-mile-per-hour pace for a full hour? Each mile run at 10 miles per hour results in an expenditure of 90 calories, while each mile run at 5 1/2 miles per hour results in an expenditure of 118 calories. Per mile, you expend more calories in slow running. It takes longer to run a mile, but by the same token, you can also persist longer. The key is to expend as many calories as possible during each regular exercise period. Doing less vigorous activity for longer periods is better for fat control than doing very vigorous activities that can be done only for

MET METs are multiples of the amount of energy expended at rest.

Calorie A unit of energy supplied by food; the quantity of heat necessary to raise the temperature of a kilogram of water 1°C (actually a kilocalorie, but usually called a calorie for weight-control purposes).

Table 4 ▶ Calories Expended per Hour in Various Physical Activities (Performed at a Recreational Level)*

Activity	Calories Used per Hour				
	100 lbs (46 kgs)	120 lbs (55 kgs)	150 lbs (68 kgs)	180 lbs (82 kgs)	200 lbs (91 kgs)
Archery	180	204	240	276	300
Backpacking (40-lb. pack)	307	348	410	472	513
Badminton	255	289	340	391	425
Baseball	210	238	280	322	350
Basketball (half-court)	225	255	300	345	375
Bicycling (normal speed)	157	178	210	242	263
Bowling	155	176	208	240	261
Canoeing (4 mph)	276	344	414	504	558
Circuit training	247	280	330	380	413
Dance, aerobics	315	357	420	483	525
Dance, ballet (choreographed)	240	300	360	432	480
Dance, modern (choreographed)	240	300	360	432	480
Dance, social	174	222	264	318	348
Fencing	225	255	300	345	375
Fitness calisthenics	232	263	310	357	388
Football	225	255	300	345	375
Golf (walking)	187	212	250	288	313
Gymnastics	232	263	310	357	388
Handball	450	510	600	690	750
Hiking	225	255	300	345	375
Horseback riding	180	204	240	276	300
Interval training	487	552	650	748	833
Jogging (5 1/2 mph)	487	552	650	748	833
Judo/karate	232	263	310	357	388
Mountain climbing	450	510	600	690	750
Pool; billiards	97	110	130	150	163
Racquetball; paddleball	450	510	600	690	750
Rope jumping (continuous)	525	595	700	805	875
Rowing, crew	615	697	820	943	1025
Running (10 mph)	625	765	900	1035	1125
Sailing (pleasure)	135	153	180	207	225
Skating, ice	262	297	350	403	438
Skating, roller/inline	262	297	350	403	438
Skiing, cross-country	525	595	700	805	875
Skiing, downhill	450	510	600	690	750
Soccer	405	459	540	621	775
Softball (fast pitch)	210	238	280	322	350
Softball (slow pitch)	217	246	290	334	363
Surfing	416	467	550	633	684
Swimming (fast laps)	420	530	630	768	846
Swimming (slow laps)	240	272	320	368	400
Table tennis	180	204	240	276	300
Tennis	315	357	420	483	525
Volleyball	262	297	350	403	483
Walking	204	258	318	372	426
Waterskiing	306	390	468	564	636
Weight training	352	399	470	541	558

*Note: Locate your weight to determine the calories expended per hour in each of the activities shown in the table based on recreational involvement. More vigorous activity, as occurs in competitive athletics, may result in greater caloric expenditures.

Source: Corbin, C. B., and Lindsey, R.

short periods. Nevertheless, vigorous activity can be very effective for some people.

Strength training can be effective in maintaining a desirable body composition. Performing exercises from the strength and muscular endurance level of the physical activity pyramid can be effective in maintaining desirable body fat levels. People who do strength training increase their muscle mass (lean body mass). This extra muscle mass expends extra calories at rest resulting in a higher metabolic rate. Also, people with more muscle mass expend more calories when doing physical activity.

Appetite is not necessarily increased through exercise. The human animal was intended to be an active animal. For this reason, the human "appetite thermostat" (called the "appestat" by some) is set as if all people are active. Those who are inactive do not have a decreased appetite. Likewise, if a person is sedentary and then begins regular exercise, the appetite does not necessarily increase because this appetite thermostat expects activity. Very vigorous activity does not necessarily cause an appetite increase that is proportional to the calories expended in the vigorous exercise.

Strategies for Action

Making a variety of self-assessments can help you make informed decisions about body composition. www.mhhe.com/fit_well/web15 Click 08. In Lab 15A you will take various body composition self-assessments. It is important that you take all of the measurements and consider all of the information before making final decisions about your body composition. Each of the self-assessment techniques has its strengths and weaknesses, and you should be aware of these when making personal decisions. The importance you place on one particular measure may be different than the importance another person places on that measure because you are a unique individual and should use information that is more relevant for you personally.

Estimating your BMR can help you determine the number of calories you expend each day. In Lab 15C you can estimate your BMR. This will give you an idea of how much energy you expend when you are resting. You can use this information together with the information about the energy you expend to help you balance the calories you consume with the calories you expend each day.

Logging your daily activities can help you determine the number of calories you expend each day. In Lab 15C, you will also log the activities you perform in a day. You can then determine your energy expenditure in these activities. You can combine this information with the information about your basal metabolism to determine your total daily energy expenditure.

Counting the calories you consume each day can help you balance the calories you expend with the calories you consume. In the concept on nutrition, you will learn how to count the number of calories you consume each day. You can use this information with the information in Lab 15C to determine if there is a balance in calories consumed and calories expended.

Self-assessment information—especially body composition information—is personal and confidential. Body composition self-assessment information is personal and should be confidential. When performing the self-assessments in Lab 15A be aware of the following:

1. If doing a self-assessment around other people makes you self-conscious, do the measurement in private.
2. If the measurement requires the assistance of another person, choose a person you trust and feel comfortable with. If you have someone help you make measurements, identify a person who will be available over time. This will allow the same person to make the measurements each time you make assessments. For Lab 15A, get the assistance of an expert and/or a partner to do skinfold measures. Of course, doing your own measurements when possible is the best way to make sure that the same person does the measures each time you do them. Recent studies show that self-measurements can be relatively accurate if done consistently with the same caliper and you practice to become skilled.
3. The formulae used to determine body fatness from skinfolds and other procedures were based on normal distributions of people. The more a person differs from normal, the less accurate the measurements will be. For this reason, most measurements are less accurate for the very lean and people with higher than normal levels of fat. Special procedures are available for athletes, and techniques such as underwater weighing, the BodPod, or bioelectrical impedance are best for those with exceptionally high levels of body fatness.
4. Some measurements, such as the thigh skinfold, are hard to make on some people. This is one reason why two different skinfolding procedures are presented in Lab 15A.
5. Self-assessments require skill. With practice, you can become skillful in making measurements. Your first few attempts will no doubt lack accuracy.

6. Use the same measuring device each time you measure (scale, caliper, measuring tape, etc.). This will assure that any measurement error is constant and will allow you to track your progress over time. For example, your scale may be off by two pounds, but if you use the same scale every time you always know the amount of the error and you can correct for it. If you use a different scale each time you weigh, the error is variable. It is difficult to correct for variable errors.

7. Once you have tried all of the self-assessments in Lab 15A, choose the ones you want to continue to do and use the same measurement techniques each time you do the measurements.

Web Resources

American Anorexia/Bulimia Association **www.aabainc.org**

North American Association for the Study of Obesity (NAASO) **www.naaso.org**

Shape up America **www.shapeup.org**

Inexpensive Calipers (available from)
Fat Control Inc. Dept CC
19310 Dutton Rd.
Stewartstown, PA 17363
wellfarm@nfdc.net

Suggested Readings

 Additional reference materials for concept 15 are available at **www.mhhe.com/fit_well/web15 Click 09.**

American College of Sports Medicine. 2001. Appropriate intervention strategies for weight loss and prevention of weight regain for adults. *Medicine and Science in Sports and Exercise* 33(12):2145–2156.

Cataldo, D., and V. H. Heyward. 2000. Pinch an inch: A comparison of several high-quality and plastic skinfold calipers. *ACSM's Health and Fitness Journal* 4(3):12–16.

Jonas, S. 2001. Weighing in on the obesity epidemic: What do we do now? *ACSM's Health and Fitness Journal* 5(5):7–10.

Kruskall, L. J. et al. 2002. Eating disorders and disordered eating—Are they the same? *ACSM's Health and Fitness Journal* 6(3):6–12.

Lohman, T. G., L. H. Houtkooper, and S. B. Going. 1997. Body fat measurement goes hi tech. *ACSM's Health and Fitness Journal* 1(1):18–21.

Manore, M. M., and J. A. Thompson. 2000. *Sport Nutrition for Health and Performance.* Champaign, IL: Human Kinetics.

Nash, J. M. 2002. Cracking the fat riddle. *Time* 160(10):46–55.

Newsweek. 3 July 2000. Fat for life. *Newsweek.* A series of articles on childhood obesity, 40–47.

Sacker, I. M., and M. A. Zimmer. 2002. *Dying to Be Thin: Understanding and Defeating Anorexia Nervosa and Bulimia—A Practical, Lifesaving Guide.* New York: Time Warner Bookmark.

Sanborn, C. F. et al. 2000. Disordered eating and the female athlete triad. *Clinics in Sports Medicine* 19(2):199–213.

Schmidt, W. D., C. J. Biwer, and L. K. Kalscheuer. 2001. Effects of long versus short bout exercise on fitness and weight loss in overweight females. *Journal of the American College of Nutrition* 20(5):497–501.

Sohn, E. 2002. The hunger artists. *U.S. News and World Report* 132(20):44–50.

Thompson, S. R., M. M. Weber, and L. B. Brown. 2001. The relationship between health and fitness magazine readings and eating-disordered weight-loss methods among high school girls. *American Journal of Health Education* 32(3):133–138.

U.S. Department of Health and Human Services. Nov. 2002. *Healthy People 2010.* 2nd ed. With *Understanding and Improving Health and Objectives for Improving Health.* 2 vols. Washington, DC: U.S. Government Printing Office.

Wei, M. et al. 1999. Relationship between low cardiorespiratory fitness and morbidity in normal weight, overweight, and obese men. *Journal of the American Medical Association* 282:1547–1553.

Welk, G. J., and S. N. Blair. 2000. Physical activity protects against the health risk of obesity. *President's Council on Physical Fitness and Sports Research Digest* 3(12):1–8.

Wong, G., and W. H. Dietz. 2002. Economic burden of obesity in youths aged 6 to 17 years: 1979–1999. *Pediatrics* 109:381.

World Health Organization. 2000. *Obesity: Preventing and Managing the Global Epidemic.* Geneva: World Health Organization.

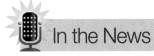

In the News

Physical activity is critical in maintaining the weight loss over time. For optimal results, weight loss programs should combine a lower caloric intake with a good physical activity program. The ACSM has recently released recommendations for weight loss treatment that indicate when weight loss would be appropriate and what guidelines should be followed in treatment. The recommendations are intended more for clinical use by physicians, dietitians, and exercise specialists. Guidelines for non-professionals based on the ACSM recommendations are outlined in Table 5. Concept 17 includes more specific information on diet and physical activity for weight control as well as guidelines on increasing lean body weight.

Table 5 ▶ Guidelines for Weight Loss Treatment

Questions about Weight Loss	Recommendations
Who should consider weight loss?	Individuals with a BMI of > 25 or in the marginal or overfat zones *should consider* reducing their body weight—especially if it is accompanied by abdominal obesity. Individuals with a BMI of > 30 *are encouraged to seek* weight loss treatment.
What types of goals should be established?	Overweight and obese individuals should target reducing their body weight by a minimum of 5–10% and should aim to maintain this long-term weight loss.
What about maintenance?	Individuals should strive for long-term weight maintenance and the prevention of weight regain over the long-term, especially when weight loss is not desired or when attainment of ideal body weight is not achievable.
What should be targeted in a weight loss program?	Weight loss programs should target both eating and exercise behaviors as sustained changes in both behaviors has been associated with significant long-term weight loss.
How should diet be changed?	Overweight and obese individuals should reduce their current intake by 500–1000 kcal/day to achieve weight loss (< 30% of calories from fat). Individualized level of calorie intake should be established to prevent weight regain after initial loss.
How should activity be changed?	Overweight and obese individuals should progressively increase to a minimum of 150 minutes of moderate intensity physical activity per week for health benefits. However, for long-term weight loss, the program should progress to higher amounts of activity (e.g., 200–300 minutes per week or > 2000 kcal/week).
What about resistance exercise?	Resistance exercise should supplement the endurance exercise program for individuals who are undertaking modest reductions in energy intake to lose weight.
What about pharmacotherapy for weight loss?	Pharmacotherapy for weight loss should only be used by individuals with a BMI > 30 or those with excessive body fatness. Weight loss medications should only be used in combination with a strong behavioral intervention that focuses on modifying eating and exercise behaviors.

Source: Based on ACSM recommendations, see suggested readings.

Lab Resource Materials: Evaluating Body Fat

General Information about Skinfold Measurements

It is important to use a consistent procedure for "drawing up" or "pinching up" a skinfold and making the measurement with the caliper. The following procedures should be used for each skinfold site.

1. Lay the caliper down on a nearby table. Use the thumbs and index fingers of both hands to draw up a skinfold or layer of skin and fat. The fingers and thumbs of the two hands should be about 1 inch apart, or half an inch on either side of the location where the measurement is to be made.
2. The skinfolds are normally drawn up in a vertical line rather than a horizontal line. However, if the natural tendency of the skin aligns itself less than vertical, the measurement should be done on the natural line of the skinfold, rather than on the vertical.
3. Do not pinch the skinfold too hard. Draw it up so that your thumbs and fingers are not compressing the skinfold.
4. Once the skinfold is drawn up, let go with your right hand and pick up the caliper. Open the jaws of the caliper and place it over the location of the skinfold to be measured and one-half inch from your left index finger and thumb. Allow the tips, or jaw faces, of the caliper to close on the skinfold at a level about where the skin would be normally.
5. Let the reading on the caliper settle for two or three seconds, then note the thickness of the skinfold in millimeters.
6. Three measurements should be taken at each location. Use the middle of the three values to determine your measurement. For example, if you had values of 10, 11, and 9, your measurement for that location would be 10. If the three measures vary by more than 3 millimeters from the lowest to the highest, you may want to take additional measurements.

Skinfold Locations for Women

Triceps skinfold— Make a mark on the back of the right arm, one-half the distance between the tip of the shoulder and the tip of the elbow. Make the measurement at this location.

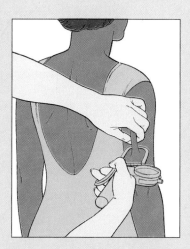

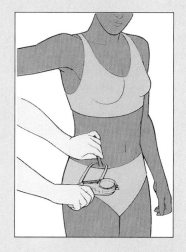

Iliac crest skinfold— Make a mark at the top front of the iliac crest. This skinfold is taken slightly diagonally because of the natural line of the skin.

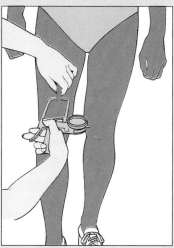

Thigh skinfold— Make a mark on the front of the thigh midway between the hip and the knee. Make the measurement vertically at this location.

*Abdominal skinfold—*Make a mark on the skin approximately one inch to the right of the navel. Make a horizontal measurement at this location for the Fitness-gram Method and a vertical measure for the Jackson-Pollock Method. (See page 290.)

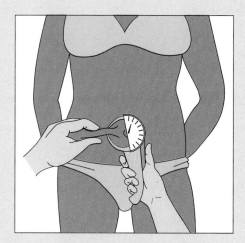

*Calf skinfold—*Same as for men.

Skinfold Locations for Men

Chest skinfold—Make a mark above and to the right of the right nipple (one-half the distance from the midline of the side and the nipple). The measurement at this location is often done on the diagonal because of the natural line of the skin.

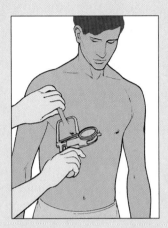

Abdominal skinfold—Make a mark on the skin approximately 1 inch to the right of the navel. Make a vertical measurement at that location for the Jackson-Pollock Method and horizontally for the Fitnessgram Method. (See page 289.)

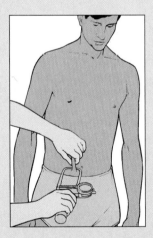

Thigh skinfold—Same as for women (see previous page).

Calf skinfold—Make a mark on the inside of the calf of the right leg at the level of the largest calf size (girth). Place the foot on a chair or other elevation so that the knee is kept at approximately 90 degrees. Make a vertical measurement at the mark.

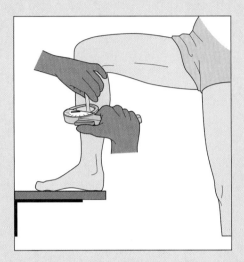

Self-Measured Tricep Skinfold for Both Men and Women

This measurement is made on the left arm so that the caliper can easily be read. Hold the arm straight at shoulder height. Make a fist with the thumb faced upward. Place the fist against a wall. With the right hand place the caliper over the skinfold as it "hangs freely" on the back of the tricep (half way from the tip of the shoulder to the elbow).

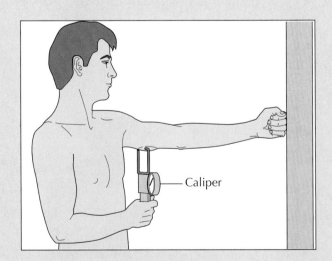

Caliper

Calculating Fatness from Skinfolds (Jackson-Pollock Method)

1. Sum three skinfolds (triceps, iliac crest, and thigh for women; chest, abdominal (vertical), and thigh for men).
2. Use the skinfold sum and your age to determine your percent fat using Chart 1 for men and Chart 2 for women. Locate your sum of skinfold in the left column and your age at the top of the chart. Your estimated body fat percentage is located where the values intersect.
3. Use the Standards for Body Fatness (Chart 4) to determine your fatness rating.

Chart 1 ▶ Percent Fat Estimates for Men (Sum of Thigh, Chest, and Abdominal Skinfolds)

Sum of Skinfolds (mm)	Age to the Last Year								
	22 and Under	23 to 27	28 to 32	33 to 37	38 to 42	43 to 47	48 to 52	53 to 57	Over 58
8–10	1.3	1.8	2.3	2.9	3.4	3.9	4.5	5.0	5.5
11–13	2.2	2.8	3.3	3.9	4.4	4.9	5.5	6.0	6.5
14–16	3.2	3.8	4.3	4.8	5.4	5.9	6.4	7.0	7.5
17–19	4.2	4.7	5.3	5.8	6.3	6.9	7.4	8.0	8.5
20–22	5.1	5.7	6.2	6.8	7.3	7.9	8.4	8.9	9.5
23–25	6.1	6.6	7.2	7.7	8.3	8.8	9.4	9.9	10.5
26–28	7.0	7.6	8.1	8.7	9.2	9.8	10.3	10.9	11.4
29–31	8.0	8.5	9.1	9.6	10.2	10.7	11.3	11.8	12.4
32–34	8.9	9.4	10.0	10.5	11.1	11.6	12.2	12.8	13.3
35–37	9.8	10.4	10.9	11.5	12.0	12.6	13.1	13.7	14.3
38–40	10.7	11.3	11.8	12.4	12.9	13.5	14.1	14.6	15.2
41–43	11.6	12.2	12.7	13.3	13.8	14.4	15.0	15.5	16.1
44–46	12.5	13.1	13.6	14.2	14.7	15.3	15.9	16.4	17.0
47–49	13.4	13.9	14.5	15.1	15.6	16.2	16.8	17.3	17.9
50–52	14.3	14.8	15.4	15.9	16.5	17.1	17.6	18.1	18.8
53–55	15.1	15.7	16.2	16.8	17.4	17.9	18.5	18.2	19.7
56–58	16.0	16.5	17.1	17.7	18.2	18.8	19.4	20.0	20.5
59–61	16.9	17.4	17.9	18.5	19.1	19.7	20.2	20.8	21.4
62–64	17.6	18.2	18.8	19.4	19.9	20.5	21.1	21.7	22.2
65–67	18.5	19.0	19.6	20.2	20.8	21.3	21.9	22.5	23.1
68–70	19.3	19.9	20.4	21.0	21.6	22.2	22.7	23.3	23.9
71–73	20.1	20.7	21.2	21.8	22.4	23.0	23.6	24.1	24.7
74–76	20.9	21.5	22.0	22.6	23.2	23.8	24.4	25.0	25.5
77–79	21.7	22.2	22.8	23.4	24.0	24.6	25.2	25.8	26.3
80–82	22.4	23.0	23.6	24.2	24.8	25.4	25.9	26.5	27.1
83–85	23.2	23.8	24.4	25.0	25.5	26.1	26.7	27.3	27.9
86–88	24.0	24.5	25.1	25.5	26.3	26.9	27.5	28.1	28.7
89–91	24.7	25.3	25.9	25.7	27.1	27.6	28.2	28.8	29.4
92–94	25.4	26.0	26.6	27.2	27.8	28.4	29.0	29.6	30.2
95–97	26.1	26.7	27.3	27.9	28.5	29.1	29.7	30.3	30.9
98–100	26.9	27.4	28.0	28.6	29.2	29.8	30.4	31.0	31.6
101–103	27.5	28.1	28.7	29.3	29.9	30.5	31.1	31.7	32.3
104–106	28.2	28.8	29.4	30.0	30.6	31.2	31.8	32.4	33.0
107–109	28.9	29.5	30.1	30.7	31.3	31.9	32.5	33.1	33.7
110–112	29.6	30.2	30.8	31.4	32.0	32.6	33.2	33.8	34.4
113–115	30.2	30.8	31.4	32.0	32.6	33.2	33.8	34.5	35.1
116–118	30.9	31.5	32.1	32.7	33.3	33.9	34.5	35.1	35.7
119–121	31.5	32.1	32.7	33.3	33.9	34.5	35.1	35.7	36.4
122–124	32.1	32.7	33.3	33.9	34.5	35.1	35.8	36.4	37.0
125–127	32.7	33.3	33.9	34.5	35.1	35.8	36.4	37.0	37.6

*Percent fat calculated by the formula by Siri. Percent fat = $[(4.95/BD) - 4.5] \times 100$, where BD = body density.

Source: Baumgartner, T. A., and Jackson, A. S.

Chart 2 ▶ Percent Fat Estimates for Women (Sum of Triceps, Iliac Crest, and Thigh Skinfolds)

Sum of Skinfolds (mm)	22 and Under	23 to 27	28 to 32	Age to the Last Year 33 to 37	38 to 42	43 to 47	48 to 52	53 to 57	Over 58
23–25	9.7	9.9	10.2	10.4	10.7	10.9	11.2	11.4	11.7
26–28	11.0	11.2	11.5	11.7	12.0	12.3	12.5	12.7	13.0
29–31	12.3	12.5	12.8	13.0	13.3	13.5	13.8	14.0	14.3
32–34	13.6	13.8	14.0	14.3	14.5	14.8	15.0	15.3	15.5
35–37	14.8	15.0	15.3	15.5	15.8	16.0	16.3	16.5	16.8
38–40	16.0	16.3	16.5	16.7	17.0	17.2	17.5	17.7	18.0
41–43	17.2	17.4	17.7	17.9	18.2	18.4	18.7	18.9	19.2
44–46	18.3	18.6	18.8	19.1	19.3	19.6	19.8	20.1	20.3
47–49	19.5	19.7	20.0	20.2	20.5	20.7	21.0	21.2	21.5
50–52	20.6	20.8	21.1	21.3	21.6	21.8	22.1	22.3	22.6
53–55	21.7	21.9	22.1	22.4	22.6	22.9	23.1	23.4	23.6
56–58	22.7	23.0	23.2	23.4	23.7	23.9	24.2	24.4	24.7
59–61	23.7	24.0	24.2	24.5	24.7	25.0	25.2	25.5	25.7
62–64	24.7	25.0	25.2	25.5	25.7	26.0	26.2	26.4	26.7
65–67	25.7	25.9	26.2	26.4	26.7	26.9	27.2	27.4	27.7
68–70	26.6	26.9	27.1	27.4	27.6	27.9	28.1	28.4	28.6
71–73	27.5	27.8	28.0	28.3	28.5	28.8	28.0	29.3	29.5
74–76	28.4	28.7	28.9	29.2	29.4	29.7	29.9	30.2	30.4
77–79	29.3	29.5	29.8	30.0	30.3	30.5	30.8	31.0	31.3
80–82	30.1	30.4	30.6	30.9	31.1	31.4	31.6	31.9	32.1
83–85	30.9	31.2	31.4	31.7	31.9	32.2	32.4	32.7	32.9
86–88	31.7	32.0	32.2	32.5	32.7	32.9	33.2	33.4	33.7
89–91	32.5	32.7	33.0	33.2	33.5	33.7	33.9	34.2	34.4
92–94	33.2	33.4	33.7	33.9	34.2	34.4	34.7	34.9	35.2
95–97	33.9	34.1	34.4	34.6	34.9	35.1	35.4	35.6	35.9
98–100	34.6	34.8	35.21	35.3	35.5	35.8	36.0	36.3	36.5
101–103	35.3	35.4	35.7	35.9	36.2	36.4	36.7	36.9	37.2
104–106	35.8	36.1	36.3	36.6	36.8	37.1	37.3	37.5	37.8
107–109	36.4	36.7	36.9	37.1	37.4	37.6	37.9	38.1	38.4
110–112	37.0	37.2	37.5	37.7	38.0	38.2	38.5	38.7	38.9
113–115	37.5	37.8	38.0	38.2	38.5	38.7	39.0	39.2	39.5
116–118	38.0	38.3	38.5	38.8	39.0	39.3	39.5	39.7	40.0
119–121	38.5	38.7	39.0	39.2	39.5	39.7	40.0	40.2	40.5
122–124	39.0	39.2	39.4	39.7	39.9	40.2	40.4	40.7	40.9
125–127	39.4	39.6	39.9	40.1	40.4	40.6	40.9	41.1	41.4
128–130	39.8	40.0	40.3	40.5	40.8	41.0	41.3	41.5	41.8

*Percent fat calculated by the formula by Siri. Percent fat = $[(4.95/BD) - 4.5] \times 100$, where BD = body density.

Source: Baumgartner, T. A., and Jackson, A. S.

Chart 3 ▶ Percent Fat Estimates for Sum of Triceps, Abdominal, and Calf Skinfolds

Men		Women	
Sum of Skinfolds	Percent Fat	Sum of Skinfolds	Percent Fat
8–10	3.2	23–25	16.8
11–13	4.1	26–28	17.7
14–46	5.0	29–31	18.5
17–19	6.0	32–34	19.4
20–22	6.0	35–37	20.2
23–25	7.8	38–40	21.0
26–28	8.7	41–43	21.9
29–31	9.7	44–46	22.7
32–34	10.6	47–49	23.5
35–37	11.5	50–52	24.4
38–40	12.5	53–55	25.2
41–43	13.4	56–58	26.1
44–46	14.3	59–61	26.9
47–49	15.2	62–64	27.7
50–52	16.2	65–67	28.6
53–55	17.1	68–70	29.4
56–58	18.0	71–73	30.2
59–61	18.9	74–76	31.1
62–64	19.9	77–79	31.9
65–67	20.8	80–82	32.7
68–70	21.7	83–85	33.6
71–73	22.6	86–88	34.4
74–76	23.6	89–91	35.5
77–79	24.5	92–94	36.1
80–82	25.4	95–97	36.9
83–85	26.4	98–100	37.8
86–88	27.3	101–103	38.6
89–91	28.2	104–106	39.4
92–94	29.1	107–109	40.3
95–97	30.1	110–112	41.1
98–100	31.0	113–115	42.0
101–103	31.9	116–118	42.8
104–106	32.8	119–121	43.6
107–109	33.8	122–124	44.5
110–112	34.7	125–127	45.3
113–115	35.6	128–130	46.1
116–118	36.6	131–133	47.0
119–121	37.5	134–136	47.8
122–124	38.4	137–139	48.7
125–127	39.3	140–142	49.5

Chart 4 ▶ Standards for Body Fatness (Percent Body Fat)

Classification	Males	Females
Essential fat	No less than 5%	No less than 10%
Borderline	5%–9%	10%–16%
High performance	5%–15%	10%–23%
Good fitness (healthy)	10%–20%	17%–28%
Marginal	21%–25%	29%–35%
Overfat	25%+	35%+

Calculating Fatness from Skinfolds (Fitnessgram Method)

1. Sum the three skinfolds (triceps, abdominal, and calf) for men and women. Use horizontal abdominal measure.
2. Use the skinfold sum and your age to determine your percent fat using Chart 3. Locate your sum of skinfold in the left column and your age at the top of the chart. Your estimated body fat percentage is located where the values intersect.
3. Use the Standards for Body Fatness (Chart 4) to determine your fatness rating.

Calculating Fatness from Self-Measured Skinfolds

1. Use either the Jackson-Pollock or Fitnessgram method but make the measures on yourself rather than have a partner do the measures. When doing the tricep measure use the self-measurement technique for men and women. (See page 290.)
2. Calculate fatness using the methods described previously.
3. Use Chart 4 to determine ratings.

Height-Weight Measurements

1. *Height*—Measure your height in inches or centimeters. Take the measurement without shoes, but add 2.5 centimeters or 1 inch to measurements, as the charts include heel height.

2. *Weight*—Measure your weight in pounds or kilograms without clothes. Add 3 pounds or 1.4 kilograms because the charts include weight of clothes. If weight must be taken with clothes on, wear indoor clothing that weighs 3 pounds or 1.4 kilograms.

3. Determine your frame size using the elbow breadth. The measurement is most accurate when done with a broad-based sliding caliper. However, it can be done using a skinfold caliper or can be estimated with a metric ruler. The right arm is measured when it is elevated with the elbow bent at 90 degrees and the upper arm horizontal. The back of the hand should face the person making the measurement. Using the caliper, measure the distance between the epicondyles of the humerus (inside and outside bony points of the elbow). Measure to the nearest millimeter (1/10 of a centimeter). If a caliper is not available, place the thumb and the index finger of the left hand on the epicondyles of the humerus and measure the distance between the fingers with a metric ruler. Use your height and elbow breadth in centimeters to determine your frame size (Chart 5); you need not repeat this procedure each time you use a height and weight chart.

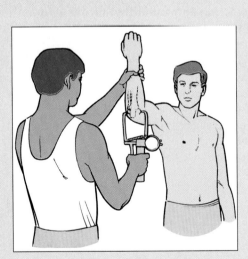

4. Use Chart 6 to determine your healthy weight range. The new healthy weight range charts do not account for frame size. However, you may want to consider frame size when determining a personal weight within the health weight range. People with a larger frame size typically can carry more weight within the range than those with a smaller frame size.

Chart 5 ▶ Frame Size Determined from Elbow Breadth (mm)

Height	Elbow Breadth (mm)		
	Small Frame	Medium Frame	Large Frame
Males			
5′2″ or less	<64	64–72	>72
5′3″–5′6 1/2″	<67	67–74	>74
5′7″–5′10 1/2″	<69	69–76	>76
5′11″–6′2 1/2″	<71	71–78	>78
6′3″ or less	<74	74–81	>81
Females			
4′10 1/2″ or less	<56	56–64	>64
4′11″–5′2 1/2″	<58	58–65	>65
5′3″–5′6 1/2″	<59	59–66	>66
5′7″–5′10 1/2″	<61	61–68	>69
5′11″ or less	<62	62–69	>69

Height is given including 1-inch heels.

Source: Metropolitan Life Insurance Company.

Chart 6 ▶ Healthy Weight Ranges for Adult Women and Men

Feet	Women Height Inches	Pounds	Feet	Men Height Inches	Pounds
4	10	91–119	5	9	129–169
4	11	94–124	5	10	132–174
5	0	97–128	5	11	136–179
5	1	101–132	6	0	140–184
5	2	104–137	6	1	144–189
5	3	107–141	6	2	148–195
5	4	111–146	6	3	152–200
5	5	114–150	6	4	156–205
5	6	118–155	6	5	160–211
5	7	121–160	6	6	164–216
5	8	125–164			

Source: U.S. Department of Agriculture and Department of Health and Human Services.

Chart 7 ▶ Body Mass Index (BMI)

Height																															
5'0"	20	21	21	22	23	24	25	26	27	28	29	30	31	32	33	34	35	36	37	38	39	40	41	42	43	44	45	46	47	48	49
5'1"	19	20	21	22	23	24	25	26	26	27	28	29	30	31	32	33	34	35	36	37	38	39	40	41	42	43	43	44	45	46	47
5'2"	18	19	20	21	22	23	24	25	26	27	27	28	29	30	31	32	33	34	35	36	37	37	38	39	40	41	42	43	44	45	46
5'3"	18	19	19	20	21	22	23	24	25	26	27	27	28	29	30	31	32	33	34	35	35	36	37	38	39	40	41	42	43	43	44
5'4"	17	18	19	20	21	21	22	23	24	25	26	27	27	28	29	30	31	32	33	33	34	35	36	37	38	39	39	40	41	42	43
5'5"	17	17	18	19	20	21	22	22	23	24	25	26	27	27	28	29	30	31	32	32	33	34	35	36	37	37	38	39	40	41	42
5'6"	16	17	18	19	19	20	21	22	23	23	24	25	26	27	27	28	29	30	31	31	32	33	34	35	36	36	37	38	39	40	40
5'7"	16	16	17	18	19	20	20	21	22	23	23	24	25	26	27	27	28	29	30	31	31	32	33	34	34	35	36	37	38	38	39
5'8"	15	16	17	17	18	19	20	21	21	22	23	24	24	25	26	27	27	28	29	30	30	31	32	33	33	34	35	36	36	37	38
5'9"	15	16	16	17	18	18	19	20	21	21	22	23	24	24	25	26	27	27	28	29	30	30	31	32	32	33	34	35	35	36	37
5'10"	14	15	16	17	17	18	19	19	20	21	22	22	23	24	24	25	26	27	27	28	29	29	30	31	32	32	33	34	34	35	36
5'11"	14	15	15	16	17	17	18	19	20	20	21	22	22	23	24	24	25	26	26	27	28	29	29	30	31	31	32	33	33	34	35
6'0"	14	14	15	16	16	17	18	18	19	20	20	21	22	22	23	24	24	25	26	26	27	28	28	29	30	31	31	32	33	33	34
6'1"	13	14	15	15	16	16	17	18	18	19	20	20	21	22	22	23	24	24	25	26	26	27	28	28	29	30	30	31	32	32	33
6'2"	13	13	14	15	15	16	17	17	18	19	19	20	21	21	22	22	23	24	24	25	26	26	27	28	28	29	30	30	31	31	32
6'3"	12	13	14	14	15	16	16	17	17	18	19	19	20	21	21	22	22	23	24	24	25	26	26	27	27	28	29	29	30	31	31
6'4"	12	13	13	14	15	15	16	16	17	18	18	19	19	20	21	21	22	23	23	24	24	25	26	26	27	27	28	29	29	30	30
	100	105	110	115	120	125	130	135	140	145	150	155	160	165	170	175	180	185	190	195	200	205	210	215	220	225	230	235	240	245	250

Weight

☐ Low   ☐ Good fitness zone   ☐ Marginal   ☐ Obese

Body Mass Index (BMI)

Use the steps listed below or use Chart 7 to calculate your BMI.

1. Divide your weight in pounds by 2.2 to determine your weight in kilograms.
2. Multiply your height in inches by 0.0254 to determine your height in meters.
3. Square your height in meters (multiply your height in meters by your height in meters).
4. Divide the value you obtain in step 3 (square of height in meters) into the value you obtain in step 1 (weight in kilograms).
5. If you use these steps to determine your BMI, use the Rating Scale for Body Mass Index (Chart 8) to obtain a rating for your BMI.

Chart 8 ▶ Rating Scale for Body Mass Index (BMI)

Classification	BMI
Obese (high risk)	Over 30
Marginal	25–30
Good fitness zone	17–24.9
Low	Less than 17

Note: An excessively low BMI is not desirable. Low BMI values can be indicative of eating disorders and other health problems. The government rating for marginal is overweight.

Determining the Waist-to-Hip Circumference Ratio

The waist-to-hip circumference ratio is recommended as the best available index for determining risk and disease associated with fat and weight distribution. Disease and death risk are associated with abdominal and upper body fatness. When a person has high fatness and a high waist-to-hip ratio, additional risks exist. The following steps should be taken in making measurements and calculating the waist-to-hip ratio.

1. Both measurements should be done with a nonelastic tape. Make the measurements while standing with the feet together and the arms at the sides, elevated only high enough to allow the measurements. Be sure the tape is horizontal and around the entire circumference. Record scores to the nearest millimeter or 1/16th of an inch. Use the same units of measure for both circumferences (millimeters or 1/16th of an inch). The tape should be pulled snugly but not to the point of causing an indentation in the skin.

2. *Waist measurement*—Measure at the natural waist (smallest waist circumference). If no natural waist exists, the measurement should be made at the level of the umbilicus. Measure at the end of a normal inspiration.

3. *Hip measurement*—Measure at the maximum circumference of the buttocks. It is recommended that you wear thin-layered clothing (such as a swimming suit or underwear) that will not add significantly to the measurement.

4. Divide the hip measurement into the waist measurement or use the waist-to-hip nomogram (Chart 9) to determine your waist-to-hip ratio.

5. Use the Waist-to-Hip Ratio Rating Scale (Chart 10) to determine your rating for the waist-to-hip ratio.

Chart 9 ▶ Waist-to-Hip Ratio Nomogram

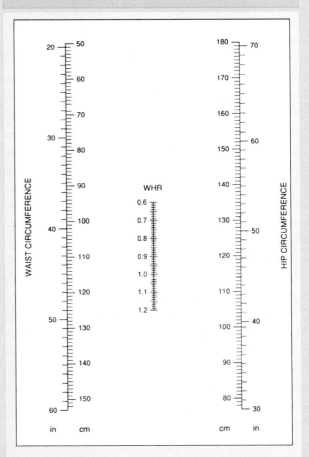

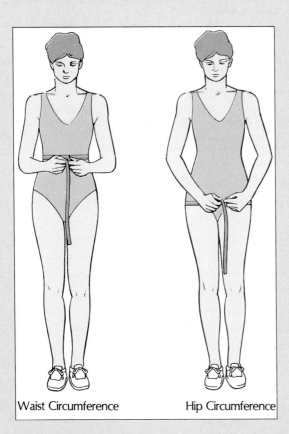

Waist Circumference   Hip Circumference

Note: Using a partner or a mirror will aid you in keeping the tape horizontal.

Chart 10 ▶ Waist-to-Hip Ratio Rating Scale

Classification	Men	Women
High risk	1.0	0.85
Moderately high risk	0.90–1.0	0.80–0.85
Lower risk	<0.90	<0.80

Lab 15A: Evaluating Body Composition: Skinfold Measures

Name	**Section**	**Date**

Purpose: To estimate body fatness using two different skinfold procedures; to compare measures made by an expert, by a partner, and by self-measurements; to learn the strengths and weaknesses of each technique; and to use the results to establish personal standards for evaluating body composition.

General Procedures: Follow the specific procedures for the two different self-assessment techniques. If possible, have one set of measurements made by an expert (instructor) for each of the two techniques. Next, work with a partner you trust. Have the partner make measurements at each site for both techniques. Finally, make self-measurements for each of the sites. If you are just learning a measurement technique, it is important to practice the skills of making the measurement. If you do measurements over time, use the same instrument (if possible) each time you measure. If your measurements vary widely, take more than one set until you get more consistent results.

If you have had an underwater weighing, an electric impedance measurement, a near-infrared interactance measure, or some other body fatness measurement done recently, record your results below.

Measurement Technique	% Body Fat	Rating
1.		
2.		

Skinfold Measurements (Jackson-Pollock Method)

Procedures:

1. Read the directions for the Jackson-Pollock Method measurements in the Lab Resource Materials.
2. If possible, observe a demonstration of the proper procedures for measuring skinfolds at each of the different locations before doing partner or self-measurements.
3. Make expert, partner, and self-measurements (see Lab Resource Materials). When doing the self-measure of the triceps use the self-measurement technique described in the Lab Resource Materials (women only).
4. Record each of the measurements in the Results section.
5. Calculate your body fatness from skinfolds by summing the appropriate skinfold values (chest, thigh, and abdominal for men; triceps, iliac crest, and thigh for women). Using your age and the sum of the appropriate skinfolds, determine your body fatness using Charts 1 and 2 in the Lab Resource Materials.
6. Rate your fatness using Chart 4 in the Lab Resource Materials.

Skinfolds by an Expert (if possible)

Male

Chest

Thigh

Abdominal

Sum

% body fat

Rating

Female

Triceps

Iliac crest

Thigh

Sum

% body fat

Rating

Skinfolds by Partner

Male

Chest

Thigh

Abdominal

Sum

% body fat

Rating

Female

Triceps

Iliac crest

Thigh

Sum

% body fat

Rating

Self-Measurements

Male

Chest

Thigh

Abdominal

Sum

% body fat

Rating

Female

Triceps

Iliac crest

Thigh

Sum

% body fat

Rating

Make a check by the statements that are true about your measurements.

☐ Person doing measurements has experience with these three skinfold measurements.

☐ Self-measurements were practiced until measurements became consistent.

☐ Results of several trials for each measure are consistent (do not vary more than 2–3 mm).

☐ You are not exceptionally low or exceptionally high in body fat.

The more checks you have, the more likely your measurements are accurate.

Skinfold Measurements (Fitnessgram Method)

Procedures:

1. Read the directions for the Fitnessgram measurements in the Lab Resource Materials.
2. Use the procedures as for the Fitnessgram Method using the triceps, abdominal, and calf sites described in the Lab Resource Materials. When doing the self-measure of the triceps use the self-measurement technique on page 290.
3. Calculate your body fatness from skinfolds by summing the appropriate skinfold values (same for both men and women). Using the sum of the appropriate skinfolds, determine your body fatness using Chart 3 in the Lab Resource Materials.
4. Rate your fatness using Chart 4 in the Lab Resource Materials.

Results:

Skinfolds by an Expert (if possible)	Skinfolds by Partner	Self-Measurements
Triceps	Triceps	Triceps
Abdominal	Abdominal	Abdominal
Calf	Calf	Calf
Sum	Sum	Sum
% body fat	% body fat	% body fat
Rating	Rating	Rating

Make a check by the statements that are true about your measurements.

☐ Person doing measurements has experience with these three skinfold measurements.

☐ Self-measurements were practiced until measurements became consistent.

☐ Results of several trials for each measure are consistent (do not vary more than 2–3 mm).

☐ You are not exceptionally low or exceptionally high in body fat.

The more checks you have, the more likely your measurements are accurate.

Conclusions and Implications:

In the space provided below, discuss your current body composition based on the two different skinfold procedures and any other measures of body fatness you may have done. Note any discrepancies in the measurements and discuss which of the measurements you think provide the most useful information. To what extent do you think you need to alter your level of body fatness?

Lab 15B: Evaluating Body Composition: Height, Weight, and Circumference Measures

Name		Section	Date

Purpose: To assess body composition using a variety of procedures, to learn the strengths and weaknesses of each technique, and to use the results to establish personal standards for evaluating body composition.

General Procedures: Follow the specific procedures for the three different self-assessment techniques. If possible, work with a partner you trust to help with measurements that you have difficulty making on yourself. If you are just learning a measurement technique, it is important to practice the skills of making the measurement. If you do measurements over time, use the same instrument (if possible) each time you measure. If your measurements vary widely, take more than one set until you get more consistent results. If possible, have an expert make measurements on you using the two procedures.

Height and Weight Measurements

Procedures:

1. Read the directions for height and weight measurements in the Lab Resource Materials.
2. Determine your healthy weight range using Chart 6 in the Lab Resource Materials. You may want to use your elbow breadth (Chart 5). People with smaller frame sizes should typically weigh less than those with a larger frame size within the healthy weight range. You may need the assistance of a partner to make the elbow breadth measurement.
3. Record your scores in the Results section.

Results:

Weight [   ]   Healthy weight range [   ]

Height [   ]

Make a check by the statements that are true about your measurements.

[ ] You are confident in the accuracy of the scale you used.

[ ] You are confident that the height technique is accurate.

The more checks you have, the more likely your measurements are accurate.
If you are a very active person with a high amount of muscle, use this method with caution.

The Body Mass Index

Procedures:

1. Use the height and weight measures from Part 1 above.
2. Determine your BMI score by using Chart 7 or the directions in the Lab Resource Materials. Determine your rating using Chart 8.
3. Record your scores and rating in the Results section.

Results:

Body mass index [   ]   Rating [   ]

If you are a very active person with a high amount of muscle, use this method with caution.

Waist-to-Hip Ratio

Procedures:

1. Measure your waist and hip circumferences using the procedures in the Lab Resource Materials.
2. Divide your hip circumference into your waist circumference or use Chart 9 in the Lab Resource Materials to calculate your waist-to-hip ratio.
3. Determine your rating using Chart 10 in the Lab Resource Materials.
4. Record your scores in the Results section.

Results:

Waist circumference [ ]

Hip circumference [ ]

Waist-to-hip ratio [ ]   Rating [ ]

Make a check by the statements that are true about your measurements.

[ ] You are confident in the accuracy of the waist and hip measurement.

Make a check by the statements that are true about you.

[ ] I am a male 5′9″ or less and have a waist girth of 34 or more.

[ ] I am a male 5′10″ to 6′4″ and have a waist girth of 36 or more.

[ ] I am a male 6′5″ or more and have a waist girth of 38 or more.

[ ] I am a female 5′2″ or less and have a waist girth of 29 or more.

[ ] I am a female 5′3″ to 5′10″ and have a waist girth of 31 or more.

[ ] I am a female 5′11″ or more and have a waist girth of 33 or more.

If you checked one of the boxes above, the waist-to-hip ratio is especially relevant for you.

Conclusions and Implications:

In the space provided below, discuss your results for the three height, weight, and circumference procedures. Note any discrepancies in the measurements. Indicate the strengths and weaknesses of the various methods. Which of the measures do you think provided you with the most useful information? If you also did the skinfold measures (Lab 15A), discuss your body composition based on all of the information you have collected (skinfolds and height, weight, and circumference measures).

Lab 15C: Determining Your Daily Energy Expenditure

Name		Section	Date

Purpose: To learn how many calories you expend in a day.

Procedures:

1. Estimate your basal metabolism using step 1 in the Results section. First determine the number of minutes you sleep.
2. Monitor your activity expenditure for one day using Chart 1. Record the number of 5-, 15-, and 30-minute blocks of time that you perform each of the different types of physical activities (e.g., if an activity lasted 20 minutes, you would use one 15-minute block and one 5-minute block). Be sure to distinguish between moderate (Mod) or vigorous (Vig) intensity in your logging. If you perform an activity that is not listed, specify the activity on the line labeled "Other" and estimate if it is moderate or vigorous. You may want to keep copies of Chart 1 for future use. One extra copy is provided.
3. Sum the total number of minutes of moderate and vigorous activity. Determine your calories expended during moderate and vigorous activity using steps 2 and 3.
4. Determine your nonactive minutes using step 4. This is all time that is not spent sleeping or being active.
5. Determine your calories expended in nonactive minutes using step 5.
6. Determine your calories expended in a day using step 6.

Results:

Daily Caloric Expenditure Estimates

Step 1:

Basal calories $= .0076 \times$ [Body wt (lbs)] $\times$ [Minutes of sleep] $=$ [Basal calories] (A)

Step 2:

Calories (moderate activity) $= .036 \times$ [Body wt (lbs)] $\times$ [Minutes of moderate activity] $=$ [Calories in moderate activity] (B)

Step 3:

Calories (vigorous activity) $= .053 \times$ [Body wt (lbs)] $\times$ [Minutes of vigorous activity] $=$ [Calories in vigorous activity] (C)

Step 4:

Minutes (nonactive) $= 1{,}440 \text{ min} -$ [Minutes of sleep] $-$ [Minutes of moderate activity] $-$ [Minutes of vigorous activity] $=$ [Nonactive minutes]

Step 5:

Calories (rest and light activity) $= .011 \times$ [Body wt (lbs)] $\times$ [Nonactive minutes] $=$ [Calories in other activities] (D)

Step 6:

Calories expended (per day) $=$ [(A)] $+$ [(B)] $+$ [(C)] $+$ [(D)] $=$ [**Daily calories**]

Answer these questions about your daily calorie expenditure estimate.

Yes **No**

☐ ☐ Were the activities you performed similar to what you normally perform each day?

☐ ☐ Do you think your daily estimated calorie expenditure is an accurate estimate?

☐ ☐ Do you think you expend the correct amount of calories in a typical day to maintain the body composition (body fat level) that is desirable for you?

Conclusions and Interpretations: In several paragraphs, discuss your daily calorie expenditure. Comment on your answers to the questions listed above. In addition, comment on whether you think you should modify your daily calorie expenditure for any reason.

Chart 1 ▶ Daily Activity Log

Day of Monitoring:

Physical Activity Category		5 Minutes	15 Minutes	30 Minutes	Minutes
Lifestyle Activity		1 2 3 4 5 6	1 2 3 4 5 6	1 2 3	
Dancing (general)	Mod				
Gardening	Mod				
Home repair/maintenance	Mod				
Occupation	Mod				
Walking/hiking	Mod				
Other:	Mod				
Aerobic Activity		1 2 3 4 5 6	1 2 3 4 5 6	1 2 3	
Aerobic dance (low impact)	Mod				
	Vig				
Aerobic eq. (rowing, stair, ski)	Mod				
	Vig				
Bicycling	Mod				
	Vig				
Running	Mod				
	Vig				
Skating (roller/ice)	Mod				
	Vig				
Swimming (laps)	Mod				
	Vig				
Other:	Mod				
	Vig				
Sport/Recreation Activity		1 2 3 4 5 6	1 2 3 4 5 6	1 2 3	
Basketball	Mod				
	Vig				
Bowling/billards	Mod				
Golf	Mod				
Martial arts (judo, karate)	Mod				
	Vig				
Racquetball/tennis	Mod				
	Vig				
Soccer/hockey	Mod				
	Vig				
Softball/baseball	Mod				
Volleyball	Mod				
	Vig				
Other:	Mod				
Flexibility Activity		1 2 3 4 5 6	1 2 3 4 5 6	1 2 3	
Stretching	Mod				
Other:	Mod				
Strengthening Activity		1 2 3 4 5 6	1 2 3 4 5 6	1 2 3	
Calisthenics (push-ups/sit-ups)	Mod				
Resistance Exercise	Mod				
Other:	Mod				

Minutes of moderate activity ☐

Minutes of vigorous activity ☐

Total minutes of activity ☐

Chart 2 ▶ Daily Activity Log

Lab 15C

Determining Your Daily Energy Expenditure

Day of Monitoring:

Physical Activity Category		5 Minutes	15 Minutes	30 Minutes	Minutes
Lifestyle Activity		1 2 3 4 5 6	1 2 3 4 5 6	1 2 3	
Dancing (general)	Mod				
Gardening	Mod				
Home repair/maintenance	Mod				
Occupation	Mod				
Walking/hiking	Mod				
Other:	Mod				
Aerobic Activity		1 2 3 4 5 6	1 2 3 4 5 6	1 2 3	
Aerobic dance (low impact)	Mod / Vig				
Aerobic eq. (rowing, stair, ski)	Mod / Vig				
Bicycling	Mod / Vig				
Running	Mod / Vig				
Skating (roller/ice)	Mod / Vig				
Swimming (laps)	Mod / Vig				
Other:	Mod / Vig				
Sport/Recreation Activity		1 2 3 4 5 6	1 2 3 4 5 6	1 2 3	
Basketball	Mod / Vig				
Bowling/billards	Mod				
Golf	Mod				
Martial arts (judo, karate)	Mod / Vig				
Racquetball/tennis	Mod / Vig				
Soccer/hockey	Mod / Vig				
Softball/baseball	Mod				
Volleyball	Mod / Vig				
Other:	Mod				
Flexibility Activity		1 2 3 4 5 6	1 2 3 4 5 6	1 2 3	
Stretching	Mod				
Other:	Mod				
Strengthening Activity		1 2 3 4 5 6	1 2 3 4 5 6	1 2 3	
Calisthenics (push-ups/sit-ups)	Mod				
Resistance Exercise	Mod				
Other:	Mod				

Minutes of moderate activity

Minutes of vigorous activity

Total minutes of activity

306

Nutrition

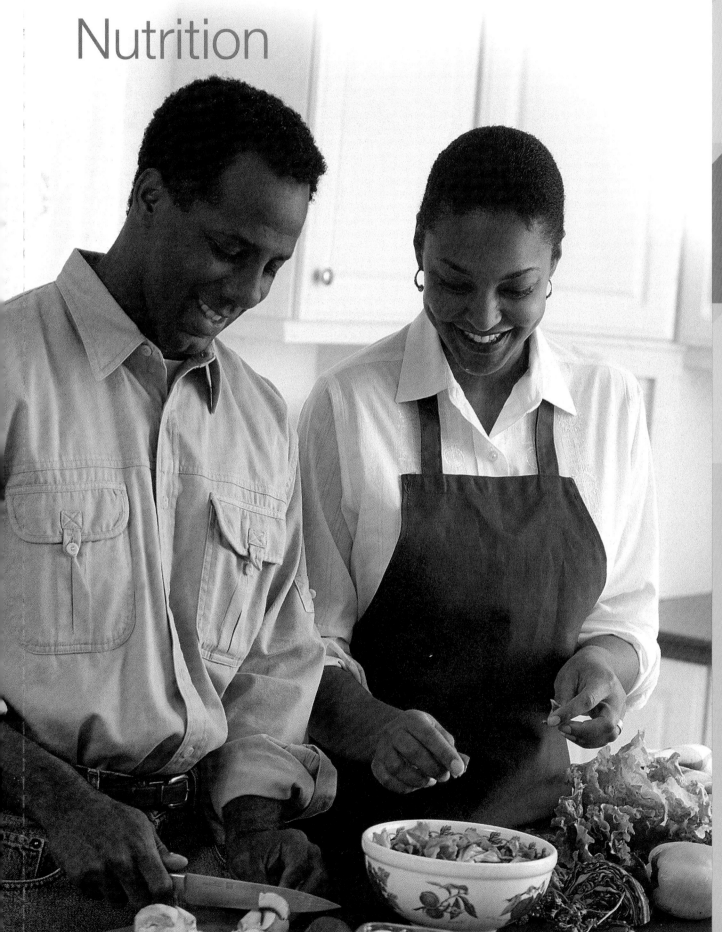

The amount and kinds of food you eat affect your health and wellness.

Health Goals

for the year 2010

- Promote health and reduce chronic disease associated with dietary factors and weight.

- Increase proportion of people who eat healthy snacks.

- Increase proportion of people who eat no more than 30 percent of calories as fat.

- Increase proportion of people who eat no more than 10 percent of calories as saturated fat.

- Increase proportion of people who eat at least five servings of vegetables and fruits daily.

- Increase proportion of people who eat at least six servings of grain products daily.

- Increase proportion of people who meet dietary recommendation for calcium.

- Reduce proportion of people who consume excess sodium.

- Reduce incidence of iron deficiency and anemia (especially children and women).

- Increase proportion of worksites that offer nutrition and/or weight management classes.

The importance of good nutrition for optimal health is well established. Eating patterns have been related to four of the seven leading causes of death and poor nutrition increases the risks for numerous diseases including heart disease, obesity, stroke, diabetes, hypertension, osteoporosis, and many cancers (i.e., colon, prostate, mouth, throat, lung, and stomach). The links to cancer are probably not fully appreciated in today's society but the American Cancer Society estimates that 35 percent of cancer risks are related to nutritional factors. In addition to these health risks, proper nutrition can enhance the quality of life by improving appearance and enhancing the ability to carry out work and leisure time activity without fatigue.

Most people believe that nutrition is important but still find it difficult to maintain a healthy diet. One reason is that foods are usually developed, marketed, and advertised for convenience and taste rather than for health or nutritional quality. Another reason is that many individuals have misconceptions about what constitutes a healthy diet. Some of these misconceptions are propagated by so-called experts with less than impressive credentials and those with commercial interests. Others are created by the confusing, and often contradictory, news reports about new nutrition research. In spite of the fact that nutrition is an advanced science, many questions remain unanswered.

In this concept, some basic nutrition guidelines are presented to inform the reader and dispel various nutrition myths. A special section is presented on nutrition and physical performance to assist those interested in sports and high-level performance. If you are interested in learning more about nutrition than is covered here you are encouraged to seek the advice of a registered dietitian or to study reliable books, journals, or government documents (see Suggested Readings and Web Resources).

Guidelines for Healthy Eating

National dietary recommendations provide a target zone for healthy eating. www.mhhe.com/fit_well/web16 Click 01. About forty-five to fifty nutrients in food are believed to be essential for the body's growth, maintenance, and repair. These are classified into six categories: carbohydrates (and fiber), fats, proteins, vitamins, minerals, and water. The first three provide energy, which is measured in calories. Specific dietary recommendations for each of the six nutrients are presented later in this concept.

Recommended Dietary Allowances values published by the Food and Nutrition Board of the National Academy of Sciences have served as the standard for nutritional adequacy for the past two decades. Recently the academy, in partnership with Health Canada, recognized the need to provide more comprehensive information about nutrient needs that better reflect the current scientific information. To accommodate this need, the RDA are gradually being changed to a more functional set of dietary intake recommendations referred to as **Dietary Reference Intakes.** These guidelines include RDA values when adequate scientific information is available, and estimated **Adequate Intake (AI)** values when sufficient data aren't available to establish a firm RDA. The DRI values also include **Tolerable Upper Intake Levels (UL)** that reflect the maximum or highest level of daily intake a person can consume without adverse effects on health. The guidelines make it clear that while too little of a nutrient can be harmful to health, so can too much. In

Excessive Nutrient Intake (levels above UL may be harmful to health)
Tolerable Upper Limit (UL)
Healthy Eating Range or **Target Zone for Nutrition**
Threshold = Recommended Dietary Allowance (RDA) or Adequate Intake (AI)
Insufficient Nutrient Intake (low levels may be harmful to health)

Figure 1 ▶ Dietary Reference Intakes: How much is enough?

many ways the RDAs can be considered threshold values similar to the threshold of training values for physical activity. The Target Zone for healthy eating would range from the RDA/AI values to the UL values (see Figure 1).

A unique aspect of the DRI values is that they are categorized by function and classification in order to facilitate awareness of the different roles that nutrients play in the diet. Guidelines have already been established for bone building nutrients, B-complex vitamins, and the antioxidant nutrients. Guidelines for micronutrients, electrolytes and fluids, energy and macronutrients, and other food components are to be released in subsequent years. Table 1 includes the DRI values (including the UL values) for most of these nutrients along with examples of food sources of the various nutrients.

The quantity of nutrients recommended varies with age and other considerations; for example, young children need more calcium than adults and pregnant women or postmenopausal women need more calcium than other women. Accordingly dietary reference intakes, including RDAs, have been established for several age/gender groups. In this book, the values used are appropriate for most adult men and women.

Some foods contain some of all six classes of nutrients (e.g., whole wheat bread) whereas others contain only one (e.g., sugar). No food is a "complete" food because none contains all of the specific essential nutrients.

The levels of the food guide pyramid provide recommendations for servings of foods. www.mhhe.com/ fit_well/web16 click 02. The food guide pyramid (Figure 2) was designed to guide people in the selection of nutritious food. The typical adult consumes too much fat and too little carbohydrate, especially complex carbohydrates. Health goals want Americans to reduce the amount of dietary fat and increase the amount of complex carbohydrates in the diet. The food pyramid provides guidelines for how to fit these foods into an overall diet

plan. According to current guidelines, carbohydrates should account for 55 to 60 percent of a person's diet and this represents foods at the bottom two layers of the pyramid. Protein should compromise about 10 to 15 percent of the calories in the diet and this is provided by meat and dairy products at the third level of the pyramid. Fat should comprise about 30 percent of the calories in the diet and is found mainly in the third and fourth levels of the pyramid.

The U.S. Center for Nutrition Policy and Promotion (CNPP), which promotes the pyramid, has provided clear guidelines on what constitutes a serving. While portions of foods that you eat may vary, dietary guidelines are based on standard serving sizes (see Figure 2). By following the dietary guidelines and serving recommendations in the pyramid, a person is more likely to obtain the recommended percentages in their diet and meet the associated nutrient recommendations included in the DRI. Be aware that the guidelines are based on the assumption that a person would be eating a 2,000 calorie diet. Individuals on a low-calorie diet would need to eat nutritionally dense foods to be sure they are getting all of the necessary nutrients needed for good health.

Recommended Dietary Allowances (RDA) A dietary guideline that specifies the amount of a nutrient needed for almost all of the healthy individuals in a specific age and gender group.

Dietary Reference Intakes (DRI) A generic term used to describe appropriate amounts of nutrients in the diet (AI, RDA, and UL).

Adequate Intakes (AI) An alternate dietary guideline that is established experimentally to estimate nutrient needs when sufficient data are not available to establish an RDA value.

Tolerable Upper Intake Level (UL) A term used to describe the maximum level of a daily nutrient that will not pose a risk of adverse health effects for most people.

Table 1 ▶ Dietary Reference Intakes (DRI), Recommended Dietary Allowances (RDA), and Tolerable Upper Limit (UL) for major nutrients.

	DRI/RDA Males	DRI/RDA Females	UL	Function
B-Complex Vitamins				
Thiamin (mg/day)	1.2	1.1	ND	Co-enzyme for carbo & amino acid metabolism
Riboflavin (mg/day)	1.3	1.1	ND	Co-enzyme for metabolic reactions
Niacin (mg/day)	16	14	35	Co-enzyme for metabolic reactions
Vitamin B-6 (mg/day)	1.3	1.3	100	Co-enzyme for amino acid and glycogen reactions
Folate (ug/day)	400	400	1000	Metabolism of amino acids
Vitamin B-12 (ug/day)	2.4	2.4	ND	Co-enzyme for nucleic acid metabolism
Pantothenic Acid (mg/day)	5*	5*	ND	Co-enzyme for fat metabolism
Biotin (ug/day)	30*	30*	ND	Synthesis of fat, glycogen and amino acids
Choline (mg/day)	550*	425*	3500	Precursor to acetylcholine
Antioxidants and Related Nutrients				
Vitamin C (mg/day)	90	75	2000	Co-factor for reactions, antioxidant
Vitamin E (mg/day)	15	15	1000	Undetermined, mainly as antioxidant
Selenium (ug/day)	55	55	400	Defense against oxidative stress
Bone Building Nutrients				
Calcium	1000*	1000*	2500	Muscle contraction, nerve transmission
Phosphorous	700	700	3000	Maintenance of ph, storage of energy
Magnesium	400–420	310–320	350	Cofactor for enzyme reactions
Vitamin D	5*	5*	50	Maintain calcium and phosphorus levels
Flouride	4*	3*	10	Stimulates new bone formation
Micronutrients and Other Trace Elements				
Vitamin K	120*	90*	ND	Blood clotting and bone metabolism
Vitamin A	900	700	3000	Required for vision, immune function
Iron	8	18	45	Component of hemoglobin
Zinc	11	8	40	Component of enzymes and proteins
Energy and Macronutrients				
Carbohydrates (45–65%)	130g	130g	ND	Energy (only source of energy for the brain)
Fat (20–35%)	ND	ND	ND	Energy, carriers of vitamins
Protein (10–35%)	.8 g/kg	.8 g/kg	ND	Growth and maturation, tissue formation
Fiber	38 g/day*	25 g/day*	ND	Digestion, blood profiles

Note: These values reflect the dietary needs generally for adults aged 19–50 years old. Specific guidelines for other age groups are available from the Food and Nutrition Board of the National Academy of Science (www.iom.edu). Values for fluids and electrolytes have not been released yet. Values labeled with an asterisk (*) are based on Adequate Intake (AI) values rather than the RDA values. ND = not determined.

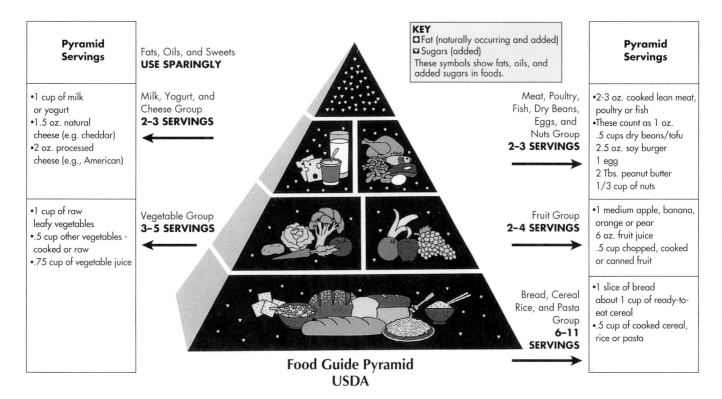

Figure 2 ▶ Food guide pyramid and sample serving sizes.

There are other models used to describe methods for helping people eat healthy nutritious diets. For example, the American Heart Association has adapted the pyramid to aid in selection of foods for heart disease prevention, a pyramid for older adults is now available, and in Canada the food guide is used to help people choose nutritious foods (see Appendix E).

🌐 **National dietary guidelines provide a sound plan for good nutrition.** www.mhhe.com/fit_well/ **web16 Click 03.** Federal law requires the publication of national dietary guidelines every five years. The most recent guidelines were published in 2000 (see Figure 3). These guidelines provide the basis for federal nutrition policy and nutrition education activities. They are also intended to provide advice to Americans about making healthy food choices. The current guidelines include more specific recommendations about maintaining a healthy weight and being physically active every day. The revised guidelines also differ from previous guidelines in making more specific suggestions about food selection. They recommend that consumers use the food pyramid to guide their food choices (as opposed to just eating a variety of foods) and also specifically recommend eating a variety of fruits and vegetables *daily*. The recommended percent of calories for each of the major food sources of dietary calories is shown in Figure 4.

*A*im for fitness...

• Aim for a healthy weight.

• Be physically active each day.

*B*uild a healthy base...

• Let the pyramid guide your food choices.

• Choose a variety of grains daily, especially whole grains.

• Choose a variety of fruits and vegetables daily.

• Keep food safe to eat.

*C*hoose sensibly...

• Choose a diet that is low in saturated fat and cholesterol and moderate in total fat.

• Choose beverages and foods to moderate your intake of sugars.

• Choose and prepare foods with less salt.

• If you drink alcoholic beverages, do so in moderation.

Figure 3 ▶ Dietary guidelines for Americans: The ABC's.
Source: U.S. Department of Agriculture.

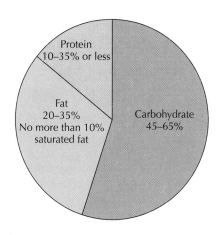

Figure 4 ▶ Recommended dietary intake.

Trends in eating patterns reveal both good and bad news about eating patterns in the United States. Over the past two to three decades, the percentage of calories from fat has decreased and the intake of fruits (up 19 percent), vegetables (up 22 percent) and grains (up 47 percent) has increased. Still, the number of servings of fruit now averages 1.5 per day, an amount lower than the recommended two servings per day. It is encouraging that vegetable

intake (3.6 per day) is above the recommended amount of three servings per day. Discouraging is the fact that nearly half of the vegetable intake is from potatoes and half of the potato intake is from French fries.

According to baseline figures from the U.S. Dietary Guidelines report, only 33 percent of people ages two and above meet the goal of eating no more than 30 percent of the diet as fat and 35 percent consume more than 10 percent saturated fat. For fruits and vegetables, the proportion of the population eating adequate servings is 40 percent and for grains 52 percent. Few Americans are eating the appropriate servings of fiber.

 Food labels provide consumers with detailed information to help make good food choices. www.mhhe.com/fit_well/web16 Click 04. Changes in food labeling laws have made it easier for consumers to know what is in the food they are eating (see Figure 5). The labels specify the amount of carbohydrates, fats, and proteins in the food and what percent contribution this food makes to the recommended daily value. The calculations are based on recommendations for people consuming about 2,000 calories per day. This is the normal calorie need for a moderately active college-age female. The

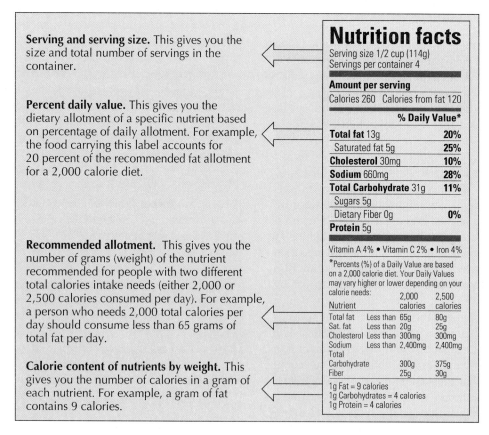

Figure 5 ▶ Using food labels.

Source: U.S. Food and Drug Administration.

tables also remind individuals that the allotments may vary if calorie needs are higher or lower. Calorie needs for active college men would tend to be higher (about 2,500–2,800 calories) so this should be considered when interpreting values from the tables.

An important aspect of the food labels is that they also provide information about the types of fats (e.g., saturated fat) and carbohydrates (e.g., simple sugars) that should be minimized in the diet as well as information on cholesterol and sodium. Food labeled as "fat-free" on the label must have less than one-half of a gram of fat per serving (50 grams). Foods labeled as "low fat" must have less than 3 grams per serving. To be labeled "low in saturated fat," a food must have less than 15 percent of its calories from saturated fat. Specific information on the different types of dietary nutrients are provided later in the concept.

Dietary Recommendations for Carbohydrates

For optimal health, carbohydrates should be the principal source of calories in the diet. www.mhhe.com/fit_well/web16 Click 05. Two major categories of carbohydrates differ in quality. Complex carbohydrates are known as starches and include fruits, vegetables, whole-grain breads, and cereals. These foods are nutritionally dense and also contain **cellulose** (a type of dietary **fiber**). Cellulose does not provide nutrition and is not digested but is considered essential for the bulk it provides for efficient digestion.

Simple carbohydrates are sugars such as sucrose, lactose, maltose, glucose, and fructose. They are low in nutritional density and are commonly found in foods considered to possess empty calories such as candy and soft drinks. The national dietary guidelines note that "the body cannot tell the difference between naturally occurring and added sugars because they are identical chemically." This statement was added to counter the public perception that some types of sugars are better than others. Foods high in simple carbohydrates do not, however, have the same benefits to health as do foods high in complex carbohydrates. Foods high in simple carbohydrates are often high in fat as well. Simple carbohydrates, especially sucrose, a sugar often found in candy and soft drinks, have also been shown to increase the incidence of dental caries. Sugar consumption, among people who have an adequate diet, is not a risk factor for diseases such as cancer and heart disease. Athletes and other active people who need supplemental calorie intake to maintain body weight may need to consume more carbohydrates, including simple carbohydrates, than people who are sedentary. Increasing carbohydrates in the diet is more desirable than supplementing proteins or consuming higher amounts of fat.

www.mhhe.com/fit_well/web16 click 06. Research evidence shows that diets high in complex carbohydrates such as whole-grain cereals, legumes, vegetables, and fruits are associated with a low incidence of lung, colon, esophagus, and stomach cancer as well as coronary heart disease. Some of this benefit may be due to the fact that complex carbohydrate diets are likely to be low in saturated fat. Water-soluble fiber, such as pectin and oat bran, has recently been shown to produce small reductions in total blood cholesterol, independent of the effects of reduced dietary fat. Long-term studies indicate that high-fiber diets may also be associated with a lower risk of diabetes mellitus, diverticulosis, hypertension, and gallstone formation. It is not known whether these health benefits are directly attributable to high dietary fiber or other effects associated with the ingestion of vegetables, fruits, and cereals in the diet. Complex carbohydrates may also be beneficial to health because they provide rich sources of vitamins and minerals. For the reasons mentioned earlier, the new dietary guidelines for Americans place a special emphasis on complex carbohydrates (see Figure 3). Since 1991, the amount of fiber in the diet has increased from 11 to 16 grams per day. This is still short of the 20 to 30 grams per day recommended by the National Cancer Institute. In concept 17, the glycemic index (GI) will be discussed. The GI can help you determine how different foods effect your blood sugar levels. Complex carbohydrates have lower GI levels than simple sugars. For example, all-bran cereal has GI of 60 and a donut has a GI of 108.

Some recommendations can be followed to assure healthy amounts of carbohydrates in the diet. The following list includes basic recommendations for carbohydrate content in the diet.

- Total carbohydrates in the diet should account for 55 percent or more of total calories consumed.
- Simple carbohydrates should be limited to 15 percent or less of total calories consumed, except for very active people.
- High-fiber foods should be included in the daily diet.

The following guidelines will help you implement these recommendations.

- Consume at least five servings of vegetables and/or fruits each day. Servings of green and yellow vegetables as well as citrus fruits are recommended. A serving of vegetables equals approximately one-half cup. A serving of fruit equals one medium-size piece.

Cellulose Indigestible fiber (bulk) in foods.

Fiber Indigestible bulk in foods that can be either soluble or insoluble in body fluids.

- Consume at least six servings a day of complex carbohydrates such as breads, cereals, and/or legumes. A serving of legumes or cereal equals approximately one-half cup. A serving of bread is one slice, one roll, or one muffin.
- Limit intake of desserts, baked goods, and other foods high in simple sugars or empty calories.
- Dietary fiber supplements other than in the form of food (such as oat bran) are not recommended unless prescribed for medical reasons.

Dietary Recommendations for Fat

Fat is an essential nutrient and provides an important energy source. www.mhhe.com/ fit_well/web16 Click 07. Humans need some fat in their diet because fats are carriers of vitamins A, D, E, and K. They are a source of essential linoleic acid, make food taste better, and provide a concentrated form of calories, which serve as an important source of energy during moderate to vigorous exercise. Fats have more than twice the calories per gram as carbohydrates.

There are several types of dietary fat. **Saturated fats** come primarily from animal sources such as red meat, dairy products, and eggs, but they are also found in some vegetable sources such as coconut and palm oils. **Unsaturated fats** are of two basic types: polyunsaturated and monounsaturated. Polyunsaturated fats are derived principally from vegetable sources such as safflower, cottonseed, soybean, sunflower, and corn oils (Omega-6 fats), and cold-water fish sources such as salmon and mackerel (Omega-3 fats). Monounsaturated fats are derived primarily from vegetable sources including olive, peanut, and canola oil.

Excess fat in the diet, particularly saturated fat, is associated with an increased risk of disease. Excessive total fat in the diet (particularly saturated fat) is associated with atherosclerotic cardiovascular diseases and breast, prostate, and colon cancer, as well as obesity. Excess saturated fat in the diet contributes to increased cholesterol, and increased LDL (low-density lipoprotein) cholesterol in the blood. For this reason, no more than 10 percent of your total calories should come from saturated fats.

Unsaturated fats are generally considered to be less likely to contribute to cardiovascular disease, cancer, and obesity than saturated fats. When polyunsaturated fats (Omega-6) are substituted for saturated fats, there is a reduction in total cholesterol and LDL cholesterol in the blood, but there may be a decrease in HDL (high-density lipoprotein) cholesterol as well. However, when monounsaturated fats are substituted for saturated fats, total cholesterol and LDL cholesterol are thought to decrease without an accompanying decrease in the desirable HDL. Limited evidence exists that Omega-3 unsaturated fats may inhibit cancers, but Omega-6 fats may not have the same effect. Fish oils have been shown to reduce triglyc-

erides, but no conclusive evidence exists that they are especially successful in reducing blood cholesterol.

Humans produce their own cholesterol even when dietary cholesterol is limited. Still, high dietary cholesterol can increase the risk of atherosclerosis and coronary heart disease. Principal sources of dietary cholesterol are organ meats, some shellfish, and egg yolks.

The 2000 Dietary Guidelines recommend a diet low in saturated fat and cholesterol but moderate in total fat. This distinction makes it clear that excess saturated fat is the main concern and also acknowledges the fact that some fat is necessary in the diet. While exceptionally low-fat diets (15 percent or lower) may be appropriate for those individuals at risk for heart disease or other health problems, such diets have been found to be harmful for the majority of the population, especially when used without supervision. For example, the evidence suggests that very low-fat diets may not provide adequate nutrients, may reduce HDL (the good cholesterol), and may increase some of the less desirable blood fats. A recent randomized clinical trial reported better long-term weight maintenance among dieters consuming moderate amounts of fat rather than low amounts. Exceptionally low-fat diets are also considered particularly unhealthy for pregnant women and young children.

Modified fats and fat substitutes in the diet can have varying health consequences. www. mhhe.com/fit_well/web16 Click 08. For decades, the public has been cautioned to avoid saturated fat. As a result, many people changed from eating butter—a product high in saturated fat—to margarine, a product typically made from vegetable products that are primarily unsaturated fat. Recent studies show that foods, such as margarine and shortening containing hydrogenated fats or **trans fatty acids** can result in greater total blood cholesterol levels and higher LDL levels. This suggests that food containing trans fatty acids should be limited in the diet. Recently, the FDA took action to require food labels to stipulate the amounts of trans fatty acids included in processed foods. Because of these developments, consumers were faced with decisions about which was the lesser of two evils, margarine or butter. A number of new margarines are on the market that contain little or no trans fatty acids (e.g., Smart Balance) and others that use all canola oil. These are probably the best options for individuals who use a spread and are concerned about cholesterol levels.

Olestra, approved several years ago by the FDA, is sometimes referred to as fake fat. It is a synthetic fat substitute in foods that passes through the gastrointestinal system without being digested. Thus, foods cooked with Olestra have fewer calories. For example, a chocolate chip cookie cooked in a normal way would have 138 calories, but an Olestra cookie would have 63. One ounce of normal potato chips contains 160 calories, but the same amount prepared using Olestra has 70. Many consumer groups opposed the approval of Olestra because it has possible side effects. A warning label must be included on this product noting these possible effects. The label reads: *"This product contains Olestra. Olestra may cause abdominal cramping and loose stools. Olestra inhibits the absorption of some vitamins and other nutrients. Vitamins A, D, E, and K have been added."* Research conducted after several years of product use led to a recent decision by the FDA that there is a "reasonable certainty of no harm" from Olestra use. Fears of significant gastrointestinal problems among large numbers of users did not materialize; however, some are still concerned about widespread use of Olestra. Some consumer groups warn that promotion of Olestra-containing products may make individuals more likely to snack on less energy-dense snack foods. They also express concern that Olestra inhibits absorption of many naturally occurring antioxidants which have been shown to have many beneficial effects on health. One thing is certain, the only potential benefit from Olestra is to reduce calories and fat in the diet. If it does not do this, as many experts expect it will not, it will not enhance your diet. Though all people do not experience side effects, some do.

Several other new products offer potential to modify the amount and effect of dietary fat in our diets. The first is a naturally occurring compound which is included in several new margarines (Benecol and Take Control). The active ingredient in this compound (sitostanol ester) comes from pine trees and has been shown to reduce total and LDL cholesterol in the blood. Several clinical trials have confirmed that these margarines are both safe and effective in lowering cholesterol levels. The products must be used regularly to be effective and may only be useful in individuals with high levels of cholesterol. Food products that

contain these specific medically beneficial compounds are often referred to as neutraceuticals or functional foods because they are a combination of pharmaceuticals and food. Debate continues as to whether this type of product will be regulated by the FDA as a drug or will be classified as a food supplement and not be regulated by FDA. Decisions on these products will, no doubt, influence the way similar neutraceuticals will be regulated in the future. If and when these products are widely used in the United States, nutrition experts will be interested to see if these products have health benefits for Americans and whether it will satisfy their tastes.

The second product that will soon appear is another fake fat. This product will be sold under the name Z-Trim. It is made exclusively from the hulls of various grains (oats, soybeans, corn, and wheat). This product has also been shown to reduce cholesterol, particularly LDL cholesterol (the bad cholesterol). Unlike other products marketed by large food or pharmaceutical companies, all proceeds will go to the federal government because it was developed by the United States Department of Agriculture. It is expected that this product will appear in foods such as cookies, cakes, and other baked items.

Some recommendations can be followed to assure healthy amounts of fat in the diet. The following list includes basic recommendations for fat content in the diet.

- Total fat in the diet should consist of no more than 30 percent of the total calories consumed.
- Saturated fat in the diet should be no more than 10 percent of total calories consumed.
- Polyunsaturated and monounsaturated fats should be substituted for saturated fat in the diet.
- Dietary cholesterol should be limited to 300 milligrams per day.

The following guidelines will help you implement the recommendations above.

- Substitute lean meat, fish, poultry, nonfat milk, and other low-fat dairy products for high-fat foods.
- Reduce intake of fried foods, especially those cooked in saturated fats (often true of fast-food restaurants),

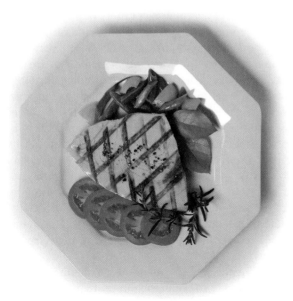

Broiled foods have less fat than fried foods.

Saturated Fat Dietary fat that is usually solid at room temperature and comes primarily from animal sources.

Unsaturated Fat Monounsaturated or polyunsaturated fat that is usually liquid at room temperature and comes primarily from vegetable sources.

Trans Fatty Acids Fats that result when liquid oil has hydrogen added to it to make it more solid. Hydrogenation transforms unsaturated fats so that they take on characteristics of saturated fats, as is the case for margarine and shortening.

desserts with high levels of fat (many cookies and cakes), and dressings with high-fat ingredients.

- Limit dietary intake of foods high in cholesterol such as egg yolks, organ meats, and shellfish.
- Use monounsaturated or polyunsaturated fats for cooking.
- Limit the amount of trans fatty acids in the diet and in cooking.
- Though two or three servings of fish per week may be prudent because of its content of Omega-3 polyunsaturated oils, there is not sufficient evidence to endorse a fish oil dietary supplement.
- Be careful of the total elimination of a single food source from the diet. For example, the elimination of meat and dairy products could result in iron or calcium deficiencies, especially among women and children.

Dietary Recommendations for Proteins

Protein is the basic building block for the body, but dietary protein constitutes a relatively small amount of daily caloric intake. Proteins are often referred to as the building blocks of your body because all body cells are made of protein. Proteins are formed from twenty different **amino acids.** More than 100 proteins are made of amino acids. Eleven of these amino acids can be synthesized from other nutrients, but nine **essential amino acids** must be obtained directly from the diet. Certain foods, called complete proteins, contain all of the essential amino acids, along with most of the others. Examples of complete proteins are meat, dairy products, and fish. Incomplete proteins contain some, but not all, of the essential amino acids. Examples of incomplete proteins are beans, nuts, and rice.

One way to identify amino acids is the *-ine* at the end of their name. For example, arginine and lysine are two of the amino acids that have received recent attention in the press. Only three of the twenty amino acids do not have the *-ine* suffix. They are aspartic acid, glutamic acid, and tryptophan.

All of the amino acids can be obtained from food, and recommended amounts are essential to good health (see Figure 6). Experts agree that there are no known benefits and some possible risks to consuming diets exceptionally high in animal protein. Certain cancers and coronary heart disease risk have been associated with high dietary intake of animal protein. Researchers are not certain whether the increased risk of contracting these diseases is because of the protein itself or because diets high in animal protein are also high in fat. High-protein diets are also damaging on the kidneys as the body must process a lot of extra nitrogen. Excessive protein intake can lead to urinary calcium loss, which can weaken bones and lead to osteoporosis.

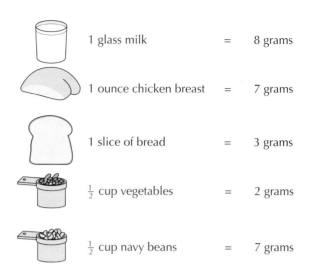

1 glass milk	=	8 grams
1 ounce chicken breast	=	7 grams
1 slice of bread	=	3 grams
½ cup vegetables	=	2 grams
½ cup navy beans	=	7 grams

Figure 6 ▶ Protein content of various foods.
Source: Williams, M.

While excessive protein is harmful, it is not our intent to suggest that animal protein should not be part of the normal diet. Rather, consumption of animal protein can be restricted somewhat, especially when fat content is high. Because of problems associated with excessive protein intake and health problems encountered by people who have used protein supplements, the latter are not recommended. In fact, many of the more serious health problems resulting from the consumption of dietary supplements are associated with excessive protein intake. More information concerning high-protein diets and protein supplements is included later in this concept and in the concept on managing diet and activity.

Vegetarian diets may provide sufficient protein but care must be used. Vegetarian diets provide ample sources of protein as long as a variety of protein-rich food sources are included in the diet. The American Dietetics Association recently published a Position Stand which documents that well-planned vegetarian diets "are appropriate for all stages of the life cycle, including during pregnancy, and lactation," and can ". . . satisfy the nutrient needs of infants, children, and adolescents." You can get enough protein as long as the variety and amounts of foods consumed are adequate." It is noted that **vegans** must supplement the diet with vitamin B$_{12}$ because this vitamin's only source is animal foods. **Lacto-ovo vegetarians** do not have the same concerns. The guidelines also emphasize the need for vegans to take care that, especially for children, adequate vitamin D and calcium are contained in the diet because most people get these nutrients from milk products.

People who eat a variety of foods including meat, dairy products, eggs, and plants rich in protein virtually always eat more protein than the body needs. Eating various foods assures that all essential amino acids are consumed.

Because of problems associated with excessive protein intake and health problems encountered by people who have used protein supplements, the latter are not recommended. In fact, many of the more serious health problems resulting from the consumption of dietary supplements are associated with excessive protein intake. More information concerning high-protein diets and protein supplements is included later in this concept and in the concept on managing diet and activity.

 Some recommendations can be followed to assure healthy amounts of protein in the diet. www.mhhe.com/fit_well/web16 Click 09. The following list includes basic recommendations for protein content.

- Protein in the diet should account for 10 to 15 percent of the total calories consumed.
- Protein in the diet should meet the RDA of 0.8 grams per kilogram (2.2 pounds) of a person's desirable weight. This is about 36 grams for a 100-pound person.
- Generally, protein in the diet should not exceed twice the RDA (1.6 grams per kilogram of a person's desirable weight).
- Vegetarians (people who severely limit the intake of animal products) must be especially careful to eat combinations of foods that assure adequate intake of essential amino acids, and vegans should supplement their diets with vitamin B_{12}.

The following guidelines will help you implement these recommendations.

- Consume at least two servings a day of lean meat, fish, poultry, and dairy products (especially those low in fat content) or adequate combinations of foods such as beans, nuts, grains, and rice in the diet.
- Dietary supplements of protein such as tablets and powders are not recommended (see section later in this concept and the concept on managing diet).

Dietary Recommendations for Vitamins

Adequate vitamin intake is necessary to good health and wellness, but excessive vitamin intake is not necessary and can be harmful. Consuming foods containing the minimum RDA of each of the vitamins is essential to the prevention of disease and maintenance of good health (see Table 1). Consuming foods high in carotinoid and retinoid is recommended because these foods are associated with the reduced risk of some forms of cancer. Carotinoid- and retinoid-rich foods such as green and yellow vegetables (carrots and sweet potatoes) contain high amounts of vitamin A. Diets high in vitamin C (citrus fruits and vegetables) and vitamin E (green leafy vegetables) are also associated with reduced risk of cancer. One recent study indicated that diets high in vitamin E are associated with reduced risk of heart disease. It has been hypothesized that vitamins C, E, and carotenoid-rich foods act as **antioxidants,** which help prevent cancer and other forms of disease. Most experts point out that selecting more servings from the second level of the food pyramid is wise, but they express caution concerning the use of vitamin supplements.

Nevertheless, a number of respected health and wellness publications and popular books have advocated antioxidant supplements, including beta-carotene (a plant product that is converted to vitamin A in the body) and vitamins C and E, to protect the body from cell-damaging free radicals resulting from environmental pollution. These publications also assumed that supplements of these vitamins had the same health effect as consuming good food high in vitamin content. Several very recent large-scale studies have shown either no benefit from beta-carotene supplements or have shown that the supplements may have negative effects. Another recent study of over 20,000 people failed to find health benefits associated with taking a daily mixture of antioxidants including vitamin E (600 IU), vitamin C (250 mg), and beta-carotene (20 mg). Individuals in the study had no lower risk for heart disease than participants taking the placebo. Additional studies are needed to confirm these findings in other populations so some experts still recommend vitamin E supplements.

While supplements have not proven to be highly effective, the benefits of antioxidants for good health are still clear. It is now accepted that there may be other beneficial substances in foods that have not been isolated or that must be consumed naturally. The initial studies suggesting

Amino Acids Twenty basic building blocks of the body that make up proteins.

Essential Amino Acids Nine basic amino acids that the human body cannot produce and that must be obtained from food sources.

Vegan A strict vegetarian who not only excludes all forms of meat from the diet but also excludes dairy products and eggs.

Lacto-ovo Vegetarians A vegetarian who includes dairy and eggs in the diet.

Antioxidants Vitamins that are thought to inactivate "activated oxygen molecules," sometimes called free radicals. Free radicals are naturally created by human cells but are also caused by environmental factors such as smoke and radiation. Free radicals may cause cell damage that leads to diseases of various kinds. Antioxidants may inactivate the free radicals before they do their damage.

Table 2 ▶ Top Ten Antioxidant All-Stars

	C (mg)	Beta Carotine (mg)	E (mg)	Folacin (mg)
Broccoli (1/2 cup cooked)	49	0.7	0.9	53
Cantaloupe (1 cup cubed)	68	3.1	0.3	17
Carrot (1 medium)	7	12.2	0.3	10
Kale (1/2 cup cooked)	27	2.9	3.7	9
Mango (1 medium)	57	4.8	2.3	31
Pumpkin (1/2 cup canned)	5	10.5	1.1	15
Red bell pepper (1/2 cup raw)	95	1.7	0.3	8
Spinach (1/2 cup cooked)	9	4.4	2.0	131
Strawberries (1 cup)	86	—	0.3	26
Sweet potato (1 medium, cooked)	28	14.9	5.5	26
Adult RDA or suggested intake	60	5–6	8–10	180–200

Runners-up: Brussels sprouts, all citrus fruits, tomatoes, potatoes, other berries, other leafy greens (dandelion, turnip, and mustard greens, swiss chard, arugula), cauliflower, green pepper, asparagus, peas, beets, and winter squash.

Source: *University of California at Berkeley Wellness Letter*

possible benefits of antioxidants were based on studies that compared the amounts of fruits and vegetables consumed so the best bet is just to include more fruits and vegetables in your diet. This is the recommendation in the Dietary Guidelines for Americans which emphasize "good food" rather than food supplements. Some foods that are especially rich in vitamins and minerals are considered nutrition "all-stars" and make good dietary choices (see Table 2).

Fortification of foods has been used to ensure adequate vitamin intake in the population. National policy requires many foods to be fortified. National policy dictates that milk be fortified with vitamin D, low-fat milk with vitamins A and D, and margarine with vitamin A. These foods were selected because they are common food sources for growing children. Many common grain products are now fortified with folic acid because low folic acid levels increase the risk of birth defects in babies. Fortification was considered essential since more than half of all women do not consume adequate amounts of folic acid in the diet during the first months of gestation (before most women even realize they are pregnant). A recent national study published in *Journal of the American Medical Association (JAMA)* reported that the prevalence of neural tube defects decreased by 19 percent compared to prefortification years (before 1996). Though factors other than fortification may have contributed to this decline, the study supports the benefits of fortification for improving nutritional intakes.

Taking a daily multiple vitamin supplement may be a good idea. Sometimes supplements are needed to meet specific nutrient requirements for specific groups. For example, older people may need a vitamin D supplement if they get little exposure to sunlight, and iron supplements are often recommended for pregnant women. Daily vitamin supplements at or below the RDA are considered safe; however, excess doses of vitamins can cause health problems. For example, excessively high amounts of vitamin C are dangerous for the 10 percent of the population who inherit a special gene related to health problems. Excessively high amounts of vitamin D are toxic, and mothers who take too much vitamin A risk birth defects to unborn children.

www.mhhe.com/fit_well/web16 Click 10. Eating a variety of foods (as recommended in the food guide pyramid) should ensure an adequate amount of vitamins in the diet but the majority of the population has an inadequate diet. Vitamin intake would be especially poor in individuals who avoid certain foods (e.g., limit fats or carbohydrates) or who make poor food choices (e.g., eating a lot of processed foods or few fruits and vegetables). Therefore, a daily multivitamin may be a good way to ensure adequate vitamin intake. A highly publicized article in the *JAMA* recently encouraged physicians to recommend daily multivitamin supplements as a normal part of their counseling. Some guidelines for selecting supplements is presented in Table 3.

Table 3 ▶ Issues to Consider Regarding the Use of Vitamin and Mineral Supplements
• Limit the use of supplements unless warranted because of a health problem or a specific lack of nutrients in the diet.
• If you decide that supplementation is necessary, select a multivitamin/mineral supplement that contains micronutrients in amounts close to the recommended levels (e.g., "One-a-day" type supplements).
• If your diet is specifically deficient in a particular mineral (e.g., calcium or iron), it may be necessary to also incorporate dietary sources or an additional mineral supplement since most multivitamins do not contain the recommended daily amount of minerals.
• Choose supplements that provide between 50 to 100 percent of the AI or RDA and avoid those that provide many times the recommended amount. The use of supplements that hype "mega-doses" or vitamins and minerals can increase the risk of some unwanted nutrient interactions and possible toxic effects.
• Buy supplements from a reputable company and look for supplements that carry the U. S. Pharmocopoeia (USP) notation (www.usp.org).

Guidelines are based on recommendations by Manore (2001).

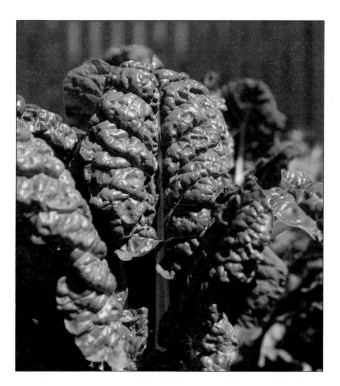

Green leafy vegetables and low-fat milk are good sources of calcium.

Some recommendations can be followed to assure healthy amounts of vitamins in the diet. The following list includes basic recommendations for vitamin content in the diet.

- Vitamins in the amounts equal to the RDAs should be included in the diet each day.

The following guidelines will help you implement these recommendations.

- A diet containing the food servings recommended for carbohydrates, proteins, and fats will more than meet the RDA standards.
- Extra servings of green and yellow vegetables, citrus and other fruits, and other non-animal food sources high in fiber, vitamins, and minerals are wise (especially foods from the nutrition all-stars).
- People who eat a sound diet as described in this concept do not need a vitamin supplement. When UL values are established for all vitamins it will be easier to determine how much is too much for any and all vitamins. Daily vitamin supplements may be appropriate for those who restrict calories. In the meantime, those who choose to take a supplement are advised not to take daily amounts larger than the RDA. The guidelines suggested in Table 3 should be considered before taking any supplement.
- People with special needs should seek medical advice before selecting supplements and should inform medical personnel as to amounts and content of all supplements (vitamin or other).

Dietary Recommendations for Minerals

Adequate mineral intake is necessary for good health and wellness, but excessive mineral intake is not necessary and can be harmful. Like vitamins, minerals have no calories and provide no energy for the body. They are important in regulating various bodily functions. Two particularly important minerals are calcium and iron. Calcium is important to bone, muscle, nerve, blood development and function, and has been associated with reduced risk of heart disease. Iron is necessary for the blood to carry adequate oxygen. Other important minerals are the following: phosphorus, which builds teeth and bones; sodium, which regulates water in the body; zinc, which aids in the healing process; and potassium, which is necessary for proper muscle function.

RDAs for minerals are established to determine the amounts of each necessary for healthy daily functioning. A sound diet provides all of the RDA for minerals. Evidence indicating that some segments of the population may be mineral-deficient have led to the establishment of health goals identifying a need to increase mineral intake for some segments of the population.

A recent National Institutes of Health (NIH) consensus statement indicates that a large percentage of Americans fail to get enough calcium in their diet and emphasizes the need for increased calcium—particularly for women who are pregnant, post-menopausal women, and people over sixty-five who need 1,500 mg/day, which is higher than previous RDA amounts. The NIH has indicated that a total intake of 2,000 mg/day of calcium is safe and that adequate vitamin D in the diet is necessary for optimal calcium absorption to take place. Though getting these amounts in a calcium-rich diet is best, calcium supplementation for those not eating properly seems wise. Many multivitamins do not contain enough calcium for some special classes of people so some may want to consider additional calcium. Check with your physician or a dietitian before you consider a supplement because individual needs vary.

One national health goal is to reduce the proportion of people who consume more than recommended amounts of sodium (2,400 mg per day) and sodium chloride or table salt (6 grams a day). Some researchers have questioned the relationship between sodium intake and health especially among apparently healthy adults. The conventional wisdom is that excessive sodium intake is especially problematic among people with high blood pressure. Salt intake up to recommended amounts is necessary for good health. Beyond those amounts, no apparent benefit exists, so restriction of salt consistent with national goals seems wise. Because many fast foods have high salt, many people in our culture consume amounts well above the recommended levels. Currently, 79 percent of the population exceeds these amounts.

Another concern is iron deficiency among very young children and women of child-bearing age. Low iron may be a special problem for women taking birth control pills because the combination of low iron levels and birth control pills has been associated with depression and generalized fatigue. Eating the appropriate number of servings from the food pyramid provides all the minerals necessary for meeting the RDA for minerals. Nutrition goals for the nation emphasize the importance of adequate servings of foods rich in calcium, such as green leafy vegetables and milk products; adequate servings of foods rich in iron, such as beans, peas, spinach, or meat; and reduced salt in the diet.

Some recommendations can be followed to assure healthy amounts of minerals in the diet. The following list includes basic recommendations for mineral content in the diet.

- Minerals in amounts equal to the RDAs should be consumed in the diet each day.
- In general, a calcium dietary supplement is not recommended for the general population; however, supplements may be appropriate for adults who do not eat well (up to 1,000 mg/day). For post-menopausal women, a calcium supplement is recommended (up to 1,500 mg/day for those who do not eat well). A supplement may also be appropriate for people who restrict

calories but RDA values should not be exceeded unless the person consults with a registered dietitian or a physician.
- Salt should be limited in the diet to no more than 4 to 6 grams per day, and even less would be desirable (3 grams). Three grams equals one teaspoon of table salt.

The following guidelines will help you implement these recommendations.

- A diet containing the food servings recommended for carbohydrates, proteins, and fats will more than meet the RDA standards.
- Extra servings of green and yellow vegetables, citrus and other fruits, and other non-animal sources of foods high in fiber, vitamins, and minerals are recommended as a substitute for high-fat foods.

Dietary Recommendations for Water and Other Fluids

Water is a critical component in the healthy diet. Though water is not in the food pyramid because it contains no calories, provides no energy, and provides no key nutrients, it is crucial to health and survival. Water is a major component of most of the foods you eat, and more than half of all body tissues are composed of it. Regular water intake maintains water balance and is critical to many important bodily functions. Though a variety of fluid replacement beverages are available for use during and following exercise, replacing water is the primary need.

Beverages other than water are a part of many diets. Some beverages can have an adverse effect on good health. Coffee, tea, soft drinks, and alcoholic beverages are often substituted for water in the diet. Too much caffeine consumption has been shown to cause symptoms such as irregular heartbeat in some people. Tea has not been shown to have similar effects, though this may be because tea drinkers typically consume less volume than coffee drinkers, and tea has less caffeine per cup than coffee. Both beverages contain caffeine, as do many soft drinks, though drip coffee typically contains two to three times the caffeine of a typical cola drink.

Excessive consumption of alcoholic beverages can have negative health implications because the alcohol often replaces nutrients. Excessive alcohol consumption is associated with the increased risk of heart disease, high blood pressure, stroke, and osteoporosis. Long-term excessive alcoholic beverage consumption leads to cirrhosis of the liver and to the increased risk of hepatitis and cancer. Alcohol consumption during pregnancy can result in low birth weight, fetal alcoholism, and other damage to the fetus. The National Dietary Guidelines indicate that alcohol used in moderation can "enhance the enjoyment of meals" and is associated with a lower risk of coronary heart disease for some individuals.

Some recommendations can be followed to assure healthy amounts of water and other fluids in the diet. The following list includes basic recommendations for water and other fluids in the diet.

- In addition to foods containing water, the average adult needs about eight glasses (8 ounces each) of water every day. Water intake must be increased even more for active people and those who exercise in hot environments.
- Coffee, tea, and soft drinks should not be substituted for water and/or other beverages or foods such as low-fat milk, fruit juices, or foods rich in calcium, which provide sources of key nutrients.
- Limit daily servings of beverages containing caffeine to no more than three.
- If you are an adult and you choose to drink alcohol, do so in moderation. The latest dietary guidelines for Americans indicate that moderation includes no more than one drink per day for women and no more than two drinks per day for men (one drink equals 12 ounces of regular beer, 5 ounces of wine—small glass, or one average-size cocktail—1.5 ounces of 80 proof alcohol).

Technology Update

Public interest in nutrition and computer technology has led to the development of many computerized nutrition analysis programs. Most early programs were either too expensive or not comprehensive enough to be of use. The (CNPP) has recently made their interactive healthy eating index (HEI) available online for free use by consumers. This online dietary assessment uses the most comprehensive database of foods available and features an easy to use interface to enter your foods. After providing a day's worth of dietary information, you will receive a "score" on the overall quality of your diet for that day. This score looks at the types and amounts of food you ate as compared to those recommended by the food guide pyramid. It also tells you how much total fat, saturated fat, cholesterol, and sodium you have in your diet. Each HEI score gives you an idea of the quality of your diet from what you ate: for one day or for up to twenty days. The HEI program is based on the Healthy Eating Index developed by the USDA to study how well the American diet complies with the recommendations of the Dietary Guidelines for Americans and the food guide pyramid. To access this resource and information, go to the CNPP website and click on Interactive Eating Index.

Sound Eating Practices

Healthy snacks can be an important part of good nutrition. Snacking is not necessarily bad. For people interested in losing or maintaining their current weight, small snacks of appropriate foods can help fool the appetite. For people interested in gaining weight, snacks can provide additional calories. For people trying to maintain or lose weight, the calories consumed in snacks will probably necessitate limiting the calories consumed at meals. The key is proper selection of the foods for snacking.

As with your total diet, the best snacks are nutritionally dense. Too often, snacks are high in calories, fats, simple sugar, and salt. Check the content of snacks. Even foods sold as "healthy snacks," such as granola bars, are often high in fat and simple sugar. Some common snacks such as chips, pretzels, and even popcorn may be high in salt and may be cooked in fat.

Some suggestions for healthy snacks include ice milk (instead of ice cream), fresh fruits, vegetable sticks, popcorn not cooked in fat and with little or no salt, crackers, and nuts with little or no salt.

Consistency (with variety) is a good general rule of nutrition. Eating regular meals every day, including a good breakfast, is wise. Many studies have shown breakfast to be an important meal. One-fourth of the day's calories should be consumed at breakfast. Skipping breakfast impairs performance because blood sugar levels drop in the long period between dinner the night before and lunch the following day. Eating every four to six hours is wise.

Moderation is a good general rule of nutrition. Just as too little food can cause problems, excessive intake of various nutrients can cause problems. More is not always better. Moderation (neither too much nor too little) in choices of foods is advised.

You do not have to permanently eliminate foods that you really enjoy, but some of your favorite foods may not be among the best of choices. Enjoying special foods on occasion is part of moderation. The key is to limit choices of foods high in "empty calories."

Considerable evidence has accumulated to indicate that the size of portions has increased in recent years. Large portions are featured in advertising campaigns to lure customers. Cafeteria-style restaurants (and others) sometimes offer all you can eat for a specific price encouraging large portions. Reducing the size of portions is very important when eating out and at home (see concept 17 for more information).

Careful selection of food choices is important for people who rely on fast foods as a significant part of their diet. More Americans rely on fast foods as part of their normal diet. Unfortunately, many fast foods are poor nutritional choices. Many hamburgers are high in fat. French fries are high in fat because they are usually cooked in saturated fat. Even choices deemed to be more nutritious, such as chicken or fish sandwiches, are often high in fat and calories because they are cooked in fat and covered with special high-fat/high-calorie sauces. Become informed about the content of fast foods before you make your selection. Some guidelines for selection of foods are provided in the concept on managing diet. Nutritional analyses for various fast foods are presented in Appendix E. Also fast foods are discussed in more detail in concept 17.

Nutrition and Physical Performance

Some basic dietary guidelines exist for active people. In general, the nutrition rules described in this concept apply to all people, whether active or sedentary, but some additional nutrition facts are important for exercisers and athletes. Because active people often expend calories in amounts considerably above normal, extra calories are needed in the diet. To avoid excess fat and protein, complex carbohydrates should constitute as much as 70 percent of total calorie intake. A higher amount of protein is generally recommended for active individuals (1.2 grams per kg of body weight) because some protein is used as an energy source during exercise. This extra amount is easily obtained through the additional calories that are consumed. Protein levels above 15 percent of the diet are typically not necessary.

Carbohydrate loading and carbohydrate replacement during exercise can enhance sustained aerobic performances. www.mhhe.com/fit_well/web16 Click 11. Athletes and vigorously active people must maintain a high level of readily available fuel, especially in the muscles. Adequate complex carbohydrate consumption is the best way to assure this.

Prior to an activity that will require extended duration of physical performance (more than one hour in length, such as a marathon), **carbohydrate loading** can be useful. Carbohydrate loading is accomplished by resting one or two days before the event and eating a higher than normal amount of complex carbohydrates. This helps to build up maximum levels of stored carbohydrate (**glycogen**) in the muscles and liver so they can be used during exercise. The key in carbohydrate loading is not necessarily to overeat but rather to eat a higher percentage of carbohydrates than normal.

Ingesting carbohydrate solutions during long, sustained exercise can also aid performance by preventing or forestalling muscle glycogen depletion. Drinking fluids that have no more than 6 to 8 percent sugar helps prevent dehydration and replenishes energy stores. Fluid replacement drinks containing 6 to 8 percent carbohydrates are helpful in preventing dehydration and replacing energy stores. A number of companies also make concentrated carbohydrate gels that deliver carbohydrates (generally ~ 80 percent complex, 20 percent simple) in a format that your body can absorb quickly for energy. Examples are PowerGel and Gu. Energy bars such as Powerbars or Clif bars are also commonly used during or after exercise to enhance energy stores. The Powerbar version provides about 100 calories of carbohydrates derived from maltodextrin, brown rice, and oat bran to provide a slow release of energy during exercise. The various carbohydrate supplements have been shown to be effective for exercise sessions lasting over an hour and also are good for replacing glycogen stores after exercise. Studies show that consuming carbohydrates 15 to 30 minutes following exercise can aid in rapid replenishment of muscle glycogen which may enhance future performance or training sessions.

These supplements would have little benefit for shorter bouts of exercise. Because they contain considerable calories they would not be recommended for individuals primarily interested in weight control.

The timing may be more important than the makeup of the pre-event meal. If you are racing or doing high-level exercise early in the morning, eat a small meal prior to starting. Eat about three hours before competition or

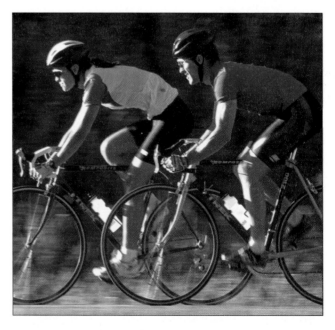

Good nutrition is essential for active people.

Table 4 ▶ Some Commonly Misrepresented Dietary Supplements Alleged to Enhance Performance

Product	Claim	The Facts
Plant steroids	• Alleged to promote muscle development similar to animal steroids.	• Plant steroids do not promote muscle mass gains in humans. One plant product is a steroid precursor (androstenedione*).
Trace elements (e.g., chromium picolinate)	• Alleged to promote muscle development.	• No evidence of effectiveness. It could lead to anemia if taken in excess. One recent study indicates possible link to cancer and chromosome damage.
Amino acids (e.g., arginine, lysine)	• Alleged to promote increases in human growth hormone that lead to increased muscle mass.	• Some evidence that increased HGH* results from intake of amino acids, but little evidence of resulting muscle mass increases. • There is risk in taking the high doses recommended by sellers. Banned in Canada.
Protein supplements	• Alleged muscle mass gains.	• No evidence of effectiveness; some are not digestible. Not superior to dietary protein as some claim, and far more costly. Overuse can lead to excess loss of body water, diarrhea, abdominal cramps, and altered kidney function.
Caffeine	• Alleged to enhance endurance performance.	• Inconsistent results. Banned by Olympic rules. Some negative health consequences. Can cause dehydration.
Vitamin supplements (e.g., B complex, B_{15})	• Alleged stress reduction and performance enhancement.	• No evidence of benefits to those who are not vitamin deficient. B_{15} (pangamic acid) is not a vitamin and can be harmful. No evidence of stress-reducing effects.
Minerals (e.g., iron)	• Alleged that athletes and active people need more than other people.	• Some evidence that active people have increased need, but the consensus is that a sound diet provides for those needs.
Hormones (e.g., melatonin)	• Claims to enhance sex life, combat aging, and reduce disease risk.	• Effects not known, especially long term. All sales banned in some European countries; a prescription is required in Canada. Hormones are powerful substances that can produce unexpected results. Actual content of product is not regulated, so there is no certainty of content. Users are considered to be "human guinea pigs" by some experts.

Note: FDA standards have not been set for many advertised products. For this reason, consumer cannot be assured of the exact content of products, and product safety cannot be assured. This is illustrated by the recall of products containing the amino acid L-tryptophan after the deaths of 32 people were linked to its use.

*For more information on these supplements, see the concept on muscle fitness.

heavy exercise to allow time for digestion. Generally, the athlete can make his or her food selection on the basis of past experience but easily digested carbohydrates are best. Generally, fat intake should be minimal because it digests more slowly; proteins and high-cellulose foods should be kept to a moderate amount prior to prolonged events to avoid urinary and bowel excretion. Drinking two or three cups of liquid will ensure adequate hydration.

Consuming simple carbohydrates (sugar, candy) within an hour or two of an event is not recommended because it may cause an insulin response that results in weakness and fatigue, or may cause stomach distress, cramps, or nausea.

High-protein diets for active people and athletes have been questioned by leading organizations in the areas of health, physical activity, and nutrition. In recent years, several books have recommended high-protein/low-carbohydrate diets for active people and for those interested in improving athletic performance. A common high-protein diet is often referred to as the 40/30/30 diet because it recommends 40 percent carbohydrates, 30 percent proteins, and 30 percent fat. The 40/30/30 plan is well above the national recommendation for protein of 10 to 15 percent and well below the 55 to 60 percent recommendation for carbohydrates.

The American College of Sports Medicine (ACSM), the American Dietetic Association (ADA), and several other groups (see Suggested Readings) have challenged the soundness of the 40/30/30 diet. They note that claims of books promoting high-protein diets are often based on unfounded ideas and oversimplification of the

Carbohydrate Loading Extra consumption of complex carbohydrates in the days prior to a long, sustained performance.

Glycogen A source of energy stored in the muscles and liver that is necessary for sustained physical activity.

facts. Some false claims and correct facts about high-protein diets are described in greater detail in the concept on managing diet. Most athletes need more carbohydrates in the diet, not fewer. As noted earlier, athletes get the extra protein they need by consuming extra calories; thus, 10 to 15 percent of the diet as protein is adequate to meet their needs. Contrary to popular opinion, extra protein (more than 15 percent) does not result in extra muscle development.

People who are interested in enhancing physical performance are especially subject to nutrition quackery. A food or nutrition product thought to enhance performance is considered to be an **ergogenic aid.** Many so-called ergogenic aids can be classified as quack products because they do not enhance performance as promised and are often exceptionally expensive. In some cases, so-called performance-enhancing supplements are dangerous to health and wellness. Examples of products that are misrepresented in terms of potential performance-enhancing benefits are dietary supplements such as vitamins, minerals, proteins and amino acids, and plant steroids. Among the most-often misrepresented products are protein and amino acid supplements, sometimes referred to as "steroid alternatives." Table 4 lists some of these.

Recent legislation designed to regulate food supplements has not been effective in protecting the consumer. The Dietary Supplements Health and Education Act was passed in 1994. It was considered by many experts to be a compromise between health food manufacturers who wanted no regulation of dietary supplements (such as vitamins, minerals, proteins, and herbs) and those who wanted strict control of these substances. Many nutrition experts now feel that the act is responsible for an explosion in sales of products that have not been proven to be effective. A more detailed discussion of nutrition supplements is included in the concept on quackery.

Strategies for Action

An analysis of your current diet is a good first step in making future decisions about what you eat. In Lab 16A, you will have an opportunity to analyze your current diet. Many experts recommend keeping a log of what you eat for at least a week if you are to get a good picture of your typical eating patterns. You will be given the opportunity to analyze your diet for one or two days.

You may want to do a longer assessment in the future. In Lab 16B, you will be given the opportunity to compare a "nutritious diet" to a "favorite diet." Doing the analyses of two different daily meal plans will help you get a more accurate picture as to whether foods you think are nutritious actually meet current healthy lifestyle goals.

Web Resources

American Dietetic Association **www.eatright.org**
Berkeley Nutrition Services **www.nutritionquest.com**
Center for Science in the Public Interest **www.cspinet.org**
Diet Analysis Web Page **http://dawp.anet.com**
Food and Drug Administration (FDA) **www.fda.gov**
Food Safety Database **www.foodsafety.gov**
Information about Glycemic Index of Foods
    www.mendosa.com/gilist.htm
National Academy of Sciences **www.nas.edu**
Center for Nutrition Policy and Promotion
    www.usda.gov/cnpp
National Nutrition Summit Database
    www.nlm.nih.gov/pubs/cbm/nutritionsummit.html
Office of Dietary Supplements **http://ods.od.nih.gov**
U.S. Department of Agriculture (USDA) **www.usda.gov**
USDA Food and Nutrition Information Center
    www.nal.usda.gov/fnic

Suggested Readings

 Additional reference materials for concept 16 are available at **www.mhhe.com/fit_well/web16 Click 12.**

American College of Sport Medicine, the American Dietetics Association, the Women's Sports Foundation, and the Cooper Institute for Aerobics Research, 1997. *Questioning 40/30/30: A Guide to Understanding Sports Nutrition Advice.*

American Dietetic Association 1997. Vegetarian diets: Position of the American Dietetic Association. *Journal of the American Dietetics Association* 97:1317–1321.

American Dietetic Association. 1998. Fat replacers: Position of the American Dietetic Association. *Journal of the American Dietetics Association* 98:463–468.

American Dietetic Association. 2000. *The Health Professional's Guide to Popular Dietary Supplements.* Chicago, IL: American Dietetic Association.

Clark, K. 1999. Replacing fat: Have we managed a miracle? *ACSM's Health and Fitness Journal* 3(2):22–26.

Coleman, E. 2000. AHA dietary guidelines. *Sports Medicine Digest* 22:133.

Fletcher, R. H., and K. M. Fairfield. 2002. Vitamins for chronic disease prevention in adults: Clinical applications. *Journal of the American Medical Association* 287(23):3127–3130.

Food and Nutrition Board, Institute of Medicine. 2002. *Dietary Reference Intakes for Energy, Carbohydrates, Fiber, Fat, Protein, and Amino Acids (Macronutrients).* Washington, DC: National Academy Press, 2002.

Jacobson, M. F., and J. Hurley. 2002. *Restaurant Confidential.* New York: Workman Publishing.

Krauss R. M. et al. 2000. AHA dietary guidelines revision 2000: A statement for health-care professionals from the Nutrition Committee of the American Heart Association. *Circulation* 102:2284–2299.

Manore, M. M. 2001. Vitamins and minerals. Part I: How much do you need? *ACSM's Health and Fitness Journal* 5(1):33–36.

Manore, M. M. 2001. Vitamins and minerals. Part II: Who needs supplements? *ACSM's Health and Fitness Journal* 5(3):33–36.

Manore, M. M. 2001. Vitamins and minerals. Part III: Can you get too much? *ACSM's Health and Fitness Journal* 5(5):26–28.

Manore, M. M., and J. A. Thompson. 2000. *Sport Nutrition for Health and Performance.* Champaign, IL: Human Kinetics.

Manore, M. M., S. I. Barr, and G. E. Butterfield. 2001. Position of the American Dietetic Association: Nutrition and athletic performance. *Journal of the American Dietetic Association* 5(1):1543–1556.

Nash, J. M. 2002. Cracking the fat riddle. *Time* 160(10):46–55.

People. 12 June 2000. Diet Riot. *People* 104–110.

Schlosser, E. 2001. *Fast Food Nation: The Dark Side of the All-American Meal.* New York: Houghton Mifflin.

Thompson, S. R., M. M. Weber, and L. B. Brown. 2001. The relationship between health and fitness magazine readings and eating-disordered weight-loss methods among high school girls. *American Journal of Health Education* 32(3):133–138.

U.S. Department of Agriculture and U.S. Department of Health and Human Services. 2000. *Report of the Dietary Guidelines Advisory Committee.* Washington, DC: U.S. Department of Agriculture and U.S. Department of Health and Human Services.

U.S. Department of Health and Human Services. 2000. *Healthy People 2010.* 2nd ed. With Understanding and Improving Health and Objectives for Improving Health, 2 vols. Washington, DC: U.S. Government Printing Office.

Van Loan, M. D. 2001. Do you restrict your food intake? The implications of food restriction on bone health. *ACSM's Health and Fitness Journal* 5(1):11–14.

Wardlaw, G. M. 2002. *Contemporary Nutrition.* 5th ed. St. Louis: McGraw-Hill.

Williams, M. H. 2002. *Nutrition for Health, Fitness, and Sports.* 6th ed. St. Louis: McGraw-Hill.

 In the News

In the Fall of 2002, Food and Nutrition Board of the Institute of Medicine (IOM) released its latest set of dietary guidelines for healthy eating. This document titled *Dietary Reference Intakes for Energy, Carbohydrate, Fiber, Fat, Fatty Acids, Cholesterol, Protein, and Amino Acids* provides guidelines for the consumption of carbohydrates, fats, and protein in the diet, as well as other nutrients in the diet. This document is the sixth in a series of reviews each of which has helped to establish Dietary Reference Intakes (DRIs) for the various nutrients essential for good health. Previous documents covered the category of micronutrients which includes various vitamins and minerals. This document now provides guidelines for the class of macronutrients such as carbohydrates (including fiber), fats (including fatty acids and cholesterol), and proteins (including specific amino acids). Like the previous editions, Recommended Dietary Allowances (RDAs) are established only if clear evidence is available to warrant a specific level.

The new IOM report establishes Acceptable Macronutrient Distribution Ranges (AMDRs) that define the range of nutrient intakes that are associated with a reduced risk of chronic disease. The document recommends that adults get 45 to 65 percent of their calories from carbohydrates, 20 to 35 percent from fat, and 10 to 35 percent from protein.

The IOM macronutrient ranges are broader than those included on pages 309 through 312 of this text that are based on recommendations of the United States Department of Agriculture's (USDA) Dietary Guidelines

Ergogenic Aid In this concept, this term will refer to a nutritional supplement claimed by its promoters to improve performance.

for Americans. The IOM provides a broader range of carbohydrate intake (45–65 percent) than the USDA (55–60 percent) guideline but both ranges are similar. The IOM recommends a broader (and slightly lower) range of fat intake (20–35 percent) than the USDA which recommends no more than 30 percent. The IOM also recommends a broader (and slightly higher) range of protein intake (20–35 percent) than the USDA (10–15 percent). Both reports are designed to help people make healthy food choices. The reason the IOM provided slightly broader range of values is to "help people make healthy and more realistic choices based on their own food preferences."

The USDA and IOM now recommend that physical activity be included as part of balancing energy to maintain a healthy body fat level throughout life. The recommendation for physical activity from the IOM document is described in the concept 4 (In the News). The report of the Food and Nutrition Boards of the IOM report is available at www.iom.edu and the USDA dietary recommendations are available at www.usda.gov.

Lab 16A: Nutrition Analysis

Name	**Section**	**Date**

Purpose: To learn to keep a dietary log, to determine the nutritional quality of your diet, to determine your average daily caloric intake, and to determine necessary changes in eating habits.

Procedure:

1. Record your dietary intake for two days using the Daily Diet Record sheets. Record intake for one weekday and one weekend day. You may wish to make copies of the Record sheet for future use.
2. Include the actual foods eaten, the amount (size of portion in teaspoons, tablespoons, cups, ounces, or other standard units of measurement). Be sure to include all drinks (coffee, tea, soft drinks, etc.). Include *all* foods eaten, including sauces, gravies, dressings, toppings, spreads, etc. Determine your calorie consumption for each of the two days. Use the Calorie Guide to Common Foods in the appendix or the Guides to Food available on the Web.
3. List the number of servings from each food group by each food choice.
4. Estimate the proportion of complex carbohydrate, simple carbohydrate, protein, and fat in each meal and in snacks, as well as for the total day.
5. Answer the questions in Chart 1 using information for a typical day based on the dietary record sheets. Score one point for each "yes" answer on Chart 1. Use Chart 2 to rate your dietary habits. Circle the appropriate rating.

Results:

Record the number of calories consumed for each of the two days.

Weekday [ ] calories   Weekend [ ] calories

Conclusions and Implications: In several sentences, discuss your diet as recorded in this lab. Explain any changes in your eating habits that may be necessary. Comment on whether the days you surveyed are typical of your normal diet.

Chart 1 ▶ Dietary Habits Questionnaire

Yes	No	Answer questions based on a typical day (use your Daily Records to help).
◯	◯	1. Do you eat three normal-sized meals?
◯	◯	2. Do you eat a healthy breakfast?
◯	◯	3. Do you eat lunch regularly?
◯	◯	4. Does your diet contain about 55–60 percent carbohydrates with a high concentration of fiber?
◯	◯	5. Are less than one-fourth of the carbohydrates you eat simple carbohydrates?
◯	◯	6. Does your diet contain 10–15 percent protein?
◯	◯	7. Does your diet contain no more than 30 percent fat?
◯	◯	8. Do you limit the amount of saturated fat in your diet (no more than 10 percent)?
◯	◯	9. Do you limit salt intake to acceptable amounts?
◯	◯	10. Do you get adequate amounts of vitamins in your diet without a supplement?
◯	◯	11. Do you typically eat 6 to 11 servings from the bread, cereal, rice, and pasta group of foods?
◯	◯	12. Do you typically eat 3 to 5 servings of vegetables?
◯	◯	13. Do you typically eat 2 to 4 servings of fruits?
◯	◯	14. Do you typically eat 2 to 3 servings from the milk, yogurt, and cheese group of foods?
◯	◯	15. Do you typically eat 2 to 3 servings from the meat, poultry, fish, beans, eggs, and nuts group of foods?
◯	◯	16. Do you drink adequate amounts of water?
◯	◯	17. Do you get adequate minerals in your diet without a supplement?
◯	◯	18. Do you limit your caffeine and alcohol consumption to acceptable levels?
◯	◯	19. Is your average calorie consumption reasonable for your body size and for the amount of calories you normally expend?
		Total number of "Yes" answers

Chart 2 ▶ Dietary Habits Rating Scale

Score	Rating
18–19	Very good
15–17	Good
13–14	Marginal
12 or less	Poor

Daily Diet Record

Day 1

Breakfast Food	Amount (cups, tsp., etc.)	Calories	Food Servings				Estimated Meal Calorie %
			Bread/Cereal	Fruit/Veg.	Milk/Meat	Fat/Sweet	
							☐ % Protein
							☐ % Fat
							☐ % Complex carbohydrate
							☐ % Simple carbohydrate
							100% Total
Meal Total							

Lunch Food	Amount (cups, tsp., etc.)	Calories	Food Servings				Estimated Meal Calorie %
			Bread/Cereal	Fruit/Veg.	Milk/Meat	Fat/Sweet	
							☐ % Protein
							☐ % Fat
							☐ % Complex carbohydrate
							☐ % Simple carbohydrate
							100% Total
Meal Total							

Dinner Food	Amount (cups, tsp., etc.)	Calories	Food Servings				Estimated Meal Calorie %
			Bread/Cereal	Fruit/Veg.	Milk/Meat	Fat/Sweet	
							☐ % Protein
							☐ % Fat
							☐ % Complex carbohydrate
							☐ % Simple carbohydrate
							100% Total
Meal Total							

Snack Food	Amount (cups, tsp., etc.)	Calories	Food Servings				Estimated Snack Calorie %
			Bread/Cereal	Fruit/Veg.	Milk/Meat	Fat/Sweet	
							☐ % Protein
							☐ % Fat
							☐ % Complex carbohydrate
							☐ % Simple carbohydrate
							100% Total
Meal Total							Estimated Daily Total Calorie %
Daily Totals							☐ % Protein
		Calories	Servings	Servings	Servings	Servings	☐ % Fat / ☐ % Complex carbohydrate / ☐ % Simple carbohydrate / 100% Total

Daily Diet Record

Day 2

Breakfast Food	Amount (cups, tsp., etc.)	Calories	Food Servings				Estimated Meal Calorie %
			Bread/Cereal	Fruit/Veg.	Milk/Meat	Fat/Sweet	
							☐ % Protein
							☐ % Fat
							☐ % Complex carbohydrate
							☐ % Simple carbohydrate
							100% Total
Meal Total	✕						

Lunch Food	Amount (cups, tsp., etc.)	Calories	Food Servings				Estimated Meal Calorie %
			Bread/Cereal	Fruit/Veg.	Milk/Meat	Fat/Sweet	
							☐ % Protein
							☐ % Fat
							☐ % Complex carbohydrate
							☐ % Simple carbohydrate
							100% Total
Meal Total	✕						

Dinner Food	Amount (cups, tsp., etc.)	Calories	Food Servings				Estimated Meal Calorie %
			Bread/Cereal	Fruit/Veg.	Milk/Meat	Fat/Sweet	
							☐ % Protein
							☐ % Fat
							☐ % Complex carbohydrate
							☐ % Simple carbohydrate
							100% Total
Meal Total	✕						

Snack Food	Amount (cups, tsp., etc.)	Calories	Food Servings				Estimated Snack Calorie %
			Bread/Cereal	Fruit/Veg.	Milk/Meat	Fat/Sweet	
							☐ % Protein
							☐ % Fat
							☐ % Complex carbohydrate
							☐ % Simple carbohydrate
							100% Total
Meal Total							Estimated Daily Total Calorie %
Daily Totals	✕	Calories	Servings	Servings	Servings	Servings	☐ % Protein ☐ % Fat ☐ % Complex carbohydrate ☐ % Simple carbohydrate 100% Total

Lab 16B: Selecting Nutritious Foods

Name		Section	Date

Purpose: To learn to select a nutritious diet, to determine the nutritive value of favorite foods, and to compare a nutritious foods values to a favorite foods values.

Procedure:

1. Select a breakfast, lunch, and dinner from the foods list in Appendix D. Include between-meal snacks with the nearest meal. If you cannot find foods you would normally choose, select those most similar to choices you might make.
2. Select a breakfast, lunch, and dinner from foods you feel would make the most nutritious meals. Include between-meal snacks with nearest meal.
3. Record your "favorite foods" and "nutritious foods" on page 332. Record the calories for proteins, carbohydrates, and fats for each of the foods you choose.
4. Total each column for the "favorite" and the "nutritious" meal.
5. Determine the percentages of your total calories that are protein, carbohydrate, and fat by dividing each column total by the total number of calories consumed.
6. Answer the questions in the Conclusions and Implications section.

Results: Record your results below. Calculate percent of calories from each source by dividing total calories into calories from each food source (protein, fat, or carbohydrate).

Source	Favorite Foods		Nutritious Foods	
	Calories	% of Total Calories	Calories	% of Total Calories
Protein				
Carbohydrates				
Fat				
Total 100%		100%		100%

Adapted from the *Surgeon General's Report on Physical Activity and Health.*

Conclusions and Implications: In several sentences, discuss differences you found between your nutritious diet and your favorite diet. Discuss the quality of your nutritious diet as well as other things you learned from doing this lab.

"Favorite" versus "Nutritious" Food Choices for Three Daily Meals

Breakfast Favorite	Food Choices				Breakfast Nutritious	Food Choices			
Food No.	Cal.	Pro. Cal.	Car. Cal.	Fat Cal.	Food No.	Cal.	Pro. Cal.	Car. Cal.	Fat Cal.
Totals					Totals				

Lunch Favorite	Food Choices				Lunch Nutritious	Food Choices			
Food No.	Cal.	Pro. Cal.	Car. Cal.	Fat Cal.	Food No.	Cal.	Pro. Cal.	Car. Cal.	Fat Cal.
Totals					Totals				

Dinner Favorite	Food Choices				Dinner Nutritious	Food Choices			
Food No.	Cal.	Pro. Cal.	Car. Cal.	Fat Cal.	Food No.	Cal.	Pro. Cal.	Car. Cal.	Fat Cal.
Totals					Totals				
Daily Totals (Calories)					Daily Totals (Calories)				
Daily % of Total Calories					Daily % of Total Calories				

Managing Diet and Activity
for Healthy Body Fat

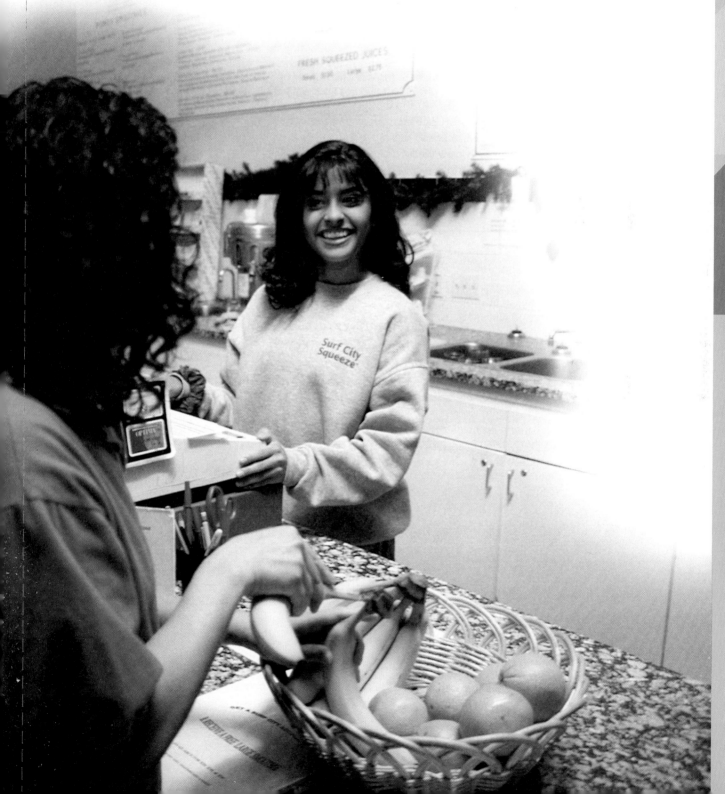

There are various management strategies for eating and performing physical activity that are useful in achieving and maintaining optimal body composition.

Health Goals

for the year 2010

- Increase prevalence of a healthy weight.
- Reduce prevalence of overweight.
- Increase proportion of people who meet national dietary guidelines.
- Increase the adoption and maintenance of daily physical activity.
- Increase teaching about nutrition and physical activity.

Most people express an interest in health and nearly everyone is concerned about their appearance. Despite the interest, the majority of the population has difficulty maintaining a healthy weight (and fat level). A 2001 poll found that 63 percent of American adults wanted to lose 20 pounds or more. Another survey reported that about 29 percent of men and 44 percent of women who are dieting are actually attempting to lose weight. Though weight and fat control are clearly important for health, experts suggest that movies, television, and magazines have created an obsession with weight loss among many teens and adults. In many cases, the concern is with losing weight rather than fat, and with appearance rather than good health. Caution is necessary so that we do not create more problems than we solve.

Because of the misplaced concern with weight loss among large numbers of people, the emphasis of this concept will be on fat loss for good health. When properly done, fat control can be safe and effective. This concept will make suggestions for losing, maintaining, and gaining body fat.

Factors Influencing Weight and Fat Control

Environmental influences can make it hard to manage body fat levels. The obesity epidemic is due as much to the environment we live in as to our individual

attitudes and beliefs. People can have good intentions. If they find themselves in environments that are not conducive to good health, they may be unable to adopt healthy lifestyles. Figure 1 presents a model that shows how various environmental factors influence the energy balance equation. The essence of the model is that we are continually confronted with environments that make it easy to consume large quantities of energy dense food. We also live in an environment in which most physical tasks are no longer necessary and people have less apparent time available for active recreation. Small increases in energy intake combined with decreases in energy expenditure lead to the storage of fat. Awareness of these environmental influences is important if you desire to maintain a healthy body fat level and weight.

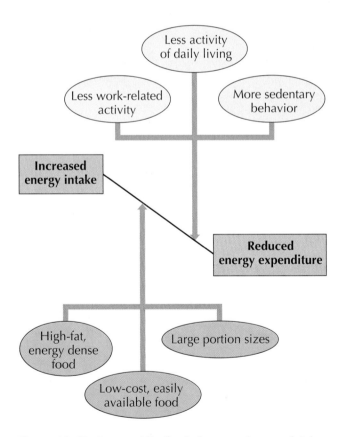

Figure 1 ▶ Factors contributing to increased energy intake and reduced energy expenditure.

Source: Model adapted from Hill et al. 1999.

The first step in fat control is establishing realistic goals. Too many teens and adults, both men and women, establish unrealistic goals for their physical appearance. Fat, weight, and body proportions are all factors that can be changed, but people often set standards for themselves that are difficult, if not impossible, to achieve. Starting with small goals is preferable to establishing goals that seem impossible to accomplish. This necessitates developing an understanding of your own body proportions as well as your body fatness. Unrealistic goals may result in eating disorders, failure to meet goals, or failure to maintain fat loss over time.

Regular physical activity is essential for long-term weight control. As described in concept 15, much of the weight gain that takes place with age (creeping obesity) can be attributed to reductions in physical activity. By maintaining an active lifestyle, you can burn off extra calories, keep your body's metabolism high, and prevent the decline in basal metabolic rate that typically occurs with aging (due to reduced muscle mass). All types of physical activity can be beneficial for weight control. Since aerobic exercise can be maintained for a long period, it allows you to expend large numbers of calories and therefore is the best type of physical activity for fat loss and maintenance. Strength training can contribute to weight control by increasing muscle mass and helping to increase metabolic rate.

Despite the documented benefits of physical activity for weight control, few people trying to lose weight report being physically active. A recent state-based survey determined that approximately one-half of individuals trying to lose weight did not engage in any physical activity and only 15 percent reported exercising regularly. The challenges many people experience with weight control may be an indirect reflection of the challenges people face in trying to be more physically active. While being physically active cannot ensure that you will become as thin as you desire, it will allow you to probably attain a body size that is appropriate for your genetics and body type.

Getting regular activity in our society is sometimes more difficult than it would seem. Numerous labor-saving devices including garage openers, escalators, moving sidewalks, motorized lawn mowers, and golf carts have made life, work, and play easier with little or no activity. Even the increase in e-mail in offices has limited the amount of activity that office workers obtain. For effective weight management, you must find ways to keep activity as a regular part of your lifestyle.

Awareness and dietary restraint are needed to avoid excess calorie intake. www.mhhe.com/fit_well/17 Click 01. Consumers are able to buy food almost anywhere. For example convenience stores and food

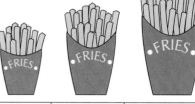

Size	Small	Large	Super Size
Calories (kcal)	450	540	610

Figure 2 ▶ Comparison of added calories in different sizes of French fries.

courts in malls allow people to snack more readily during the day. To provide more apparent value to consumers, restaurants and convenience stores have continued to provide larger portion sizes. Supersizing and Value-Meals are commonly used terminology to denote ways to get more food for your money. In the 1960s, the average serving of McDonald's French fries was about 200 calories. Today, a large serving provides 540 calories and the "super size" approximately 610 calories. Similarly, consumers can now purchase soft drinks in volumes up to 64 ounces rather than a standard 12- to 16-ounce drink. While consumers should be value conscious with gasoline and other commodities, food is one area where consumers should show some restraint. Choosing normal-sized meals and drinks is one way to avoid excess calories in your diet (see Figure 2).

Behavioral goals are more effective than outcome goals. Researchers have shown that setting **outcome goals** or goals that set a specific amount of weight or fat loss (gain), can be discouraging. If a **behavioral goal** of eating a reasonable number of calories per day and expending a reasonable number of calories in exercise is met, outcome goals will be achieved. Most experts believe that behavioral goals work better than weight or fat loss goals, especially in the short term.

Outcome Goal A statement of intent to achieve a specific test score or a specific standard associated with good health or wellness. An example would be, "I will lower my body fat level by 3 percent."

Behavioral Goal A statement of intent to perform a specific behavior (changing a lifestyle) for a specific period of time. An example would be, "I will reduce the fat in my diet to 30 percent or less of my total calories."

Short-term goals can help you reach long-term goals. Individuals wanting to lose weight often want to accomplish their goals too quickly. Losing 20 or 30 pounds can seem impossible but breaking this long-term goal down into manageable short-term goals is more effective. Guidelines from the ACSM and other organizations recommend maximum weight loss goals of 1 to 2 pounds per week. Efforts to lose weight faster than that will typically lead to frustration or the cessation of the program. The best way to determine if your goals are reasonable is if they can be maintained for a lifetime. Because your weight can fluctuate with the amount of water lost or retained, daily monitoring of weight can also be discouraging. Weight may drop dramatically one day because of water loss and increase the next. Care must be taken not to worry too much about daily weight or fat losses or gains.

To get accurate assessments of true changes in body fatness, weight and body fatness assessments should not be done too frequently. Drinking adequate amounts of water is important to people who are restricting calories and will reduce the risk of false changes in body fat. Measuring weight is best done early in the morning before you have eaten breakfast.

Diet and activity can contribute to more body fat loss than diet alone. If weight loss is accomplished solely through dietary changes, a significant part of the weight lost will be from muscle. Studies have shown that a program that includes diet and physical activity will lead to a greater loss of body fat than a program based solely on diet. The total weight loss from the programs may be about the same, but a larger fraction of the weight comes from fat when physical activity is included in the program.

Guidelines for Losing Body Fat

Changes in eating patterns can be effective in fat loss. www.mhhe.com/fit_well/web17 Click 02.

- Restrict calories in moderate amounts per day rather than make large reductions in daily caloric intake.
- Eat less fat. Research shows that reduction of the fat in the diet not only results in fewer calories consumed (fats have more than twice the calories per gram as carbohydrates or proteins) but in greater body fat loss as well.
- Severely restrict **empty calories** which provide little nutrition and can account for an excessive amount of your daily caloric intake. Examples of these foods are candy (often high in simple sugar) and potato chips (often fried in saturated fat).
- Increase complex carbohydrates. Foods high in fiber, such as fresh fruits and vegetables, contain few calories for their volume. They are nutritious and filling, and are especially good foods for a fat loss program.

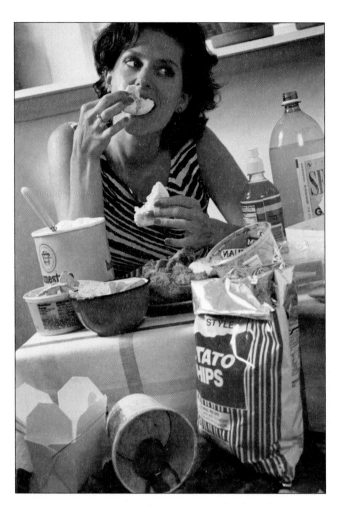

Foods with "empty calories" have few nutrients and often are relatively high in calorie content.

- Learn the difference between craving and hunger. Hunger is a physiological phenomenon that is a result of the body's need to supply energy to sustain life. A craving is simply a desire to eat something, sometimes a food you do not particularly like. When you feel the urge to eat, you may want to ask yourself: Is this real hunger or a craving? Hunger is accompanied by growling of the stomach and is most likely to occur after long periods without food. If you have the urge to eat soon after a meal, it is probably from craving, not hunger.
- Develop personal habits that can help you make better dietary choices when eating at restaurants, work, and special occasions. Making good selections when purchasing and preparing food are also important. See Table 1 for suggestions.

Extreme diets are not likely to be effective. Diets that require severe caloric restriction or exercise programs that require exceptionally large caloric expenditure can be effective in fat loss over a short period, but are seldom maintained for a lifetime. Studies show that extreme programs for fat and weight control, designed to "take it off fast,"

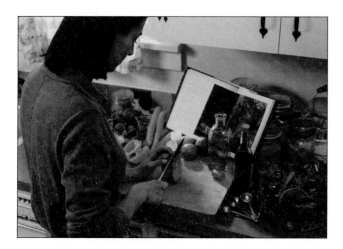

If you snack, consider foods high in complex carbohydrates.

result in long-term success rates of less than 5 percent. Research shows that one reason extremely low-calorie diets are ineffective is that they may promote "calorie sparing." When calorie intake is 800 to 1,000 or less, the body protects itself by reducing basal and resting metabolism levels (sparing calories). This results in less fat loss, even though the calorie intake is very low.

A healthy lifestyle includes a healthy diet and regular exercise. For some people, it may be necessary to develop a daily habit of eating several hundred calories less than other people or maintaining an exercise schedule that expends more calories than the normal person if desirable body fat levels are to be maintained. These habits of moderation can realistically become part of your normal lifestyle.

Fad diets are not a satisfactory means of long-term weight reduction and may adversely affect your health. Hundreds of fad diets and diet books exist, but dietitians warn that drastic juggling of food constituents has little scientific basis. Such diets are usually unbalanced and may result in serious illness or even death, especially for the obese person who is already apt to be suffering from a number of health disorders. Fad diets cannot be maintained for long periods; therefore, the individual usually regains any lost weight. Less than 5 percent of people who lose weight maintain the loss for more than a year. Constant losing and gaining, known as the yo-yo syndrome, may be as harmful as the original obese condition.

Total fasting is dangerous, as are crash (fast) diets. Pill popping, hormone injections, and powder and liquid diets have little value in long-term weight-control programs and present many health hazards. When in doubt, avoid diets that:

- Promise fast, easy solutions.
- Promise to help you achieve ideal weight without mental inspiration and perspiration.
- Favor one food as the answer to weight problems.
- Promise that your fat will melt away.

Despite their popularity, high-protein diets have not been shown to be effective for fat loss. www.mhhe.com/fit_well/web17 Click 03. High-protein diets are one of the most common types of fad diets promoted in magazines and books. Examples of these diets include Sugar Busters, the Zone, Dr. Atkins New Diet Revolution, Protein Power, the Stillman Diet, and The Carbohydrate Addicts Diet. Recommending a high-protein diet is basically the same as recommending a low carbohydrate diet because the increase in proteins is typically at the expense of carbohydrates. These diets are sometimes referred to as 40/30/30 diets because they recommend lower carbohydrate intake (40 percent rather than 55 percent or 60 percent) and high-protein intake (30 percent rather than 10 to 15 percent). The diets vary in content but all implicate carbohydrate as the source of obesity.

They base this premise on the incorrect logic that anything that increases insulin levels is bad since insulin causes the body to take up and store energy as fat. It is true that carbohydrates cause your body to release insulin but this fact by itself does not make carbohydrates bad. Insulin is a necessary hormone that helps the body regulate blood sugar. Insulin is released when the body takes in carbohydrates so that blood sugar can be kept at stable levels (just like the body regulates core temperature). Simple sugars such as candy and soda lead to quick increases in blood sugar so the body releases insulin to bring the blood sugar values back down to normal. They contain few nutrients and excess calories to the diet. Complex carbohydrates (e.g., bread, pasta, rice, potatoes), on the other hand, are broken down slowly and do not cause the same effect on blood sugar. They contribute valuable nutrients and fiber in the diet and should constitute the bulk of a person's diet. Lumping simple carbohydrates together with complex carbohydrates is not appropriate since they are processed differently and have different nutrient values. Experts agree that simple sugars should be consumed in moderation but evidence does not show that the consumption of complex carbohydrates contributes to obesity or any negative health problem.

The main reason that fad diets exclusively warn not to eat carbohydrates is that the body does lose water weight when carbohydrate intake is low. Water is required to store carbohydrates in the body, so if people consume fewer calories than they expend they will lose weight no matter what they eat.

High-protein diets can be harmful on the kidneys and liver and may add excess saturated fat to the diet. The popularity of high-protein diets is troubling to

Empty Calories Calories in foods considered to have little nutritional value.

Table 1 ▶ Guidelines for Healthy Shopping and Eating in a Variety of Settings

Guidelines for shopping	• Shop from a list to avoid the purchase of foods that contain empty calories and other foods that will tempt you to overeat. • Shop with a friend to avoid buying unneeded foods. For this technique to work, the other person must be sensitive to your goals. In some cases, a friend can have a bad, rather than a good, influence. • Shop on a full stomach to avoid the temptations of snacking on and buying junk food. • Check the label for contents of foods to avoid foods that are excessively high in fat or saturated fat.
Guidelines for how you eat	• When you eat, do nothing else but eat. If you watch television, read, or do some other activity while you eat, you may be unaware of what you have eaten. • Eat slowly. Taste your food. Pause between bites. Chew slowly. Do not take the next bite until you have swallowed what you have in your mouth. Periodically take a longer pause. Be the last one finished eating. • Do not eat food you do not want. Some people do not want to waste food so they clean their plate even when they feel full. • Follow an eating schedule. Eating at regular meal times can help you avoid snacking. If meals are spaced equally throughout the day, it can help reduce appetite. • Leave the table after eating to avoid taking extra unwanted bites and servings. • Eat meals of equal size. Some people try to restrict calories at one or two meals to save up for a big meal. • Eating several *small* meals helps you to avoid hunger (fools the appetite) and helps you keep from losing control at one meal. • Avoid second servings. Limit your intake to one moderate serving. If second servings are taken, make them one-half the size of first servings. • Limit servings of salad dressings and condiments (e.g., catsup). These are often high in fat and calories, and can sometimes amount to greater calorie consumption than is expected.
Guidelines for controlling the home environment	• Store food out of sight. Avoid containers that allow you to see food. It is especially important to limit the accessibility of foods that tempt you and foods with empty calories. "Foods that are out of sight, are out of mouth." • Do your eating in designated areas only. Designate areas such as the kitchen and dining room as eating areas so you do not snack elsewhere. It is especially easy to eat too much while watching television. • If you snack, eat foods high in complex carbohydrates and low in fats, such as fresh fruits and carrot sticks. • Freeze leftovers. Leftover foods are often tempting to eat. Freezing them so that it takes preparation to eat them will help you avoid temptation.
Guidelines for controlling the work environment	• Take food from home rather than eating from vending machines or catering trucks. • Do not eat while working but take your lunch as a break. Do something active during other breaks. For example, take a walk. • Avoid sources of food provided by coworkers, for example, food in work rooms, such as birthday cakes, or candy in jars. • Have drinking water or low-calorie drinks available to substitute for snacks.
Guidelines for eating on special occasions	• Practice ways to refuse food. Knowing exactly what to say will help you not get talked into eating something you do not want. • Eat before you go out so you are not as hungry at parties and events. • Do not stand near food sources and distract yourself if tempted to eat when you are not really hungry. • Limit servings of non-basic parts of the meal. It is easy to consume large numbers of calories on alcohol, soft drinks, appetizers and desserts. Limit these items.
Guidelines for eating out at restaurants	• Try to make healthy selections from the menu. Choose chicken without skin, fish, or lean cuts of meat. Grilled or broiled options are better than fried. Choose healthier options for dessert as many decadent desserts can have more calories than the whole dinner. • Limit the use of sauces and condiments such as butter, margarine, catsup, mayonnaise, and salad dressings. Asking for the condiments "on the side" would allow you to determine how much to put on. • Do not feel compelled to eat everything on your plate. Many restaurants serve exceptionally large portions to try to please the customers. • Order à la carte rather than full meals to avoid multiple courses and servings. • Avoid supersizing your meals if eating at fast food restaurants as this can add unwanted calories.

physicians and public health officials. The American Heart Association (AHA) recently released a science advisory statement on high-protein diets to warn health-care professionals about the potential risks. They point out high-protein diets may not be harmful in the short term but may lead to some long-term problems if maintained. Extra protein in the diet is not used efficiently in the body and may impose a metabolic burden on the kidneys and liver. High-protein intakes can also be accompanied by high consumption of saturated fat and cholesterol that can increase risks of coronary heart disease. With low levels of carbohydrate intake, the body enters into a state of metabolic ketosis in which the body starts to break down other substrates for energy. This state has been shown to lead to a loss of appetite but the long-term effects have not been determined.

The AHA document compared the various high-protein diets against other AHA and public health guidelines. The Sugar Busters and Zone diets were actually in compliance with the AHA guidelines for total fat and saturated fat consumption but still were viewed as too restrictive and high in protein. The Atkin's diet is one of the most controversial of the high-protein diets because it specifically recommends a high consumption of animal fat. This diet runs against guidelines from the AHA and the overall U.S. Dietary Guidelines. Two recent studies widely cited in the popular press showed that those on the Atkins' diet actually lost more weight than those on a more balanced diet. The studies also showed that, over the short term, cholesterol and other blood fats were not increased as many have suggested. The AHA issued a statement noting that these studies are quite small and lasted for only a short time. The AHA points out that the Atkins' diet was not compared to the balanced diet it recommends and that there was no evidence showing that the diet improves health. At the same time, a recent report in *the Journal of the American Medical Association* points to the substantial evidence that diets high in whole grains, fruits, and vegetables, low in saturated and hydrogenated fat, and that contain an adequate Omega-3 fatty acid can provide significant protection against heart disease. To stem the confusion among consumers concerning high-protein diets, the National Institute of Health has initiated a clinical trial to systematically evaluate long-term health outcomes of high-protein diets.

Artificial sweeteners and fat substitutes may help but cannot be considered a "sure cure" for body fat problems. www.mhhe.com/fit_well/web17 Click 04. Artificial sweeteners are frequently used in soft drinks and food to reduce the calorie content. Because they have few or no calories, these supplements were expected to help people with weight control. However, since they were introduced the general public has not eaten fewer calories and more people are now overweight than before they were introduced. Studies suggest that people consuming these products end up consuming just as many calories per day as people consuming products with real sugar or sweeteners.

New products often referred to as "fake fat" are used as a fat substitute in baking and cooking. Potato chips and other fried foods cooked in these products as well as baked goods using these products have less fat and fewer calories. If you eat no more food than usual and substitute foods made with these products you will consume fewer calories and less fat. Experts worry that consumers will not eat the same amount of foods with these fake fats but will feel they can eat more because the fake fats contain fewer calories and less fat.

Dietary supplements or products containing ephedra should be avoided. www.mhhe.com/fit_well/web17 Click 05. Because long-term weight control is difficult, many individuals seek simple solutions from various nonprescription weight loss products. These products include laxatives and various appetite suppressants. Many products contain the stimulant ephedra (or the herbal version Ma Huang). The Federal Drug Administration (FDA) has proposed restrictions on ephedra use because of numerous adverse events and even deaths attributed to its use. A synthetic version of ephedrine (phenylpropanolalamine) found in many appetite suppressants (e.g., Dexatrim and Acutrim) was previously thought to be safe but the FDA Nonprescription Drug Advisory Committee has recommended that all nonprescription products containing this compound be taken off the market. The stronger restriction of this product (which is regulated as an over-the-counter drug) may actually increase the use of ephedra-containing products which are considered dietary supplements. As described in concept 25, the Dietary Supplement Health and Education Act puts the burden of proof on the FDA to determine if products are unsafe and this is a daunting challenge. A report in *JAMA* indicated that over 50 percent of the ephedra supplements tested by the FDA failed to list the ephedra content or had amounts 20 percent or higher than listed on the label. Consumers should be wary of dietary supplements due to the unregulated nature of the industry.

Guidelines for Gaining Muscle Mass

Young people often have difficulty in gaining weight or muscle mass. Typically, those most likely to have difficulty in gaining weight are age ten to twenty. The reason for this is that more calories are required to maintain weight during the growing years than in adulthood. They have probably been told more than once that they will not have trouble gaining weight when they grow older. This is true for most people, but it is of little consolation to those who want to gain weight now. During adolescence, most people begin to gain weight, including muscle mass that can be enhanced with regular exercise. Excessive eating to gain weight (especially during adolescence) is not without its problems. The body requires more caloric intake during the teen years because the body is growing. A person who develops a

Technology Update

Scientists and medical researchers have actively sought medical solutions to the obesity epidemic. While changes in lifestyle offer the best long-term solution, the risks of obesity and the associated burden on the public health-care system warrant efforts to identify useful pharmacologic treatments. Currently, there are only two prescription drugs that are approved for use in the United States for long-term use by the FDA. All current pharmacotherapies are considered to be adjuncts to lifestyle modification and are only used with obese patients (BMI > 30) or overweight individuals with other "comorbidities" (e.g., diabetes, hypertension). The two medications that are currently being prescribed are described below for educational purposes only—they should only be used under direct supervision by a physician.

Sibutramine Sibutramine acts by inhibiting the reuptake of serotonin and noradrenaline. In research studies, weight loss has been found to be greater among sibutramine-treated participants compared with those receiving a placebo. Maintenance of weight loss has also been enhanced for 6 to 18 months following initial weight loss if the person continued with the medication. Side effects include sharp increases in blood pressure and resting heart rate. Several negative drug interactions are also possible so this should only be used with physician guidance.

Orlistat Orlistat acts to enhance weight loss by inhibiting the body's absorption of fat. Results from well-controlled studies have shown that patients taking orlistat lost significantly more weight than patients taking a placebo medication. The weight loss was typically accompanied by reductions in total and LDL-cholesterol, blood pressure, and glucose/insulin levels, indicating that the changes are related to improvements in metabolic function. A major limitation of the drug is that it also blocks the absorption of fat soluble vitamins (A, D, E, K, as well as beta-carotene). Therefore, prolonged use can lead to vitamin deficiencies unless supplementation is included in the diet.

habit of high-caloric intake during this time may have a difficult time controlling fatness when the demands on the body are less. Most people who want to gain weight want to gain lean body tissue. Only those who have body fat percentages less than what is considered to be essential for good health need to gain body fat.

Changes in frequency and composition of meals is important to gain muscle mass. To increase muscle mass the body requires a greater caloric intake. The challenge is to provide enough extra calories for the muscle without excess amounts going to fat. An increase of 500 to 1000 calories a day will help most people gain muscle mass over time. Studies indicate that smaller, more frequent meals may be beneficial for weight gain since it would tend to keep the metabolic rate high. The majority of extra calories should come from complex carbohydrates. Breads, pasta, rice, fruits such as bananas, and potatoes are good sources. Granola, nuts, juices (grape and cranberry), and milk also make good high-calorie, healthy snacks. High-protein diets or diet supplements are not particularly effective if you maintain a normal diet. High-fat diets can result in weight gain but may not be best for good health, especially if they are high in saturated fat. If weight gain does not occur over a period of weeks and months with extra caloric consumption, medical assistance may be necessary.

Physical activity is important in gaining muscle mass. Regular strength training can aid in weight gain. The stimulus from this form of exercise causes the body to increase protein synthesis which allows the body to gain muscle mass. Of course, the body requires higher levels of caloric intake to form this new muscle tissue.

Excessive aerobic exercise may actually make it difficult to gain weight. Although some regular aerobic exercise is necessary for health and cardiovascular fitness, it may be necessary to limit aerobic exercise if weight gain is the goal. Studies have shown that extensive aerobic training can even cause a reduction in muscle mass. When training to gain weight, aerobic exercise expending no more than 3,500 calories per week is probably best.

Strategies for Action

Knowing about guidelines for controlling body fat is not as important as following them. The guidelines presented in this concept are only of value if you use them. In Lab 17A, you will have the opportunity to identify some of the guidelines that you feel will help you the most in the future.

Recordkeeping is important to meeting fat-control goals and making moderation a part of your normal lifestyle. Studies have shown that it is easy to fool yourself when determining the amount of food you have eaten or the amount of exercise you have done. Once fat-control goals have been set, whether for weight loss, maintenance, or gain, it is important to keep records of your behavior. People often underestimate the amount of food they have eaten, particularly the number of calories consumed. They also tend to overestimate the amount of exercise they do. Keeping a diet log and an exercise log can help you monitor your behavior and maintain the lifestyle necessary to meet your goals. A log can also help you monitor changes in weight and body fat levels. But remember, care should be taken to avoid too much emphasis on short-term weight changes. Lab 17B will help you learn about the actual content of fast foods so you learn to make better choices when eating out.

The support of family and friends can be of great importance in balancing calorie intake and calorie expenditure. The importance of family and friends for successful adherence to a regular physical activity program can't be overemphasized. Family and friends can also help you in changing and adhering to healthy eating practices. Parents who overeat often have children who eat more than normal. In these cases, the entire family must participate in a program to control fatness. Family and friends should provide support for the person wanting to gain or lose fat by helping them follow the guidelines presented in this concept, rather than tempting the person to eat improperly. Unfortunately, sometimes friends and family members can put too much emphasis on the person's fat loss. This can have the opposite effect of that intended if it is perceived as an attempt to control one's behavior. The use of extrinsic rewards such as money or special gifts for achieving goals may be effective in the short term, but it may result in resentment rather than adherence over the long term. Encouragement and support rather than control of behavior is the key!

Group support can be one of the best reinforcers of proper eating and exercise behavior. Group support has been found to be beneficial to many individuals who are attempting to change their behavior. Alcoholics have found that the support of others is critical to their rehabilitation. (Alcoholics Anonymous grew as a result of this need.) If you want to alter your body composition, especially to lose body fat, group support is important if you are to make permanent lifestyle changes in diet and exercise. Groups such as Overeaters Anonymous and Weight Watchers have been organized to help those who need the support of peers in attaining and maintaining desirable fat levels for a lifetime.

Some psychological strategies can be of assistance in eating and exercising to attain and maintain a desirable level of body fat.

- Avoid food fantasies. Sometimes the thought of food is what causes overeating. Practice restructuring your thought process to something other than food fantasies. Use mental imagery to create a mind's-eye view of something you enjoy other than food. When food fantasies occur, you may want to exercise or engage in some activity that refocuses your attention.
- Avoid weight fantasies. Sometimes the thought of being excessively thin or muscular occurs. By itself, this may not be bad. If, however, it causes you to become discouraged and makes your goals seem unattainable, it is bad. When weight fantasies occur, do some other activity to redirect your focus of attention or imagine something other than the weight fantasy. Altering mental fantasies takes practice.
- Avoid **negative self-talk.** One type of negative self-talk occurs when a person starts self-criticism for not meeting a goal. For example, if a person is determined not to eat more than one serving of food at a party but fails to meet this goal, he or she might say, "It's no use stopping now; I've already blown it." It is not too late. Failing to meet goals can happen to anyone. Negative self-talk makes it easy to fail in the future. A more appropriate response would involve **positive self-talk** such as, "I'm not going to eat anything else tonight; I can do it."

Web Resources

American Dietetic Association **www.eatright.org**
Berkeley Nutrition Sciences **www.nutritionquest.com**
Center for Science in the Public Interest **www.cspinet.org**
Fast Food Facts: Interactive Food Finder **www.olen.com/food**
Internal Revenue Service **www.irs.gov**
Meals Online **www.my-meals.com**
Office of Dietary Supplements **http://ods.od.nih.gov**
USDA Food and Nutrition Information Center
    www.nal.usda.gov/fnic

Negative Self-Talk Self-defeating discussions with yourself focusing on your failures rather than your successes.

Positive Self-Talk Telling yourself positive, encouraging things that help you succeed in accomplishing your goals.

Suggested Readings

Additional reference materials for concept 17 are available at **www.mhhe.com/web17 Click 06.**

American College of Sports Medicine. 2001. Appropriate intervention strategies for weight loss and prevention of weight regain for adults. *Medicine and Science in Sports and Exercise* 33(12):2145–2156.

 Blanck, H. M., L. K. Khan, and M. Serdula. 2001. The use of nonprescription weight loss products: Results from a multistate survey. *Journal of the American Medical Association* 286:930–935.

Bryant, C. X., J. A. Peterson, and J. M. Conviser. 2001. High-protein, low-carbohydrate diets: Fact vs. fiction. *Fitness Management* 40–45.

Food and Nutrition Board, Institute of Medicine. 2002. *Dietary Reference Intakes for Energy, Carbohydrates, Fiber, Fat, Protein and Amino Acids (Macronutrients).* Washington, DC: National Academy Press.

Goodman, W. C. 2002. *The Invisible Woman: Confronting Weight Prejudice in America.* Carlsbad, CA: Gurze Books.

Jacobson, M. F., and J. Hurley. 2002. *Restaurant Confidential.* New York: Workman Publishing.

Manore, M. M., and J. A. Thompson. 2000. *Sport Nutrition for Health and Performance.* Champaign, IL: Human Kinetics.

Manore, M. M., S. I. Barr, and G. E. Butterfield. 2001. Position of the American Dietetic Association: Nutrition and athletic performance. *Journal of the American Dietetic Association* 5(1):1543–1556.

Meacham, S. L. et al. 2002. Nutrition suggestions for the cancer survivor. *ACSM's Health and Fitness Journal* 6(1):6–12.

Morgan, J. F. 2000. From Charles Atlas to Adonis complex: Fat is more than a feminist issue. *Lancet* 356:1372–1373.

Nash, J. M. 2002. Cracking the fat riddle. *Time.* 160(10): 46–55.

People. 12 June 2000. Diet Riot. *People* 104–110.

Sacker, I. M., and M. A. Zimmer. 2002. *Dying to Be Thin: Understanding and Defeating Anorexia Nervosa and Bulimia—A Practical, Lifesaving Guide.* New York: Time Warner Bookmark.

Schlosser, E. 2001. *Fast Food Nation: The Dark Side of the All-American Meal.* New York: Houghton Mifflin.

Serdula, M. K. et al. 1999. Prevalence of attempting weight loss and strategies for controlling weight. *Journal of the American Medical Association* 282:1353–1358.

St. Joer, S. T. et al. 1999. Dietary protein and weight reduction: A statement for healthcare professionals from the nutrition committee of the Council on Nutrition, Physical Activity and Metabolism of the American Heart Association. *Circulation* 104:1869–1874.

Tate, D. F., R. R. Wing, and R. A. Winett. 2001. Using internet technology to deliver a behavioral weight loss program. *Journal of the American Medical Association* 285(9):1172–1177.

Van Loan, M. D. 2001. Do you restrict your food intake? The implications of food restriction on bone health. *ACSM's Health and Fitness Journal* 5(1):11–14.

Wardlaw, G. M. 2002. *Contemporary Nutrition.* 5th ed. St. Louis: McGraw-Hill.

Williams, M. 2002. *Nutrition for Health, Fitness and Sports.* 6th ed. St. Louis: McGraw-Hill.

Wong, G., and W. H. Dietz. 2002. Economic burden of obesity in youths aged 6 to 17 years: 1979–1999. *Pediatrics* 109:e81.

In the News

In recent years there has been considerable interest in a nutritional parameter known as the glycemic index (GI). It is an index that attempts to quantify how different foods influence our blood sugar levels. Many fad diets base recommendations on the notion that foods with a high GI cause the body to overeat, store extra energy as fat, or lead to diabetes. Though some evidence shows the glycemic index may influence how carbohydrates are metabolized and used in the body, the possible effects on diseases such as diabetes and heart disease are not clear. One issue is that the GI value tells you only how rapidly a particular carbohydrate turns into sugar but does not tell you how much of that carbohydrate is in a serving of a particular food. An extension of the GI called the glycemic load (GL) reflects the GI of a food multiplied by its carbohydrate content. According to new tables published in the July 2002 issue of the *American Journal of Clinical Nutrition*, foods can actually have a high GI value but a low GL value (watermelon is a good example). While some evidence indicates that foods with high GI and GL values should be avoided, a leading obesity expert recently indicated it is currently *"premature to recommend that the general population avoid foods with a high glycemic index."* Information in subsequent years may help to clarify this issue. A complete listing of GI and GL for various foods is available online at **www.mendosa.com/gilists.htm**

Lab 17A: Selecting Strategies for Managing Eating

Name		Section	Date

Purpose: To help you select strategies for managing eating to control body fatness.

Procedures:

1. Read the strategies listed in Chart 1.
2. Make a check in the box beside five to ten of the strategies that you think will be most useful to you.
3. Answer the questions in the Conclusions and Implications section.

Chart 1 ▶ Strategies for Managing Eating to Control Body Fatness

✔	Check 5 to 10 strategies that you might use in the future.
	Shopping Strategies
	Shop from a list.
	Shop with a friend.
	Shop on a full stomach.
	Check food labels.
	Consider foods that take some time to prepare.
	Methods of Eating
	When you eat, do nothing but eat. Don't watch television or read.
	Eat slowly.
	Do not eat food you do not want.
	Follow an eating schedule.
	Do your eating in designated areas such as kitchen or dining room only.
	Leave the table after eating.
	Avoid second servings.
	Limit servings of condiments.
	Limit servings of nonbasics such as dessert, breads, and soft drinks.
	Eat several meals of equal size rather than one big meal and two small ones.
	Eating in the Work Environment
	Take your own food to work.
	Avoid snack machines.
	If you eat out, plan your meal ahead of time.
	Do not eat while working.
	Avoid sharing foods from coworkers including birthday cakes, etc.
	Have activity breaks during the day.
	Have water available to substitute for soft drinks.
	Have low-calorie snacks to substitute for office snacks.

✔	Check 5 to 10 strategies that you might use in the future.
	Eating on Special Occasions
	Practice ways to refuse food.
	Avoid tempting situations.
	Eat before you go out.
	Don't stand near food sources.
	If you feel the urge to eat, find someone to talk to.
	Strategies for Eating Out
	Limit deep-fat fried foods.
	Ask for information about food content.
	Limit use of condiments.
	Choose low-fat foods (e.g., skim milk, low-fat yogurt).
	Choose chicken, fish, or lean meat.
	Order á la carte.
	If you eat desserts, avoid those with sauces or toppings.
	Eating at Home
	Keep busy at times when you are at risk of overeating.
	Store food out of sight.
	Avoid serving food to others between meals.
	If you snack, choose snacks with complex carbohydrates such as carrot sticks or apple slices.
	Freeze leftovers to avoid temptation of eating them between meals.

Conclusions and Implications:

1. In several sentences, discuss your need to use strategies for effective eating. Do you need to use them? Why or why not?

2. In several sentences, discuss the effectiveness of the strategies contained in Chart 1. Do you think they can be effective for people who have a problem controlling their body fatness?

Lab 17B: Evaluating Fast Food Options

Name		Section	Date

Purpose: The purpose of this lab is to learn about the energy and fat content of fast food and how to make better choices when eating at these restaurants.

Procedures:

1. Using Appendix E, select a fast food restaurant and select a typical meal you might order there.
2. Record the total calories, fat calories, saturated fat intake, and cholesterol for each food item.
3. Sum up the totals for the meal in Chart 2.
4. Record recommended daily values by selecting an amount from Chart 1. Estimate should be based on your estimated needs for the day.
5. Compute the percentage of the daily recommended amounts that you consume in the meal by dividing recommended amounts (step 4) into meal totals (step 3). Record percent of recommended daily amounts in Chart 2.
6. Answer the questions in the Conclusions and Implications section.

Chart 1 ▶ Recommended Daily Amounts of Fat, Saturated Fat, Cholesterol, and Sodium

	2000 kcal	3000 kcal
Total Fat:	65 grams	97.5 grams
Saturated Fat:	20 grams	30 grams
Cholesterol:	300 mg	450 mg
Sodium:	2400 mg	3600 grams

Results:

Chart 2 ▶ Listing of Foods Selected for the Meal

Food item	Calories	Total fat (g)	Saturated fat (g)	Cholesterol(mg)
1.				
2.				
3.				
4.				
5.				
6.				
Total for meal (sum up each column)				
Recommended Daily Amount (record values in Chart 1)				
% of recommended daily amt. (% total/recommended 100)				

Conclusions and Implications: In several sentences, answer the following questions.

Describe how often you eat at fast food restaurants and indicate whether you would like to reduce how much fast food you consume.

Were you surprised at the amount of fat, saturated fat, and cholesterol in the meal that you selected?

What could you do differently at fast food restaurants to reduce your intake of fat, saturated fat, and cholesterol?

Stress and Health

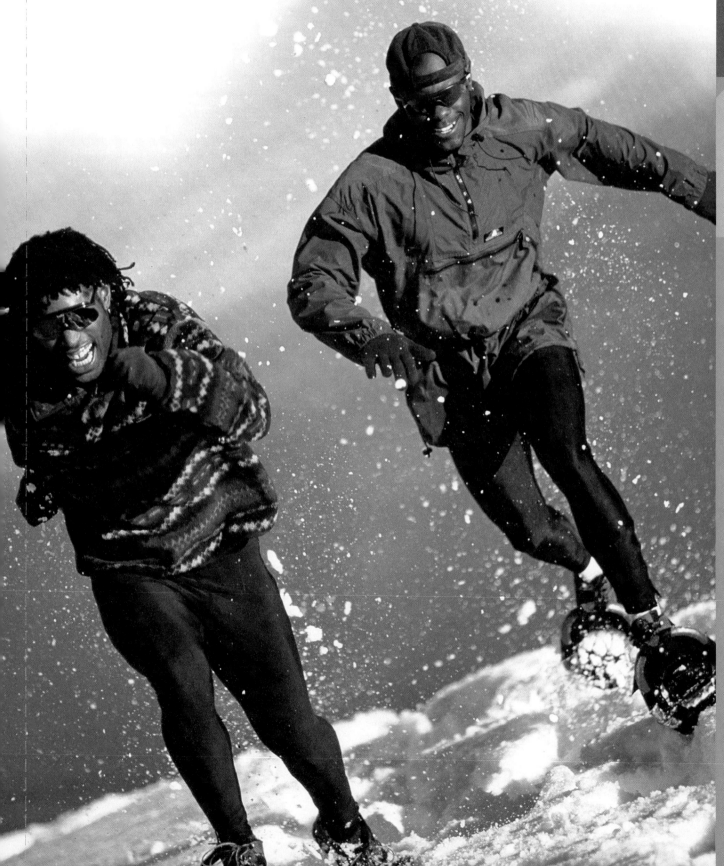

Mental and physical health are affected by an individual's ability to avoid or adapt to stress.

Health Goals
for the year 2010

- Improve mental health and ensure access to appropriate, quality mental health services.

- Increase mental health treatment, including treatment for depression and anxiety disorders.

- Increase mental health screening and assessment.

- Reduce suicide and suicide attempts, especially among young people.

- Increase availability of worksite stress reduction programs.

Stress has been linked to between 50 and 70 percent of all illnesses. Some mental and physical conditions that can be psychosomatic (or stress-related) include the following: high blood pressure and heart disease; psychiatric disorders, such as depression and schizophrenia; indigestion; colitis; poor posture; headaches; insomnia; diarrhea; constipation; increased blood clotting time; increased cholesterol concentration; diuresis; edema; and low back pain. Other serious diseases, such as cancer, can be influenced by a person's state of mind. In many cases, there is considerable time between a major stressor and the onset of a disease, so we do not always associate the two. Because of this, the effect of stress on our body's function has likely been underestimated.

Stress affects nearly everyone to some degree. In fact, approximately 67 percent of adults indicate that they feel "great stress" at least one day a week. Because stress is such a common problem in our society, stress management is viewed as a priority lifestyle similar to physical activity and a healthy diet. This concept will review the cause and consequences of stress and will provide practical guidelines on how to manage stress more effectively.

Reactions to Stress

All people have a similar general reaction to stress. We all share the same physiological system for responding to **stress,** leading to certain commonalities in experience. The autonomic nervous system is associated with a fight or flight response that mobilizes bodily resources when a **stressor** is identified. Sometimes, this alarm reaction of the body may be essential to survival, but when evoked inappropriately or excessively, it may be more harmful than the effects of the original stressor. Activation of this response impacts a variety of systems including physiological, emotional, cognitive, and behavioral. Hans Selye described the General Adaptation Syndrome demonstrating how the autonomic system reacts to stressful situations, and the conditions under which the system may break down (see Table 1). The term "general" highlights the similarities in responses to stressful situations across individuals.

Another constant is a "general" preference for some optimal, generally moderate level of stress (see Figure 1). We all need sufficient stress to motivate us to engage in activities that make our lives meaningful. Otherwise, we might become apathetic and bored, leading to less than optimal health and wellness. In fact, a certain level of stress, called **eustress,** is experienced positively. For example, running in a 10K race stresses the body but is generally experienced as enjoyable by the runner. In contrast, **distress** refers to levels of stress that compromise performance and well-being. So, each of us possesses a system that allows us to mobilize resources when necessary and that seeks to find some homeostatic level of arousal (see Figure 1).

Table 1 ▶ The Three Stages in Hans Selye's General Adaptation Syndrome

Stage 1: Alarm Reaction
Any physical or mental trauma will trigger an immediate set of reactions that combat the stress. Because the immune system is initially depressed, normal levels of resistance are lowered, making us more susceptible to infection and disease. If the stress is not severe or long lasting, we bounce back and recover rapidly.

Stage 2: Resistance
Eventually, sometimes rather quickly, we adapt to stress, and we actually have a tendency to become more resistant to illness and disease. Our immune system works overtime for us during this period, keeping up with the demands placed upon it.

Stage 3: Exhaustion
Because our body is not able to maintain homeostasis and the long-term resistance needed to combat stress, we invariably experience a drop in our resistance level. No one experiences the same resistance and tolerance to stress, but everyone's immunity at some point collapses following prolonged stress reactions. Stress-fighting reserves finally succumb to what Selye called "diseases of adaptation."

Source: Health News Network.

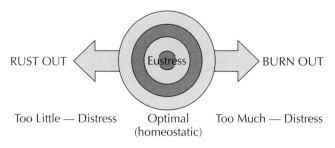

Figure 1 ▶ Stress target zone.

Individuals respond differently to stress. Despite the similarities, each individual experiences stressful situations differently. This is partly due to inherited predispositions and partly due to our unique histories of experiencing and attempting to cope with stress. Recognizing these individual differences has important implications for our well-being because knowledge of our own unique ways of reacting can increase our awareness of the personal impact of stress. For example, some people experience the physiological reactions to stress saliently. Such individuals may notice severe muscular tension during times of high stress. Others may experience the emotional effects of stress more strongly, reporting subjective experiences of anxiety or depressed mood. This information can help you know when to take active measures to manage stress, and which stress management techniques are likely to be most effective.

The optimal level of arousal of stress also varies significantly from person to person. What one person finds stressful may not be stressful to another. Stress mobilizes some to greater efficiency, while it confuses and disorganizes others. For example, sky diving or riding a roller coaster would be thrilling for some people, but for others it would be a stressful and unpleasant experience. Knowing your own optimal level of arousal can help you to manage stress more effectively to optimize health and wellness.

Sources of Stress

The first step in managing stress is to recognize the causes and to be aware of the symptoms. You need to recognize the situations in your life that are the stressors. Identify the things that make you feel "stressed-out." Everything from minor irritations, such as traffic jams, to major life changes, such as births, deaths, or job loss, can be stressors. A stress overload of too many demands on your time can make you feel that you are no longer in control. You may feel so overwhelmed that you become depressed.

Make yourself aware of how your body feels when you are under stress. Are your muscles beginning to tighten? Are you gritting your teeth, gripping the steering wheel tightly, drumming your fingers, tapping your foot, or hunching your shoulders? Can you feel your heart beating faster, your breathing rate becoming faster and more shallow? Are you perspiring, shaking, or getting a headache? By being aware of your most common stressors you will have a better chance of avoiding them or learning how to cope with them. In Lab 18C you will have the opportunity to evaluate muscle tension.

Stress can come from a variety of sources. There are many kinds of stressors. Environmental stressors include heat, noise, overcrowding, climate, and terrain. Physiological stressors may be such things as drugs, caffeine, tobacco, injury, infection or disease, and physical effort.

Emotional stressors are the most frequent and important stressors affecting humans. Some people refer to these as psychosocial stressors. These include life-changing events, such as a change in work hours or line of work, family illnesses, problems with superiors, deaths of relatives or friends, and increased responsibilities. In school, pressures such as grades, term papers, and oral presentations may induce stress. A recent national study of daily experiences indicated that more than 60 percent of all stressful experiences fall in a few areas. These areas are listed in Table 2.

Stressors vary in severity. Because stressors vary in magnitude and duration, many experts categorize them by severity. Major stressors create major emotional turmoil or require tremendous amounts of adjustment. This category includes personal crises (e.g., major health problems or death in family, divorce/separation, financial problems, legal problems) and job/school-related pressures or major age-related transitions (e.g., college, marriage, career, retirement). Minor stressors are generally viewed as shorter term or less severe. This category includes events or problems such as traffic hassles, peer/work relations, time pressures, or family squabbles, just to name a few. Major stressors can alter our daily patterns of stress and

Stress The nonspecific response (generalized adaptation) of the body to any demand made upon it in order to maintain physiological equilibrium. This positive or negative response results from emotions that are accompanied by biochemical and physiological changes directed at adaptation.

Stressor Anything that places a greater than routine demand on the body or evokes a stress reaction.

Adaptation The body's efforts to restore normalcy.

Eustress Positive stress, or stress that is mentally or physically stimulating.

Distress Negative stress, or stress that contributes to health problems.

Table 2 ▶ Ten Common Stressors in the Lives of College Students and Middle-Aged Adults

College Students	Middle-Aged Adults
1. Troubling thoughts about the future	1. Concerns about weight.
2. Not getting enough sleep	2. Health of a family member
3. Wasting time	3. Rising prices of common goods
4. Inconsiderate smokers	4. Home maintenance (interior)
5. Physical appearance	5. Too many things to do
6. Too many things to do	6. Misplacing or losing things
7. Misplacing or losing things	7. Yard work or outside home maintenance
8. Not enough time to do the things you need to do	8. Property, investments, or taxes
9. Concerns about meeting high standards	9. Crime
10. Being lonely	10. Physical appearance

Source: Kanner, A. D. et al.

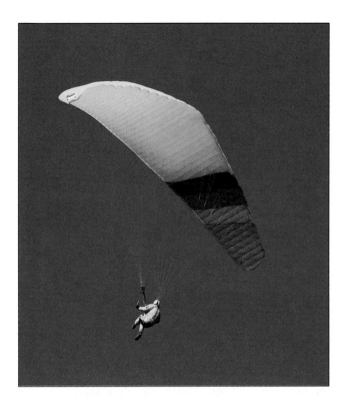

One person's stress is another's pleasure.

impair our ability to handle the minor stressors or hassles of life. Minor stressors can accumulate and create more significant problems. It is important to be aware of both types of stressors.

The nature and magnitude of stressors change during the life span. Depending on your perspective, some periods in life may be more stressful than others, but each phase provides its own challenges and experiences. Some argue that adolescence represents the most stressful time of life. Drastic changes in a person's body and numerous psychosocial challenges must be overcome. College provides additional mental challenges as well as financial pressures and the pressures of living independently. During the early adult years, tremendous pressures and responsibilities force you to juggle career and family obligations. Late adulthood presents still other new challenges such as coping with declining functioning or illness. While the nature of the stressor changes, the presence of stress remains consistent. Learning to manage stress can make it easier to handle the changing stresses in life.

 Financial problems, school work, and employment are significant sources of stress for college students. www.mhhe.com/fit_well/web18 Click 01. Today, the average age of college students is estimated to be in the upper twenties. This is because many people go back to school while working or change careers later in life. No matter what your age, financial problems are stressful. However, students who are not self-sufficient or who have to work as well as attend school are especially likely to experience stress associated with money. Students

are often given access to credit cards even though they may have little experience managing money. To avoid financial problems and their associated stresses, all people would be advised to adhere to the following guidelines:

- Prepare a budget and stick to it. A budget should include an itemized list of planned expenditures. The amount budgeted for all expenses should be less than total income.
- Avoid using credit or credit cards. Credit allows you to buy things you cannot afford but it also reduces your buying power by 5 to 25 percent. Saving to buy the things you want and need allows you to get more for your money.
- Communicate with significant others about spending. Lack of communication is associated with many money problems.

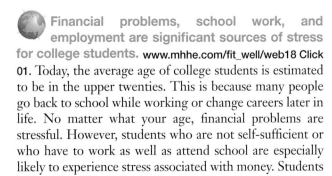

Technology Update

A website prepared by a coalition of colleges and universities is now available to help students and potential students prepare for and cope with the college experience. The site gives information concerning many different topics typical students find stressful including finding financial aid, responsible borrowing, and avoiding scholarship scams. Consult Web Resources for more information.

For college students, schoolwork can be a full-time job and those who have to work outside of school must handle the stresses of both jobs. Although the college years are often thought of as a break from the stresses of the real world, college life has its own unique stressors. Obvious sources of stress include exams, public speaking requirements, and becoming comfortable with talking to professors. Students are often living independent of family for the first time and at the same time negotiating new relationships—with roommates, dating partners, and so on. Young people entering college are also faced with a less structured environment and simultaneously with the need to control their own schedules. Though this environment has a number of advantages, students are faced with a greater need to manage their time effectively. Concept 19 will introduce a number of ways to effectively cope with the unique stresses of the college environment.

Stress can be self-induced and pleasurable, or it can be unpleasurable. www.mhhe.com/ fit_well/web18 Click 02. While many people blame external sources for their stress, much of our stress is self-induced. For example, athletes deliberately place themselves in stressful, competitive situations, lawyers and surgeons attempt the challenge of difficult cases or operations, and pregnant women willingly accept the psychological and physiological stress of bearing children. For some, stress can be addictive. Many **Type A personalities** seek out stressful situations and seemingly thrive on the pressure. Other individual characteristics associated with increased exposure to and enjoyment of highly stimulating situations include sensation seeking, novelty seeking, and impulsivity. Although individuals high in these characteristics may be able to withstand higher levels of stress, they are also at increased risk for unhealthy lifestyles (e.g., alcohol, nicotine and other drug use, unprotected sexual behavior) and associated negative health consequences. Self-induced stress may also be an unpleasant but necessary interlude that cannot be avoided. For example, the risk of falling is necessary in learning to ride a bicycle.

At one time, all people with Type A personalities were thought to be at special risk of health problems, especially heart disease. More recent studies indicate that many Type A personalities adapt to stress well, while others do not. Those who do not express their anger and have hostility associated with stressful situations are more likely to be at risk. A recent study found that these emotions may increase risk for heart disease by increasing cholesterol levels and contributing to the development of obesity. In addition to the physical health risks, recent research suggests that individuals who are high in hostility are likely to have poor social support and greater susceptibility to chronic depression.

Negative, ambiguous, and uncontrollable events are usually the most stressful. While stress can come from both positive and negative events, negative ones generally cause more distress because negative stressors usually have harsher consequences and little benefit. Positive stressors on the other hand usually have enough benefit to make them worthwhile. So, while the stress of getting ready for a wedding may be tremendous, it is not as bad as the negative stress associated with losing a job.

Ambiguous stressors are harder to accept than more clearly defined problems. In most cases, if the cause of a stressor or problem can be identified, then active measures can be taken to improve the situation. For example, if you are stressed about a project at work or school, you can employ specific strategies to help you complete the task on time. Stress brought on by a relationship with friends or coworkers, on the other hand, may be harder to understand. In some cases, it may not be possible to determine the primary source or cause of the problem. These situations are more problematic because fewer clear-cut solutions exist.

Another factor that makes events stressful is a lack of control. Stress brought on by illness, accidents, or natural disasters fit into this category. Because little can be done to change the situation, these events leave us feeling powerless. If the stressor is something that can be dealt with more directly, then efforts at minimizing the stress are likely to be effective. This helps us to feel more in control. As important as the true level of control over stressful events is the individual's perceived level of control. Individual perceptions regarding the controllability of events are often referred to as one's locus of control. People with an internal locus of control generally believe that they have the capacity to impact the outcomes of stressful events. In contrast, individuals with an external locus of control generally believe that outcomes are determined by factors other than personal control (i.e., luck, fate, powerful others). People with a history of exposure to uncontrollable stressful events are particularly likely to develop an external locus of control.

Appraising Stress

Your appraisal of a stressful situation influences its severity. Stressors by themselves generally do not cause problems unless they are perceived or appraised as stressful. Appraisal usually involves a consideration of the consequences of the situation and an evaluation of the

---

Type A Personality A personality type characterized by impatience, ambition, and aggression; Type A personalities may be more prone to the effects of stress but may also be more able to cope with stress.

resources that are available to help you cope with the situation. Stressors that have major consequences and little hope of resolution pose the greatest threat. By maintaining an optimistic view of stressful situations, you can minimize the effect of stress on your lifestyle. In fact, having a positive attitude can create a self-fulfilling prophecy. Individuals with positive thoughts and expectations for recovery show higher recovery rates from illness, and evidence shows that people with a positive outlook will live longer on average. You will have a chance to learn more about the importance of appraisals in concept 19.

Certain personality characteristics have been found to be associated with the ability to deal with stressful situations. www.mhhe.com/ fit_well/web18 **Click 03.** While all people are exposed to stress, some people handle it better than others. Much of the difference lies in how people appraise a stressful situation. Certain characteristics (collectively referred to as **hardiness**) have been found to influence a person's reaction to stressful situations. Individuals possessing hardiness have been found to appraise and respond to stress in more favorable ways than people without it. Research in a college population indicates that individuals who are high in hardiness are at reduced risk for illness, due to the way they perceive stress and the coping mechanisms they use in response to stressful situations. The dimensions of hardiness are:

Commitment: The stressors of everyday life can be overwhelming to many people. While stress cannot be avoided, a sense of commitment to your life and your aspirations can make stress more tolerable. Hardy individuals possess a strong sense of commitment and are willing to put up with adversity to keep pushing toward their desired goals.

Challenge: Many people experience considerable stress from the high-pressure demands of school and work. Much of the stress is caused by concern about being able to meet these new demands and the fear associated with failure. Hardy individuals see new responsibilities and situations as challenges rather than stressors. With this perspective, new situations become opportunities for growth rather than chances for failure.

Control: As previously mentioned, situations tend to be more stressful when they are out of our control. Rather than easily giving up when situations seem out of control, hardy individuals find ways to assume control over their problems. Being proactive rather than reactive is an effective strategy to combating stress. It is important to acknowledge that many stressors may be out of your control. In these situations, it is important to "go with the flow." Depending on the degree of control that is available, some coping strategies may be more effective than others. Specific recommendations are provided in the next concept.

Stress Responses and Health

Chronic or repetitive acute stress can cause or exacerbate a variety of health problems. Some stress persists only as long as the stressor is present. For example, job-related stress caused by a challenging project would generally subside once that project is complete. In contrast, exposure to chronic stress or repeated exposure to acute stress may lead to a host of long-term negative physical and mental health consequences. Stress has been linked to chronic health maladies that plague individuals on a daily basis such as headaches, indigestion, insomnia, and the common cold. In fact, a recent study concluded that "out-of-control" stress was the leading preventable source of increased health-care cost in the workforce, roughly equivalent to the costs of health problems related to smoking.

Even illnesses with a substantial genetic component such as cardiovascular disease and depression have been linked to stress. The diathesis stress model suggests that individuals with a genetic or biological predisposition for a particular illness will express that illness only when environmental stresses are sufficient. Schizophrenia provides a good example of this model. Stress can impact health outcomes through multiple response modalities including physical, cognitive, emotional, and behavioral.

Stress can have physical effects on the body. Many of the commonly observed symptoms of stress are physical in nature. Increases in heart rate and blood pressure and sweaty palms are some of the many physical changes that are commonly observed following acute stress (see Figure 2). It is important to recognize that these physiological responses to stress are a normal part of the body's response. How one interprets these sensations significantly impacts how one will react emotionally and behaviorally. For example, public speaking is a situation that leads to autonomic arousal for most people. Those who handle these situations well probably recognize that these sensations are normal and may even interpret them as excitement about their upcoming speech. In contrast, those who experience severe and sometimes debilitating anxiety are probably interpreting these same sensations as indicators of fear, panic, and loss of control.

Chronic exposure to stress can lead to other physical symptoms such as headaches, indigestion, and stomach cramps. Muscle tension is another common result of stress. One form of this tension is seen in the unnecessary "bracing" or "splinting" action of muscles, for example, the clinched jaw, hunched shoulders, white knuckles, or muscles contracting when not needed. They may stay contracted for long periods without your being aware of it. This tension can cause muscle spasms and pain that, in turn, becomes an additional stressor.

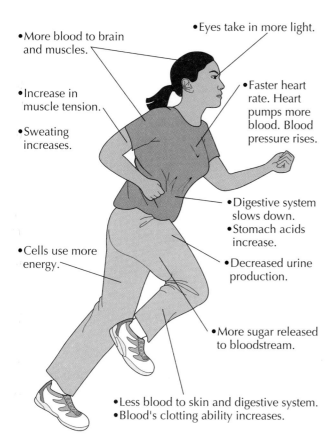

- More blood to brain and muscles.
- Eyes take in more light.
- Increase in muscle tension.
- Faster heart rate. Heart pumps more blood. Blood pressure rises.
- Sweating increases.
- Cells use more energy.
- Digestive system slows down.
- Stomach acids increase.
- Decreased urine production.
- More sugar released to bloodstream.
- Less blood to skin and digestive system.
- Blood's clotting ability increases.

Figure 2 ▶ Physical symptoms of stress.

You can evaluate tension by learning to recognize signs of muscle tension. In Lab 18C, you will have the opportunity to practice evaluating signs of neuromuscular hypertension.

Fatigue is often a symptom of chronic stress. It can result from lack of sleep, emotional strain, pain, disease, or a combination of these factors. Fatigue can be classified as either **physiological fatigue** or **psychological fatigue,** but both can result in a state of exhaustion or **chronic fatigue syndrome.**

Stress can have mental and emotional effects on the body. The challenges caused by psychosocial stress may lead to a variety of mental and emotional effects. In the short term, stress can impair concentration and attention span. Anxiety is an emotional response to stress that is characterized by apprehension. Because the response usually involves expending a lot of nervous energy, anxiety can lead to fatigue and muscular tension.

Anxiety may persist long after a stressful experience. For example, getting physically or sexually assaulted is an incredibly stressful experience and one that tends to stay with a person long after the crime. In some cases, traumatic experiences may lead to Post-Traumatic Stress Disorder (PTSD). Symptoms of PTSD include re-experiencing or "flashbacks" of the traumatic event, avoidance of situations that remind the person of the event, emotional numbing, and increased level of arousal.

People who are excessively stressed are more likely to be depressed than people who have optimal amounts of stress in their lives. Health-care costs for depressed people are 70 percent higher than for those who are not, and costs for people reporting high levels of stress are 50 percent higher than their less-stressed counterparts. Recent research has shown that drugs commonly prescribed to reduce depression can be effective in many cases but that they often do not get to the source of the life stressors that cause depression and often have side effects that are not positive.

Stress can lead to changes in behavior. Stress can cause people to adopt nervous habits like biting their nails. It can also cause normally calm people to become irritable and short-tempered. Other behavioral responses to stress include altered eating and sleeping patterns, smoking, and use of alcohol and other drugs.

In addition to increased tendencies for negative behavior, stress can result in a reduced tendency toward positive behaviors such as regular physical activity and sufficient sleep. The combination of more negative behaviors and less positive behaviors can lead to additional health problems.

Excessive stress reduces the effectiveness of the immune system. Research on the immune system indicates that stress compromises the function of your body's immune system. With an inefficient immune system, it is more difficult to fight off bacterial infections and to recover from medical treatments. An altered immune function also increases a person's susceptibility to allergens. Therefore, allergies and asthma attacks may be more severe under periods of high stress. Other autoimmune disorders such as rheumatoid arthritis are also worsened by stress.

Hardiness A collection of personality traits thought to make a person more resistant to stress.

Physiological Fatigue A deterioration in the capacity of the neuromuscular system as the result of physical overwork and strain; also referred to as true fatigue.

Psychological Fatigue A feeling of fatigue usually caused by such things as lack of exercise, boredom, or mental stress that results in a lack of energy and depression; also referred to as subjective or false fatigue.

Chronic Fatigue Syndrome A clinical condition characterized by a pronounced fatigue or debilitating tiredness.

Strategies for Action

Self-assessments of stressors in your life can be useful in managing stress. In Lab 18A, you will have the opportunity to evaluate your stress levels using the Life Experience Survey. In Lab 18B, you will assess your hardiness, a characteristic associated with effectively coping with stress. In Lab 18C you will evaluate your neuromuscular tension. If you find that you are high in stress, you can use the techniques described in the next concept to help reduce your stress levels.

Web Resources

American Institute of Stress **www.stress.org**
American Psychological Association **www.apa.org**
Health News Network **www.healthnewsnet.com**
International Stress Management Association
    www.stress-management-isma.org
National Center for Post Traumatic Stress Disorder
    www.ncptsd.org

Suggested Readings

Additional reference materials for concept 18 are available at **www.mhhe.com/fit_well/web18 Click 04.**

Benson, H. 1 June 2001. Mind-body pioneer. *USA Today.*
Burns, D. D. 1999. *The Feeling Good Handbook.* New York: Plume.

Diener, E. et al. 2002. Subjective well-being: The science of happiness and life satisfaction. In Snyder, C. R. and S. J., Lopez. *Handbook of Positive Psychology.* New York: Oxford University Press.
Edwards, K. J. 2001. Stress, negative social exchange, and health symptoms in university students. *Journal of American College Health* 50(2):57–80.
Fredrickson, B. 2000. Cultivating positive emotions to optimize health and well-being. *Prevention and Treatment.* http://journals/prevention/vol3/pre0030001a.html.
Girdano, D., and G. Everly. 2000. *Controlling Stress and Tension.* 6th ed. Needham, MA: Allyn and Bacon, Inc.
Greenberg, J. S. 2002. *Comprehensive Stress Management.* 7th ed. St. Louis: McGraw-Hill.
Hudd, S. et al. 2000. Stress at college: Effects on health habits, health status, and self-esteem. *College Student Journal* 34(2):217–227.
Kubzansky, L. D. et al. 2001. Is the glass half empty or half full? A prospective study of optimism and coronary heart disease in the normative aging study. *Psychosomatic Medicine* 63:910–916.
Seligman, M. E. 1998. *Learned Optimism: How to Change Your Mind and Your Life.* New York: Pocket Books.
Snyder, C. R., and S. J. Lopez. 2002. *Handbook of Positive Psychology.* New York: Oxford University Press.
U.S. Department of Health and Human Services. Nov. 2000. *Healthy People 2010.* 2nd ed. With *Understanding and Improving Health and Objectives for Improving Health.* 2 vols. Washington, DC: U.S. Government Printing Office.

In the News

The landscape of college life has changed significantly. According to the American Council on Education, only 40 percent of today's college students enroll full-time immediately after high school. Once in college, more students now work to support their studies and many go back to school after spending time in the working world. These students are likely to have additional pressures not characteristic of the typical college student. Further, more of today's students are the first in their families to go to college. This may place additional pressure on these students to succeed. As a result of these factors, rates of mental health problems among college students have increased dramatically (see Figure 3.) One study indicated that 10 percent of college students are clinically depressed. In another study, 53 percent of students reported feeling depressed at some point during their college careers and 9 percent reported considering suicide. Although more people are receiving care for mental health problems than have in the past, the vast majority are still not receiving adequate care.

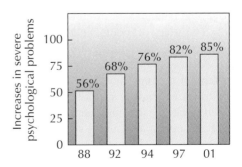

Figure 3 ▶ Colleges reporting increased psychological problems.
Source: Robert Gallagher.

Lab 18A: Evaluating Your Stress Level

Name	Section	Date

Purpose: To evaluate your stress during the past year and determine its implications.

Procedure:

1. Complete the Life Experience Survey based on experiences during the past year. Place a number in the boxes beside events you experienced.
2. Add all of the negative numbers and record your score (distress) in the Results section. Add the positive numbers and record your score (eustress) in the Results section. Use all of the events in the last year.
3. Find your scores on the Rating Scale (Chart 1) and record your ratings.
4. Interpret the results by answering the questions, and discussing the conclusions and implications in the space provided.

Results:

Sum of negative scores   `17`   (distress)   Rating on negative scores [ ]

Sum of positive scores   `7`   (eustress)   Rating on positive scores [ ]

Chart 1 ▶ Scale for Life Experiences and Stress

	Sum of Negative Scores (Distress)	Sum of Positive Scores (Eustress)
May need counseling	14+	
Above-average	9–13	11+
Average	6–9	9–10
Below-average	<6	<9

Scoring the Life Experience Survey:

1. Add all of the negative scores to arrive at your own distress score (negative stress).
2. Add all of the positive scores to arrive at a eustress score (positive stress).

The Life Experience Survey. This survey lists a number of life events that may be distressful or eustressful. Read all of the items. If you did not experience an event leave the box blank. In the box after each event that you did experience, write a number ranging from −3 to +3 using the scale described in the directions. Extra blanks are provided to write in positive or negative events not listed. Some items apply only to males or females. Items 48 to 56 are only for current college students.

Conclusions and Implications: In several sentences, discuss your current stress rating and its implications.

Life Event

Directions: If you did not experience an event, leave the box next to the event empty. If you experienced an event, enter a number in the box based on how the event impacted your life. Use the scale below:

Extremely Negative Impact	= –3
Moderately Negative Impact	= –2
Somewhat Negative Impact	= –1
Neither Positive or Negative	= 0
Somewhat Positive Impact	= +1
Moderately Positive Impact	= +2
Extremely Positive Impact	= +3

1. Marriage — +1
2. Detention in jail or comparable institution — 0
3. Death of spouse — 0
4. Major change in sleeping habits (much more or less sleep) — 0
5. Death of close family member:
   a. mother — 0
   b. father — 0
   c. brother — 0
   d. sister — 0
   e. child — 0
   f. grandmother — –1
   g. grandfather — 0
   h. other (specify) _____ — 0
6. Major change in eating habits (much more or much less food intake) — 0
7. Foreclosure on mortgage or loan — 0
8. Death of a close friend — 0
9. Outstanding personal achievement — +3
10. Minor law violation (traffic ticket, disturbing the peace, etc.) — –1
11. *Male:* Wife's/girlfriend's pregnancy — –2
    Female: Pregnancy —
12. Changed work situation (different working conditions, working hours, etc.) — –1
13. New job — 0
14. Serious illness or injury of close family member:
    a. father — 0
    b. mother — 0
    c. sister — 0
    d. brother — 0
    e. grandfather — 0
    f. grandmother — –2
    g. spouse — 0
    h. child — –1
    i. other (specify) _____ — 0
15. Sexual difficulties — –1
16. Trouble with employer (in danger of losing job, being suspended, demoted, etc.) — –2
17. Trouble with in-laws — –1
18. Major change in financial status (a lot better off or a lot worse off) — –1
19. Major change in closeness of family members (decreased or increased closeness) — –1

20. Gaining a new family member (through birth, adoption, family member moving in, etc.) — 0
21. Change of residence — 0
22. Marital separation from mate (due to conflict) — 0
23. Major change in church activities (increased or decreased attendance) — –1
24. Marital reconciliation with mate — 0
25. Major change in number of arguments with spouse (a lot more or a lot less arguments) — +1
26. *Married Male:* Change in wife's work outside the home (beginning work, ceasing work, changing to a new job) — 0
    Married Female: Change in husband's work (loss of job, beginning new job, retirement, etc.) —
27. Major change in usual type and/or amount of recreation — –1
28. Borrowing more than $10,000 (buying a home, business, etc.) — –1
29. Borrowing less than $10,000 (buying car, TV, getting school loan, etc.) — 0
30. Being fired from job — 0
31. *Male:* Wife/girlfriend having abortion — 0
    Female: Having abortion —
32. Major personal illness or injury — 0
33. Major change in social activities; e. g., parties, movies, visiting (increased or decreased participation) — –1
34. Major change in living conditions of family (building new home, remodeling, deterioration of home, neighborhood, etc.) — 0
35. Divorce — 0
36. Serious injury or illness of close friend — –1
37. Retirement from work — 0
38. Son or daughter leaving home (due to marriage, college, etc.) — 0
39. Ending of formal schooling — 0
40. Separation from spouse (due to work, travel, etc.) — 0
41. Engagement — 0
42. Breaking up with boyfriend/girlfriend — 0
43. Leaving home for the first time — 0
44. Reconciliation with boyfriend/girlfriend — 0

Other recent experiences that have had an impact on your life. List and rate.

45. _____ —
46. _____ —
47. _____ —

For Students Only

48. Beginning new school experience at a higher academic level (college, graduate school, professional school, etc.) — +2
49. Changing to a new school at same academic level (undergraduate, graduate, etc.) — –1
50. Academic probation — 0
51. Being dismissed from dormitory or other residence — 0
52. Failing an important exam — 0
53. Changing a major — 0
54. Failing a course — 0
55. Dropping a course — 0
56. Joining a fraternity/sorority — 0

Source: Sarason, G., Johnson, J. H., and Siegel, J. M.

Lab 18B: Evaluating Your Hardiness

Name	Section	Date

Purpose: To evaluate your level of hardiness and to help you identify the ways in which you appraise and respond to stressful situations.

Procedure:

1. Complete the Hardiness Questionnaire. Make an X over the circle that best describes what is true for you personally.
2. Summarize your score using the scoring chart.
3. Evaluate your score using the Hardiness Rating Chart and record your ratings.
4. Interpret the results by answering the questions, and discussing the conclusions and implications in the space provided.

Hardiness Questionnaire

Questions	Not True	Rarely True	Sometimes True	Often True	Score
1. I look forward to school and work on most days.	1	2	3	4	
2. Having too many choices in life makes me nervous.	4	3	2	1	
3. I know where my life is going and look forward to the future.	1	2	3	4	
4. I prefer to not get too involved in relationships.	4	3	2	1	
Commitment Score Sum 1–4					
5. My efforts at school and work will pay off in the long run.	1	2	3	4	
6. I just have to trust my life to fate to be successful.	4	3	2	1	
7. I believe that I can make a difference in the world.	1	2	3	4	
8. Being successful in life takes more luck and good breaks than effort.	4	3	2	1	
Control Score Sum 5–8					
9. I would be willing to work for less money if I could do something really challenging and interesting.	1	2	3	4	
10. I often get frustrated when my daily plans and schedule get altered.	4	3	2	1	
11. Experiencing new situations in life is important to me.	1	2	3	4	
12. I don't mind being bored.	4	3	2	1	
Challenge Score Sum 9–12					

Results:

Commitment score [ ]

Commitment rating [ ]

Control score [ ]

Control rating [ ]

Challenge score [ ]

Challenge rating [ ]

(Sum the three scores)

Hardiness score [ ]

Hardiness rating [ ]

Chart 1 ▶ Hardiness Rating:

Rating	Individual Hardiness Scale Scores	Total Hardiness Scores
High hardiness	14–16	40–48
Moderate hardiness	10–13	30–39
Low hardiness	Less than 10	Less than 30

Conclusions and Implications:

1. In several sentences, discuss your three hardiness scores. Commitment scores reflect a dedication toward personal goals and life in general. Control scores reflect a belief that events in your life are within your control. Challenge scores reflect an ability to see stressful situations as opportunities for growth. Do you think these scores have implications for you? Are there changes you can make?

2. In several sentences, discuss your total hardiness score. This collection of traits has been referred to as the "stress-resistant personality" since hardy individuals have been found to respond better to stressful situations. Do you think your score is accurate for you? Do you think the score has implications for you?

Lab 18C: Evaluating Neuromuscular Tension

Name	Section	Date

Purpose: To learn to recognize signs of excess muscle tension.

Procedure:

1. Choose a partner. Designate one partner as the subject and the other as the tester.
2. The subject should lie supine in a comfortable position and consciously try to relax.
3. The tester should kneel beside the subject's right hand and remain very still and quiet while the subject is concentrating.
4. After five minutes have elapsed, the tester should observe the subject for signs of visual tension in Chart 1. Check "yes" or "no" for symptoms of visual tension.
5. Quietly and gently, the tester should grasp the subject's right wrist with his or her fingers, and slowly raise it about 3 inches from the floor, letting it hinge at the elbow, then let the hand drop. Observe for the manual symptoms in Chart 1. *Caution:* Make no movement or sound to disturb your partner's concentration and relaxation. Check "yes" or "no" for manual symptoms of tension.
6. You may wish to repeat this after another minute or two.
7. Arouse the subject at the end of the testing and total the number of "yes" checks.
8. Find the rating in Chart 2 and record your score and rating.
9. Change roles and repeat the evaluation with a new subject and tester.
10. Answer the questions in the Results (below) and Conclusions and Implications sections.
11. If time permits, perform the exercises from Table 1 in this concept.

Results:

Check one circle for each of the following questions.

Yes   No

○   ○   Were you aware of your own tension?

○   ○   Was it more difficult to relax than you expected?

○   ○   Did your awareness of your partner make it more difficult to concentrate?

○   ○   Could you concentrate on your breathing without altering its rhythm?

○   ○   Could you learn to release muscular tension and help manage your stress with additional practice?

○   ○   Could you learn to release tension while sitting or standing with your eyes open?

○   ○   Do you think your score today is typical of your normal tension level?

Chart 1 ▶ Signs of Tension Observed by Tester

Visual Symptoms	No	Yes
Frowning	○	○
Twitching	○	○
Eyelids fluttering	○	○
Breathing	○	○
shallow	○	○
rapid	○	○
irregular	○	○
Mouth tight	○	○
Swallowing	○	○

Manual Symptoms	No	Yes
Assistance (subject helps lift arm)	○	○
Resistance (subject resists movement)	○	○
Posturing (subject holds arm in raised position)	○	○
Perseveration (subject continues upward movement)	○	○
Total score equals sum of "yes" checks		

Chart 2 ▶ Tension-Relaxation Rating Scale

Classification	Total Score
Excellent (relaxed)	0
Very good (mild tension)	1–3
Good (moderate tension)	4–6
Fair (tense)	7–9
Poor (marked tension)	10–12

Record Your Tension-Relaxation Rating

Conclusions and Implications:

In several sentences, describe the implications this lab has for you in terms of your daily life (e.g., sleeping, studying, taking exams, performing on stage).

Stress Management, Relaxation, and Time Management

While stress cannot be avoided, proper stress management techniques can help to reduce the impact of stress in your life.

Health Goals

for the year 2010

- Improve mental health and ensure access to appropriate, quality mental health services.

- Increase mental health treatment, including treatment for depression and anxiety disorders.

- Increase mental health screening and assessment.

- Reduce suicide and suicide attempts, especially among young people.

- Increase availability of worksite stress reduction programs.

As outlined in concept 18, we all experience stress on a daily basis and must find ways to manage stress effectively. We can do many things to prevent excessive levels of stress. Examples include exercising regularly, getting sufficient sleep, building a strong social support network, allowing time for recreation, and engaging in effective time management. Despite our best efforts, stressful situations will occur and we must find a way to deal with them. Later in this concept three effective methods for managing stress will be described.

Physical Activity and Stress Management

Regular activity and a healthy diet can help you adapt to stressful situations. An individual's capacity to adapt is not a static function but fluctuates as situations change. The better your overall health, the better you can withstand the rigors of tension without becoming susceptible to illness or other disorders. Physical activity is especially important because it conditions your body to function effectively under challenging physiological conditions.

Physical activity can provide relief from stress and aid in muscle tension release. Physical activity has been found to be effective at relieving stress, particularly white-collar job stress. Studies show that regular exercise decreases the likelihood of stress disorders and reduces the intensity of the stress response. It also shortens the time of recovery from an emotional trauma. Its effect tends to be short term, so one must continue to exercise regularly for it to have a continuing effect. Aerobic exercise is believed to be especially effective in reducing anxiety and relieving stress (though other activities are also good). Whatever your choice of exercise, it is likely to be more effective as an antidote to stress if it is something you find enjoyable.

Physical activity can improve mental health. www.mhhe.com/fit_well/web19 Click 01. The physical health benefits of exercise have been well established for some time. Recent research suggests that the benefits of exercise extend beyond the physical and into the realm of mental health. Studies have demonstrated that exercise can reduce anxiety, aid in recovery from depression, and assist in efforts to eliminate negative health behaviors such as smoking.

- **Physical activity can reduce anxiety.** Evidence shows that physical activity leads to reductions in anxiety in non-clinical samples. One recent study found that exercise may also be effective in reducing anxiety among individuals with panic disorder. An aerobic exercise program led to reductions in panic symptoms relative to a control group. Although exercise was not as effective as medication, it may be a useful addition to other treatment methods for anxiety disorders.

- **Physical activity can reduce depression.** A randomized clinical trial compared antidepressant medication with aerobic exercise to a combined antidepressant and exercise condition in the treatment of major depressive disorder. Results indicated that the aerobic exercise group fared as well as the other two at the end of treatment. In addition, patients who only exercised were less likely to have a remission to depression at a six-month follow-up. Individuals in the exercise condition possibly felt more responsible for the improvements in their condition and this increase in self-efficacy led to better long-term outcomes.

- **Physical activity can aid in changing behaviors related to health.** A recent study tested vigorous physical activity as an adjunct to a cognitive-behavioral smoking cessation program for women. The results indicated that women who received the exercise intervention were able to sustain continuous abstinence from smoking for a longer period of time relative to those who did not receive the exercise intervention. Women in the exercise condition also gained less weight during smoking cessation.

Stretching exercises and rhythmical exercises especially aid in relaxation. People who work long hours at a desk can release tension by getting up frequently and stretching, by taking a brisk walk down the hall, or by performing "office exercises."

Exercising to music or to a rhythmic beat has been found to be relaxing and even "hypnotic." Some exercises designed specifically for relaxation are illustrated in Table 1.

Sleep and Stress

Various techniques can reduce muscle tension. One of the symptoms of stress is muscle tension. Muscle tension can lead to pain, which in turn can negatively influence quality of life, especially for older adults. Various procedures typically used by physical therapists (e.g., ultrasound, heat, cold, and massage) can be helpful in relieving muscle tension. Care should be taken to ensure that these procedures are used properly, typically by experts. Recently, the National Institutes of Health (NIH) concluded that acupuncture has value in relieving muscle tension and associated pain. Again, it is important that the person administering the treatment has appropriate credentials. Most of the treatments described here are for the relief of already existing muscle tension. They are passive techniques that may give relief to symptoms but may do little to eliminate the cause of the problem.

Stress can impair sleep and lack of sleep can be a source of stress. One of the effects of negative stress is insomnia or inability to sleep. Business pressures, worries about college exams, concerns for loved ones who are ill, and other stressors can cause insomnia. On the other hand, lack of sleep is a stressor itself. Using the coping strategies described in this concept can help people who have insomnia. A common myth is that older people need less sleep than younger people. The amount of sleep you need does not change with age. Other factors should also be considered. Some guidelines follow:

- Check with your doctor about medications. Some medicines, such as weight loss pills and decongestants, contain caffeine, ephedrine, or other ingredients that interfere with sleep.
- Avoid tobacco use. Nicotine is a stimulant and can interfere with sleep.
- Avoid excess alcohol use. Alcohol may make it easier to get to sleep but may be a reason why you wake up at night and stay awake.

- Exercise late in the day but do not do vigorous activity right before bedtime.
- Sleep in a room that is cooler than normal.
- Avoid hard-to-digest foods late in the day. Fatty and spicy foods should be avoided.
- Avoid large meals late in the day or right before bedtime. A light snack before bedtime should not be a problem for most people.
- Avoid too much liquid before bedtime.
- Avoid naps during the day.
- Go to bed and get up at the same time each day.
- Do not study, read, or engage in other activities in your bed. You want your brain to associate your bed with sleep, not with activity.
- If you are having difficulty falling asleep, do not stay in bed. Get up and find something to do until you begin to feel tired and then go back to bed.

Social Support and Stress Management

Social support is important for effective stress management. **Social support** has been found to play an important role in coping with stress. Social support has been linked to faster recovery from various medical procedures. One study of athletic injuries has shown that people who were the most stressed were injured more often, and those who had the poorest support system were the most likely to be injured. While the mechanism for this effect is not understood, it is clear that social support plays a major role in stress management. Social support can assist in problem-focused and emotion-focused forms of coping. Friends and family can provide concrete advice that can help solve a problem, and they can also provide moral support and encouragement.

Social support can come from various sources. Everyone needs someone to turn to for support when feeling overwhelmed. Support can come from friends, family members, clergy, a teacher, a coach, or a professional counselor. Different sources may provide different forms of support. Even pets have been shown to be a good source of social support with consequent health and quality of life benefits. The goal is to identify and nurture relationships that can provide this type of support. In turn, it is important to look for ways to support and assist others.

Social Support Any behavior that assists another person in addressing a specific need.

Table 1

Table 1 Relaxation Exercises

1. Neck Stretch

Roll the head slowly in a half-circle from 9:00 to 8:00 to 7, 6, 5, 4, 3, and then reverse from 3 to 9. Close your eyes and feel the stretch. Do *not* make a full circle by tipping the head back. Repeat several times.

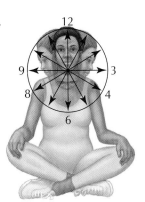

2. Shoulder Lift

Hunch the shoulders as high as possible (contract) and then let them drop (relax). Repeat several times. Inhale on the lift; exhale on the drop.

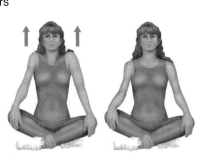

3. Trunk Stretch and Drop

Stand and reach as high as possible; tiptoe and stretch every muscle, then collapse completely, letting knees flex and trunk, head, and arms dangle. Repeat two or three times. Inhale on the stretch and exhale on the collapse.

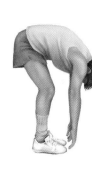

4. Trunk Swings

Following the trunk stretch and drop (see illustration 3), remain in the "drop" position and with a minimum of muscular effort, set the trunk swinging from side to side by shifting the weight from one foot to the other, letting the heels come off the floor alternately. Keep the entire body (especially the neck) limp.

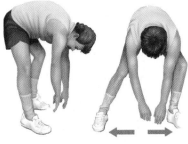

5. Tension Contrast

With arms extended overhead, lie on your side. Tense the body as stiff as a board, then let go and relax, letting the body fall either forward or backward in whatever direction it loses balance. Continue letting go for a few seconds after falling and allow yourself to feel like you are still sinking. Repeat on the other side.

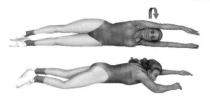

There are many types of social support. Social support can generally be divided into three main components: informational, material, and emotional. Informational (technical support) refers to tips, strategies, or advice that can help a person get through a specific stressful situation. For example, a parent, friend, or coworker may offer insight into how they once resolved similar problems. Material support refers to direct assistance to get a person through a stressful situation. An example would be providing a loan to help pay off a short-term debt. Lastly, emotional support refers to encouragement or sympathy that a person provides to help another cope with a particular challenge.

Obtaining good social support requires close relationships. Although we live in a social environment, it is often difficult to ask people for help. Sometimes the nature and severity of our problems may not be apparent to others. Other times, friends may not want to offer suggestions or insight because they do not want to appear too pushy. To obtain good support, it is important to develop quality personal relationships with several individuals. Research on the effects of social support indicates that the quality of social support, not the quantity, leads to better health outcomes.

Work and Leisure

The amount of time the average person spends at work has increased rather than decreased in the last two decades. Since 1860, the amount of hours typically spent in work decreased dramatically. The most recent statistics (see Figure 1), however, indicate a trend toward increased work time. A major reason for this recent increase is that more people now hold second jobs than in the past. Also, some jobs of modern society have increasing rather than decreasing time demands. For example, medical doctors and other professionals often work more hours than the 35 to 44 hours that the majority of people work. Nearly three times as many married women with children work full time now as compared with 1960.

Experts have referred to young adults as the "overworked Americans" because they work several jobs, maintain dual roles (full-time employment coupled with normal family chores), or they work extended hours in demanding professional jobs. A recent Gallup poll shows that the great majority of adults have "enough time" for work, chores, and sleep but not enough time for friends, self, spouse, and children. When time is at a premium, the factors most likely to be negatively

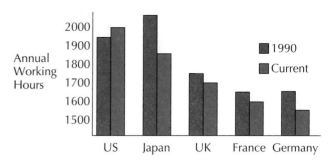

Figure 1 ▶ Average annual working hours of five nations.
Source: Organization for Economic Cooperation and Development.

affected are personal health, relationships with children, and marriage or romantic relationships.

Work pressures can be stressful. This suggests a need to manage time effectively and to find activities that are enjoyable during free time.

Free time is important to the average person. Most people say that **free time** is important, but surveys indicate that more than half of all adults feel that they get too little of it. Many adults report that they get too little time for **recreation** or to simply relax and "do nothing" (leisure).

Recreation and leisure are important contributors to wellness (quality of life). www.mhhe.com/fit_well/web19 Click 02. **Leisure** is time spent "doing things I just want to do" or "doing nothing." Recreation, on the other hand, is often purposeful. Leisure and recreation can contribute to stress reduction and wellness, though leisure activities are not done specifically to achieve these benefits.

The value of recreation and leisure in the busy lives of people in Western culture is evidenced by the emphasis public health officials place on availability and accessibility of recreational facilities in the future.

Free Time Time not committed to work or other duties of the day.

Recreation Recreation means creating something anew. In this book, it refers to something that you do for your amusement or for fun to help you divert your attention and to refresh yourself (re-create yourself).

Leisure Time that is free from the demands of work is often called leisure time. Leisure is more than free time; it is also an attitude. Leisure activities need not be means to ends (purposeful) but are ends in themselves.

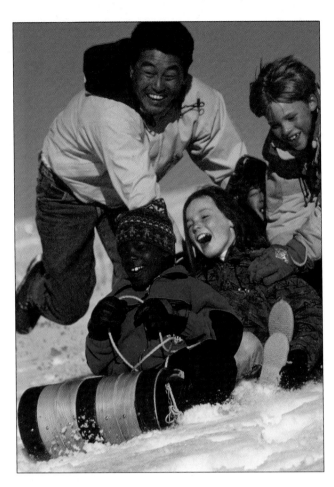

It is important to take time for recreation.

To achieve wellness and stress-reduction benefits, recreation should provide a sense of play. **Play** is done of one's own free will and most often done for fun or intrinsic rather than extrinsic reasons. Activities performed for material things such as trophies and medals can be considered recreational as long as the principal reason for doing the activity is a sense of fun and playfulness. If the activity is done primarily for extrinsic reasons, it may not provide wellness benefits and is probably not true recreation. For example, playing golf to impress the boss is an extrinsic reason that may increase life stress rather than decrease it.

There are many meaningful types of recreation. Many recreational activities involve moderate to vigorous physical activity. If fitness is the goal, these activities should be chosen. Involvement in nonphysical activities also constitutes recreation. For example, reading is a participation activity that can contribute significantly to other wellness dimensions, such as emotional/mental and spiritual. Passive involvement (spectating) is a third type of participation.

Passive participation has been criticized by some people who feel that active participation is an important ingredient of meaningful recreation. Experts point out that spectating can be refreshing and meaningful. For example, watching a good play at the theater qualifies as meaningful recreation and could be true leisure. Likewise, active participation in community theater can be meaningful recreation. To achieve the wellness benefits of recreation, liberal participation and meaningful passive involvement (spectating) are encouraged.

Television viewing has its limitations but is not without its advantages as a recreational activity. Television is a free-time activity that deserves special mention. Evidence presented elsewhere in this book shows that people who spend a great deal of time watching television tend to be fatter and less physically active than people who spend less time watching television. On the other hand, 58 percent of adults feel that watching television is a "good" use of free time. Nevertheless, as many as four in ten people feel that they watch too much television. According to a recent Gallup poll, television is still the favorite way to spend an evening for most Americans, and more people feel that television is good rather than bad for society. Like other activities, it can qualify as leisure and recreation and, for many people, can be useful in stress reduction.

Time Management

Effective time management aids in adapting to the stresses of modern living. Many people in our culture lead stress-filled lives and see the need for lifestyle changes but fail to carry out their plans for various reasons. Most often mentioned is the lack of time. "I would like to exercise, but I don't have the time." "My two jobs don't allow me as much time as I would like to spend with my family." "I know I need to relax and enjoy myself, but I just can't find the time." You may never find time to do all of the things you want to do, but you can learn to manage time more effectively to help you cope with the stresses of daily living. In Lab 19C you will get the opportunity to practice the time-management skills outlined in the section that follows.

There are some steps that can be followed to help you manage your time effectively.

Step 1—Establish Priorities

Analyze what you value in life. Most Americans indicate that they want to reduce time spent in work-related activities and spend more time in recreation, at leisure, and with family or friends. Make a list of your priorities. Are you meeting these priorities? Would you like to have more time for certain activities? Would you like to spend more time with certain people?

Step 2—Monitor Your Current Time Use

What we say we value does not always provide the basis for the way we spend our time. Keep a daily log of actual time expenditures to help you see how you could save time to devote to activities you value.

Step 3—Analyze Your Current Time Use

In each day, the time available for daily activities is fixed. To have more time for priorities, you must modify your schedule. Analysis of daily logs can help you determine how you spend your time. Ask yourself these questions:

- *In what activities can I spend less time?* Be honest. It's easy to say you'll spend less time on work, but can you really do it? Sometimes committed time other than work can be the problem. For example, some joggers spend so much time running that they have less time to spend with family.
- *What can I do to reduce time spent in these activities?* Maybe you can "kill two birds with one stone." For example, recreational time could be used to build fitness. Recreational time could also be family time (e.g., jog with the family). The key is finding activities that truly fulfill priorities for everyone involved. Finding work or recreational activities closer to home may save time.

Step 4—Make a Schedule

Writing a daily schedule can help you use time more effectively. This will allow you to enjoy life as a result of meeting priorities and spending time doing the things that enrich life for you and others important to you. A schedule should not be a rigid plan; it should be flexible enough to allow spontaneous activities.

If you cannot adhere to your time schedule, you should modify it. Your plan may not be realistic, and adhering to it could cause you stress. In that case, the schedule is a problem rather than a solution to a problem.

Committed time can also be free time. You should make a commitment to reserve time for important activities. Taking the time to "re-create" yourself or to enjoy family and friends is important. Sometimes the only way to "find the time" is to plan for it. Charts for helping you manage time effectively are provided in Lab 19C accompanying this concept.

Evaluating Stress and Potential Coping Strategies

Stress appraisals help you decide on a strategy. When faced with a stressful situation, the first thing one must do is assess the situation and determine how best to proceed. How you make this assessment has a major impact on your stress response and the methods used to cope. This is readily apparent from the different reactions that people have to the same or similar stressors. The events of September 11, 2001, provide a vivid example. Everyone who witnessed these events, in person, or on television was profoundly impacted. At the same time, individual reactions varied dramatically. Most felt overwhelming sadness, many felt extreme anger, others felt hopeless or desperate, and yet others felt lost or confused. Undoubtedly, some were simply too shocked to process their emotional experience at all. With time, most Americans began to experience a wave of additional emotions such as hope, patriotism, community, courage, and determination. Others were slower to experience these positive emotions and many developed anxiety, depression, or post-traumatic stress disorder. All of these emotions were reactions to the same stressful events. Although a number of factors contributed to these individual differences (e.g., proximity to New York City and Washington, DC, personal relationship with someone who lost their life), differences in appraisals of the events were probably responsible for much of the variability. Factors that comprise evaluations or appraisals of stressful events and potential coping mechanisms include locus of control, self-efficacy, and outcome expectancies.

Your locus of control influences your coping responses. As described in concept 18, an individual's locus of control can have a significant impact on how one responds to a stressful situation. Research has consistently found that people with an internal locus of control have better health outcomes. These individuals are more likely to take active steps to address problems that created stress, rather than avoiding a problem. Those with an external locus of control are more likely to use passive methods for managing stress. At the same time, an internal locus of control is not always beneficial. A pessimistic explanatory style is characterized by internal, global, and stable attributions about failure. In other words, when these individuals fail, they believe it is their fault and their failure is characteristic of their past and future performance in all areas of their lives. Thus, for an internal locus of control to be beneficial to your well-being, you must combine it with the belief that you are capable of making changes to prevent future problems.

Play Play is something one does of his/her own free will. The play experience is fun, intrinsically rewarding, and a self-absorbing means of self-expression. It is characterized by a sense of freedom or escape from life's normal rules.

Your self-efficacy influences your stress management strategy. Self-efficacy refers to the belief that one is capable of performing a particular task. For example, a professional golfer would generally have high self-efficacy for making a five-foot putt. The rest of us would probably have considerably lower self-efficacy for performance on this same task. Of relevance to health and wellness are people's beliefs about their ability to engage in effective coping strategies or make changes in their lifestyles that will prevent future risk. They must believe that they can successfully engage in problem solving or stick with an exercise program in order to succeed. One way to increase self-efficacy is to increase your knowledge of the options available for managing stress. We hope that the information you learn in this concept will serve this purpose.

Your outcome expectancies influence your stress management strategy. In addition to believing in your own ability to manage stress, you must believe that the response will lead to the desired outcome, in this case stress reduction. These beliefs are called "outcome expectancies," because they represent what you expect to happen as a result of your response. In this concept, you will learn about a number of empirically validated approaches for managing stress. Knowing that these approaches are supported by research should increase your confidence that using these skills will lead to the outcomes you are seeking.

Coping with Stress

Unresolved stress poses the greatest physical and emotional danger. While some stressors are short-lived, many stressors persist over a long period of time. The ability to adapt, or cope with these stressors, largely determines their ultimate effect. If effective coping strategies are used, the effects of a stressful situation can be more tolerable. In many cases, reasonable solutions or compromises can be found. On the other hand, if ineffective coping strategies are used, problems may become even worse. This can lead to more stress and more severe outcomes. Although stress cannot be avoided, it can be managed. Effective stress management is a skill that contributes to both health and quality of life.

Coping strategies can be classified into three basic categories. Individuals deal with stress in a variety of ways; however, the methods of **coping** can generally be classified as **emotion-focused, problem-focused,** or **appraisal-focused** (see Table 2). Emotion-focused coping strategies attempt to regulate the emotions resulting from stressful events. In contrast, problem-focused strategies are aimed at changing the source of the stress. Appraisal-focused coping strategies are based on changing the way one perceives the stressor or changing one's perceptions of

Table 2 ▶ Strategies for Stress Management	
Category	**Description**
Emotion-focused Strategies	**Strategies that minimize the emotional and physical effects of the situation.**
• Relaxing	• Using relaxation techniques to reduce the symptoms of stress.
• Exercising	• Using physical activity to reduce the symptoms of stress.
• Seeking passive social support	• Talking with someone about what you are experiencing or accepting sympathy and understanding.
• Praying	• Looking for spiritual guidance to provide comfort.
Problem-focused Strategies	**Strategies that directly seek to solve or minimize the stressful situation.**
• Systematic problem solving	• Making a plan of action to solve the problem and following through to make the situation better.
• Being assertive	• Standing up for your own rights and values while respecting the opinions of others.
• Seeking active social support	• Getting help or advice from others who can provide specific assistance for your situation.
Appraisal-focused Strategies	**Strategies that alter perceptions of the problem or your ability to effectively cope with the problem.**
• Cognitive restructuring	• Changing negative or automatic thoughts leading to unnecessary distress.
• Seeking knowledge or practicing skills	• Finding ways to increase your confidence in your ability to cope.
Avoidant Coping Strategies	**Strategies that attempt to distract the individual from the problem.**
• Ignoring	• Refusing to think about the situation or pretending no problem exists.
• Escaping	• Looking for ways to feel better or to stop thinking about the problem, including eating or using nicotine, alcohol, or other drugs.

resources for effectively managing stress. While each of these strategies may be effective in various circumstances, **avoidant coping** strategies, like ignoring or escaping the problem, are likely to be ineffective for almost everyone.

A key in stress management is to select coping strategies appropriate for the type of stress that you are experiencing. If you are confronting a situation largely out of your control, the problem-focused efforts to change the situation will unlikely be effective. For these situations, use emotion-focused coping strategies that help to minimize the effects of the stress. On the other hand, if you are experiencing stress from issues or events that you can control, then more problem-focused efforts will likely improve the situation. Appraisal-focused coping strategies may set the stage for you to more effectively use either emotion- or problem-focused strategies.

Coping with most stress requires a variety of thoughts and actions. Stress forces our bodies to work under less than optimal conditions, yet this is the time when we need to function at our best. Effective coping may require some efforts to regulate the emotional aspects of the stress and other efforts directed toward solving the problem. For example, if you are experiencing stress over grades in school, you have to accept your current grades and also take active steps to improve them. Your appraisal of your past performance and the likelihood of improving your performance in the future will significantly impact how you respond to the situation. It does no good to worry about past events. Instead, it is important to look ahead for ways to solve the problems at hand. Coping with this situation may, therefore, require the use of all three effective coping strategies.

Emotion-Focused Coping Strategies: Relaxation, Prayer, and Positive Thinking

Relaxation technique and/or coping strategies can help in relieving stress. When you are aware of what stress does to your body, you can do something to relieve those symptoms immediately as well as on a regular and more long-term basis. While there is no magical cure for stress or tension, various therapeutic approaches may be effective in helping you handle stress. These approaches can slow your heart and respiration, relax tense muscles, clear your mind, and help you relax mentally and emotionally. Perhaps most importantly, these techniques can improve your outlook and help you better cope with the stressful situation. In Lab 19A you will perform a progressive relaxation program. Performing Lab 19A only once will not prepare you to use relaxation techniques effectively. Remember, you must practice learning to relax.

Some treatments are less desirable than others because they act only as "crutches" or "fire extinguishers" and do not get at the root of the problem. Hypnosis may lead to fantasy and dependency. Alcoholic beverages, tranquilizers, and painkillers may give temporary relief and may be prescribed by a physician as part of the treatment, but they do not resolve the problem and may even mask symptoms or cause further problems such as addiction. Drugs do not provide a long-term solution to chronic stress or tension. Contrary to vitamin and mineral advertisements, supplementing the diet with vitamin C or so-called "stress" vitamin formulations has no proven benefits.

Various conscious relaxation techniques exist. Conscious relaxation techniques reduce stress and tension by directly altering the symptoms. When you are stressed, heart rate, blood pressure, and muscle tension all increase to help your body deal with the challenge. Conscious relaxation techniques act to reduce these normal effects and bring the body back to a more relaxed state. Most techniques employ the "three Rs" of relaxation to help the body relax: (1) reduce mental activity, (2) recognize tension, and (3) reduce respiration. Because these techniques do not change the nature or impact of a stressor, they are considered to be a passive or emotion-focused coping strategy.

Several examples of these techniques are described here:

- *"The Quick Fix"*—To get relief from a stressful situation during the day, take a timeout for five to ten minutes by finding a quiet place away from the situation with as few distractions as possible. Sit, loosen your clothes, take off your shoes, and close your eyes. Then follow these steps: (1) Inhale deeply for about four seconds and exhale, letting the air out slowly for about eight seconds (twice as long as the inhalation). Do this several times. (2) Mentally visualize a pleasant image, such as a peaceful lake or stream. Continue to relax and breathe deeply. (3) When your time is up, breathe deeply and stretch luxuriously. Go back to your work refreshed and with a changed attitude. You may need to do this several times a day.

- *Jacobson's Progressive Relaxation Method*—You must be able to recognize how a tense muscle feels before you can voluntarily release the tension. In this technique, contract the muscles strongly, and relax. Each of the large muscles is relaxed first and later the small ones. The contractions are gradually reduced in intensity until no movement is visible. Always, the emphasis is placed on detecting the feeling of tension as the first step in "letting go," or "going negative." Jacobson, a pioneer in muscle relaxation research, emphasized the importance

Coping A person's constantly changing cognitive and psychological efforts to manage stressful situations. Coping strategies can be either active or passive.

Problem-focused Coping A method of adapting to stress that is based on changing the source or cause of stress.

Emotion-focused Coping A method of adapting to stress that is based on regulating the emotions that cause stress.

Appraisal-focused Coping A method of adapting to stress that is based on changing your perceptions of stress and finding resources for coping.

Avoidant Coping Seeking immediate, temporary relief from stress through distraction or self-indulgence.

Technology Update

In concept 8, heart rate watches were described. While the intended purpose of the watches is to help you monitor your heart rate during exercise, they can also be used to help you manage stress. Heart rate can be used in biofeedback (autogenic relaxation training) training for relaxation. When you are in a relaxed state, the heart rate is low. Instead of using the monitor to see if you can get your heart rate in the target zone and keep it there, you can use the heart rate monitor to obtain feedback concerning the effectiveness of your relaxation techniques.

of relaxing eye and speech muscles, because he believed these muscles trigger reactions of the total organism more than other muscles. A sample contract-relax exercise routine for relaxation is presented in Lab 19A.

- *Autogenic (Self-generated) Relaxation Training*—Several times daily, sit or lie in a quiet room with eyes closed. Block out distracting thoughts by passively concentrating on preselected words or phrases. This technique has been used to focus on heaviness of limbs, warmth of limbs, heart rate regulation, respiratory rate and depth regulation, and coolness in the forehead. It evokes changes opposite to those produced by stress. Research has shown that people who are skilled in this technique can decrease oxygen consumption, change the electrical activity of the brain, slow the metabolism, decrease blood lactate, lower body temperature, and slow the heart rate.

- *Biofeedback—Autogenic Relaxation Training*—Biofeedback training utilizes machines that monitor certain physiological processes of the body and provide visual or auditory evidence of what is happening to normally unconscious bodily functions. The evidence of "feedback" is then used to help you decrease these functions. When combined with autogenic training, subjects have learned to relax and reduce the electrical activity in their muscles, lower blood pressure, decrease heart rate, change their brain waves, and decrease headaches, asthma attacks, and stomach acid secretion.

- *Imagery*—Thinking autogenic phrases, you can visualize such feelings as "sinking into a mattress or pillow," or you can think of being a "limp, loose-jointed puppet with no one to hold the strings." You can imagine being a "half-filled sack of flour resting on an uneven surface" or pretend to be "a sack of granulated salt left out in the rain, melting away." Some people seem to respond better to the concept of "floating" than to feeling "heavy." It also includes visualizing pleasant, relaxing scenes as mentioned in the description of The Quick Fix. You attempt to place yourself in the scene and experience all of the sounds, colors, and scents.

Whatever the image you wish to conjure, imagery can help take your mind off anxieties and distractions and, at the same time, release unwanted tension in the muscles using the principle of mind over matter.

Prayer and positive thinking can help you cope with stress and daily problems.

- *Prayer*—Recent studies have shown that prayer can decrease blood pressure for many people and can be a source of internal comfort. It can have other calming effects that are associated with reduced distress. It can also provide confidence to function more effectively, thereby reducing stresses associated with ineffectiveness at work or in other situations.

- *Positive Thinking*—Research supports the idea that optimism relates to psychological well-being. Recent research suggests that positive emotion may also be an effective coping mechanism for managing acute stress. Positive moods seem to help undo the effects of negative emotions. For example, positive moods have been shown to undo some of the cardiovascular effects associated with negative emotions. Positive moods may also help individuals effectively use additional coping strategies to manage stress. The practical implications are relatively simple. Do whatever you need to do to

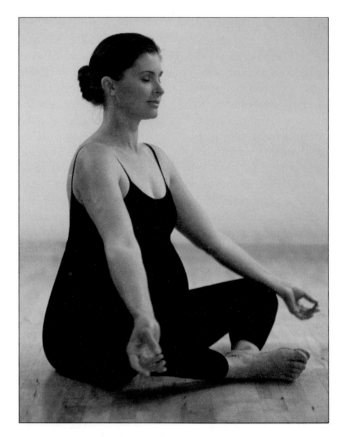

Prayer and meditation can reduce physical symptoms of stress and can help you cope.

create a positive mood when you are stressed or upset. The one thing you do not want to do is dwell on your negative mood. This is likely to prolong the negative mood state and the negative physical, cognitive, and behavioral consequences.

Problem-Focused Coping Strategies: Systematic Problem Solving and Assertiveness

Problem solving and assertiveness can help you cope. Each stressful situation has its own unique circumstances and meaning to the individual. Thus, providing specific information on how to actively cope with each stressor you may face becomes impossible. However, you can develop a consistent way of responding to difficult situations. A technique called systematic problem solving provides an excellent framework. This approach has been shown to improve the likelihood of problem resolution.

The first step is called brainstorming. This is when you generate every possible solution to the problem. During this stage, you should not limit the solutions you generate in any way. Even silly or impractical solutions should be included. After you have generated a comprehensive list, you can narrow your focus by eliminating any solutions that do not seem reasonable. When you have reduced the number of solutions to a reasonable number (four or five), carefully evaluate each option. You should consider the potential costs and benefits of each approach to aid in making a decision. Once you decide on an approach, it is time to carefully plan the implementation of the strategy.

This includes anticipating anything that might go wrong and being prepared to alter your plan as necessary.

In some cases, directly addressing the source of stress involves responding assertively. For example, if the source of stress is an employer placing unreasonable demands on your time, the best solution to the problem may involve talking to your boss about the situation. This type of confrontation is difficult for many people concerned about being overly aggressive. However, you can stand up for yourself without infringing on the rights of others.

Many people confuse assertiveness with aggression leading to passive responses in difficult situations. An aggressive response intimidates others and fulfills one's own needs at the expense of others. In contrast, an assertive response protects your own rights and values while still respecting the opinions of others.

Once you are comfortable with the idea of responding assertively, you may want to practice or role play assertive responses before trying them in the real world. Find a friend you trust and practice responding assertively. Your friend may provide valuable feedback about your approach, and the practice may increase your self-efficacy for responding and your expectancies for a positive outcome.

Appraisal-Focused Coping Strategies: Cognitive Restructuring

Changing your way of thinking can help you cope. Research suggests you can reduce stress by "changing the way you think." At one time or another, virtually all people have "distorted thinking" that can create unnecessary

Table 3 ▶ Checklist of Cognitive Distortion

Type of Cognitive Distortion	Description
1. All or None Thinking	You look at things in absolute, black-and-white categories.
2. Overgeneralization	You view a negative event as a never-ending pattern of defeat.
3. Mental Filter	You dwell on the negatives and ignore the positives.
4. Discounting the Positives	You insist that your accomplishments and positive qualities don't count.
5. Jumping to Conclusions	(A) Mind reading—You assume that others are reacting negatively to you when there is no definite evidence of this; (B) Fortune telling—You arbitrarily predict that things will turn out badly.
6. Magnification or Minimization	You blow things out of proportion or shrink their importance inappropriately.
7. Emotional Reasoning	You reason from how you feel: "I feel like an idiot, so I must be one." Or "I don't feel like doing this, so I'll put it off."
8. "Should Statements"	You criticize yourself or other people with "shoulds" or "shouldn'ts." "Musts," "oughts," and "have tos" are similar offenders.
9. Labeling	You identify with your shortcomings. Instead of saying, "I made a mistake," you tell yourself, "I am a jerk," or "a fool," or "a loser."
10. Personalization and Blame	You blame yourself for something that you weren't entirely responsible for, or you blame other people and overlook ways that your own attitudes and behaviors might contribute to the problem.

Source: Burns, D. D.

Table 4 ▶ Ten Ways to Untwist Your Thinking

The Ten Ways	Description
1. Identify the Distortion	Write down your negative thoughts so you can see which of the ten cognitive distortions you are involved in. This will make it easier to think about the problem in a more positive and realistic way.
2. Examine the Evidence	Instead of assuming that your negative thought is true, if you feel you never do anything right, you could list several things that you have done successfully.
3. The Double Standard Method	Instead of putting yourself down in a harsh, condemning way, talk to yourself in the same compassionate way you would talk to a friend with a similar problem.
4. The Experimental Technique	Do an experiment to test the validity of your negative thought. For example, if during an episode of panic, you become terrified that you are about to die of a heart attack, you could jog or run up and down several flights of stairs. This will prove that your heart is healthy and strong.
5. Thinking in Shades of Gray	Although this method might sound drab, the defects can be illuminating. Instead of thinking about your problems in all-or-none extremes, evaluate things on a range from zero to 100. When things do not work out as well as you hoped, think about the experience as a partial success rather than a complete failure. See what you can learn from the situation.
6. The Survey Method	Ask people questions to find out if your thoughts and attitudes are realistic. For example, if you believe that public speaking anxiety is abnormal and shameful, ask several friends if they ever felt nervous before they gave a talk.
7. Define Terms	When you label yourself "inferior," "a fool," or "a loser," ask, "What is the definition of 'a fool'?" You will feel better when you see that there is no such thing as a fool or a loser.
8. The Semantic Method	Simply substitute language that is less colorful or emotionally loaded. This method is helpful for "should" statements. Instead of telling yourself "I *shouldn't* have made that mistake," you can say, "It would be better if I hadn't made that mistake."
9. Re-attribution	Instead of automatically assuming you are "bad" and blaming yourself entirely for a problem, think about the many factors that may have contributed to it. Focus on solving the problem instead of using up all your energy blaming yourself and feeling guilty.
10. Cost-Benefit Analysis	List the advantages and disadvantages of a feeling (like getting angry when your plane is late), a negative thought (like "No matter how hard I try, I always screw up"), or a behavior pattern (like overeating and lying around in bed when you are depressed). You can also use the Cost-Benefit Analysis to modify a self-defeating belief such as, "I must always be perfect."

Source: Burns, D. D.

stress. Distorted thinking is also referred to as negative or automatic thinking. To alleviate stress, it can be useful to recognize some of the common types of distorted thinking. If you can learn to recognize distorted thinking, you can change the way you think and often reduce your stress levels. Some common types of distorted thinking are listed in Table 3.

If you have ever used any of the ten types of distorted thinking described in Table 3, you may find it useful to consider different methods of "untwisting" your thinking. Using the strategies for untwisting your thinking can be useful in changing negative thinking to positive thinking (see Table 4).

If you really want to change your way of thinking to avoid stress, you may have to practice the guidelines outlined in Table 4. To do this, you can think of a recent situation that caused stress. Describe the situation on paper, and see if you used distorted thinking in the situation (see Table 3). If so, write down which types of distorted thinking you used. Finally, determine if any of the guidelines in Table 4 would have been useful. If so, write down the strategy you could have used. When a similar situation arises, you will be prepared to deal with the stressful situation. Repeat this technique, using several situations that have recently caused stress.

Strategies for Action

This entire concept is dedicated to strategies and skills for preventing, managing, and coping with stress. It is important to understand that for strategies to be effective they must be used regularly. Likewise techniques such as progressive relaxation require practice and consistent use. You are encouraged to consider all of the strategies

in Table 2 and then focus on using those that best meet your needs. The four labs that accompany this concept offer you the chance to practice relaxing tense muscles (19A), evaluate your levels of social support (19B), plan to manage time effectively (19C), and evaluate your current coping strategies (19D).

Web Resources

American Institute of Stress **www.stress.org**
American Psychological Association **www.apa.org**
International Stress Management Association
  www.stress-management-isma.org
National Institute of Mental Health **www.nimh.nih.gov**

Suggested Readings

 Additional reference materials for concept 19 are available at www.mhhe.com/fit_well/web19 Click 03.

Babyak, M. et al. 2000. Exercise treatment for major depression: Maintenance of therapeutic benefit at 10 months. *Psychosomatic Medicine* (62)(5):633–638.

Bernardi, L. et al. 2001. Effect of rosary prayer and yoga mantras on autonomic cardiovascular rhythms: Comparative study. *British Medical Journal* 323:1446–1449.

Blonna, R. 2000. *Coping with Stress in a Changing World.* 2nd ed. St. Louis: McGraw-Hill.

Burns, D. D. 1999. *The Feeling Good Handbook.* rev. ed. New York: Plume/Penguin Books.

Girdano, D., and G. Everly. 2001. *Controlling Stress and Tension.* 6th ed. Needham Heights, MA: Allyn and Bacon, Inc.

Greenberg, J. S. 2002. *Comprehensive Stress Management.* 7th ed. St. Louis: McGraw-Hill.

Jacobson, E. 1978. *You Must Relax.* New York: McGraw-Hill.

Maddux, J. E. 2002. Self efficacy: The power of believing you can. In Snyder, C. R. and S. J. Lopez, (eds.). *Handbook of Positive Psychology.* New York: Oxford University Press.

Pargament, K. L., and A. Mahoney. 2002. Spirituality: Discovering and conserving the sacred. In Snyder, C. R., and S. J. Lopez, (eds.). *Handbook of Positive Psychology.* New York: Oxford University Press.

Paterson, R. J. 2000. *The Assertiveness Workbook: How to Express Your Ideas and Stand Up for Yourself at Work.* Oakland, CA: New Harbinger Publications.

Rutherford, M. et al. November 13, 2000. Pal power: If friends are gifts we give ourselves, it's good to be greedy. Hold on to what you've got—and grab some more. *Time.*

Selye, H. 1978. *The Stress of Life.* 2nd ed. New York: McGraw-Hill.

Seward, B. L. 2001. *Health and the Human Spirit.* Boston: Allyn and Bacon.

Shapiro, S. L. et al. 2002. Meditation and positive psychology. In Snyder, C. R., and S. J. Lopez, (eds.). *Handbook of Positive Psychology.* New York: Oxford University Press.

Snyder, C. R. (ed.). 2001. *Coping with Stress: Effective People and Processes.* New York: Oxford University Press.

Snyder, C. R., and S. J. Lopez, (eds.). 2002. *Handbook of Positive Psychology.* Oxford, UK: University Press.

U.S. Department of Health and Human Services. Nov. 2000. *Healthy People 2010.* 2nd ed. With *Understanding and Improving Health and Objectives for Improving Health.* 2 vols. Washington, DC: U.S. Government Printing Office.

Williams, R., and V. Williams. 1999. *Anger Kills: 17 Strategies for Controlling Hostility That Can Harm You.* New York: Harper Collins Publishers, Inc.

In the News

Earlier in this concept, you learned that social support is a protective factor that reduces the impact of stress on health and wellness. Although this is generally the case, a recent study showed that it depends upon your level of stress. For people under low levels of stress, having a diverse social network is associated with a lower rate of upper respiratory infections (URI) such as colds. On the other hand, high social network diversity was associated with increased incidence of colds for those experiencing a high level of stress. Self-reported symptoms of colds were verified by a physician who performed a thorough examination. So, you may want to focus on the quality and limit the quantity of social support when you are feeling stressed.

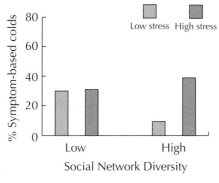

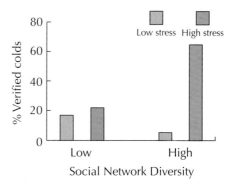

Source: Hamrick, N., Cohen, S., & Rodriguez, M. S. 2002.

Lab 19A: Relaxing Tense Muscles

Name	Section	Date

Purpose: To learn how to relax tense muscles.

Procedure:

Part I

1. Lie on your back in a quiet, nondistracting atmosphere while you are learning this relaxation technique. (Later, you will want to be able to use the technique in public, everyday situations, while you are at work, or any time you are under stress.) Get as comfortable as possible. Close your eyes.
2. Do the Contract-Relax Exercise Routine for Relaxation. Contract the muscles to a moderate level of tension (do not use maximum contractions) as you inhale for five to seven seconds. Study where you are feeling the tension. Try to keep the tension isolated to the designated muscle group without allowing it to spill over to other muscles. Use the dominant side of the body first; repeat on the nondominant side.
3. Next, release the tension completely, instantly relaxing the muscles, and exhale. Extend the feeling of relaxation throughout your muscles for 20 to 30 seconds before contracting again. Think of relaxation words like warm, calm, peaceful, and serene.
4. If time permits, you should practice each muscle group two to five times (until tension is gone) before proceeding to the next group. In a class, you may only have time for one trial. For home practice, do the routine twice a day for 15 minutes.

Contract-Relax Exercise Routine for Relaxation

1. Hand and forearm—Contract your right hand, making a fist; hold 3 counts. Relax and keep letting go 6–10 counts. Repeat, then do left fist, then both fists.
2. Biceps—Flex elbows and contract your biceps; hold 3 counts. Relax and continue relaxing 6–10 counts. Repeat.
3. Triceps—Extend elbows, contract the triceps on the back of the arms. Hold 3 counts. Relax 6–10 counts. Repeat.
4. Relax hands, forearms, and upper arms.
5. Forehead—Raise your eyebrows and wrinkle your forehead; hold 3 counts. Relax and continue relaxing 6–10 counts.
6. Cheeks and nose—Make a face. Wrinkle your nose and squint. Hold 3 counts. Relax and continue relaxing 6–10 counts.
7. Jaws—Clench your teeth 3 counts. Relax 6–10 counts.
8. Lips and tongue—With teeth apart, press lips together and press tongue to roof of mouth. Hold 3 counts. Relax 6–10 counts.
9. Neck and throat—Push head backward while tucking chin, pushing against floor or pillow if lying down. If sitting, push against high chairback. Hold 3 counts. Relax for 6–10 counts.
10. Relax forehead, cheeks, nose, jaws, lips, tongue, neck, and throat. Relax hands, forearms, and upper arms.
11. Shoulder and upper back—Hunch shoulders to ears. Hold 3 counts. Relax 6–10 counts.
12. Relax lips, tongue, neck, throat, shoulders, and upper back.
13. Abdomen—Suck in abdomen. Hold 3 counts. Relax 6–10 counts.
14. Lower back—Contract and arch the back. Hold 3 counts. Relax 6–10 counts.
15. Thighs and buttocks—Squeeze your buttocks together and push your heels into the floor (if lying down) or against a chair rung (if sitting). Hold 3 counts. Relax 6–10 counts.
16. Relax shoulders and upper back, abdomen, lower back, thighs, and buttocks.
17. Calves—Pull instep and toes toward shins. Hold 3 counts. Relax 6–10 counts.
18. Toes—Curl toes; hold 3 counts. Relax 6–10 counts.
19. Relax every muscle in your body.

Note: Eventually, you should progress to a combination of muscle groups and gradually eliminate the "contract" phase of the program.

Part II Perform each of the relaxation exercises that follow (see page 364 for pictures).

1. **Neck Stretch**—Roll the head slowly in a half-circle from 9:00 to 8:00 to 7, 6, 5, 4, and 3. Then reverse from 3 to 9. Close your eyes and feel the stretch. Do *not* make a full circle by tipping the head back. Repeat several times.

2. **Shoulder Lift**—Hunch the shoulders as high as possible (contract) and then let them drop (relax). Repeat several times. Inhale on the lift; exhale on the drop.

3. **Trunk Stretch and Drop**—Stand and reach as high as possible; tiptoe and stretch every muscle, then collapse completely, letting knees flex and trunk, head, and arms dangle. Repeat two or three times. Inhale on the stretch and exhale on the collapse.

4. **Trunk Swings**—Following the trunk stretch and drop, remain in the "drop" position and with a minimum of muscular effort, set the trunk swinging from side to side by shifting the weight from one foot to the other, letting the heels come off the floor alternately. Keep the entire body (especially the neck) limp.

5. **Tension Contrast**—With arms extended overhead, lie on your side. Tense the body as stiff as a board, then let go and relax, letting the body fall either forward or backward in whatever direction it loses balance. Continue letting go for a few seconds after falling and allow yourself to feel like you are still sinking. Repeat on the other side.

Results:

(Yes) (No) Did you find the relaxation exercises effective?

(Yes) (No) Do you think you would find them useful as part of your normal daily routine or as a "quick fix" for stress?

(Yes) (No) Did you find the contract-relax exercise routine relaxing?

(Yes) (No) Do you think you would find it useful as part of your normal daily routine or as a quick fix for stress?

Conclusions and Implications:

In several sentences, discuss whether or not you feel that relaxation exercises will be a part of your wellness program.

Lab 19B: Evaluating Levels of Social Support

Name	Section	Date

Purpose: To evaluate your level of social support and to identify ways that you can find additional support.

Procedures:

1. Use Chart 1 to get personal social support scores. Answer each question. Place number of answers in score box. Sum these questions for each score.
2. In the Results section, record your scores and rate your social support (use Chart 2 for ratings).
3. Use Chart 2 to evaluate the quality and nature of your social support network.
4. Answer the questions in the Conclusions and Implications section.

Chart 1 ▶ Social Support Questionnaire

The following questions assess various aspects of social support. Base your answer on your actual degree of support, not on the type of support that you would like to have. Place a check in the space that best represents what is true for you.

	Not True 1	Somewhat True 2	Very True 3	Score
1. I have close personal ties with my relatives.	✓			
2. I have close relationships with a number of friends.	✓			
3. I have a deep and meaningful relationship with a spouse or close friend.		✓		
Access to social support score:				4
4. I have parents and relatives who take the time to listen and understand me.		✓		
5. I have friends or co-workers whom I can confide in and trust when problems come up.		✓		
6. I have a nonjudgmental spouse or close friend who supports me when I need help.		✓		
Degree of social support score:				6
7. I feel comfortable asking others for advice or assistance.			✓	
8. I have confidence in my social skills and enjoy opportunities for new social contacts.			✓	
9. I am willing to open up and discuss my personal life with others.			✓	
Getting social support score:				9

Scores and Ratings   (Use Chart 2 to obtain ratings).

Access to social support score	4	Rating	Low
Degree of social support score	6	Rating	Moderate
Getting social support score	9	Rating	High
Total social support score (sum of three scores)	19	Rating	Moderate

Results:

Chart 2 ▶ Rating Scale for Social Support		
Rating	**Item Scores**	**Total Score**
High	8–9	24–27
Moderate	6–7	18–23
Low	Below 6	Below 18

Conclusions and Implications:

1. In several sentences, discuss your overall social support. Do you think your scores and ratings are a true representation of your social support?

2. In several sentences, describe any changes you think you should make to improve your social support system. If you do not think change is necessary, explain why.

Lab 19C: Time Management

Name	**Section**	**Date**

Purpose: To help you learn to manage time to meet personal priorities.

Procedure:

1. Follow the four steps outlined below.
2. Answer the questions in the Conclusions and Implications section.

Results:

Step 1: Establishing Priorities

1. Check circles that reflect your priorities from the list below. Add priorities as necessary.

2. Rate each of the priorities you checked. Use a 1 for highest priority, a 2 for moderate priority, and 3 for low priority.

Check Priorities	Rating	Check Priorities	Rating	Check Priorities	Rating
② more time with family		○ more time with boy/girlfriend		② more time with spouse	
① more time for leisure		② more time to relax		① more time to study	
② more time for work success		① more time for physical activity		① more time to improve myself	
○ more time for other recreation		○ other _____		○ other _____	

Step 2: Monitor Current Time Use

1. On the daily calendar, keep track of daily time expenditure.
2. Write in exactly what you did for each time block.

7–9 a.m.	9–11 a.m.	11 a.m.–1 p.m.	1–3 p.m.

3–5 p.m.	5–7 p.m.	7–9 p.m.	9–11 p.m.

Step 3: Analyze Your Current Time Use

Where can I spend less time? (write below)   Where do I need to spend more time? (write below)

Step 4: Make a Schedule: Write in Your Planned Activities for the Day

7–9 a.m.	9–11 a.m.	11 a.m.–1 p.m.	1–3 p.m.
3–5 p.m.	5–7 p.m.	7–9 p.m.	9–11 p.m.

Conclusions and Implications:

In several sentences, discuss how you might modify your schedule to find more time for important priorities.

Lab 19D: Evaluating Coping Strategies

Name		Section	Date

Purpose: To learn how to use appropriate coping strategies that work best for you.

Procedures:

1. Think of five recent stressful experiences that caused you some concern, anxiety, or distress. Describe these situations in Chart 1. Then use Chart 2 to make a rating for changeability, severity, and duration. Assign one number for each category for each situation.
2. In Chart 3 place a check for each coping strategy that you used in coping with each of the five situations you described.
3. Answer the questions in the Conclusions and Implications section.

Results:

Chart 1 ▶ Stressful Situations

Think of five different stressful situations. Appraise each situation and assign a score (changeable, severity, duration) using the scale in Chart 2.

Briefly describe the situation.	Changeable	Severity	Duration
1.			
2.			
3.			
4.			
5.			

Chart 2 ▶ Appraisal of the Stressful Situations

Use this chart to rate the five situations you described above. Assign a number for changeability, severity, and duration for each situation in Chart 1.

	1.	2.	3.	4.	5.
Was the situation changeable?	Completely within my control	Mostly within my control	Both in and out of my control	Mostly out of my control	Completely outside of my control
What was the severity of the stress?	Very minor	Fairly minor	Moderate	Fairly major	Very major
What was the duration of the stress?	Short-term (weeks)	Moderately short	Moderate (months)	Moderately long	Long (months to year)

Chart 3 ▶ Coping Strategies

Directions: Place a check for each coping strategy you used for each of the five situations you described.

Think about your response to the five stressful situations you recently experienced and check the strategies that you used in each situation.	Situation	Situation	Situation	Situation	Situation
Coping Strategy	**1**	**2**	**3**	**4**	**5**
1. I apologized or corrected the problem as best I could.					
2. I ignored the problem and hoped that it would go away.					
3. I told myself to forget about it and grew as a person from the experience.					
4. I tried to make myself feel better by eating, drinking, or smoking.					
5. I prayed or sought spiritual meaning from the situation.					
6. I expressed anger to try to change the situation.					
7. I took active steps to make things work out better.					
8. I used music, images, or deep breathing to help me relax.					
9. I tried to keep my feelings to myself and kept moving forward.					
10. I pursued leisure or recreational activity to help me feel better.					
11. I talked to someone who could provide advice or help me with the problem.					
12. I talked to someone about what I was feeling or experiencing.					

Conclusions and Implications:

1. In several sentences, discuss the coping strategies you used. Were they the ones you used the most? The ones you typically use? Were they effective? Would you consider other strategies in the future?

The Use and Abuse of Tobacco

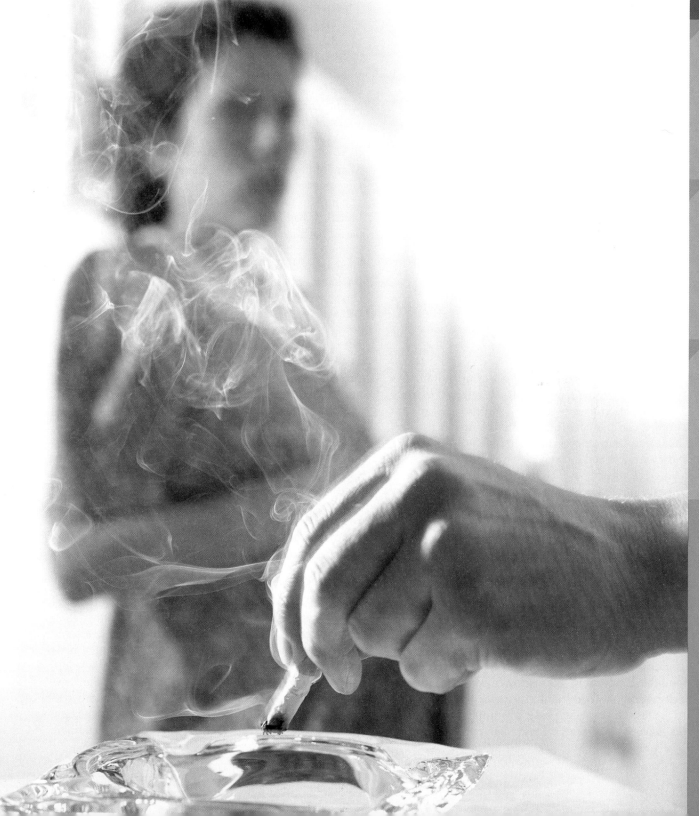

Tobacco use is the number one cause of preventable disease and is associated with the leading causes of death in our culture.

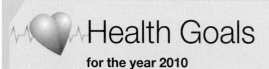

Health Goals

for the year 2010

- Reduce disease, disability, and death related to tobacco use and exposure to secondhand smoke.

- Reduce initiation of tobacco use among youth.

- Reduce tobacco use.

- Reduce exposure to secondhand smoke.

- Increase tobacco-free environments.

- Increase tobacco-use cessation attempts.

- Eliminate tobacco ads that influence youth and young adults.

- Increase average age of first tobacco use by adolescents and young adults.

Tobacco is the number one cause of preventable mortality in the United States. It is linked to most of the leading causes of death and also leads to various other chronic conditions. Rates of smoking in the United States have decreased in recent decades due to better awareness and a changed social norm concerning smoking and tobacco use. Despite the progress, smoking is still a major public health problem. Today, 46.5 million adults in the United States were current smokers (25.7 percent of men and 21.5 percent of women). The majority of smokers would prefer to quit but find freeing themselves from the grip of nicotine addiction too difficult. This concept will review the health risks of tobacco use and provide practical guidelines for quitting.

Tobacco and Nicotine

Tobacco and its smoke contain over 400 noxious chemicals, including 200 known poisons and 50 carcinogens. Tobacco smoke contains both gases and particulates. During one phase of burning tobacco (the gaseous phase), a variety of gases dangerous to humans are released. The most dangerous is carbon monoxide. This gas binds onto hemoglobin in the bloodstream and thereby limits how much oxygen can be carried in the bloodstream. The regular exposure to carbon monoxide by smokers contributes to the "winded" feeling that smokers experience during physical activity. While not likely from smoking, overexposure to carbon monoxide can be fatal.

The other phase of burning tobacco is the particulate phase. This phase releases a variety of particulates that contain a variety of carbon-based compounds referred to as tar. Many of these compounds are known to be **carcinogens.** Cigarettes have nearly 2,000 times more benzene contamination than the Perrier water that was recalled years ago because it had benzene levels that were above health standards. Nicotine is also inhaled during the particulate phase of smoking. Nicotine is a highly addictive and poisonous chemical (often used in insecticides). It has a particularly broad range of influence and is a potent and powerful psychoactive **drug** that affects the brain and alters mood and behavior (see next fact).

Nicotine is the addictive component of tobacco. When smoke is inhaled, the nicotine reaches the brain in seven seconds, where it acts on highly sensitive receptors and provides a sensation that brings about a wide variety of responses throughout the body. At first, the heart and breathing rates increase. Blood vessels constrict, peripheral circulation (especially to the hands and feet) slows down, and blood pressure increases. New users may experience dizziness, nausea, and headache. Then, feelings of tension and tiredness are relieved.

After a few minutes, the feeling wears off and a rebound or **withdrawal** effect occurs. The smoker may feel depressed and irritable and have the urge to smoke again. **Addiction** occurs with continued use. Nicotine is one of the most addictive drugs known, even more addictive than heroin or alcohol.

Smokeless chewing tobacco is as addictive (and maybe more so) as smoking and produces the same kind of withdrawal symptoms upon quitting. Chewing tobacco comes in a variety of forms including loose leaf, twist, or plug form. Rather than being smoked, the chaw, wad, or quid stays in the mouth for several hours, where it mixes with saliva and is absorbed into the bloodstream. Smokeless tobacco contains about seven times more nicotine than cigarettes, and more of it is absorbed because of the length of time the tobacco is in the mouth. It also contains a higher level of carcinogens than cigarettes.

Snuff, a form of smokeless tobacco, comes in either dry or moist forms. Dry snuff is powdered tobacco mixed with flavorings, designed to be sniffed, pinched, or dipped. Moist snuff is used the same way, but it is moist, finely cut tobacco in a loose form or in a teabag-like packet. It comes in a variety of flavors. Experts believe that the flavoring of smokeless tobacco is designed to attract young users.

The Health and Economic Costs of Tobacco

 Smoking is the most preventable cause of death in our society. www.mhhe.com/fit_well/web20 **Click 01.** Smoking is the leading known cause of lung cancer associated with an estimated 124,813 deaths in the United States over a recent four year period. Smoking is also associated with seven other cancers and a variety of other diseases (see Table 1). After lung cancer, the leading causes of death associated with smoking are ischemic heart disease (81,976) and chronic airway obstruction (64,735). Overall, smoking causes 440,000 deaths per year, and adult males and females lose an average of 13.2 and 14.5 years, respectively, because they smoke. Smoking is not just an American problem. Worldwide, 2.5 to 3 million people die annually from smoking.

Smoking has tremendous economic costs. In addition to the cost of human life, smoking is associated with tremendous economic costs to society. It is estimated that each pack of cigarettes sold in the United States costs $7.18 in medical costs and lost productivity. Overall, smoking caused over $150 billion in annual health-related economic losses from 1995 to 1999. The economic costs of smoking are estimated to be about $3,391 per smoker per year.

The health risks from tobacco are directly related to overall exposure. In past years, tobacco companies denied there was conclusive proof of the harmful effects of tobacco products. Now, in the face of overwhelming medical evidence, tobacco officials have finally conceded that tobacco is harmful to health. It is now clear that the more you use the product (the more doses), the greater the health risk. Several factors determine the dosage: (1) the number of cigarettes smoked; (2) the length of time one has been smoking; (3) the strength (amount of tar, nicotine, etc.) of the cigarette; (4) the depth of the inhalation; and (5) the amount of exposure to other lung damaging substances (e.g., asbestos). The greater the exposure to smoke, the greater the risk.

Table 1 ▶ Unhealthy Effects of Smoking

- It is the number one avoidable cause of mortality in the United States.
- It is the number one cause of lung cancer deaths in the United States.
- It is the number one cause of cancer in women.
- It is the number one cause of cancer of the esophagus (especially when combined with alcohol).
- It is the number one cause of cancer of the kidney.
- It is the number one cause of pancreatic cancer.
- It increases risk of cancer of the oral cavity.
- It increases risk of cancer of the larynx.
- It increases risk of fatal breast cancer.
- It increases risk of leukemia.
- It increases risk of cancer of the urinary bladder.
- It increases risk of heart attack and heart disease.
- It increases risk of atherosclerosis.
- It increases risk of Type II diabetes.
- It increases risk of stomach ulcers.
- It increases risk of chronic bronchitis and emphysema.
- It increases risk of miscarriage, infant death, and other complications in pregnant women.
- It causes 88 million more days of sickness per year than for nonsmokers.
- Every cigarette shortens a smoker's life by one minute.
- It decreases the HDL in the blood.

Cigar and pipe smokers have lower death rates than cigarette smokers but still are at great risk. Cigar and pipe smokers usually inhale less and, therefore, have less risk of heart and lung disease, but cigarette smokers who switch to cigars and pipes tend to continue inhaling the same way. As the number of cigars smoked and the depth of smoke inhalation increases, the risk of death from cigar smoking approaches that of cigarette smoking. Cigar and pipe smoke contains most of the same harmful ingredients as cigarette smoke, sometimes in higher amounts. They may also have high nicotine content, leading to no appreciable difference between cigarette and pipe/cigar smoking with respect to the

Carcinogen A substance thought to promote or facilitate the growth of cancerous cells.

Drug Any biologically active substance that is foreign to the body and is deliberately introduced to affect its functioning.

Withdrawal A temporary illness precipitated by the lack of a drug in the body of an addicted person.

Addiction A drug-induced condition in which a person requires frequent administration of a drug in order to avoid withdrawal.

development of nicotine dependence. Cigar and pipe smokers also have higher risks of cancer of the mouth, throat, and larynx relative to cigarette smokers. Pipe smokers are especially at risk for lip cancer.

Although rates of pipe smoking are relatively low, concern about cigar use has increased. Cigar smoking has become quite trendy in recent years, and many associate cigar smoking with power and influence. Perhaps as a result of positive portrayals of cigar smoking in American culture, adolescents and adults have recently increased their use of cigars at the same time that cigarette smoking has been decreasing. Efforts similar to those aimed at changing the social norm for cigarette smoking may be necessary to reduce the prevalence of cigar smoking.

All smokers pollute the air that everyone must breathe. When a smoker lights up, individuals around him or her are exposed to **secondhand** smoke. Secondhand smoke is a combination of **mainstream** and **sidestream** smoke. Sidestream smoke is considered more dangerous than mainstream smoke because it contains higher concentrations of thirteen carcinogens, plus other harmful substances, including nicotine, tar, and carbon monoxide. Its carbon monoxide levels are reported to be from two to fifteen times greater than in the mainstream smoke. Carbon monoxide robs the blood of oxygen. Offices where smoking is allowed may have triple the amount of nicotine level considered hazardous. Emphysema, hypertension, and chronic bronchitis have been related to large doses of cadmium (a carcinogen).

The odor of tobacco smoke presents an additional environmental irritant. It clings to hair, skin, and clothes. Smokers are generally less aware of the health consequences and other negative characteristics of cigarette smoke. They have generally become accustomed to the effects of smoking on their bodies and the environment, and their impaired sense of smell may make it difficult for them to detect the odor caused by secondhand smoke.

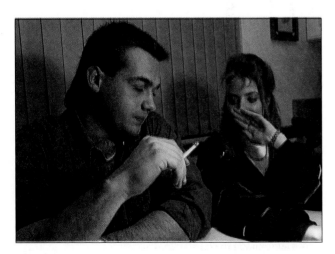

Secondhand smoke makes us all involuntary smokers.

Increasing the awareness of smokers about the effects of secondhand smoke may serve to benefit both the smoker and those they interact with. A recent study showed that awareness by smokers of the impact of secondhand smoke was a significant predictor of the likelihood of quitting.

Secondhand smoke poses a significant health risk. www.mhhe.com/fit_well/web20 Click 02. Nonsmokers who must breathe secondhand smoke are in fact "involuntary" or "passive" smokers and can suffer serious health problems, especially if they are repeatedly exposed to tobacco smoke over long periods of time. The Environmental Protection Agency (EPA) estimated as many as 3,800 lung cancer deaths per year could be attributed to secondhand smoke. Passive smoking has also been found to increase the risk of heart attacks, causing 35,000 to 40,000 deaths per year in the United States. The EPA suggested a direct link between secondhand smoke and asthma. It is believed that smoke accounts for serious respiratory ailments in as many as 200,000 children. The National Center for Health Statistics found that children in nonsmoking households are likely to be healthier and miss fewer days of school than children who live with smokers. Evidence also indicates that the divorce rate is significantly higher among smokers than nonsmokers. Because of these effects, the EPA has classified secondhand smoke as a serious environmental problem.

Even short-term exposure to secondhand smoke can negatively impact health. A recent study showed that as little as 30 minutes of exposure to secondhand smoke decreases the functioning of endothelial cells in the coronary arteries, and endothelial cell function is believed to be central to the development of atherosclerosis. The authors estimated that exposure to secondhand smoke conferred approximately 30 percent risk relative to actually smoking.

While not technically considered as secondhand exposure, smoking during pregnancy can also harm a developing fetus or newborn baby. Studies suggest that smoking contributes to increased rates of premature births. Mothers who smoke are also found to be less likely to nurse their baby, and if they do nurse, the duration of nursing tends to be less than for nonsmoking women.

Smokeless tobacco has similar health risks to other forms of tobacco. Some smokers switch to smokeless tobacco because of the misconception that it is a safe substitute for cigarette, cigar, and pipe smoking. While smokeless tobacco does not lead to the same respiratory problems as smoking, the other health risks may be even greater because smokeless tobacco has more nicotine and higher levels of carcinogens. Because it comes in direct contact with body tissues, the health consequences are far more immediate than those from smoking cigarettes. One-third of teenage users have receding gums, and about half have precancerous lesions, 20 percent of

Table 2 ▶ Health Risks of Smokeless Tobacco

Smokeless tobacco increases the risk of the following:

- Oral cavity cancer (cheek, gum, lip, palate). It increases the risk by 4 to 50 times, depending on length of time used.

- Cancer of the throat, larynx, and esophagus.

- Precancerous skin changes.

- High blood pressure.

- Rotting teeth, exposed roots, premature tooth loss, worn-down teeth.

- Ulcerated, inflamed, infected gums.

- Slow healing of mouth wounds.

- Decreased resistance to infections.

- Arteriosclerosis, myocardial infarction, and coronary occlusion.

- Widespread hormonal effects, including increased lipids, higher blood sugar, and more blood clots.

- Increased heart rate.

which can become oral cancer within five years. Some of the health risks of smokeless tobacco are listed in Table 2.

The Facts about Tobacco Usage

Smoking was an accepted part of our culture, but the social norm has changed in recent years. www.mhhe.com/fit_well/web20 Click 03. While smoking has always been a part of our culture, the industrialization and marketing in the middle of the twentieth century led to tremendous social acceptance of smoking. As odd as it may sound, cigarettes were once provided free to airline passengers when they boarded planes. The release of the Surgeon General's Report on smoking in 1964 and aggressive and well-funded anti-smoking campaigns from various public health agencies have contributed to reductions in smoking in the United States. Since the 1950s, the prevalence of smoking has steadily declined from a high of 50 percent. Although slower, the decline has continued over the past ten years. Based on recent data from the National Health Interview Survey, rates of smoking in the United States have dropped from 25 percent to 23.5 percent since 1993. More recent preliminary data suggest that this trend will continue to near 20 percent in this decade. Decreases in smoking rates are at least partly attributable to the recent 49 percent increase in the price of cigarettes. The bad news is that this rate of decline is too slow to meet the *Healthy People 2010* objective of 12 percent.

Efforts to reduce smoking among young people are likely to have the biggest impact, given that over 55 percent of smokers are under the age of forty-five. The Surgeon

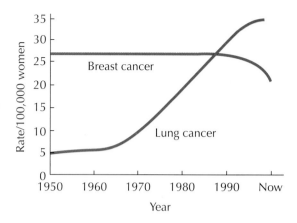

Figure 1 Age-adjusted death rates for lung cancer and breast cancer among women, United States, 1950 to present.

Note: Death rates are age-adjusted to the 1970 population.

Sources: National Center for Health Statistics.

General also called attention to the problem of smoking among women in the 2002 report. Decreases in rates of smoking have been more dramatic for men. As a result, the gender gap in smoking prevalence has now decreased to less than 5 percent, representing a major decrease over the past fifty years. Due to persistent rates of smoking among women, lung cancer has now taken over as the leading cause of death from cancer among women (see Figure 1). About 90 percent of all lung cancer deaths among women are attributable to smoking. The Surgeon General's Report outlines a number of steps that should be taken to decrease smoking among women.

The use of smokeless tobacco is not as prevalent as smoking, but the National Institute of Drug Abuse estimates that 22 million Americans (mostly males) have used it. Young people are also among the most frequent users. Efforts to reduce the use of smokeless tobacco in these high-risk populations continues.

Most tobacco users begin "using" during adolescence and find it hard to quit. www.mhhe.com/fit_well/web20 Click 04. The initiation of smoking is viewed as a pediatric problem by most public health experts. According to a recent report from the Centers for Disease Control, 6,000 people every day under the age of nineteen try their first cigarette. At least 3,000 adolescents

Secondhand Smoke A combination of mainstream and sidestream smoke.

Mainstream Smoke Smoke that is exhaled after being filtered by the smoker's lungs.

Sidestream Smoke Smoke that comes directly off the burning end of the cigarette/cigar/pipe.

Technology Update

The Food and Drug Administration regulates products designed to help people kick the nicotine habit. Several of these prescription products have been approved by the FDA. Other products such as nicotine water have been sold as food supplements. The FDA recently determined "nicotine water" to be an unregulated drug that cannot be sold as a supplement. The FDA also ruled that the sale of nicotine lollipops and lip balm is illegal. The attorney generals of more than forty states would like to have the FDA regulate tobacco flavored nicotine lozenges. They indicate that the lozenges have never been tested for safety and the sweet candy taste will appeal to children. The product manufacturers feel that the lozenges are neither food nor drug and fall outside of FDA regulation. The Supreme Court ruled that the FDA has no regulatory powers over tobacco so the future of the product depends on how they are classified—as tobacco product, food, or drug.

a day reach adulthood (over the age of nineteen) as confirmed cigarette smokers. Overall, 90 percent of smokers began before the age of nineteen. This is the group that finds it most difficult to break the habit later in life.

In a recent study, more than one-third of high school students reported using some form of tobacco in the past month and more than one-fourth of high school students were current cigarette smokers. Much of the blame for tobacco use among adolescents has been attributed to the tobacco industry. Reports from internal tobacco documents released during lawsuits indicate that much of the more than 5-billion-dollar-a-year marketing budget of the tobacco industry is targeted toward youth. Substantial evidence suggests that cartoon characters such as Joe Camel used in tobacco advertising are more effective in marketing to children than adults. One study found that nearly a third of three-year-olds could match Joe Camel to cigarettes.

On the positive side, smoking rates have decreased. A number of factors including increased tobacco taxes, stricter smoking regulations, and increased spending on prevention programs have been cited as contributors to the recent decrease. Several states have initiated programs where tobacco tax money is used to fund prevention programs. If teenage smoking continues to decrease at this rate, the United States could meet the 2010 national health objective of reducing smoking in high school students to 16 percent.

Smokeless tobacco use also begins early in life. Fifty percent of the users report that they started before the age of thirteen and early use is increasing. The nationwide use of smokeless tobacco among eighth to twelfth graders is three to four percent.

Health problems associated with tobacco use have resulted in legal settlements for damages. Over forty states have sued the tobacco industry to recoup funds spent by Medicaid for people with smoking-related diseases. Several states have reached settlements of hundreds of millions of dollars. A federal settlement has not been reached, so individual states are continuing with their lawsuits. In the Minnesota case, millions of pages of tobacco industry documents were made public, and they revealed that in many instances the tobacco industry was targeting youth in their marketing, despite years of denial.

Various factors influence a person's decision to begin or quit smoking. www.mhhe.com/fit_well/web20 Click 05. The reasons for starting smoking are varied, but strikingly similar to reasons given for using alcohol and other drugs (see Table 3). Once a person starts, he or she will typically find it difficult to quit. While a variety of smoking cessation programs are available, several studies have found that increasing the price of cigarettes is the most successful method of reducing smoking among youth. A recent survey revealed that 38 percent of high school students felt that higher prices would help to reduce teen smoking.

Many young women who begin smoking believe that it helps them to control their weight and negative mood states. For example, models and dancers have a high incidence of smoking, and the desire to keep weight down is given as a common reason. Some smokers feel they are unable to quit because they fear gaining weight. The evidence shows people who smoke do not have a lower weight over the long term than nonsmokers. People who fear weight gain should especially not begin smoking, and those who currently smoke may need psychological help when quitting smoking to help overcome fears about weight gain.

People who smoke cigarettes have a tendency to also use alcohol, marijuana, and hard drugs. More smokers use other drugs than do nonsmokers. This is particularly true of the college age (18–25). The reasons are unclear, but it may be that people who do not smoke have a better understanding of the health risks, have better self-esteem, and have better support systems of family and friends. Also they may have

Table 3 ▶ Why Young People Start Using Tobacco

- Peer influence
- Social acceptance
- Desire to be "mature"
- Desire to be "independent"
- Desire to be like their role models
- It looks appealing in advertisements

learned how to say no without giving in to the pressures and lures that make the smokers use tobacco in the first place (Table 3).

The association between smoking and other drug use may account for some third variable. For example, people high in certain personality factors like sensation seeking or impulsivity may be at increased risk of both smoking and other drug use. A recent study supports this possibility, finding no causal association between cigarette smoking and alcohol use.

The addictive nature of nicotine makes it difficult to quit using tobacco. When a person first stops using tobacco, withdrawal symptoms occur. Symptoms can include cravings for tobacco, anxiety, headaches, gastrointestinal discomfort, mood changes, irritability, difficulty with sleeping, difficulty concentrating, tremors, changes in appetite, and cravings for sweets. Because people react differently, a person may experience only a few or all of the symptoms. The length of time it takes to recover from the symptoms varies from days, weeks, or months. Most people do not succeed the first time they try to quit. A recent study estimated that 15.7 million adult smokers had stopped smoking for at least 1 day during the past year in an attempt to quit. The important thing is to keep trying to quit, because most people will eventually succeed (45.7 million adults were former smokers).

Strategies for Action

Some techniques and strategies increase the probability of breaking the nicotine addiction. www.mhhe.com/fit_well/web20 Click 06. The U.S. Public Health Service (USPHS) recently published a consumer's guide to quitting smoking. It determined that the following five factors are associated with your likelihood of success:

1. Get ready.
2. Get support.
3. Learn new skills and behaviors.
4. Get medication and use it correctly.
5. Be prepared for relapse or difficult situations.

Listed below are some more specific strategies that are consistent with these five basic keys to quitting:

- You must want to quit. The reasons could be for health, family, money, etc.
- Remind yourself of the reasons. Each day, repeat to yourself the reasons for not using tobacco.
- Decide how to stop. Methods to stop include counseling, attending formal programs, quitting with a friend, "cold turkey" (abruptly), and quitting gradually. More succeed "cold turkey" than with the gradual approach.
- Remove reminders and temptations (ashtrays, tobacco, etc.).
- Use substitutes and distractions. Substitute low-calorie snacks or chewing gum, change your routine, try new activities, and sit in nonsmoking areas.
- Do not worry about gaining weight. If you gain a few pounds, it is not as detrimental to your health as continuing to smoke.
- Get support. Try a formal "quit smoking program." Examples include "Freedom from Smoking" (American Lung Association) and "Fresh Start" (American Cancer Society). Many state, county, and local health

departments, as well as colleges and universities, have programs. Seek support from friends and relatives.
- Assess your current behavior (see Lab 20A).
- Consider a "crutch." If you choose to taper off, you may want to consider a product that requires a prescription, such as a nicotine transdermal patch (Zyban) or nicotine chewing gum.
- Alternative tobacco products *may* help. Low-tar or ultra-low-tar cigarettes have helped some people stop smoking. They can, however, be just as harmful as regular cigarettes if use continues. Realistically, it is likely that repeated and prolonged exposure to any type of smoke would be harmful to human health.
- Develop effective stress management techniques. The single most frequently cited reason for difficulty in quitting smoking is stress.
- Set up a system of rewards for your success (e.g., use the money you would have spent on cigarettes to do something nice for yourself).

The USPHS consumer guide also provides a list of questions you may want to ask yourself as you prepare to quit. This exercise may help you increase your motivation to change and decrease the likelihood of a relapse. You may want to talk about your answers with your health-care provider.

1. Why do you want to quit?
2. When you tried to quit in the past, what helped and what did not?
3. What will be the most difficult situations for you after you quit? How will you plan to handle them?
4. Who can help you through the tough times? Your family? Friends? Your health-care provider?
5. What pleasures do you get from smoking? In what ways can you still get pleasure if you quit?

The good news is that when you quit, you may feel better right away and your body will eventually heal most of the damage. You will feel more energetic, the coughing will stop, you will suddenly begin to taste food again, and your sense of smell will return. Your lungs will eventually heal and look like the lungs of a nonsmoker. Your risk of lung cancer will return to that of the nonsmoker in about 15 to 20 years. There is life after smoking!

Web Resources

Agency for Health Care Policy and Research **www.ahcpr.gov**
American Cancer Society **www.cancer.org**
American Dental Association **www.ada.gov**
American Heart Association **www.americanheart.org**
American Lung Association **www.lungusa.org**
Dr. Koop-Tackling Tobacco Abuse **www.drkoop.com/tobacco**
National Center for Chronic Disease Prevention and Health Promotion: Tobacco Information and Prevention Source **www.cdc.gov/tobacco**
Quitnet—A Free Resource to Quit Smoking **www.quitnet.org**
Surgeon General Report on Smoking and Health **www.surgeongeneral.gov/tobacco**
You Can Quit Smoking, Consumer Guide, June 2000. U.S. Public Health Service **www.surgeongeneral.gov/tobacco/consquits.htm**

Suggesting Readings

Additional reference materials for concept 20 are available at **www.mhhe.com/fit_well/web20** Click 07.

CDC. 2001. Current cigarette smoking among adults. *Morbidity and Mortality Weekly Reports* 50(49): 1101–1106.

CDC. 2002. Trends in cigarette smoking among high school students—United States. *Morbidity and Mortality Weekly Reports* 51(19):409–412.

Karnath, B. 2002. Smoking cessation. *American Journal of Medicine* 112(5):399–400.

Murray, R. P. et al. 2002. Longitudinal analysis of the relationship between changes in smoking and changes in drinking in a community sample: The Winnipeg health and drinking survey. *Health Psychology* 21(3):237–243.

Payne, W. A., and D. B. Hahn. 2002. *Understanding Your Health*. 7th ed. St. Louis: WCB/McGraw-Hill.

Rigotti, N. A., J. E. Lee, and H. Wechsler. 2000. U.S. college students' use of tobacco products: Results of a national survey. *JAMA* 284(6):699–705.

U.S. Department of Health and Human Services. 2000. *Reducing Tobacco Use: A Report of the Surgeon General*. Atlanta: U.S. Department of Health and Human Services, CDC, National Center for Chronic Disease Prevention and Health Promotion, Office on Smoking and Health.

U.S. Department of Health and Human Services. Nov. 2000. *Healthy People 2010*. 2nd ed. With *Understanding and Improving Health and Objectives for Improving Health*. 2 vols. Washington, DC: U.S. Government Printing Office.

🎙 In the News

As the health risks of smoking have become more widely known and social norms regarding smoking have become less favorable, government has begun to get involved more actively in efforts to curb smoking. At the state level, California recently passed legislation making all restaurants and bars smoke free. Regardless of the impact on the prevalence of smoking, it will undoubtedly have a major public health impact due to decreased exposure to secondhand smoke. The Canadian national government also recently took steps to reduce smoking. Canadian cigarettes now have graphic warnings depicting the negative consequences that can occur from smoking (see the picture below). The ads appear to be having the desired effects. A recent survey by the Canadian Cancer Society found that:

- 43 percent of smokers are more concerned about the health effects of smoking because of the new warnings

- 44 percent of smokers said the new warnings increased their motivation to quit smoking, and of those who attempted to quit, 38 percent said the warnings were a factor in motivating them in their quit attempt

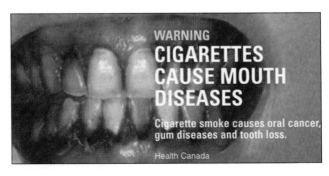

Source: Health Canada.

Lab 20A: Use and Abuse of Tobacco

Name	Section	Date

Purpose:
To help you understand the risks of diseases (such as heart disease and cancer) associated with the use of tobacco or exposure to tobacco by-products.

Procedure:
1. Read the Tobacco Use Risk Questionnaire (Chart 1).
2. Answer the questionnaire based on your tobacco use or exposure.
3. Record your score and rating (from Chart 2) in the Results section.

Results:

What is your Tobacco Risk score? [   ] (total from Chart 1)

What is your Tobacco Risk rating? [   ] (see Chart 2)

Chart 1 ▶ Tobacco Use Risk Questionnaire

Circle one response in each row of the questionnaire. Determine a point value for each response using the point values in the first row of the chart. Sum the numbers of points for the various responses to determine a Tobacco Use Risk score.

Categories	Points 0	1	2	3	4
Cigarette Use	Never smoked		1–10 cigarettes a day	11–40 cigarettes a day	40+ cigarettes a day
Pipe and Cigar Use	Never smoked	Pipe occasional use	Cigar infrequent daily use	Cigar or pipe frequent daily use	Cigar heavy use
Smoking Style	Don't smoke		No inhalation	Slight to moderate inhalation	Deep inhalation
Smokeless Tobacco Use	Do not use	Occasional use: not daily	Daily use: one use per day	Daily use: multiple use per day	Heavy use: repetitious multiple use daily
Secondhand or Sidestream Smoke	No smokers at home or in workplace	Smokers at workplace but not at home	Smokers at home but not workplace	Smokers at home and at workplace	
Years of Tobacco Use	Never used	1 or less	2–5	5–10	10+

NOTE: Different forms of tobacco use pose different risks for different diseases. This questionnaire is designed to give you a general idea of risk associated with use and exposure to tobacco by-products.

Chart 2 ▶ Tobacco Use Risk Questionnaire Rating Chart

Rating	Score
Very high risk	16+
High risk	7–15
Moderate risk	1–6
Low risk	0

Conclusions and Implications:

1. In several sentences, discuss your personal risk. If your risk is low, discuss some implications of the behavior of other people that affect your risk, including what can be done to change these risks. If your risk is above average, what changes can be made to reduce your risk?

2. In several sentences, discuss how you feel about public laws designed to curtail tobacco use. Discuss your point of view, either pro or con.

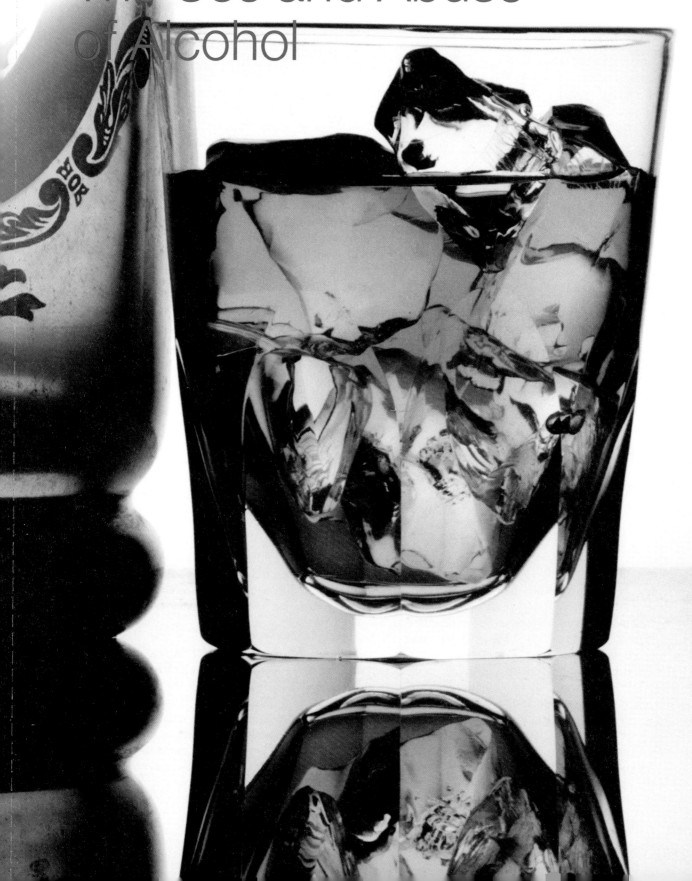

The Use and Abuse of Alcohol

Alcohol is among the most widely used and destructive drugs and ranks high among causes of health problems and death in our culture.

Health Goals

for the year 2010

- Reduce substance abuse to protect the health, safety, and quality of life for all, especially children.

- Reduce deaths and injuries caused by alcohol-related motor vehicle crashes.

- Reduce cirrhosis deaths.

- Reduce alcohol-related injuries and hospital emergency room visits.

- Reduce number of young people who ride with a driver who has been drinking alcohol.

- Increase number of young people who are alcohol free.

- Reduce binge drinking and average alcohol consumption.

- Extend legal requirements for maximum blood alcohol content (BAC) levels to .08 percent for drivers.

Alcohol is the most widely used and destructive drug in the United States. If all of the deaths caused by this drug are counted, it is the third major health problem in the United States. It is second only to tobacco as a cause of premature death in this country. It is considered to be more destructive than tobacco because of the devastating results of drinking and driving (or operating other vehicles) and because of the consequences of increased crime, physical and sexual abuse, and destroyed family relationships that are often associated with overindulgence in alcohol. It is estimated that about 14 million people in the United States, representing over 7 percent of the total population, meet criteria for some type of alcohol-related diagnosis.

Alcohol and Alcoholic Beverages

Alcoholic beverages contain ethanol (ethyl alcohol), an intoxicating and addictive drug that is most often misused in the United States. The active **drug** in alcoholic beverages (ethanol) is a toxic chemical, but unlike methanol (wood alcohol) and isopropyl (rubbing alcohol), it can be consumed in small doses. As a drug, it is classified as a depressant. By depressing the central nervous system, alcohol often makes people more relaxed and uninhibited. For this reason, alcohol is often referred to as a social lubricant.

Alcoholic beverages have been consumed by humans for thousands of years—written records in Egyptian hieroglyphics warned against the overconsumption of alcohol. Unfortunately, many people in our culture (particularly college students) view drunkenness as a rite of passage and an expectation. Indeed, there are more synonyms for the word drunk or **intoxication** than for any other word in the English language. This illustrates the importance that we give to overconsumption. Fortunately, as people mature, they tend to reduce their consumption, as responsibilities such as work and family become more important.

Alcoholic beverages have varying concentrations of alcohol but often have similar amounts per serving. Beverages are usually served in proportions such that a drink of any one of the three categories (beer, wine, or liquor) contains the same amount of alcohol. Beer is usually served in a 12-ounce can, bottle, or mug. A typical glass of wine holds 4 ounces, and a shot of liquor is 1.25 ounces. Even though the percentage of alcohol in the beverages differs, the drinks would be equivalent in alcohol because each would contain about 15 ml of alcohol (see Figure 1).

The effect of alcohol on the body depends on many factors. Alcohol is absorbed directly into the bloodstream through the walls of the stomach and the small intestines. It then concentrates in various organs in proportion to the amount of water each contains. The brain has a high water content, so much of the alcohol goes there, where it depresses the central nervous system. The rate and magnitude of the effects on an individual depend upon the drinker's level of fatigue; his/her mood; what and how much food is in the stomach; other

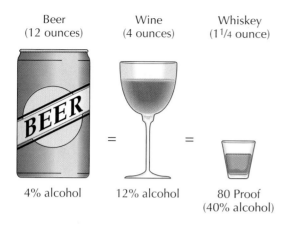

Beer
(12 ounces)

Wine
(4 ounces)

Whiskey
(1 1/4 ounce)

4% alcohol

12% alcohol

80 Proof
(40% alcohol)

Figure 1 ▶ Alcohol content of drinks.

Source: Data from the U.S. Surgeon General and the Government Printing Office.

drugs/medications consumed; body size/weight; rate of consumption; whether blood alcohol content (BAC) levels are increasing or decreasing; individual body chemistry/genetic predisposition; individual beliefs about the effects of alcohol; and context in which drinking occurs. In general, the more and faster one drinks, the greater the effect. Differences in effects are apparent between genders even when differences in body size are considered. One reason for this is that women have lower amounts of body water so a given amount of alcohol will represent a greater percentage of the volume of the blood in their bloodstream. Another factor is that women have lower amounts of the enzymes needed to process alcohol. Thus, alcohol stays in the bloodstream longer before being broken down.

With exposure to alcohol, people develop **tolerance** to alcohol's effects. Tolerance is something that many people (especially men) boast about, with statements like "I can hold my liquor." They may also ridicule others who have not developed tolerance with statements like "you're a lightweight." The reality is that tolerance has mostly negative indications. Practically speaking, the more tolerance one develops, the more he or she has to drink (and spend) to get the same effects. Tolerance is also one of the signs of alcohol abuse and dependence. Recent studies suggest that individuals with an "innate" tolerance to alcohol's effects are also at increased risk for developing problems with alcohol. These people are able to drink heavily without experiencing strong effects, even before extensive exposure to the drug. So, if you are able to drink a lot without feeling the effects, you should recognize that you are at high risk for problems.

The body cannot usually process alcohol as quickly as it is consumed. Alcohol in the bloodstream is eventually oxidized in the liver. Under normal conditions, the liver can process up to 0.25 ounces of alcohol

an hour. Because the average alcoholic beverage contains 0.5 ounces of alcohol, it takes approximately two hours to completely process a drink. If the rate of alcohol consumption is greater than the rate at which it is processed, the alcohol content in the bloodstream begins to increase. The amount of alcohol in the blood is measured as a percentage and is referred to as blood alcohol content (BAC). This figure is used by law enforcement officials to determine if a driver is legally intoxicated.

Studies show the risk in driving increases when the BAC is between 0.01 and 0.04 percent. A BAC of .04 percent is approximately half a drink if you weigh 120 pounds and one drink if you weigh 160. A BAC of .10 percent used to be the level at which driving became illegal in most states. Due to evidence of impairment at much lower doses and the extreme social and economic costs associated with drinking and driving, most states have reduced the legal limit to .08 percent. According to the Insurance Institute for Highway Safety, thirty-two states and the District of Columbia have implemented the .08 standard, and several other states have passed legislation that will adopt this standard in the future.

 Technology Update

A new product from Guardian Angel aims to prevent drinking and driving by providing feedback about blood alcohol levels. People can bring the small strips with them when they are drinking and test themselves before getting behind the wheel. Although it will be some time before the impact of these products can be adequately assessed, Guardian Angel has been commended by those involved in the fight to reduce drunk driving. The president of the National Commission against Drunk Driving stated "The NCADD is extremely pleased to see the efforts of companies like Guardian Angel, who are developing instruments to aid in the fight against drinking and driving, as well as promote responsible living."

Drug Any biologically active substance that is foreign to the body and is deliberately introduced to affect its functioning.

Intoxication Also referred to as drunkenness; a blood alcohol of .08 or .10 depending on the state. National health goals recommend a .08 standard.

Tolerance The phenomenon of requiring more and more alcohol over time to achieve the desired effect.

Health and Behavioral Consequences of Alcohol

The health effects of alcohol consumption depend on the amount that is consumed. Alcohol consumed in moderation (i.e., two or fewer drinks per day for men and one or fewer drinks per day for women) can reduce risks of cardiovascular disease. The reason for this is that alcohol consumed in these moderate amounts can raise the levels of high-density lipoproteins (HDLs), which are referred to as "good cholesterol." Alcohol consumption beyond these levels can lead to a host of physical consequences. Alcohol use is the leading cause of disease and death from liver dysfunction with an estimated 2 million people suffering from alcohol induced liver disease. In addition to impacting liver function, excessive alcohol consumption is associated with increased risk for cardiovascular disease, cancer, and stroke. Heavy drinking may also impair immune functioning leading to increased risk for infectious diseases including pneumonia and tuberculosis (Figure 2 shows the association between alcohol use and various causes of death).

Women appear to be especially susceptible to the negative health consequences of heavy drinking. Assuming similar levels of alcohol consumption, women are more likely to experience liver, cardiovascular, and brain damage from drinking. Alcohol also increases risk for the development of breast cancer and negatively impacts the reproductive system. Excessive alcohol use may lead to infertility, hormonal imbalance, and menstrual disturbance. Women who are pregnant or trying to become pregnant must also consider the impact of alcohol use on the fetus. Drinking during pregnancy can lead to Fetal Alcohol Syndrome, which is associated with low birth weight, physical defects, mental retardation, and stunted growth.

The greatest danger of alcohol occurs when the drinker gets behind the wheel of a motor vehicle. www.mhhe.com/fit_well/web21 Click 01. Alcohol-related traffic crashes are the leading cause of death and spinal cord injury for young Americans. The driver's likelihood of causing a highway accident increases significantly at a BAC of 0.04 percent (approximately the level reached by a 150-pound man who has one to two drinks in an hour) (see Figure 2). When the BAC reaches 0.10 percent, the chances have increased by 600 percent. In a government survey, 70 percent of college students reported driving while under the influence at least once in the past year, and 22 percent said they had done it five times or more. Two out of five Americans will be involved in an alcohol-related auto crash at some time in their lives. In the United States, someone is killed in an alcohol-related crash every 30 minutes. The effects of alcohol on driving performance are listed in Table 1.

Alcohol Consumption and Alcohol Abuse

The Surgeon General has expressed serious concern about the amount of alcohol consumed in the United States and the consequences of alcohol consumption. www.mhhe.com/fit_well/web21 Click 02. In the year 2000, 47 percent of Americans over the age of twelve indicated that they consumed alcohol during the past month. This makes alcohol the most widely used drug of abuse in this country. Twenty-one percent of the population reported engaging in binge drinking as defined by five or more drinks on one occasion in the past month. In addition, one out of every ten people age twelve or older reported drinking and driving in the past 12 months. Unfortunately, the national health goal of reducing per capita consumption to 2 gallons is far from being reached.

The consequences of alcohol abuse touch the lives of the majority of U.S. citizens. About half of those surveyed reported that they have a close family member who has a problem with alcohol. For those who are victims of crime, roughly one-fourth reported that the perpetrator was drinking at the time. Nearly half of all traffic fatalities are alcohol

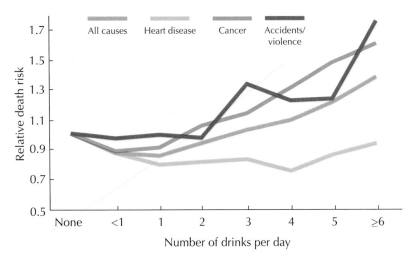

Figure 2 ▶ Alcohol consumption and death risk.

*Adjusted for age and smoking habits
Source: American Cancer Society.

Table 1 ▶ The Effects of Blood Alcohol Content (BAC) on Driving

BAC 0.02%

- Vision impaired: less ability to see objects in motion; less ability to monitor multiple objects
- Lowered attention span
- Reaction time slows
- Less critical of own actions

BAC 0.05–0.06%

- Reduced inhibitions (taking unnecessary chances)
- Visual abilities decrease; side vision impaired approximately 30%
- Superficial feelings of relaxation
- Judgment is the first function to be impaired
- Braking distance is extended
- Diminished ability to maneuver through narrow spaces
- Coordination impaired
- Information processing impaired
- Impaired driving performance at moderate speed

BAC 0.08%

- Seriously impaired vision, especially at night
- Overconfidence in driving ability
- Emotions are exaggerated
- Thinking and reasoning powers impaired
- Less ability to concentrate
- Judgments dulled: careless
- Hinders muscle control and coordination
- Distances are misjudged
- Impaired driving performances at low speeds
- Possible steering inaccuracy
- Increased use of accelerator and brake

Source: MAAD.

Table 2 ▶ Social Problems Associated with Alcohol Abuse

Problems	Percentage of Alcohol-Related Cases
Suicides	33
All deaths from auto accidents	40
All deaths from accidents, suicides, murders	50
All deaths from boating accidents	60
Deaths from drownings	69
Deaths from falls	17–53
Sexual assaults	72
Child abuse	60
Family violence	80
College academic problems	34
Deaths from college sorority/fraternity hazings	90
College undergraduates reporting unplanned sexual activity (at least one instance)	29

Binge drinkers pose risks to others as well as themselves. www.mhhe.com/fit_well/web21 Click 04. A recent report from the National Institute on Alcohol Abuse and Alcoholism (NIAAA) has further raised awareness of the college drinking problem. This report outlined some of the negative consequences associated with heavy drinking in college. Potential negative consequences to the drinker include academic impairment, memory loss, injuries, alcohol poisoning, and death. Behaviors of binge drinkers that pose risks to others as well as themselves include vandalism, drunk driving, unprotected sex, physical aggression, and sexual assault.

Given the high rates of binge drinking, the benefit of efforts to curb heavy college drinking could be considerable. The NIAAA task force made specific recommendations for prevention indicating that changes at the individual, college/university, and community levels would be necessary to meet the *Healthy People 2010* goals. With respect to prevention and treatment at the individual or group level, the task force identified brief motivational enhancement and cognitive-behavioral skills training as the most effective. These relatively brief interventions (as short as 1 one-hour session) help students motivate themselves to make changes and teach them basic skills they can use to meet their goals.

Having a family member with an alcohol problem places you at increased risk for developing a problem yourself. Experts have known for some time that the development of alcohol abuse and dependence has a genetic component. Alcohol problems run in families and it is now estimated that genetics may account for as

related, and the estimated economic cost of alcohol abuse is nearly 185 billion. This is equivalent to $635 per year for every man, woman, and child. A list of some of the alcohol-related problems that contribute to the costs to society are listed in Table 2.

College students drink more than the rest of society and are more at risk for alcohol problems than other segments of the population. www.mhhe.com/fit_well/web21 Click 03. The problem of college drinking has gained increased attention over the past ten years due to the high prevalence of binge drinking (44 percent in 2001) and a number of college student deaths related to excessive alcohol consumption. Binge drinking is defined as five or more drinks in a row for men and four or more drinks in a row for women. Although rates of binge drinking have remained relatively stable during the past ten years, rates of frequent binge drinking appear to be increasing. As a result, the Surgeon General and the United States Department of Health and Human Services (USDHHS) have singled out college binge drinking in *Healthy People 2010*.

much as half of the risk for alcoholism. In the future, we may find out exactly how genetic differences contribute to risk, but for now we know that genetics are important. So, if you have a family history of alcoholism, you should be especially careful about your drinking behavior.

Environment also plays a role in the initiation and escalation of alcohol use. During childhood, parents play an important role in the socialization process which includes socialization regarding alcohol use. Parents who talk to their kids about alcohol use, provide social support, and monitor the behavior of their children are less likely to have children who drink excessively during adolescence. This is important, because early onset of drinking increases the risk for later problems. During adolescence, peers take on a powerful role in the development of alcohol problems. One of the best predictors of adolescent alcohol use patterns is the pattern of alcohol use among their close friends. Peer influences continue into the college years when heavy drinking becomes more normative. Research shows that college students significantly overestimate how much their peers drink. Efforts to alter these inaccurate perceptions have led to decreases in alcohol use and related problems.

Beliefs about the effects of alcohol develop early and play an important role in later drinking behavior. The promotion of alcohol as a social lubricant leads to the development of positive beliefs about the effects of alcohol, referred to as alcohol expectancies. These beliefs have been shown to develop even prior to personal experience with alcohol. Furthermore, positive alcohol expectancies in childhood are associated with alcohol consumption and the development of alcohol-related problems later in life. Once drinking has begun, positive alcohol expectancies typically increase, leading to the maintenance or progression of drinking behavior. Efforts to combat unrealistic expectations about the effects of alcohol have shown promise in reducing alcohol consumption and related negative consequences. Table 3 lists some of the environmental factors that promote drinking.

Different types of alcohol problems have different types of symptom patterns. The term **alcoholism** is widely used to define individuals with alcohol problems, but this label does not adequately define the range of alcohol-related problems. Current diagnostic categories for alcohol-related problems include alcohol dependence and alcohol abuse (see Tables 4 and 5 for signs of each). Those who meet criteria for alcohol dependence are what most people think of when they use the term alcoholic. These people are physically dependent on alcohol and will experience withdrawal symptoms if they are without alcohol for even a relatively short period of time.

Although alcohol dependence is a major problem because of serious health concerns, the vast majority of

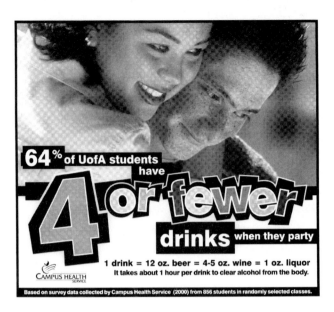

Knowledge of peer behavior can reduce peer pressure.
University of Arizona, Campus Health Service, used by permission.

people with alcohol problems are not in this category. One study indicated that only one out of every four hazardous drinkers is alcohol dependent. That means that about 75 percent of those who drink too much fall into the category of alcohol abuse. Alcohol abuse is less severe than alcohol dependence and generally does not include strong craving for alcohol, loss of control drinking (inability to stop once you begin), or physical dependence. Although alcohol abuse is less severe than dependence, much of the individual and societal costs associated with alcohol are attributable to alcohol abusers (see Tables 4 and 5 for signs of alcohol abuse and dependence).

Table 3 ▶ Why People Start Drinking

- Peer pressure
- Need to belong and to be accepted
- Media depiction of drinking
- Advertising depiction of drinking
- Lack of knowledge about its effects
- Easy access (especially at home)
- Absence of strong religious attachment
- Male bonding (especially in college)
- Cultural traditions at college
- Social lubrication
- It makes them feel good

Alcoholism The loss of control over drinking behavior and/or the lack of ability to refrain from becoming intoxicated.

Table 4 ▶ What Is Alcohol Dependence?

Alcoholism, also known as alcohol dependence, is a disease that includes four symptoms:

Craving A strong need, or compulsion, to drink.

Loss of control The inability to limit one's drinking on any given occasion.

Physical dependence Withdrawal symptoms, such as nausea, sweating, shakiness, and anxiety, occur when alcohol use is stopped after a period of heavy drinking.

Tolerance The need to drink greater amounts of alcohol in order to get high.

Table 5 ▶ What Is Alcohol Abuse?

- Failure to fulfill major work, school, or home responsibilities.
- Drinking in situations that are physically dangerous, such as while driving a car or operating machinery.
- Having recurring alcohol-related legal problems, such as being arrested for driving under the influence of alcohol or for physically hurting someone while drunk.
- Continued drinking despite having ongoing relationship problems that are caused or worsened by the drinking.

Source: National Institute on Alcohol Abuse and Alcoholism.

Strategies for Action

Some people should not drink at all and most people who drink should drink less. Moderate alcohol consumption is safe for many people and may even have some health benefits. However, most people who drink do so beyond safe levels. If you do drink, experts recommend no more than one drink per day for women and no more than two drinks per day for men.

For some people, even moderate levels of alcohol consumption place them at undue risk. Dr. Ernest Noble (former director of the NIAAA) believes that some people should abstain completely (see Table 6).

If you currently exceed safe levels of consumption, you can take steps to control your drinking.

- Make a list of the reasons to stop drinking or cut down.
- Set a goal for yourself and make a plan to meet that goal.
- Monitor your drinking so you know exactly when, where, and how much you are drinking.
- Use the self-monitoring to identify situations that trigger strong urges to drink.
- Eliminate or limit the amount of alcohol in your home.
- Limit the amount of time you spend drinking by drinking slowly, alternating between alcoholic and nonalcoholic drinks, or spending less time in drinking settings like bars or parties.
- Practice drink refusal skills by designating certain non-drinking days. If friends offer you a drink explain to them that you are not drinking that day. You can offer to be the designated driver on your non-drinking days.
- Don't try to keep up with your friends and avoid drinking games that promote excessive use.

If you think you may have a problem with alcohol, help is available. If you think you or someone you know has a problem with alcohol, look for certain signs (see Table 5). If a problem does exist, there are a number of options available. Self-help groups like Alcoholics Anonymous (AA) and Rational Recovery are widespread in the United States. Treatment centers are also readily available. Most treatment centers focus on abstinence-based treatment, but some will help non-alcohol-dependent drinkers control their drinking. The options for treating alcohol-dependence have expanded in recent years (see In the News).

If you are giving a party at which alcohol will be served, be a responsible host/hostess.

- Encourage guests to bring a designated driver.
- Secure safe transportation for those who are intoxicated. Do not let them drive.
- Have plenty of nonalcoholic beverages and high-protein and starchy foods available for the guests.
- Tactfully remove alcoholic beverages from the hands of guests who overindulge.
- Close the bar an hour or two before the party ends.

Table 6 ▶ People Who Should Not Drink

- People under age twenty-one (legal age)
- Athletes striving for peak performance
- Women trying to get pregnant or who are pregnant or nursing
- Alcoholics or recovering alcoholics
- People with a family history of alcoholism
- People with a medical or surgical problem and/or on medications
- Psychiatric patients or persons experiencing severe psychosis
- People driving vehicles or operating dangerous machinery or involved in public safety
- People conducting serious business transactions or study

Web Resources

Alcoholics Anonymous **www.alcoholics-anonymous.org**

The Drink Wheel from Intoximeters, Inc.
www.intox.com/wheel/drinkwheel.asp

Higher Education for Alcohol and Other Drug Prevention (Department of Education) **www.edc.org/hec**

National Clearinghouse for Alcohol and Drug Information (NCADI) **www.health.org**

National Institute on Alcohol Abuse and Alcoholism
www.niaaa.nih.gov

Rational Recovery **www.rational.org**

Suggested Readings

Additional reference materials for concept 21 are available at **www.mhhe.com/fit_well/web21 Click 05.**

Jones, B.T., W. Corbin, and K. Fromme, 2000. A review of expectancy theory and alcohol consumption. *Addiction* 96(1):57–72.

Johnston, L. D., P. M. O'Malley, and J. G. Bachman. 2000. *The Monitoring the Future National Survey Results on Adolescent Drug Use: Overview of Key Findings, 1999.* Rockville, MD: National Institute on Drug Abuse.

Larimer, M. E., and J. M. Cronce. 2002. Identification, prevention and treatment: A review of individual-focused strategies to reduce problematic alcohol consumption by college students. *Journal of Studies on Alcohol* Supplement No. 14:148–163.

NIAAA. 2000. *Tenth Special Report to the U.S. Congress on Alcohol and Health from the Secretary of Health and Human Services.* Bethesda, MD: National Institute on Alcohol Abuse and Alcoholism.

Payne, W. A., and D. B. Hahn. 2002. *Understanding Your Health.* 7th ed. St. Louis: WCB/McGraw-Hill.

Task Force of the National Advisory Council on Alcohol Abuse and Alcoholism. 2002. *High-Risk Drinking in College: What We Know and What We Need to Learn.* Bethesda, MD: National Institutes of Health.

U.S. Department of Health and Human Services. 2000. *Healthy People 2010* 2nd ed. With *Understanding and Improving Health and Objectives for Improving Health.* 2 vols. Washington, DC: U.S. Government Printing Office.

Wechsler, H. et al. 2000. College binge drinking in the 1990s: A continuing problem. Results of the Harvard School of Public Health 1999 College Alcohol Study. *Journal of American College Health* 48:199–210.

Wechsler, H. et al. 2000. What colleges are doing about student binge drinking: A survey of college administrators. *Journal of American College Health* 48:219–226.

 In the News

Historically, the primary aid to recovery from alcoholism has been AA, a self-help organization with groups throughout the country. Until recently, evidence for the success of AA has come from anecdotal reports from people who used AA to maintain sobriety. Recently, the NIAAA conducted a multisite clinical trial demonstrating the effectiveness of 12-step programs (based on the principles of AA). This type of empirical evidence provides greater confidence in the effectiveness of this approach. Still, there are many for whom certain aspects of AA are poorly received. For example, there is a strong spiritual component to AA which may prevent some people from seeking out AA or following through with the program.

Fortunately, there are now alternatives to 12-step programs. The same multisite trial mentioned previously (Project MATCH) also demonstrated that two other behavioral programs were effective in treating alcoholism.

These programs (motivational enhancement and cognitive-behavioral therapy) were just as effective as the 12-step programs and can often be implemented in a shorter period of time. They also place more emphasis on personal control over behavior. Regardless of which approach appeals to a particular person, there is now something for everyone.

Another NIAAA trial called Project COMBINE is under way. This study will test the combined effectiveness of psychosocial interventions and medication. Acamprosate and Naltrexone, (already been approved for use by the FDA) are the medications being tested. Acamprosate has been approved for use in Europe with promising results. It is currently undergoing clinical trials for approval in the United States. The hope is that the combination of psychosocial and medical intervention will provide even better outcomes for those suffering from alcohol dependence.

Lab21A: Blood Alcohol Level

Name		**Section**	**Date**

Purpose: To learn to calculate your (or a friend's) blood alcohol content (BAC).

Procedures:

1. Assume a drink is a 12-ounce can or bottle of 4 percent beer or a 4-ounce glass (a small glass) of 12 percent alcohol (wine), or a mixed drink with a 1-ounce shot glass (jigger) of 100 proof liquor (or one and one-fourth of a jigger of 80 proof).

    Case A: Assume you consumed two drinks within 40 minutes.

    Case B: Assume you consumed two drinks over a period of one hour and twenty minutes.

    Case C: Assume you had two six-packs of beer (twelve cans) over five hours.

    Case D: Same as C, but if you weigh fewer than 150 pounds, assume you weigh 50 pounds more than you now weigh, and if you weigh more than 150 pounds, assume you weigh 50 pounds less.

2. Divide 3.8 by your weight in pounds to obtain your "BAC maximum per drink," or refer to Chart 1. You should obtain a number between 0.015 and 0.04 (based on one drink in 40 minutes). Use the formula below to determine BAC over time.

$$\text{Approximate BAC over time} = \frac{(3.8 \times \text{\# of drinks})}{(\text{body weight})} - \frac{[0.01 \times (\text{\# min.} - 40)]}{40}$$

3. After 40 minutes have passed, your body will begin eliminating alcohol from the bloodstream at the rate of about 0.01 percent for each additional 40 minutes. Multiply the number of drinks you've had by your "BAC maximum per drink" and subtract 0.01 percent from the number for each 40 minutes that have passed since you began drinking—but don't count the first 40 minutes. Compute your BAC for cases A, B, C, and D.

    Example: Case A. Mary weighs 100 pounds. $\dfrac{3.8 \times 2}{100} = \dfrac{7.6}{100} = 0.076\%$ BAC

    Case B. Mary takes 80 minutes. $0.076\% - \dfrac{[0.01 \times (80 - 40)]}{40} = 0.066\%$ BAC

4. Record your results below by writing the formula and computing the BAC for each case.

Results:

Case A $\dfrac{(3.8 \times \underline{\quad} \text{ \# drinks})}{\underline{\quad} \text{lbs}} = \underline{\quad}\% \, \text{BAC}$

Case B $\dfrac{(3.8 \times \underline{\quad} \text{ \# drinks})}{\underline{\quad} \text{lbs}} - \dfrac{[0.01 \times (\underline{\quad} \text{ \# min.} - 40)]}{40} = \text{BAC} \left(\quad \right) - \left(\quad \right) = \underline{\quad}\% \, \text{BAC}$

Case C $\dfrac{(3.8 \times \underline{\quad} \text{ \# drinks})}{\underline{\quad} \text{lbs}} - \dfrac{[0.01 \times (\underline{\quad} \text{ \# min.} - 40)]}{40} = \text{BAC} \left(\quad \right) - \left(\quad \right) = \underline{\quad}\% \, \text{BAC}$

Case D $\dfrac{(3.8 \times \underline{\quad} \text{ \# drinks})}{\underline{\quad} \text{lbs}} - \dfrac{[0.01 \times (\underline{\quad} \text{ \# min.} - 40)]}{40} = \text{BAC} \left(\quad \right) - \left(\quad \right) = \underline{\quad}\% \, \text{BAC}$

1. Would you (or your friend) be able to drive legally according to your state laws? Place an X over your answer.

Case A. (Yes) (No)

Case B. (Yes) (No)

Case C. (Yes) (No)

Case D. (Yes) (No)

2. Would you (or your friend) be able to drive legally if the Health Goals for the Year 2010 (.08) were put into effect? Place an X over your answer.

Case A. (Yes) (No)

Case B. (Yes) (No)

Case C. (Yes) (No)

Case D. (Yes) (No)

Conclusions and Implications: In several sentences, discuss what you have learned from doing this activity.

Chart 1 ▶ Determining Blood Alcohol Level (%)

Your Weight in Pounds	Drinks Consumed in One Hour				
	1	2	3	4	5
100	0.038	0.076	0.114	0.152	0.190
120	0.032	0.064	0.096	0.128	0.160
140	0.027	0.054	0.081	0.108	0.135
160	0.024	0.048	0.072	0.096	0.120
180	0.021	0.042	0.063	0.084	0.105
200	0.019	0.038	0.057	0.076	0.095
220	0.017	0.034	0.051	0.068	0.085
240	0.016	0.032	0.048	0.064	0.080

Using Chart 1
- Find body weigh on left.
- Find drinks consumed at top.
- Connect row and column to determine BAL.

Lab 21B: Perceptions about Alcohol Use

Name	**Section**	**Date**

Purpose: To help you better understand perceptions about drinking behaviors.

Procedures:

1. Think of a person you care about. Do not identify this person on this lab report.
2. Answer each of the questions in the questionnaire below as honestly as possible, evaluating the behavior of the person you have identified. Calculate a total score and determine a rating (see Chart 1).
3. At another time, when you do not have to submit your results, you should answer the questions about yourself.
4. Answer the questions in the Conclusions and Implications section.

Results:

	Never	Sometimes	Frequently	Too Often	Add Score
1. How often does the person drink?	0	1	2	3	
2. How often does the person have six or more drinks on one occasion?	0	1	2	3	
3. How often do friends of the person drink?	0	1	2	3	
4. How often has the person been unable to stop after starting to drink?	0	1	2	3	
5. How often does the person need a drink to get started in the morning.	0	1	2	3	
6. How often has the person been unable to remember previous events after drinking?	0	1	2	3	
7. How often does the person miss class or work associated with drinking?	0	1	2	3	
8. How often does the person have social or personal problems associated with drinking?	0	1	2	3	
9. How often does the person deny drinking too much? (only for those who you consider to drink too much)	0	1	2	3	

Total Score:

Chart 1 ▶ Drinking Behavior Rating Scale

Rating	Score
Alcohol abuse*	18+
Drinking problem	12–17
Potential problem	8–11
Low risk of problem	<8

*Professional help recommended

Rating

Conclusions and Implications:

1. In several sentences, discuss the drinking behavior of the person you identified. Do you think your ratings give an accurate picture of the person? Do you think the person you rated has a problem with alcohol?

2. In several sentences, discuss the drinking behavior of the person's friends. Do the friends promote drinking or not?

3. In several sentences, discuss things that you could do to help a friend or loved one solve a drinking problem.

The Use and Abuse of Other Drugs

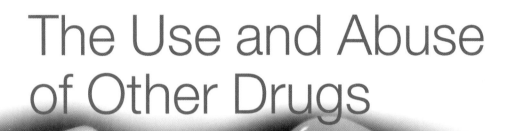

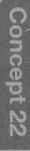

Drug abuse has serious health consequences and enormous personal, social, and economic costs.

Health Goals
for the year 2010

- Reduce substance abuse to protect the health, safety, and quality of life for all, especially children.

- Reduce deaths and injuries caused by drug-related motor vehicle crashes.

- Reduce drug-induced deaths and intentional injuries from drug-related violence.

- Reduce loss of productivity in workplace and increase availability of treatment programs for drug abusers.

- Increase number of young people who stay drug free.

- Reduce steroid use among young people.

- Increase proportion of young people who disapprove of substance abuse.

About a third of college students currently use illegal drugs, up from a low of 29 percent in 1991, but far below the 56.2 percent who used illicit drugs in 1980. Millions of people are arrested each year for drug offenses—including sale, distribution, and possession. This has a tremendous cost to society. Tobacco and alcohol are the most commonly used drugs in the United States (see concepts 20 and 21). This concept discusses **drug abuse** and misuse with emphasis on the illegal, so-called street drugs.

Drugs

Drugs may be classified in several ways, but the mood-altering or psychoactive drugs are the ones we hear about most. Mood-altering and **psychoactive drugs** may be placed in five major groups: depressants, opiates, stimulants, hallucinogens, and designer drugs. Drugs in the same group have similar effects. Narcotics (opiates) are actually depressants, but because the word *narcotics* is so widely used in law enforcement and in society in general, they are generally given their own category. Each of the five categories of drugs is discussed in this concept, and the effects are described in Tables 1 through 5. The effects are classified as either physiological or psychological (meaning primarily affecting the body versus primarily affecting behavior). Because the effects of drugs can vary with each individual and with different doses, it is only possible to generalize about the effects in the tables that follow.

Depressant drugs include alcohol, benzodiazepines, and barbiturates. Depressants come in the form of pills, liquids, or injectables (see Table 1). In small doses, they slow the heart rate and respiration. In larger doses (for example, alcohol), they act as a poison and damage every organ system in the body. In large enough doses they can depress heart beat and respiration resulting in death, if quick intervention is not available. In terms of their effect on behavior, the user might at first feel stimulated, despite the actual depressant effect. Depression, loss of coordination, drop in energy level, mood swings, and confusion occur after prolonged use.

Opiates include heroin, codeine, morphine, and methadone. www.mhhe.com/fit_well/web22 Click 01. Narcotics are either smoked, injected, sniffed, or

Table 1 ▶ Depressants ("Downers," Sedatives)

Examples	Physiological Effects	Psychological Effects
• Alcohol	• In small doses, slow the heart and respiration	• Initial effect: stimulation, lowered inhibitions, excited talking, sense of well-being
• Anxiolytics (e.g., Valium, Xanax, meprobamate, sleeping pills, methaqualone)	• In large doses, act as a poison and damages every organ system	• After prolonged use: depression, loss of coordination, drop in energy level, mood swings, confusion, euphoria
• Barbiturates (Mebaral, Nembutal)	• Quick sedation: vomiting; loss of motor and neurological control, combined with alcohol can lead to coma and death	• Amnesia

Table 2 ► Opiates

Examples	Physiological Effects	Psychological Effects
• Codeine • Morphine • Synthetic opiates (e.g., Percoset, Oxycontin) • Methadone	• Narcotics: blockage of pain, chronic constipation, depressed respiration, redness and irritation of nostrils, nausea, lowered sexual drive, impaired immune system.	• Narcotics: euphoria and feeling of pleasure. Nontherapeutic doses may result in mental distress, such as fear and nervousness. In heavy users, drowsiness and apathy may occur.
• Heroin (also called smack)	• Heroin: blood clots, bacterial endocarditis, serum hepatitis, brain abscess, HIV infection (from shared needles). In pregnant users, high risk of miscarriage, stillbirths, birth defects, toxemia, addicted babies.	

swallowed (see Table 2). Heroin has no legal medical use in the United States and has a high rate of addiction. It is three times stronger than morphine and the other medicinal narcotics. Narcotics are all opium poppy derivatives or synthetics that emulate them. The *narco-* part of the word derives from the Greek word for sleep, because of its sleep-inducing properties.

Every narcotic, legal or illegal, is a potential poison. Although rare, a single dose can be fatal. A large percent of all deaths related to narcotic abuse is caused by overdose, impurities of the drug, or mixing the drug with other depressants such as alcohol. The mixing of drugs in the same or similar categories can produce a heightened physiological effect known as synergism or the **synergistic effect.** The combined use makes drug taking far more dangerous. The same is true among some prescription and over-the-counter drugs; when used in combination, they can be dangerous.

Stimulants include nicotine, cocaine, and amphetamines. Some effects of stimulants are described in Table 3. One of these stimulants—cocaine—comes in powder form (coke) and a rocklike form (crack). It is inhaled, injected, or smoked. If crack is snorted, it might be used several months or even years before the user becomes addicted. In contrast, when it is smoked it produces a very intense and instant high that lasts only 8 to 20 minutes. The user can become addicted much more rapidly. The low cost of crack has contributed to its abuse.

Purified methamphetamine (also known as ice, meth, or crystal) comes in rock form or powder. As a powder, it is usually smoked in a glass pipe or cigarette. It is a powerful stimulant with a high that lasts from 8 to 30 hours. No other drug damages the body as much as ice. It may be sold as pure methamphetamine or as a mixture of heroin, crack, and methadrine. Nicotine is a stimulant that is discussed in more detail in the concept on tobacco.

Designer drugs are made in laboratories and have many of the same properties as the drugs they simulate, such as pain relievers, anesthetics, or amphetamines. Designer drugs (see Table 4) are modifications of illegal or restricted drugs, made by underground chemists who create street drugs that are not specifically listed as controlled. They are created by changing the molecular structure of an existing drug to create a new substance. Since these drugs are being created all of the time, the effect that they might have is unknown. In the past, some have killed the people who take them, some have paralyzed people, and some have been innocuous. The people who take these drugs are human guinea pigs. Designer drugs are a class of drugs often associated with all-night underground dance parties frequented by teens and college students, so-called raves.

There are thousands of variations of amphetamines alone, and new drugs are continuously being concocted in illegal labs. These drugs are often extremely potent and can be contaminated, or botched, in the laboratory so that one dose can seriously damage or kill the user. The risk of overdose or adverse side effects is high.

Drug Abuse The use of a drug to an extent that it produces impairment of social, psychological, or physiological functioning.

Psychoactive Drug Any drug that produces a temporary change in the physiological functions of the nervous system, affecting mood, thoughts, feelings, or behavior.

Synergistic Effect The joint actions of two or more drugs that greatly increase the effects of each.

Table 3 ▶ Stimulants

Examples	Physiological Effects	Psychological Effects
• Cocaine (also called coke or crack)	• Cocaine: sore throat, hoarseness, shortness of breath (leads to bronchitis and emphysema), eyes dilate, seeing "lights" around objects. May become addicted the first time.	• Cocaine: initial rush of energy, feeling confident; as it wears off: depression, moodiness, irritability, severe mental disorders. • Crack: intense euphoria, then crushing depression, intense feeling of self-hate; as it wears off: depression and sadness, intense anxiety about where to get more drugs, vicious, aggressive, paranoid.
• Amphetamines and methamphetamines (also called speed, crank); diet and pep pills, ritalin	• Stimulants: excite central nervous system; increase blood pressure, respiration, and heart rate (sometimes resulting in convulsions and stroke); reduce appetite; highly addictive; overdose is fatal; with increased use: dizziness, headaches, sleeplessness; with long-term use: progressive brain damage, malnutrition, HIV infection (from shared needles).	• Stimulants: initially, feeling of being invincible, alertness, outgoing, excited; with increased use: feeling of anxiety; with long-term use: hallucinations, psychosis.
• Ice (also called crystal or meth)	• Ice: extreme energy, sleeplessness, seizures, flushed skin, constricted pupils.	• Ice: major effect is toxic psychosis; euphoria, delusions of grandeur, think they are invincible, violent when provoked.
• Nicotine	• See concept 20	• See concept 20

Table 4 ▶ Designer Drugs

Examples	Effects

Date Rape Drugs
  Rohypnol
  Gamma Hydroxy Butyrate (GHB)
  Ketamine (also called Special K)
	Predominantly central nervous system depressants. Rohypnol incapacitates, may cause amnesia; GHB can cause comas, seizures, insomnia, anxiety, tremors, nausea, and sweating; Ketamine can cause delirium, amnesia, impaired motor function, high blood pressure, depression, and potentially fatal respiratory problems.

3-4 methylenedioxymethamphetamine (MMDA, also called Ecstacy or X)	May cause irregular heart beat, intensified heart problems, exhaustion, liver and brain damage, nervousness, muscle tension, and dry mouth; initial feelings of calm may be followed by psychosis and/or psychological burnout.
4-methyl-2,5dimethoxyamphetamine (DOM) 4-bromo-2,5dimethoxyamphetamine (DOB) 4-bromo-2,5dimethoxyphenethylamine (NEXUS or 2-CB)	Causes effects similar to mescaline/amphetamines. Causes mood and perceptual alterations and increases potential for panic reaction. In higher doses may cause aggressive behavior. DOM can trigger spasms in blood vessels, shutting down blood flow to the arms and legs.

Drugs that cause the user to have hallucinations are called hallucinogens or psychedelics. www.mhhe.com/fit_well/web22 Click 02. Among the psychedelic drugs that cause **hallucinations** are LSD, PCP, and marijuana (see Table 5). Dosages of these drugs are so potent that they are measured in micrograms (a microgram is one-millionth of a gram, and a gram is approximately equivalent to the weight of a standard paper clip). Less-known drugs in this category include peyote cactus buttons, and mushrooms or "shrooms" which are chewed. They are used legally by some American Indians in religious rites.

Marijuana use became widespread in the 1960s and despite decreases since that time, marijuana is still the most widely used illicit drug in the United States The active ingredient in marijuana is delta-9-tetrahydrocannabinol (THC), which leads to a range of experiences that differ from person to person. A recent study

Table 5 ▶ Hallucinogens (Psychedelics)

Examples	Physiological Effects	Psychological Effects
• Hallucinogens	• Hallucinogens: usually elevate blood pressure, dilate pupils, cause dizziness	• Hallucinogens: all signs and symptoms very similar to state of temporary psychosis and can lead to recurrent and even permanent psychosis. Hallucinations, distorted sense of space/time, bad trips (panic attacks, delusions, paranoia) that can return as flashbacks months later.
• GD-Lyserogic acid diethylamide (LSD also called acid)	• LSD: changes chromosomes and may result in birth defects of babies of users; bad trips, confusion, flashback.	• LSD: vivid hallucinations, feelings of overlapping/merging of the senses, expanded consciousness and mystical experiences, stimulated awareness and desire, confusion, flashback.
• Phencyclidine (PCP)	• PCP: accumulates in fat cells and may remain in body longer than most drugs; impairs immune system, poor coordination, weight loss, speech problems, heart and lung failure, irreversible brain damage, convulsions, coma, and death.	• PCP: insensitivity to pain can lead to death; euphoria, depersonalization, hallucinations, delirium, amnesia, tunnel vision, loss of control, and violent behavior.
• Marijuana (also called pot, grass, weed, herb)	• Marijuana: long-term use includes bronchitis, emphysema and lung cancer, bloodshot eyes, heart disease, infertility, and sexual dysfunction, permanent memory loss (brain damage).	• Marijuana: may not hallucinate; pleasant relaxed feeling; giddiness; self-preoccupation; less precise thinking; task performance impaired; inertia develops; with prolonged use: may be withdrawn and apathetic, have anxiety reactions, paranoia. Eventually, decreased motivation and enthusiasm, reduced ability to absorb and integrate effectively, scholastic performance profoundly impaired.
• Inhalants (solvents, aerosols, and nitrites, also known as poppers, rush)	• Inhalants: slow reaction time; maybe headache, nausea, and vomiting; can cause seizure, brain damage, suffocation, heart attack, and death; double vision; sensitivity to light; dizziness; loss of coordination; weakness; numbness; irregular heartbeat; maybe liver and kidney failure; maybe bone marrow damage.	• Inhalants: giddiness, overexcitement, less inhibition, feelings of being all-powerful; powerfulness soon fades and leaves irritability.

indicated that the types of effects people experience may be due in part to genetic differences. Marijuana is generally smoked in a pipe, joint or bong, though it may also be eaten and is increasingly smoked in hollowed out cigars called blunts. Blunts often contain other drugs like PCP as well as marijuana.

Inhalants are sometimes listed separately because their effects are so serious. They reach the brain in seconds, and the effect lasts only a few minutes. They come in three types: (1) solvents, such as glue, gasoline, paints, paint thinner, typewriter correction fluid, lighter fluid, shoe polish, and liquid wax; (2) aerosols, such as hair spray, air fresheners, insect spray, and spray paint; and (3) nitrites, including amyl nitrite, nitrous oxide (laughing gas), and butyl nitrite (a room odorizer or liquid incense).

The Consequences of Drug Use

The use of drugs takes a human toll in terms of increased morbidity and mortality and lost productivity. In recent years, drug-related visits to the emergency room have increased. Over 500,000 drug-related visits are reported annually with more than half due to drug overdoses. ER visits associated with cocaine, heroin, and marijuana use have increased, whereas visits related to methamphetamine use have decreased. Annually, over 19,000 people died of drug induced causes, including poisonings and deaths related to prescription drug use. This

Hallucinations Seeing, feeling, and/or hearing imaginary things or seeing things in a distorted way.

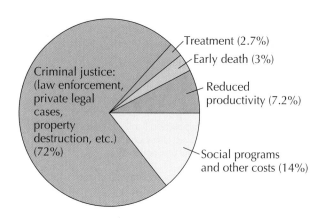

Figure 1 ▶ The estimated cost of drug abuse (percent of total costs).

Source: National Institute on Drug Abuse.

does not even take into account indirect effects of drug use on mortality including deaths from accidents, homicides, or AIDS (acquired via intravenous drug use). Because of problems with low productivity at the worksite, a large percentage of American businesses now conduct employee drug tests. Among the problems of drug-abusing employees are more frequent absences, erratic performance, increased violence and stealing, bad judgment, and increased accidents that often endanger others.

Drug use also has significant economic costs. The economic costs of illicit drug abuse are estimated at approximately $100 billion a year. Approximately 3.5 million people are dependent on illicit drugs, but the majority of the national economic burden is not related to treatment (3 percent). More than half of the costs are associated with drug-related crime. In addition, Americans spent an estimated $60 billion on drugs, with $38 billion spent on cocaine, $9.6 billion spent on heroin, $7 billion spent on marijuana, and $2.7 billion spent on other illegal drugs and on the misuse of legal drugs. Figure 1 illustrates the portion of costs resulting from factors such as law enforcement expenditures, social programs, and reduced productivity.

Use and Abuse of Drugs

Drug use generally begins with smoking cigarettes. The graduation from one drug (such as tobacco or alcohol) to another drug (such as cocaine or heroin) is commonly called the gateway concept, and tobacco, alcohol, and marijuana are referred to as the gateway drugs. Of course, most people who smoke or drink will not go on to use illegal drugs, but it is rare for people who do not smoke or drink to use illegal drugs. The average age for starting to smoke cigarettes is twelve, and for alcohol and marijuana about thirteen. In general, the younger a person is when he or she starts using drugs, including nicotine and alcohol, the more

likely that person is to use illegal drugs and the more likely he or she is to become physically dependent on drugs. Genetics or individual differences in personality may make some more likely to smoke, drink, and use illicit drugs. Regardless, the evidence is clear that early initiation of any substance use places one at risk for later problems.

The reasons given for using drugs are similar to the reasons given for using alcohol and tobacco. www.mhhe.com/fit_well/web22 Click 03. Typically, the reasons people give when asked why they use drugs or how they got started include the following:

- Peer pressure (i.e., "Everyone is doing it" even though in most cases the majority of people aren't using drugs).
- It makes young people feel more "adult."
- "I just wanted to see what it was like (to experiment)."
- To have fun.
- "It makes me feel good."
- As a rebellion against parents or authority.
- To cope with pressure/stress.
- To take a risk (thrill seeking).

Some risk factors make one more likely to misuse or abuse drugs. www.mhhe.com/fit_well/web22 Click 04. The potential for **addiction** depends on genetic vulnerability, the type of drug used, method of administration used, attitudes toward drug use, peer group use, expectations regarding drug effects, and ease of access. Genetics account for as much as 50 percent of alcohol and nicotine addiction and the same is likely true for other drugs of abuse. This does not mean that one is destined to become an addict because the remaining 50 percent is within your control. Some drugs are more addictive than others, so dependence on narcotics and sedatives is more likely than dependence on hallucinogens or designer drugs (though addiction to these substances occurs as well). The route of administration also affects risk for addiction. For example, the likelihood of becoming addicted to cocaine is much higher if it is smoked as crack than if it is inhaled as powder. People who believe drug use is acceptable and affiliate with others with similar views are more likely to use drugs and to develop problems. Those who believe drugs will have strong positive effects and few negative effects are also at greater risk, especially if they use drugs as a way to cope with stress. People who live in areas where drugs are readily available are also at increased risk.

Marijuana is the most widely used illegal drug in the United States and many favor legalization. In the year 2000, nearly 11 million Americans, or nearly 5 percent of people over the age of twelve reported use of marijuana (see Figure 2). A recent study indicated that public support for the legalization of marijuana has increased in recent years. Thirty-four percent of respondents indicated

Technology Update

One of the most frequent uses of the Internet is to obtain health information. The website of the National Institute on Drug Abuse (NIDA) (see Web Resources) is one excellent source that provides information about drugs and health. The website has sections for students, teachers and parents, and the general public relating to science and practice, trends and statistics, treatment and prevention, and current drugs of abuse. Online documents are available on such topics as "club drugs" (**www.clubdrugs.org**), marijuana (**www.marijuana-info.org**), and steroids (**www.steroidabuse.org**).

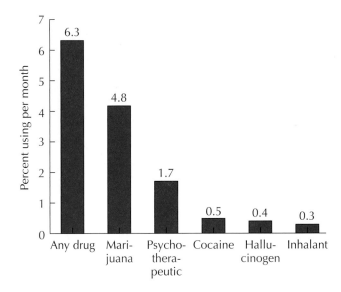

Figure 2 ▶ Illicit drug use among persons aged twelve and older, by drug (% per month).

Source: Substance Abuse and Mental Health Services Administration. 2001.

they favored legalization of marijuana, the highest percentage since the poll began in 1969. Proponents and opponents agree that legalization of marijuana for medical use in some states has increased public support for decriminalization. Advocates argue that the negative consequences of marijuana are far less than the consequences associated with the use of legal drugs like alcohol and tobacco, and that marijuana is less addictive. Although there may be some truth to this argument, marijuana still has risks.

Many marijuana users are psychologically dependent, and marijuana has a host of physical and social consequences (unrelated to its illegality). With respect to health, chronic marijuana use leads to many of the negative consequences associated with cigarette smoking, including cardiovascular disease, and lung cancer. A recent study showed that marijuana use also increases risk for stroke. Another study found that marijuana use leads to nearly a five-fold increase in acute risk for a heart attack, especially among those with existing cardiovascular risk. Acute and chronic marijuana use is also associated with impaired cognitive abilities. Short-term marijuana use leads to a reduction in IQ scores. Long-term marijuana use leads to impairments in attention, memory, and learning. Although the debate is ongoing regarding the addictive potential of marijuana (physical dependence), it is clear that one can become psychologically addicted to the drug. Psychological dependence is characterized by craving for the drug and continued use despite negative consequences.

Cocaine is the second most commonly used illicit drug along with other stimulants like methamphetamine. During the 1990s, cocaine use decreased dramatically from its peak in the 1980s. However, cocaine use among young people has increased with 9.8 percent of high school seniors currently reporting lifetime use. Use of other stimulant drugs like methamphetamine has also increased. These drugs activate dopamine release in the brain and are therefore highly addictive. Evidence shows

long-term effects on brain chemistry and behavior. A recent study showed that methamphetamine addicts had 15 percent fewer dopamine receptors than people who had never abused the drug. Dopamine is the neurotransmitter in the brain responsible for reward and feelings of pleasure. With fewer dopamine receptors, the individual needs more dopamine in the brain to produce feelings of pleasure, and one of the few ways to increase dopamine levels is to administer more of the drug. This helps to maintain their use of the drug. The decreased density of receptors has additional consequences for memory and motor skills, which are also related to dopamine levels in the brain.

The most dramatic increases in drug use during the past five years have been for the "club" drugs. Club drugs include Ecstasy (MDMA), Rohypnol, GHB, Ketamine, DOM, DOB, and NEXUS. MDMA, a hallucinations, is inhaled, injected, or swallowed. The drug was initially popular at all-night dance parties called raves, but its use has expanded beyond the club scene. A recent national study of college students found that Ecstasy use increased 69 percent in recent years. This study was also among the first to provide information about the characteristics of young people who use the drug. Another study showed that 12 percent of teenagers have tried the drug.

Addiction A drug-induced condition in which a person requires frequent administration of a drug in order to avoid withdrawl; also refered to as physical dependence.

Table 6 ▶ Common Characteristics of Ecstasy Users
Ecstasy Users Are More Likely to Do the Following:
• use marijuana
• binge drink
• smoke cigarettes
• have multiple sexual partners
• consider arts and parties as important
• consider religion less important
• spend more time socializing with friends
• spend less time studying

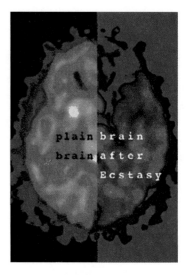

Figure 3 ▶ Toxic effects of MDMA (Ecstasy).

Only alcohol and marijuana are used by more teens. The increase in MDMA use appears to reflect the fact this drug is not just a club drug anymore. It is becoming more prevalent in other settings and in suburban and rural areas.

GHB, Rohypnol, and Ketamine use are also increasing despite the fact that these drugs do not provide the high associated with most other drugs of abuse. They are most often thought of as date rape drugs because the rapist usually slips it into his victim's drink. Women should be especially careful not to leave their drinks unattended or accept drinks from strangers. Despite being used much less often than MDMA, date rape drugs contribute to more hospital visits and deaths than Ecstasy. The characteristics of Ecstasy users are described in Table 6.

The increased use of club drugs is a concern given the strong evidence of their harmful effects. Recent evidence indicates that Ecstasy alters brain levels of serotonin, negatively impacts memory, and affects brain regions that regulate sleep, mood, and learning (see Figure 3). These effects appear to be even more pronounced among women, placing them at very high risk. Further studies in animals and humans suggest that the negative effects of MDMA may last as long as seven years.

With increased availability of prescription medications in our culture, illegal use and abuse has increased. www.mhhe.com/fit_well/web22 **Click 05.** Prescription drugs that are often used inappropriately include stimulants such as Ritalin, opiates like Percoset, and benzodiazepines like Valium and Xanax. College students at several northeastern colleges indicated that these drugs were widely used by students, who obtained the drugs illegally or from friends with prescriptions. Overuse of these medications may cause serious medical complications, and, in the case of opiates and benzodiazepines, may lead to physical dependence

and risk of severe withdrawal symptoms. Recently, there has been a lot of concern about use of the drug Oxycontin (sometimes referred to as "hill billy heroin"), a strong time-release capsule approved for use in the United States to treat severe pain. The drug has been linked to hundreds of deaths from overdose. In addition, some are concerned that the aggressive marketing of the drug has led to high levels of abuse. In support of these concerns, the National Household Survey on Drug Abuse found that nonmedical use of Oxycontin nearly doubled from 1999 to 2000. Like any opiate drug, the risks associated with abuse are considerable and attempts to stop after heavy use should be done with consultation of a physician.

Accidental misuse of prescriptions and medications is common and dangerous. An unwitting abuse of drugs, particularly among the elderly, is overdosing because of forgetfulness. A particular problem is taking medicine twice. Other people take several prescriptions at the same time for different ailments, and sometimes these come from different doctors who are unaware that the patient is being treated by another physician. These drugs may interact dangerously or have a synergistic effect. A study of elderly patients (over the age of sixty-five) found that over 90 percent were taking at least one prescription medication, with an average of over four. Further, over 10 percent of emergency room visits in this group were due to medication complications. This study highlights the importance of talking to your doctor about all medications you may be taking and how they interact with one another.

Accidental misuse can also occur if drugs are taken from the medicine cabinet at night in the dark or if medications are stored in unlabeled bottles so that the wrong drug is taken. Using outdated drugs can also lead to problems. After a medication is no longer needed, any remaining part of it should be destroyed. Because people react differently to drugs, it is possible to become addicted to a prescription drug even when you follow the directions.

Anabolic steroids are prescription drugs sold on the black market that are widely abused. Anabolic steroids are known as roids, juice, and sauce. These drugs are usually taken for a specified period followed by a period of nonuse (cycling) and users often combine different types of steroids to maximize the effects (stacking). Users are also likely to misuse or abuse other drugs and frequently share needles, increasing the risk of disease transmission. Recent studies show habituation often occurs with use of this drug. The side effects of steroids are described in concept 11.

Government studies estimate that there are 1 million steroid users in the United States. About 2 percent of high school seniors report current steroid use. After a decade of decreased use, rates have begun to increase again. Steroid use is also a concern on college campuses and unfortunately, colleges and universities may not be doing their part to prevent the problem. In a survey of over 21,000 collegiate athletes, 15 to 20 percent of those who used steroids or supplements indicated that the source of the substance was a coach, trainer, team physician, or other representative of the college or university.

Women who are pregnant, nursing, or want to get pregnant should avoid drug use, including many prescription drugs. The National Institute on Drug Abuse (NIDA) conducted the National Pregnancy Health Survey, a national assessment of the extent of drug use by women during pregnancy, and estimated that 5.5 percent of the 4 million women who gave birth each year in the United States used illegal drugs while they were pregnant. Taking drugs during pregnancy can result in various conditions:

- Premature separation of the placenta from the womb and hemorrhage, threatening the lives of both the baby and the mother. Cocaine use makes mothers

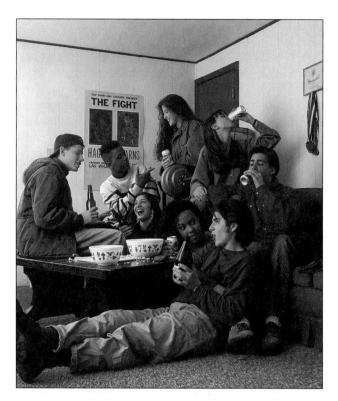

Peer pressure contributes to drug use and abuse.

twice as likely to have this problem relative to women on other drugs and four times more likely than women not on drugs.
- Miscarriage resulting from increased blood pressure causing uterine contractions. Birth defects also occur.
- Decreased oxygen to the baby and possibly a fetal stroke.
- Low birth weight and shorter babies.
- Babies born addicted who then experience withdrawal symptoms.
- Increased risk of sudden infant death syndrome (SIDS).
- Increased risk of learning disabilities, as well as delayed motor, speech, and language development.

Strategies for Action

The best way to avoid problems associated with drug use is not to try illegal drugs and to be careful in the use of legal drugs. The information presented in this concept clearly indicates that starting to take a drug for reasons other than managing your own good health increases the risk of taking more drugs in the future. Most readers of this book have already made the decision not to take illegal drugs and will follow the guidelines presented earlier concerning how to avoid misusing legal drugs. Nevertheless, at some time in the lives of most people, medication will be taken. Be continually aware of what

you are taking and why. You need to monitor the use of medications to be sure that you are using them as directed and not in combination with other medications that may result in dangerous synergistic effects.

One of the characteristics needed to resist peer pressures to use drugs is healthy self-esteem. You need to believe that you are important. Learning skills to cope with problems and stress is also essential (see the concept on stress management). Using a responsible process to make decisions is another skill that needs to be acquired. Knowing the effects and risks of drugs should help you to make more responsible decisions. To combat peer pressure, the ability to clearly and effectively say no is necessary. Be assertive. And finally, you need to choose friends whose values support, rather than undermine, your own.

 People who have a problem with drugs typically will need help to develop skills and personal characteristics to quit using them. www.mhhe.com/fit_well/web22 Click 06. For people with a problem, the first step is recognizing that help is needed. In Lab 22A you will have the opportunity to evaluate the behavior of a friend or loved one to determine if the person needs help. If a person needs help, he or she needs to talk to someone who can be trusted, perhaps a friend or relative or maybe you can help. You may be able to help the person seek help from a referral source such as an employee assistance program, family or university physician or hospital, or your city or county health department.

These sources help get the person into a rehab program or support group. Some of the better-known, nationwide programs include Alcoholics (or Narcotics or Cocaine) Anonymous and Al-Anon Family Groups. Another option is to look in the yellow pages of the telephone book for rehab programs operated by public and private agencies. Still another possibility is to call a hotline, and someone will direct you to help in your area. Three of these include:

- National Institute on Drug Abuse (NIDA) Hotline (1-800-662-HELP)
- Cocaine Helpline (1-800-COCAINE)
- Just Say No International (1-800-258-2766)

At a later time it would be wise to answer the questions in Lab 22A for yourself rather than for a friend or loved one. This will allow you to determine if you might need help.

Web Resources

Cocaine Anonymous World Services **www.ca.org**
Drug Free Resource Net **www.drugfreeamerica.org**
National Clearinghouse for Alcohol and Drug Information **www.health.org**
National Institute on Drug Abuse **www.nida.nih.gov**

Suggested Readings

 Additional reference materials for concept 22 are available at **www.mhhe.com/fit_well/web22 Click 07.**

Executive Office of the President, Office of National Drug Control Policy. 2001. *The Economic Costs of Drug Abuse in the United States.* Washington, DC: Office of National Drug Control Policy.
Fields, R. 2001. *Drugs in Perspective.* 4th ed. St. Louis, MO: McGraw-Hill.

National Institute on Drug Abuse. 2000. Publication No. 00-3721. *Research Report; Steroid Abuse and Addiction.* Bethesda, MD: NIDA.
National Institute on Drug Abuse. 2001. *Monitoring the Future: National Results on Adolescent Drug Use.* Bethesda, MD: NIDA.
Payne, W. A., and D. B. Hahn. 2002. *Understanding Your Health.* 7th ed. St. Louis, MO: McGraw-Hill.
Solowij, N. et al. 2002. Cognitive functioning of long-term heavy cannabis users seeking treatment. *Journal of American Medical Association* 287(9):1123–1131.
Strote, J., J. E. Lee, and H. Wechsler. 2002. Increasing MDMA use among college students: Results of a national survey. *Journal of Adolescent Health* 30(1): 64–72.
Substance Abuse and Mental Health Services Administration. 2001. *Summary of Findings from the 2000 National Survey on Drug Abuse.* Washington, DC: US Department of Health and Human Services.

In the News

MDMA or Ecstasy poses serious risks to health as outlined earlier. One problem is we do not know the contents of the drugs that are being marketed as Ecstasy. Evidence shows dealers are passing off other drugs as Ecstasy that are likely to be even more dangerous. One such drug is the amphetamine paramethoxyamphetamine (PMA). This drug was banned by the federal government in 1973 and never became very popular after two deaths were tied to its use.

Unfortunately, the drug is surfacing again and is often sold as Ecstasy. Street names for the drug include Death and Mitsubishi Double-Stack. PMA has effects similar to Ecstasy, including increased pulse rate and blood pressure and a sense of well-being. Large doses can lead to irregular heart beats, heart attacks, kidney failure, convulsions, coma, and death. The recent deaths of nine young people in Illinois and Florida have been attributed to the drug.

Lab 22A: Use and Abuse of Other Drugs

Name	**Section**	**Date**

Purpose: To help you evaluate a friend or family member's behavior and potential for becoming an abuser of drugs. If this report is submitted to an instructor, be sure *not* to identify by name the person you are evaluating.

Procedure: Answer these questions to determine if the person you are evaluating could be an abuser of medications. Place an X over the answer that applies.

A. Prescription Drug Abuse

(Yes) (No) 1. Does he/she take more medicine than prescribed per dosage?

(Yes) (No) 2. Does he/she feel more nervous than ever when the medicine wears off?

(Yes) (No) 3. Does he/she hoard medicine?

(Yes) (No) 4. Does he/she gulp pills?

(Yes) (No) 5. Does he/she hide the amount of medicine taken from friends, family, or his/her doctors?

(Yes) (No) 6. Does his/her doctor know he/she has other doctors, and do they have a list of all the medications he/she is taking from all sources (dentist, family physician, specialists)?

The more questions to which you answered "yes," the more likely he/she is to be a drug abuser.

B. Risk Factors for Becoming Addicted

(Yes) (No) 1. Have any members of his/her family ever abused drugs?

(Yes) (No) 2. Was he/she abused as a child, or did he/she go through other trauma during childhood?

(Yes) (No) 3. Is he/she now undergoing unusual stress or mental pain?

(Yes) (No) 4. Does he/she have easy access to drugs?

(Yes) (No) 5. Has or does he/she used drugs recreationally?

(Yes) (No) 6. If he/she has or now uses drugs recreationally, did or does he/she choose the fastest method of getting a hit?

The more "yes" answers you have, the greater his/her risk of addiction. (Remember that alcohol is a drug, too.)

C. Signs and Symptoms That a Problem with Drugs Exists

(Yes) (No) 1. Does he/she use drugs as an escape or to help cope with a stressful situation?

(Yes) (No) 2. Does he/she become depressed easily?

(Yes) (No) 3. Does he/she use drugs the first thing in the morning?

(Yes) (No) 4. Has he/she ever tried to quit and resumed using again?

(Yes) (No) 5. Does he/she do things under the influence of a drug that he/she would not normally do?

(Yes) (No) 6. Has he/she had any drug-related "close calls" with the police, or any arrests?

(Yes) (No) 7. Does he/she think a party or social gathering isn't fun unless drugs are served?

(Yes) (No) 8. Does he/she feel proud of an increased tolerance to drugs?

Yes No 9. Does he/she use drugs when alone?

Yes No 10. Has or does he/she use a wide variety of drugs?

Yes No 11. Is he/she constantly thinking about being high?

Yes No 12. Does he/she avoid people or places that oppose usage?

Yes No 13. Has his/her friends, family, teachers, or employer expressed concern about his/her use?

Yes No 14. Is his/her usage causing him/her to neglect responsibilities?

Yes No 15. Has he/she ever had blackouts or lack of memory of drug use or other events?

Yes No 16. Has he/she stolen to get money for drugs?

Yes No 17. Has he/she seriously considered that he/she might have a drug problem?

The more questions to which you answer yes, the more likely he/she is to have a serious problem with drugs.

Results:

A. Does he/she abuse prescription drugs (medications)? Yes No
   (Questions A: 1–6)

B. Is he/she at considerable risk for addiction? Yes No
   (Questions B: 1–6)

C. Does he/she have a serious problem with drugs? Yes No
   (Questions C: 1–17)

Conclusions and Implications:

In several sentences, discuss a plan of action that could be taken by a person who has a problem with misuse of over-the-counter drugs, prescription drugs, or illegal drugs. Discuss specific things you could do to help a person with a problem.

*At some point you may want to answer the questions yourself.

Preventing Sexually Transmitted Diseases

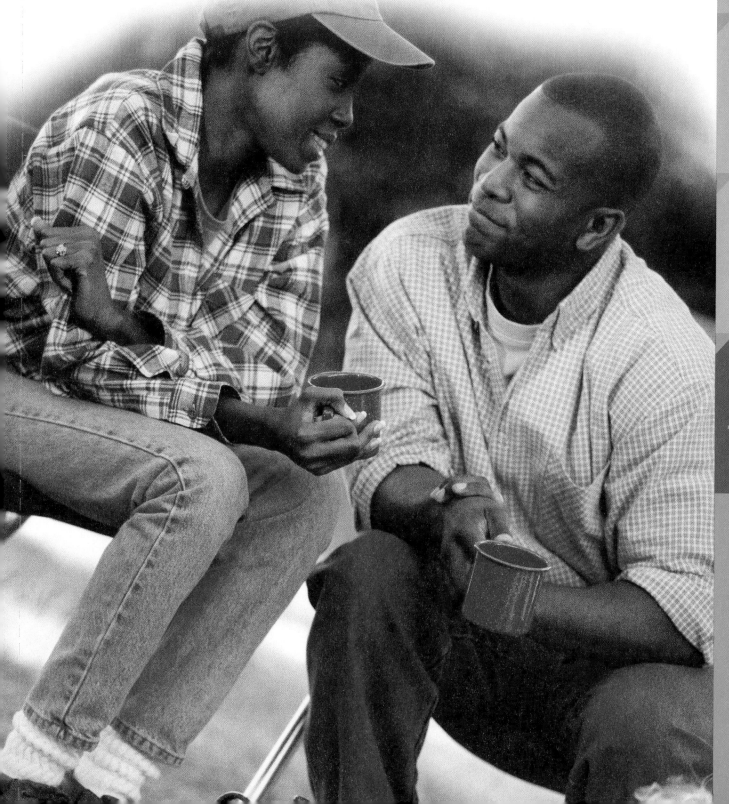

Safe sex and sound information about sexually transmitted diseases are important to health and wellness.

Health Goals

for the year 2010

- Promote responsible sexual behaviors, to prevent sexually transmitted diseases (STDs) and their complications.

- Reduce incidence of Chlamydia, gonorrhea, syphillis, genital herpes, human papillomavirus (HPV), pelvic inflammatory disease (PID), and hepatitis B.

- Reduce incidence of and death from human immunodeficiency syndrome (HIV) and acquired immunodeficiency syndrome (AIDS).

- Increase proportion of young people who abstain from sexual intercourse, use condoms during sexual activity, and avoid risky sexual behaviors.

- Increase STD, including HIV, screening and treatment.

- Via television programming, increase positive messages relating to responsible sexual behavior.

The sexual experience is an interpersonal one that influences our actions and behaviors. It is basic to family life and fundamental to the reproduction of the human species. Approached responsibly, the human sexual experience contributes to wellness and quality of life in many ways. When approached irresponsibly, it can result in disease and personal and interpersonal suffering. Responsible decision making requires sound information regarding the symptoms, causes, and treatments of sexually transmitted diseases (STDs).

General Facts

The healthy sexual experience can contribute to wellness in many ways. Because human sexual experience is interpersonal, it is a social one. It affects many more people than a sexual partner. Personal beliefs have much to do with the feelings that participants have toward the sexual experience; thus, spiritual wellness is influenced. Because the sexual experience is often emotionally charged, emotional wellness is also affected. Clearly, intellectual decisions are made concerning the experience, so intellectual well-being is a factor to consider as well. The sexual act is a physical experience that can be pleasurable but that has many long-lasting physical consequences. All five wellness dimensions are involved in decisions concerning participation in, the meaningfulness of, and the long-term consequences of the sexual experience. The healthy sexual experience requires sensitive and thoughtful consideration of the consequences.

Decisions concerning sexual behavior have lifelong consequences. Positive consequences of a sexual experience include pleasure, childbearing, and an enriched, happy family life. Negative lifelong consequences can include unwanted pregnancy, emotional and physical stress, and strained social relationships, among others. Unsafe sex also takes a toll in disease and death for large numbers of people worldwide.

Unsafe sexual activity can result in disease, poor health, and much pain and suffering. Until the 1940s, **sexually transmitted diseases (STDs)** were a leading cause of death. The discovery of penicillin and other antibiotics, and improved public health practices, lowered the death rate from STDs, but they remained a significant health problem. In 1991, STDs became one of the ten leading causes of death in the United States, principally because of the high death rate from **acquired immune deficiency syndrome (AIDS)** caused by the **human immunodeficiency virus (HIV).** In the new millennium, STDs have dropped from the top ten list, primarily because of the effectiveness of recently developed drugs in reducing the death rate from HIV/AIDS. STDs, including HIV/AIDS, will continue to be a leading health problem in the future if better prevention programs are not implemented.

In addition to the general national health goals designed to prevent, control, and reduce STDs, specific goals include increasing STD education in schools and colleges, extending regulations to protect workers, and improving services through community agencies designed to help the general public.

HIV/AIDS

Of all STDs, HIV/AIDS poses the greatest health threat to the nation and the world. www.mhhe.com/fit_well/web23 **Click 01.** Health experts indicate that we are in the midst of a worldwide HIV/AIDS epidemic. Many experts say that the AIDS epidemic has become larger than the plague. Each year, over 40,000 people in the United States are infected with HIV, and approximately 900,000 are already infected. Worldwide, the problem is even more profound, with about 14,000 people infected each day and a total of 40 million people currently living with HIV. So far, about 16 million people worldwide have died from AIDS. Although AIDS-related deaths in North America have decreased over the last decade, rates of new cases have remained stable for the past several years.

Minorities and women are populations in which the incidence of HIV/AIDS is increasing disproportionately. What was once thought to be a disease of males, especially gay men, is now increasingly a female condition. Because of recent changes in the clinical case definitions from when HIV was first discovered, many more women are classified as having AIDS than in previous years. In the past, AIDS was defined by many specific ailments among HIV-positive individuals. Because women have different ailments associated with HIV (cervical cancer, recurrent pneumonia, and pulmonary tuberculosis), some women were being denied new and experimental treatments available to men. The revised definition of AIDS includes these ailments so twenty-six conditions and a low **CD4+ cell** count are now used to define it. Although the change in definition led to increased estimates of AIDS cases among women, the genuine level of risk has also increased. The proportion of AIDS cases occurring among women in the United States rose dramatically in the 1980s and 1990s but has since leveled off. Internationally, women account for an even larger proportion of AIDS cases (48 percent). The majority of women with AIDS are infected through heterosexual intercourse, which now accounts for more than 80 percent of HIV cases worldwide. African American and Hispanic women are at especially high risk, accounting for 77 percent of cases in the United States despite accounting for less than one-fourth of the population.

Although not as dramatic as rates in minority women, rates of infection are also increasing disproportionately for men from minority groups. African-American and Hispanic men account for over half of U.S. cases, and AIDS is now the leading cause of death for African American men between the ages of twenty-five and forty-four. The disproportionate numbers are the most dramatic for pediatric cases, where African American and Hispanic children account for over 80 percent of cases with African American children alone accounting for over half. The high levels of risk among minorities have led to the development of multi-million-dollar governmental programs to fight HIV/AIDS among African American and Hispanic populations.

HIV is the virus that causes AIDS. A test of **serostatus** can indicate if a person is seropositive. When a person tests seropositive for HIV, it means that a blood test has indicated the presence in the body of the HIV. HIV invades the body's immune system cells, even killing them. This results in damage to the immune system and the body's ability to fight infections. One of the principal problems is that HIV causes immune suppression by directly invading and killing CD4+ helper cells. When too many of these cells (also called **T helper cells**) are destroyed, the body cannot fight opportunistic infections effectively.

What all of this means is that the immune system can no longer function properly, thereby making the seropositive person more susceptible to various types of diseases and disorders. **Antibodies** in the blood that normally fight infections are ineffective in stopping the HIV from invading the body. Though it is not clear exactly why HIV affects the immune system as it does, the stages of HIV are better understood than in the past. First, HIV infects the body. Over time, white blood cells are damaged, and antibodies become ineffective. Depending on time elapsed and individual variance in the progression of the disease, AIDS may develop or no symptoms may appear (see Figure 1). After HIV enters the body, it takes several months before enough antibodies are developed to be able to detect its presence. Newer tests are available, which detect a portion of the HIV virus known as P24.

Sexually Transmitted Diseases (STD) Disease for which a primary method of transmission is sexual activity.

Acquired Immune Deficiency Syndrome (AIDS) An HIV-infected individual is said to have AIDS when he/she has developed certain opportunistic infections (for example, pneumonia, tuberculosis, yeast infections, or other infections) or when their CD4+ cell count drops below 200.

Human Immunodeficiency Virus (HIV) A virus that causes a breakdown of the immune system among humans, resulting in the inability of the body to fight infections. It is a precursor to AIDS.

CD4+ Cell A type of cell that protects against infections and that instigates the body's immune response. HIV kills these cells so a high count usually means better health; also known as T helper cell.

Serostatus A blood test indicating the presence of antibodies the immune system creates to fight disease. A seropositive status indicates that a person has antibodies to fight HIV and is HIV positive.

T Helper Cells A disease-fighting blood cell that is damaged by the HIV virus; also called a CD4+ cell.

Antibodies Bodies in the bloodstream that react to overcome bacterial and other agents that attack the body.

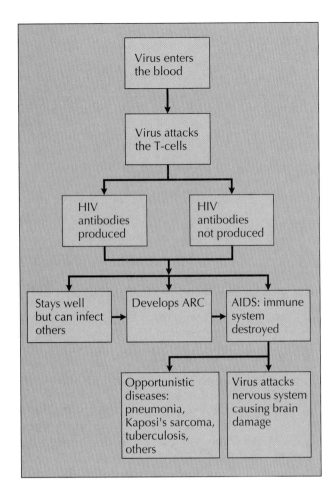

Figure 1 ▶ Stages of HIV infection.

Table 1 ▶ Drugs Approved for HIV Infection		
Nucleoside/ Nucleotide RT Inhibitors	**Non-nucleoside RT Inhibitors**	**Protease Inhibitors**
• zidovudine, AZT	• delavirdine	• ritonavir
• abacavir	• nevirapine	• saquinavir
• ddCr	• efavirenz	• indinavir
• ddI		• amprenavir
• d4T		• nelfinavir
• 3TC		• lopinavir
• ZDV		
• tenofovir		
• didanosine		

HIV among those infected does not prevent transmission, though there is less risk of transmission for those with low blood virus levels. Apparently virus "reservoirs" exist that allow transmission even when drugs have reduced HIV to undetectable levels. The recent discovery of new strains of HIV have caused concern among public health officials. More than a few of the new strains are resistant to one or more of the different classes of anti-HIV drugs (see Table 1). People with resistant strains have fewer available treatment options. Resistant strains are now being passed from those who are currently HIV-positive to those previously not infected.

These tests may prove to be an improvement over those of the past, but they are more expensive. One reason that HIV is so widely transmitted is that in the early stages, before it can be confirmed by testing, HIV can be transmitted. If untreated, five of ten people infected with HIV will develop AIDS within ten years. Four of ten who go untreated will develop **AIDS-related complex (ARC),** another illness associated with HIV, and one in ten will have no apparent ill effects.

An individual has AIDS when he or she is infected with HIV and develops various opportunistic diseases because of impairment of the immune system. Among the conditions that indicate the presence of AIDS are pneumonia, tuberculosis, **Kaposi's sarcoma,** yeast infections, and the previously described conditions for women. Other symptoms include fatigue, swollen glands, rashes, weight loss, and loss of appetite. Those HIV victims who have access to the "cocktail" of drugs used to treat HIV/AIDS can live much longer than previously thought possible. When treated with the cocktail, many have become free of detectable amounts of HIV as long as they continue the treatments. Non-detectable levels of

We haves no cure for AIDS. www.mhhe.com/ fit_well/web23 Click 02. For those infected with HIV/AIDS, there is no known cure. However, treatments have been developed to suppress or slow the progress of the disease process. As mentioned earlier, current treatments for HIV/AIDS include administration of a combination of drugs. Highly Active Retroviral Therapy (HART), often referred to as the AIDS "cocktail." The drugs that make up the cocktail are a combination of reverse transcriptase inhibitors and protease inhibitors. A total of eighteen drugs are now approved for use in the treatment of HIV (see Table 1).

Two types of reverse transcription inhibitors work in different ways to accomplish the same goal of interfering with the enzyme that HIV needs to replicate. Nucleoside and nucleotide drugs essentially trick the body by providing faulty DNA building blocks so the body is unable to produce more of the virus. Non-nucleotide drugs accomplish the same task by binding to the reverse transcriptase. Protease inhibitors work by interfering with the protease enzyme that HIV uses to produce infectious virus particles. These combination treatments can cost up to $15,000 per year, and the drugs must be taken in a complex sequence. They also have a number of adverse side effects. Of concern is the fact that 95 percent of the HIV-infected people worldwide do not currently have access to these drugs.

A number of new drugs are also being investigated, including additional reverse transcriptase inhibitors and protease inhibitors as well as entirely new classes of drugs. New drug classes include fusion inhibitors that interfere with the ability of HIV to enter a cell, entry inhibitors that prevent HIV from attaching to cells, and integrase inhibitors that interfere with HIV's ability to corrupt the normal DNA of a cell. Many of these drugs, like T-20, are now in clinical trials and should be available in a few years if the results are positive.

Although drug therapies now offer hope, they also contribute to a host of undesirable side effects. Anyone infected with HIV has to be pleased about the increased effectiveness of drug therapies. At the same time, those who are not infected may be less concerned about contracting the virus, leading to a rebound in the incidence of HIV. In fact, a recent study showed that gay men who frequently viewed ads about the effectiveness of new drug therapies were more likely to engage in unsafe sex practices. Because of this, public health officials fear another wave of new infections. Drug therapies have received a lot of media attention but little emphasis has been placed on the negative effects of these drugs. Anyone who is taking an AIDS cocktail could shed a little light on the down side. Some of the many side effects include: nausea, diarrhea, gastrointestinal symptoms, liver abnormalities, defects in blood fat metabolism, premature bone thinning, insulin abnormalities, inflammation of the pancreas, nerve damage, and death. In addition, the person can develop immunity to these drugs. This is particularly problematic for patients who have been on the drugs for a long period of time.

The search for a vaccine for HIV is well underway though no vaccine is currently available. About thirty different vaccines are currently undergoing clinical trials. A number of new vaccines have also shown great promise in animal studies. For example, one vaccine made from a cold virus was shown to produce a strong immune response to HIV in rhesus monkeys. Animals that received the experimental vaccine showed high levels of white blood cells and T-cells known to combat the infection. The treated monkeys also demonstrated better health and decreased mortality. Preliminary studies in humans have also shown promise and full scale clinical trials will begin soon. One potential problem with the delivery of the vaccine via the adenovirus (common cold) is that most people have had such extensive exposure to adenovirus that their bodies may destroy it before it can have a therapeutic effect. Preliminary evidence suggests

that increasing the dose can avoid this problem. Even if the vaccine is effective, it will likely take at least five years before it is widely available.

Another hope for an AIDS vaccine comes from studies showing that certain people seem to be genetically immune to the HIV virus. One study found that a group of women were resistant to contracting the disease despite regular sexual intercourse with infected partners. Another group of people from European ancestry have been shown to possess a genetic mutation that causes them to resist HIV. This mutation apparently occurred as an adaptation to the plague in previous centuries. There are also some individuals who possess a non-progressor or non-pathologic strain of HIV. This strain has a different genetic structure than other strains resulting in the lack of progression of the disease. Greater understanding of the genetic mechanisms that contribute to these types of resistance to HIV may eventually lead to gene therapies to prevent the transmission of the disease.

When best to treat HIV aggressively remains controversial. Experts agree that the cocktail of drugs is the most effective treatment for HIV, but two camps of experts exist when it comes to scheduling the treatment. Some recommend "hitting early and hitting hard." This means administering drugs as soon as a seropositive status is confirmed. More experts now suggest that the treatment should wait until the **viral load** is elevated. Standards for viral load have been established by public health officials. This level varies for men and women because women have less virus in their blood for the same stage and because they have greater risk of opportunistic infections than men for the same viral load.

Those who recommend waiting to treat HIV do so because they feel that early treatment may lead to resistance to the drug prematurely. This approach may become a more viable alternative with evidence that drug therapies can be effective even when CD4+ counts are quite low (as low as 200). Furthermore, the Department of Health and Human Services recently revised their recommendations suggesting that treatment begin when T-cell levels drop below 350 or viral loads reach 55,000. Although no agreement exists on the best way to treat HIV, we should have the answer within the next ten

AIDS-Related Complex (ARC) The development of HIV-related immunodeficiency conditions but not those considered to be AIDS.

Kaposi's Sarcoma A type of cancer evidenced by purple sores (tumors) on the skin.

Viral Load The level of virus (HIV) in the blood.

years. A long-term study will be conducted by Community Programs for Clinical Research on Aids (CPCRA) with funding from the National Institute of Allergy and Infectious Diseases (NIAID). The study called SMART (Strategies for Management of Anti-retroviral Therapies) will enroll 6,000 people from twenty-one sites across the United States Study participants will be randomly assigned to one of two groups. The first group will receive aggressive drug therapy from the beginning of the trial. The other group will be given drug therapy only when their CD4+ T-cell count drops below 250, and only until their CD4+ T-cell count rises above 350. SMART will follow these patients for up to nine years.

Many people with HIV do not know they are infected. A recent study found that about 40 percent of people infected with HIV are not aware of it. In a sample of about 19,000 AIDS patients, two of five people tested positive for HIV within a year of being diagnosed with AIDS. Even in a sample of people at high risk for HIV, about 30 percent reported that they had not been tested. This complicates efforts to achieve national health goals because treatment is often delayed and those who are unaware of their HIV status may transmit the virus unknowingly.

Public health efforts have begun to focus more on this problem, stressing the need for more prevention targeting those who may be unknowingly transmitting HIV. As part of a new program designed to reduce HIV cases by 50 percent, the Centers for Disease Control (CDC) has already committed $100 million and hopes to raise additional funds from the government and drug companies. One of the primary messages of this program, called project Seropositive Approach to Fighting the HIV Epidemic (SAFE), is that people need to get tested earlier to prevent the spread of the disease and to maximize the effectiveness of treatment. The goal is to increase the percentage of people who know that they are HIV positive to 95 percent. Although individuals must be responsible enough to get tested, health professionals could also facilitate testing of high-risk patients. A recent study showed that about 40 percent of HIV positive patients had information in their charts suggesting they were at high risk more than a year before they were actually tested. People with obvious risk factors like IV drug use or other STDs should be strongly encouraged to get tested.

There are two mechanisms for most HIV transmission. The two primary mechanisms responsible for the transmission of HIV are sexual activity and contact with infected blood (sharing needles or transfusion). Among men, the greatest number of new cases result from men having sex with men, though a significant number of cases result from heterosexual sex. Among women, risk of transmission is most frequent in heterosexual sex. Worldwide, 75 percent of all AIDS cases are now transmitted by heterosexual sex.

 Technology Update

The CDC officials believe that part of the reason people do not get tested for HIV is that it takes too long to get the results. The days of waiting to hear may simply be more than some people feel they can handle. According to a CDC official, one of the essential steps in reaching the goal of 95 percent awareness of HIV positive status is to develop tests that provide results more quickly. Only one rapid HIV test has been approved by the FDA. The Murex SUDS HIV-1 test manufactured by Abbott Diagnostics is capable of providing accurate results in as few as ten minutes. Unfortunately, Abbott discontinued production of the test in 2000. A number of other tests appear to provide accurate results, but patent issues have prevented them from becoming commercially available. The CDC and the FDA are continuing to encourage manufacturers to seek FDA approval, and there is hope that they will be commercially available in the next year or two. Although accuracy of these tests is comparable to those used by most physicians, a positive result should always be confirmed by a doctor. Nonetheless, this technology may lead more people to get tested sooner.

More than 25 percent of new cases are a result of injecting drugs with contaminated needles and most of the rest of the cases are among people who may combine these risk factors. Because of efforts to protect the blood supply, few cases result from contaminated blood. Some cases are transmitted from HIV-infected mothers to children during childbirth. At least one study has shown that Cesarean delivery can reduce the risk of mother-to-baby transmission if the mother is seropositive. Recent evidence has led to the recommendation that infected mothers consider alternatives to breast feeding.

Those with other STDs such as herpes and syphilis have a greater risk of transmission of HIV than those who do not have these conditions. Eight percent of HIV cases in one recent study were a result of oral sex. If future studies verify this finding, it suggests that oral sex may be a more risky behavior than previously thought.

HIV is not spread through the air or in saliva, sweat, or urine. It does not spread by hugging, sharing foods or beverages, or casual kissing. Contact with phones, silverware, or toilet seats does not cause the spread of HIV.

HIV must invade the blood in order for a person to become infected. People who had blood transfusions prior to 1985 had an increased risk of HIV transmission, but since that time the safety of the blood supply has increased dramatically. You have no danger in donating blood, only in receiving HIV-infected blood.

The risk of acquiring HIV/AIDS is reduced if exposure to HIV and to the methods of transmission are avoided. A recent National Institutes of Health consensus statement indicated that HIV transmission could be reduced if legislative barriers to needle exchange programs were lifted, if greater emphasis were given to youth education programs about HIV/AIDS, if greater funding were available for treatment of people who abuse drugs, and if educational efforts among high-risk populations were increased. Speakers at a recent World AIDS Conference spoke out in favor of similar recommendations. In this country, not all people agree with these recommendations. Nevertheless, it is important to examine the evidence and make decisions that will help meet national health goals for HIV/AIDS. Worldwide, the money expended on treatment far exceeds the amounts spent on prevention. Experts suggest that if we are to meet national health goals, more effort and money will need to be spent on prevention.

Evidence shows that relatively short-term educational sessions with trained counselors can reduce risk of HIV transmission. A seven-week program using small groups and a counselor motivated people to refrain from risky behaviors that increase risk. Other steps that can be taken to lower your risk of HIV infection are presented in Table 2. Only a small percentage of health-care workers have become infected from contact with infected blood at medical or dental facilities.

Table 2 ▶ Factors Associated with Reducing Risk of HIV/AIDS

- Abstain from sexual activity.
- Limit sexual activity to a noninfected partner. A lifetime partner who never had sex with other people and never used injected drugs (other than medically administered) is the only safe partner.
- Avoid sexual activity or other activity that puts you in contact with another person's semen, vaginal fluids, or blood.
- Use a new condom (latex) every time you have sex, especially with a partner who is not known to be safe. Know how to use it properly.
- Use a water-based lubricant with condoms, because petroleum-based lubricants increase risk of condom failure.
- Abstain from risky sexual activity, such as anal sex and sex with high-risk people (prostitutes, people with HIV or other STDs).
- Do not inject drugs.
- Never share a needle or drug paraphernalia.
- Get tested for STDs, and seek proper treatment.
- Anal and oral sex places people at higher risk of contracting STDs.
- People who have had an STD have increased risk of HIV/AIDS.

Other Sexually Transmitted Diseases

STDs infect about 12 million people each year. www.mhhe.com/fit_well/web23 Click 03. Although the consequences of STDs other than HIV/AIDS are not as severe, they contribute to significant short- and long-term health problems. They are also extremely common in young people, many of whom are unaware that they are infected with an STD. Five of the ten most commonly reported infectious diseases in the United States are sexually transmitted.

The most frequently reported STD in the United States is Chlamydia. **Chlamydia** is the most commonly reported STD. The number of cases has increased dramatically in recent years and there are currently about 3 million new cases of Chlamydia each year. Infection with *chlamydia trachomatis* may result in inflammation of the urethra, fallopian tube, and the cervix for females and inflammation of the epididymis for males (located over the testes).

In women, the health consequences of chlamydia are extensive. The disease has been linked to increased risk of **Pelvic Inflammatory Disease (PID)** as well as a number of other secondary health problems including urethritis, cervicitis, ectopic pregnancy, infertility, and chronic pelvic pain. As a result of the high levels of risk for women, new guidelines from the U.S. Preventive Services Task Force suggest that sexually active women under the age of twenty-five should undergo routine screening for chlamydia.

Another widespread STD is gonorrhea. **Gonorrhea** and hepatitis B are the next most frequently reported of all STDs. In the late 1990s, there was a rather dramatic decrease in the number of gonorrhea cases. Although this is a step in the right direction, we still need to educate people about prevention. Gonorrhea is a bacterial infection that can be treated with modern antibiotics if detected early. However, recent strains of the gonorrhea organism have become resistant to antibiotics, due to widespread overuse, causing concern among public health officials since some cases are quite difficult to treat.

Chlamydia A bacterial infection similar to gonorrhea that attacks the urinary tract and reproductive organs.

Pelvic Inflammatory Disease (PID) An infection of the urethra (urine passage) that can lead to infertility among women.

Gonorrhea A bacterial infection of the mucous membranes including the eyes, throat, genitals, and other organs.

Sexual activity is the principal method of disease transmission. Penile and vaginal gonorrhea are the most common types. Symptoms usually occur within three to seven days after bacteria enter the system. Among men the most common symptoms are painful urination and penile drip or discharge. Symptoms are less apparent among women, though painful urination and vaginal discharge are not uncommon. Other types of gonorrhea often have fewer symptoms. Chills, fever, painful bowel movements, and sore throat are the most common.

Early detection by a culture or smear test at the site or sites of sexual contact is how the disease is diagnosed. Early cure is especially important for females because gonorrhea can lead to pelvic inflammatory disease, which can result in infertility.

Syphilis is another serious but less commonly contracted STD. Syphilis was a serious national health problem in the 1940s, when it was ten times more prevalent than it is now. STDs showed a dramatic increase during the 1970s and 1980s. Fortunately, progress toward the national health goal of reducing the number of syphilis cases has been made. Syphilis was the first STD for which national control measures were initiated. Reported cases of syphilis declined 84 percent nationwide during the 1990s. CDC reports that syphilis continues to have a disproportionate effect on African Americans and people living in the South.

Like gonorrhea, syphilis is a bacterial infection that can be effectively treated with antibiotics. The symptoms of syphilis include **chancre** sores that generally appear at the primary site of sexual contact, then change from a red swelling to a hardened ulcer on the skin. Even if not treated, the sores disappear after a period of one to five weeks. It is important to get treatment even after this primary phase of the disease because the disease is still present and contagious. After several weeks or longer, secondary symptoms occur, such as a rash, loss of hair, joint pain, sore throat, and swollen glands. Even after these symptoms go away, untreated syphilis lingers in a latent phase. Serious health problems may result, including blindness, deafness, tumors, and stillbirth.

Early detection is important and can be diagnosed from chancre discharge or a blood test several weeks after the appearance of chancres. There is an association between syphilis and the spread of HIV. Apparently, the presence of chancres greatly increases the risk of transmitting HIV during sexual activity.

Of all STDs, genital herpes is among the most commonly spread because of a lack of awareness of infection. Genital herpes, one of the most commonly reported STDs, is caused by the herpes simplex

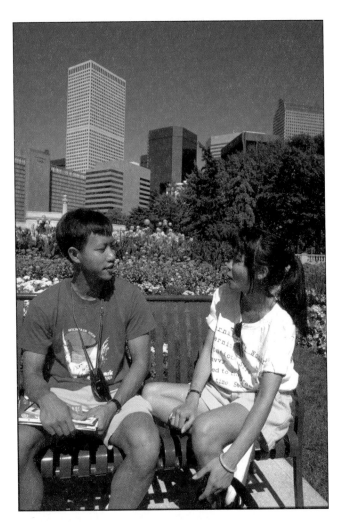

Open communication concerning sexual histories is important in preventing STDs.

virus (HSV). Estimates suggest that about 45 million people in the United States are infected with genital herpes. HSV is a family of many viruses that can produce various disorders in humans, such as shingles and chicken pox. HSV Type 1 is often called lip or oral herpes because it causes cold sores and fever blisters on the lips and the mouth. HSV Type 2 is often referred to as the STD type because it is known to cause genital lesions. These lesions or blisters on the penis, vagina, or cervix usually occur two to twelve days after infection and typically last a week to a month. Swollen glands and headache may also occur.

Though Type 2 HSV is generally referred to as the STD type, it is now known that both Types 1 and 2 HSV can cause genital sores, just as either type can cause lip and oral sores. At present no cure exists for genital sores caused by HSV, though some prescription drugs can help treat the disease symptoms. HSV can remain dormant in the body for long periods of time, and as a result, symptoms can recur at any time, especially after undergoing stress or illness.

Genital herpes is especially contagious when the blisters are present. Condom use or abstinence from sexual activity when symptoms are present can reduce the risk of transmission of the disease. Herpes is more dangerous for women than men because of the association between genital herpes and cervical cancer and the risk of transmitting the disease to the unborn.

The human papillomavirus (HPV) is a very common STD in young people. An estimated 5.5 million people become infected with HPV each year making this STD one of the most commonly transmitted. HPV is responsible for the development of genital warts, but most people do not develop them and are therefore unaware that they are infected. Although the disease is asymptomatic in the short term, it leads to significantly increased risk for cervical cancer in women. In fact, HPV is the leading cause of cervical cancer. Certain strains of HPV are particularly dangerous, accounting for approximately 80 percent of cases of cervical cancer. The risk of cervical cancer is compounded for women with a history of HPV and chlamydia. A recent study suggests that the combination of HPV and chronic use of birth control pills also compounds the level of risk. Women with a history of chlamydia and/or women who have used birth control pills for five or more years should consider being tested for HPV, due to the combined risk associated with these factors.

Some lesser known STDs are significant health problems. Pubic crab lice, chancroid, and genital warts are examples of lesser known but prevalent STDs. Some general information about these diseases is presented in Table 3. There are also a number of vaginal infections that can be sexually transmitted, including bacterial vaginosis (BV) and trichomoniasis.

Table 3 ▶ Facts about Lesser Known STDs

Genital Warts (Condylomas)

- Comprise approximately 5% of all reported STDs.
- Are most prevalent in ages fifteen to twenty-four.
- Are caused by the human papilloma virus (HPV).
- Are linked to cervical and genital cancers.
- Are hard and yellow or gray on dry skin.
- Are soft and pink, red or dark on moist skin.
- There is no known culture test.
- Early diagnosis is important (because of association with some forms of cancer).
- The prescription drug Podophyllin is one treatment.

Pubic Lice (Crabs)

- Are pinhead-sized insects (parasites) that feed on the blood of the host.
- Are transmitted by sexual contact and/or contact with contaminated clothes, bedding, and other washable items.
- Symptoms include itching; some people have no symptoms.
- Can be controlled by using medicated lotion and shampoos, and by washing contaminated bedding, etc.
- Do *not* transmit other STDs.

Chancroid

- Is caused by bacteria.
- Is more commonly seen in men than in women, particularly uncircumcised males.
- Symptoms include one or more sores or raised bumps on the genitals.
- Can result in progressive ulcers occurring on the genitals. Sometimes the ulcers persist for weeks or months.
- Can be successfully treated with certain antibiotics.

Syphilis An infection caused by a corkscrew-shaped bacteria that travels in the bloodstream and embeds itself in the mucous membranes of the body, including those of the sexual organs.

Chancre A sore or lesion commonly associated with syphilis.

Genital Herpes A viral infection that can attack any area of the body but often causes blisters on the genitals.

Pubic Lice Lice that attach themselves to the base of pubic hairs; also called crabs.

Chancroid A bacterial infection resulting in sores or ulcers on the genitals; different from chancres associated with syphilis.

Genital Warts Warts, caused by a virus, that grow in the genital/anal area (also called condyloma).

Strategies for Action

A first step in prevention is to recognize the risk. Young people are especially at risk for STDs. Nearly two-thirds of all STDs occur in people under the age of twenty-five. Both teens and college students are at high risk. In Lab 23A, you will have the opportunity to evaluate the risk of a friend or loved one. You may also want to evaluate your own risk using the STD Risk Questionnaire. Probable reasons for the high risk among young people are presented here.

- Perceived immortality. Many teens feel that disease is something that happens to other people, not to them. For example, one study indicated that a large proportion of teens do not feel that they are the kind of person who would get AIDS.
- Risky sexual activity. Evidence suggests that teens and young adults often do not follow the STD guidelines presented earlier in this concept. For example, data suggest that 70 percent are sexually active by age twenty, yet few have used condoms.
- Instant gratification. Many young people believe that sex should be entirely spontaneous. They fear what their partner might say if he/she is prepared to have sex and has protection available. They also feel that they cannot pass up an opportunity to have sex. It must be now.
- Inability to talk about sexual issues. It is easier for some young people to be sexually active than it is for them to truly communicate with each other about commitments and protection.

College students are at risk for HIV and other STDs due to the practice of serial monogamy. Many college students are sexually active, yet the majority do not use condoms on a consistent basis. This is, in part, due to perceptions that they are in committed relationships and, therefore, are at low risk for infection. Such perceptions are problematic for several reasons. First, college students typically define a regular partner as someone they have been with for as little as one month, with the majority defining a regular partner as someone they have been with for less than six months. Second, more college students do not get tested on a regular basis, if at all. Third, when students perceive that they are in a committed relationship, the likelihood of abstention from sex and condom use decreases dramatically. This is particularly true when an alternative form of birth control, primarily birth control pills, is being used. The common result is unprotected sexual intercourse between two people who have known one another for a relatively short period of time, and who are unaware of their own and each other's STD status. Many students go through multiple committed relationships during the college years. This type of serial monogamy places college students at increased risk for HIV and other STDs even though they may not believe that they are engaging in high-risk behavior.

We can help prevent STDs in the future by better educating young people about sexuality. The *Surgeon General's Call to Action to Promote Sexual Health and Responsible Behavior* stresses the need for open dialogue about sexuality. The report generated considerable controversy due to statements about homosexuality and sex education. The report stated that sexual orientation is generally determined by adolescence, and no evidence exists that sexual orientation can be changed. The report also stated that little evidence exists that abstinence-based sex education is effective, and evidence does not show that educating youth about birth control leads to increased sexual behavior. Regardless of one's opinions about these statements, the need for more open communication about sexuality is clear. America's youth are among the most sexually active in the world and among the least educated about sex.

The methods for preventing other STDs are the same as those for preventing HIV. The factors associated with reduced risk for HIV/AIDS presented in Table 2 are also important in preventing other STDs. The only true way to be protected against STDs is to have sex with a mutually exclusive partner who has never had sex with anyone else or has tested negative for all STDs. Even condoms, the primary form of protection against STDs, are not fail safe. Although they are effective in preventing gonorrhea and HIV, the National Institutes of Health concluded that there was not enough

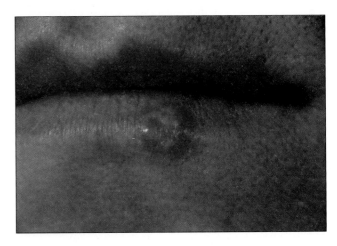

Lip (oral) herpes.

evidence to confidently say that condoms provide adequate protection against other STDs including chlamydia, trichomoniasis, and human papillomavirus.

Another method of prevention that may be available in the future is the use of topical microbicides. A microbicide is a topical preparation (foam, gel, or cream), that is applied vaginally or anally to prevent infection. These products are primarily being developed to target HIV but evidence shows they could also be effective in preventing other STDs. Several topical microbicides are currently undergoing clinical trials, but it may be several years before they become available.

Hotlines are available to help people who want information concerning STDs such as HIV/AIDS. The following national AIDS hotlines are toll-free and allow the caller to retain anonymity:

(English) 1-800-342-AIDS (342-2437)
(Spanish) 1-800-344-SIDA (344-7432)

The CDC's national STD hotline (1-800-227-8922) is a toll-free number that provides information for a variety of STDs.

Web Resources

CDC Center for STD Prevention
www.cdc.gov/nchstp/od/nchstp.html
CDC—Division of Sexually Transmitted Diseases
www.cdc.gov/nchstp/dstd/dstd.html
Harvard AIDS Institute
www.hsph.harvard.edu/organizations/hai
Healthy People 2010 **www.health.gov/healthypeople**
National Institute of Allergy and Infectious Diseases
www.niaid.nih.gov
The Office of HIV/AIDS Policy **www.surgeongeneral.gov/aids**

Suggested Readings

 Additional reference materials for concept 23 are available at **www.mhhe.com/fit_well/web23 Click 04.**

Berg, A., and U.S. Preventive Services Task Force. 2001. Screening for chlamydial infection: Recommendations and rationale. *American Journal of Preventive Medicine* 20(30):90–94.

Centers for Disease Control and Prevention. 2001. *HIV/AIDS Surveillance Report* 13(1).

Corbin, W. R., and K. Fromme. 2002. Alcohol use and serial monogamy as risks for sexually transmitted diseases in young adults. *Health Psychology* 21(3):229–236.

Cox, F. D. 2000. *The Aids Booklet.* St. Louis, MO: McGraw-Hill.

Johnston, M. I., and J. Flores. 2001. Progress in HIV vaccine development. *Current Opinion in Pharmacology* 1: 504–510.

Moreno, V. et al. 2002. Effect of oral contraceptives on risk of cervical cancer in women with human papillomavirus infection: The IARC multicentric case-control study. *Lancet* 359(9312):1085–1092.

Payne, W. A., and D. B. Hahn. 2002. *Understanding Your Health.* 7th ed. St. Louis: McGraw-Hill, Chapter 13.

Rosenfeld, I. 23 July 2000. New treatments (HIV/AIDS), renewed hope. *Parade Magazine* 4.

Rosenfeld, I. 6 Aug. 2000. Stay safe: Know your STDs. *Parade Magazine* 8.

Sterling, T. et al. 2001. Initial plasma HIV-1 RNA levels and progression to AIDS in women and men. *New England Journal of Medicine* 344(10):720–725.

U. S. Department of Health and Human Services. Nov. 2000. *Healthy People 2010.* 2nd ed. With Understanding and Improving Health and Objectives for Improving Health. 2 vols. Washington, DC: U.S. Government Printing Office.

United States Public Health Service. Office of the Surgeon General. 2001. *Surgeon General's Call to Action to Promote Sexual Health and Responsible Sexual Behavior.* Washington, DC USPHS, Office of the Surgeon General.

🎤 In the News

The topic of sex education in the schools has always been a controversial one and recent statements by the Surgeon General have fueled the debate. Advocates for both sides should be able to support one method recently shown to impact adolescent sexual behavior. An elementary school-based program designed to improve student grades and cooperative behavior led to significant reductions in the number of sexual partners and rates of pregnancy at age twenty-one. Among those who were single at age twenty-one, the intervention was associated with increased probability of condom use during the most recent sexual intercourse. The intervention was particularly effective for African American students who showed reduced probability of contracting a sexually transmitted disease. All of these positive outcomes occurred in the absence of direct efforts to target sexual behavior. In theory, increasing involvement in school and commitment to learning decreases behaviors that might jeopardize future success. Although this explanation is speculative, the results of the study may provide a promising new avenue for prevention of risky sexual behaviors.

Despite the very positive results of this study, many are concerned that it will be used to fuel arguments against sex education in the schools. The argument would be "if we can reduce sexual activity without talking about sex, why talk about it." Results indicating that some sex education programs also have a positive impact on sexual behavior would argue against this idea. Perhaps a combination of sex education, efforts to get children more involved in school, and conversations with parents will lead to even better outcomes.

Lab 23A: Sexually Transmitted Disease Risk Questionnaire

Name	Section	Date

Purpose: To help you understand the risks of contracting a sexually transmitted disease.

Procedure:

1. Read the Sexually Transmitted Disease Risk Questionnaire.
2. Answer the questionnaire based on information about someone you know who might be at high risk of contracting an STD.
3. Record the scores in the Results section for the person for whom the questionnaire was answered but do *not* include the person's name on the lab sheet. Use the scores to make a rating (Chart 2) and draw conclusions.
4. You may also wish to answer the questionnaire based on your own information but do *not* record your personal results on the lab sheet. Use these scores strictly for your own personal information.

Chart 1 ▶ Sexually Transmitted Disease Risk Questionnaire

Directions: Mark an X over one response in each row of the questionnaire. Determine a point value for each response using the values in the circles. Sum the numbers of points for the various responses to determine a STD risk score.

	Points				
Categories	**0**	**1**	**3**	**5**	**8**
Feelings about prevention	Able to talk with future partner about STDs. (0)	Find it hard to discuss STDs with a possible partner. (1)			
Behaviors	Never engages in sexual activity. (0)		Sexual activity with one partner, well-known to him/her. (3)	Sexual activity with one partner, not well-known to him/her. (5)	Sexual activity with multiple partners and/or high-risk individuals. (8)
Behavior of friends	Most friends do not engage in unsafe sexual activity. (0)	Many friends engage in unsafe sexual activity. (1)			
Contraception	Not sexually active. (0)	Would use condom to prevent STD. (1)		Would sometimes use condom to prevent STD. (5)	Would never use condom to prevent STD. (8)
Other	Does not use drugs. (0)				Uses injected drugs in unsafe manner. (8)

Chart 2 ▶ Risk Questionnaire Rating Chart	
Rating	**Score**
High risk	9+
Above average risk	7–8
Moderate risk	4–6
Low risk	0–3

Results:

What is the person's STD risk score? [   ] (Total from STD Risk Questionnaire)

What is the person's STD rating? [   ] (See STD Risk Questionnaire Rating Chart.)

Conclusions and Implications: Of course, risk varies with different types of STDs. However, this questionnaire will give you an idea of an individual's "general" risk for most STDs. Answer the following questions about the risk of the person you scored and rated.

1. In several sentences, explain which STD you think this person should be especially concerned about. Why?

2. What specific recommendations would you have for the person for whom you filled out this questionnaire?

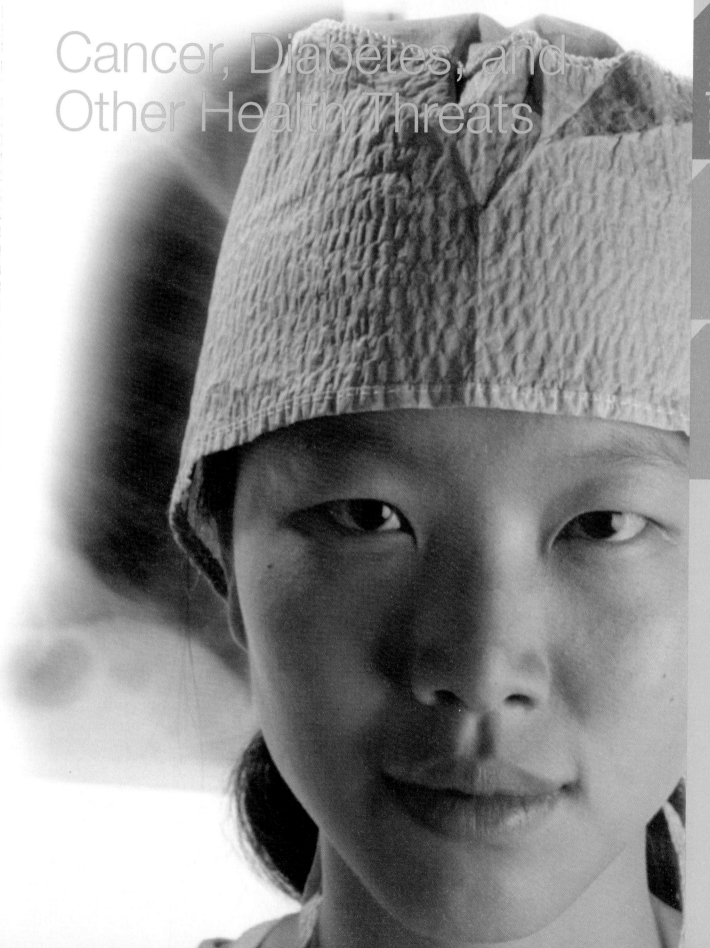

Cancer, Diabetes, and Other Health Threats

Many health problems that cause pain, suffering, and premature death are associated with unhealthy lifestyles.

Health Goals
for the year 2010

- Reduce cancer cases, as well as illness, disability, and death from it.

- Increase rate of cancer screening.

- Increase cancer survivors (five years or more).

- Increase diabetes screening and education.

- Prevent and reduce death from diabetes and disabilities associated with diabetes.

- Decrease incidence of depression.

- Increase healthy days.

- Increase screening and availability of medical treatment for a variety of health threats.

- Eliminate health disparities.

- Improve air quality, ensure safe water, and reduce environmental waste and hazards.

- Reduce unintentional injuries (focus on head and spinal cord) from all sources including firearms, drowning, pedestrian, bicycle and auto accidents, and fires.

- Reduce violence and abuse.

- Reduce the proportion of people who experience regular sadness or unhappiness.

Each year, many deaths and much pain and suffering could be prevented by altering lifestyles associated with various diseases and health threats. Heart disease, the leading cause of death, stroke (third leading cause of death), and osteoporosis were discussed in the concept on health benefits of physical activity, so they will not be discussed here. Among the conditions that are discussed in this concept are cancer, diabetes, bronchitis/emphysema, injuries, diabetes mellitus and emotional disorders (including suicide). Cancer is second only to heart disease among the leading causes of death. Deaths from heart disease have decreased in recent years, but deaths from cancer have increased. If this trend continues, cancer will soon become the leading cause of death in North America. Diabetes, injuries, and suicide all rank among the top ten leading causes of death in our society.

Cancer

Cancer is a group of more than 100 different diseases. According to the American Cancer Society, cancer is a group of many different conditions characterized by abnormal, uncontrolled cell growth that will ultimately invade the blood and lymph tissues and spread throughout the body if not treated. Throughout the human body, new cells are constantly being created to replace older ones. For reasons unknown, abnormal cells sometimes develop capable of uncontrolled growth. **Benign tumors** are generally not considered to be cancerous because their growth is restricted to a specific area of the body by a protective membrane. Treatment is important because any tumor can interfere with normal bodily functioning. Once removed, a benign tumor typically will not return.

Malignant tumors are called **carcinomas** because they are capable of uncontrolled growth that can cause death to tissue. Malignant cells invade healthy tissues and deplete them of nutrition and interfere with a multitude of tissue functions. In the early stages of cancer, malignant tumors are located in a small area and can be more easily treated or removed. In advanced cancer, the cells invade the blood or lymph systems and travel throughout the body **(metastases).** When this occurs, cancer becomes much more difficult to treat. Figure 1 illustrates how an abnormal cell can divide to form a primary tumor (a), get nourishment from new blood vessels (b), invade the blood system (c), and escape to form a new (secondary) tumor (d). Four stages of cancer range from I to IV with I being the early stage and IV being most advanced. The early stage is characterized by containment only in the layers of cells where they developed. When cancer spreads beyond the original layers (see Figure 1), it is considered to be invasive and is rated with a higher stage rating. Early detection is very important in the treatment and cure of cancer. One method of detecting a tumor is to take a **biopsy** of suspicious lumps in the breasts, testicles, or other parts of the body.

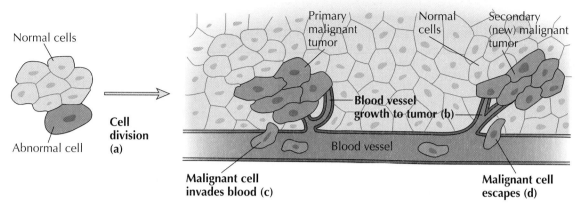

Figure 1 ▶ The spread of cancer (metastasis).

Cancer is a leading killer in our society. www.mhhe.com/fit_well/web24 Click 01. Cancer is the second leading cause of death in our society. One of every four deaths in the United States is caused by some form of cancer. Slightly more than one in three women and slightly less than one in two men will have cancer at some time in his/her life. It is the cause of much suffering and accounts for a large portion of the money spent on health care. Other diseases, such as heart disease and stroke, have decreased in recent years, but for cancer such declines have been less dramatic.

Of the more than 100 forms of cancer, four account for more than half of all illness and death. Of the 100 different kinds of cancer, a much smaller number account for 2 percent or more of cancer incidence and deaths. Some are similar for both sexes, but others are different. These most common cancers are illustrated in Figure 2.

Four forms of cancer (sometimes referred to as the Big 4) account for more than half of all illness and death (see Figure 2). Because of the high incidence of these types of cancers (lung, colon-rectal, breast, and prostate) they are discussed in more detail here. In addition, three forms of cancer for which college students have relative high-risk are also discussed (skin, ovary, and uterus). In Lab 24A you will have the opportunity to assess your risk for each of these types of cancer.

Breast Cancer

Breast cancer is the leading type of cancer and is the second leading killer for women. Breast cancer is becoming more common though it is not among the more frequent types among men. Men, like women, should do regular screening. Like colon-rectal and lung cancers, breast cancer is most prevalent among African Americans and

least prevalent among Asians and Hispanics (more than twice as frequent).

Symptoms include lumps and/or thickening or swelling of the breasts. In many cases, lumps or tumors are present before they can be detected with self-exams. This is one reason for regular **mammograms** (breast X-ray). Breast pain may also exist but is more often a symptom of benign tumors. Risk becomes greater as you grow older. Other risk factors include sex (females have higher risk), family history of disease, early menstruation, estrogen supplementation or use of oral contraceptives, late birth or no children, excessive use of alcohol, poor eating habits, and sedentary living. Recent research suggests a possible link between breast implantation and breast cancer.

Early detection steps include regular self-exams of the breasts (see Lab 24B), breast exams by a physician, and regular mammograms. Contradictory findings of studies have led to a debate concerning the effectiveness of

Benign Tumor A slow-growing tumor that does not spread to other parts of the body.

Malignant Tumor Malignant means "growing worse." A malignant tumor is one that is considered to be cancerous and will spread throughout the body if not treated.

Carcinoma A malignant or invasive form of tumor.

Metastases The spread of cancer cells to other parts of the body.

Biopsy Removal of a tissue sample that can be checked for cancer cells.

Mammogram An X-ray of the breast.

Cancer Type

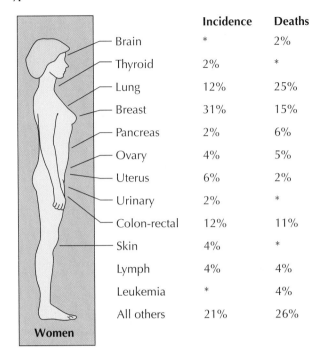

Deaths	Incidence			Incidence	Deaths
*	3%	Oral	Brain	*	2%
3%	*	Esophagus	Thyroid	2%	*
31%	14%	Lung	Lung	12%	25%
3%	*	Liver	Breast	31%	15%
5%	2%	Pancreas	Pancreas	2%	6%
3%	3%	Kidney	Ovary	4%	5%
11%	30%	Prostate	Uterus	6%	2%
3%	7%	Urinary	Urinary	2%	*
10%	11%	Colon-rectal	Colon-rectal	12%	11%
*	5%	Skin	Skin	4%	*
5%	4%	Lymph	Lymph	4%	4%
4%	3%	Leukemia	Leukemia	*	4%
22%	18%	All others	All others	21%	26%
		Men	**Women**		

Figure 2 ▶ Cancer incidence and death by site and sex (percent).

Source: American Cancer Society.

*equals less than 2%.

mammography in detecting and preventing breast cancer. Also under debate is the frequency of treatment. Recommendations in Table 1 are based on recommendations of the American Cancer Society at the time this book went to press.

Standard treatments for breast cancer include lumpectomy (removal of the tumor and surrounding lymph nodes), mastectomy (removal of breast and surrounding lymph nodes), chemotherapy, radiation, and/or hormone therapies. Tamoxifen, or other drugs, may be prescribed for those at high risk.

Colon-Rectal Cancer

Colon-rectal cancers are the second leading overall killers because they affect men and women equally. There has been a consistent, but small, decline in colon-rectal cancer among men and women over the past two decades. Like lung cancer, risk is highest among African Americans. Whites have slightly less risk. Risk among Asians and Hispanics is less than half that of blacks. It is most common among those over fifty years of age. When caught early, 90 percent of colon-rectal cancers can be cured.

Symptoms may include cramping in the lower stomach, change in shape of stool, urge to have a bowel movement when there is no need to have one, or blood in the stool. Because observable blood in the stool could indicate

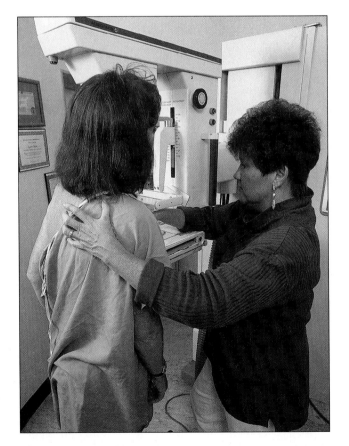

Cancer risk can be reduced by periodic medical tests and self-screening.

Table 1 ▶ Cancer Screening Guidelines			
Test or Procedure	**Sex**	**Age**	**Frequency**
General Cancer Related Checkup			
Exam for cancers of the thyroid, prostate, ovaries or testes, lymph nodes, mouth, and skin	Men/women	20–39	Every three years
Breast Cancer			
Breast self-exam	Women	20	Every month
Breast exam by physician including mammogram	Women	20–39	Every three years
	Women	40+	Every year
Colon-Rectal Cancer*			
Fecal occult blood test	Men/women	50+	Every year
Sigmoidoscopy	Men/women	50+	Every five years
Barium enema	Men/women	50+	Every five to ten years
Colonoscopy	Men/women	50+	Every ten years
Lung			
X-ray (chest)	Men/women	Any age	If other symptoms exist
Prostate			
Digital rectal exam and PSA test	Men (Normal risk)	50+	Yearly
	Men (High risk)	45+	Yearly**
Testes			
Self-exam	Men	20+	Monthly
Uterus/Cervix			
Pelvic exam and PAP test**	Women	Sexually active	Yearly
Endometrial	Women		
Screening and biopsy	Women at risk	35+	With risk or symptoms
Skin Cancer			
Self-exam	Men and women	Any age	Monthly
Exam by physician	Men and women	Any age	With symptoms

*Frequency varies based on tests done and test results; all tests may not be necessary.

**With repeated negative test, less frequent screening may be indicated.

an advanced problem, do regular screenings including a fecal blood test (see Table 1). Other screening tests include a barium enema, a sphygmoidoscopy, or a colonscopy (considered as a the gold standard by the American Cancer Society). A new painless test not currently available offers promise for the future. The APC gene test involves examination of stool samples for damaged genes that trigger cancers.

Except for the APC gene test, all of the tests are designed to detect either the presence of polyps that can turn into cancer, or polyps (or cancers) that are bleeding. Any or all of the tests may be recommended by a physi-cian, especially after age fifty. Frequency of screening recommended by the American Cancer Society is shown in Table 1. Some experts feel that the colonoscopy is better than the sigmoidoscopy because it checks the entire colon for polyps rather than the lower one-third. Recent studies show that the frequency of screening should vary depending on symptoms and heredity. For example, people with a family history of colon-rectal cancer or those who have found a polyp in previous exams should schedule a procedure more frequently than listed in Table 1. The most common treatments are surgery for cancer or polyp removal, radiation, and/or chemotherapy.

Table 2 ▶ Strategies for Preventing Cancer

- Eat a healthy diet: reduce fat to less than 30%, increase complex carbohydrates, decrease simple carbohydrates, avoid junk food, and eat green and yellow vegetables.

- Eliminate tobacco use: cigarettes, other smoking, and smokeless tobacco.

- Perform regular activity: be physically fit, do daily exercise, and avoid obesity.

- Reduce sun and ultraviolet light exposure: use sunscreen, wear protective clothing, and avoid exposure to sun and tanning lights.

- Do regular self-screening and medical testing.

- Avoid carcinogens in food (such as sodium nitrate in bacon) and in other sources (such as insecticides).

- If you drink alcohol, use moderation.

- Avoid breathing polluted air.

- Avoid excessive X-rays.

- Have a positive attitude and a fighting spirit.

Risk factors include diet, use of alcohol, family history, physical activity patterns, and smoking. Though the American Cancer Society does not recommend the use of supplements, there is some evidence that some vitamins and minerals (vitamin E, selenium, calcium, folic acid), aspirin or aspirin-like drugs, and post-menopausal hormones may reduce risk. You may assess your risk in Lab 24A.

Lung Cancer

Frequently referred to as lung cancer, it includes cancers of the lungs and bronchi and is the leading killer of men and women. Lung cancer continues to rise for women though it has decreased in the last decade for men. It is only in the last two decades that lung cancer deaths surpassed breast cancer deaths among women. Smoking has decreased more rapidly among men than women in recent years, which may explain the recent increase in lung cancer among women. In the last decade smoking rates among youth and young adults have increased suggesting that lung cancer deaths may increase in the years ahead. Incidence and death rates are much higher among African Americans than whites with considerably lower rates among Asians and Hispanics.

Symptoms include persistent cough, chest pain, reoccurring pneumonia or bronchitis, and sputum streaked with blood. By far the greatest risk factor is smoking followed by a polluted or smoke filled environment (see Lab 24A). Early detection steps include monitoring for symptoms, chest X-rays, and analyses of sputum samples. Standard treatments include radiation and chemotherapies. Other procedures include cell-targeted antibody treatment and bone marrow transplants.

Prostate Cancer

Prostate cancer is present when a tumor invades the prostate gland located in the lower abdomen. It is the most frequent form of cancer among men and accounts for one-tenth of all cancer deaths. Deaths increased from 1950 to 1990 when they peaked. Since then, the death rate associated with improved treatment and early detection has decreased. The death rate among African Americans is five times higher than among Asians, more than three times higher than Hispanics, and more than twice as high as whites. Prostate cancer is most prevalent among men over the age of fifty.

Symptoms include urination problems (weak stream, interrupted stream, inability to start or stop, pain, high frequency especially at night, and/or presence of blood) as well as persistent pain in the low back, pelvis, or thighs. Early detection techniques include a digital rectal exam by a physician (to detect an enlarged prostate gland), and a prostate-specific antigen (PSA) blood test. The frequency of the need for a PSA has been debated. Current research suggests that the results of early PSA tests will dictate the need for future tests. For some the need for a test may be more or less frequent than specified in Table 1. Risk factors include age, family history, race, and dietary fat. Depending on age, stage of the cancer, and other medical conditions, treatments vary. For some in the early stages, watchful waiting may be the prescription. Other treatments include surgery to remove the prostate, and/or radiation, chemotherapy, or hormone therapy. Hormone therapy is intended to shrink the prostate to relieve pain and symptoms. Treatments now in development include implantation of radioactive seeds in the prostate.

Uterus and Ovary Cancer

When combined, these types of cancers account for 10 percent of all cases and 7 percent of all deaths among women. Uterine cancer is of two different types: cervical cancer occurs when cancers develop in the cervix or opening to the uterus, and endometrial cancer occurs when a tumor develops in the inner wall of the uterus. Ovarian cancer occurs when a cancer develops in an ovary. Symptoms of ovarian cancer include abdominal swelling and digestive disturbances. Vaginal bleeding can be a symptom of either uterine or ovarian cancer. Other vaginal discharge may be a symptom of uterine cancer.

Cervical cancers are closely related to the presence of some types of HPV, a sexually transmitted disease.

Women who had sex at an early age, who have had sex with many partners, or with people who have had sex with many partners are at increased risk of cervical cancer. Smoking is also a risk factor for cervical cancer. Endometrial cancer is related to high exposures of estrogen over a lifetime, obesity, and having other diseases such as diabetes or high blood pressure. Risk factors for ovarian cancer include age, family history, and lack of pregnancy during the lifetime. A recent study showed that risk is considerably higher among those who have taken estrogen-progestin therapy, especially those who have taken them for ten years or more. Those who have had breast cancer or who are at high risk of breast cancer have a relative high risk of ovarian cancer.

A periodic and thorough pelvic exam is the best method of screening for cervical and ovarian cancer. A **PAP** test is an important part of the exam for detecting cervical cancer. This test, named for Dr. George Papanicolaou who pioneered it, involves taking scrapings (samples) from the cervix and analyzing them under a microscope. Because screening for HPV is also important, some experts favor a new PAP test (Thin Prep) because it allows the regular PAP test and the HPV to be done from one sample. The necessary frequency of PAP tests is under debate. A new test, PAP sure, that swabs the cervix with vinegar, then uses a light to visually check for abnormal cells, is also now available. Table 1 contains current recommendations. Vaginal ultrasound and/or use of a tumor marker CA 125 may be effective in diagnosing ovarian cancer.

Treatments include surgery to remove one or both of the ovaries and fallopian tubes (depending on age) and/or removal of the uterus (hysterectomy). Radiation therapy and chemotherapy are other options.

Skin Cancer

Each year more than 1 million people get basal or squamous cell cancer. This curable form is not included in the overall incidence statistics in Figure 2. **Melanoma,** on the other hand, is a deadly cancer if not treated early. Kaposi's sarcoma, prevalent among those with AIDS, is another form of skin cancer. Melanoma is ten times more frequent in whites than African Americans. Unlike many other forms of cancer, it is not necessarily a disease of older adults. Young people who do not take preventive measures are at risk.

Symptoms include dark pigmented growths, changes in size or color of moles, changes in other nodules on the skin, skin bleeding or scaliness, and skin pain. The principal risk factor is exposure to ultraviolet light such as sun exposure. Excessive sun exposure is common among college students. Some feel that tanning lights are safe, but recent research has shown the opposite. Other risk factors include family history, pale skin, exposure to pollutants, and radiation.

Early detection is essential to treatment so regular screening is important. Screening techniques include self-exams of the skin followed by a physician's exam of suspicious lesions. The following ABCD rule can be useful in doing self-exams. A is for asymmetry; does one half of a growth look different than the other half. B is for border irregularity; are the edges notched, rugged, or blurred. C is for color; is the color uniform, not varying in shades of tan, brown, and black. D is for any lesion with a diameter greater than 6 millimeters (about 3/8 of an inch). Beware of sudden or progressive growth of any lesion.

Non-malignant basal cell cancers can be treated in a doctor's office using freezing, heat, or laser procedures. Early melanoma involves the removal of affected cells and surrounding lymph tissues. Advanced cases require chemo and/or radiation therapies. Immunotherapy is another option.

Prevention is the key. Important preventive measures include having regular skin examinations, limiting exposure to the sun or tanning devices, reducing exposure during midday hours (10 A.M. to 4 P.M.), covering the skin when exposed to the sun (hat, long pants, long sleeve shirts, high collars on shirts, sunglasses), and using sunscreen (SPF of 15 or higher). Those with a history of severe sunburn as a child should be especially careful to follow the guidelines listed above.

Many factors are associated with increased risk of cancer; unhealthy lifestyles are among them. The malfunction of genes that control cell growth and development is responsible for all cancers. Five to 10 percent of cancers result from an inherited faulty gene. Environmental and lifestyle factors are the other contributors (see Figure 3). The importance of lifestyle factors such as sedentary living, diet, tobacco use, sexual behavior, and alcohol use were outlined for specific types of cancer in the previous section. Some general guidelines are outlined in Table 2. Examples of less obvious factors (see Figure 3), include geophysical (radiation), pollution (PCB, a by-product of the plastic industry), industrial products (asbestos, DDT, and 2-4-5-T also known as Agent Orange), and medical (X-ray). Substances contained in many of these are considered to be **carcinogens**

PAP Test A test of cells of the cervix to detect cancer or other conditions. Cancer risk can be reduced by periodic medical tests and self-screening.

Melanoma Cancer of the cells that produce skin pigment.

Carcinogen A substance that tends to produce a tumor or cancer. Examples include asbestos fibers and various substances in tobacco.

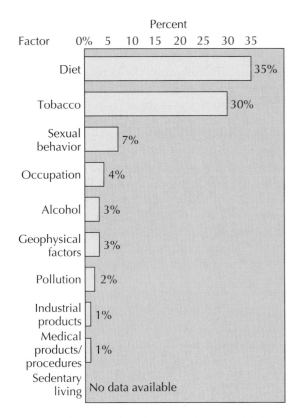

Figure 3 ▶ Lifestyle and environmental cancer risk factors.
Source: Data from the American Cancer Society.

because exposure to them causes cancer. Avoiding exposure to or consumption of carcinogens reduces risk of cancer.

Also as noted in the previous section, early screening is essential in reducing risk. Cancers that can be detected by currently available screening methods account for about one-half of all cases. Having a positive attitude is another factor that cannot be discounted. People with a fighting spirit and who hold out hope have less reoccurrence of cancer than people with less positive attitudes.

Many forms of cancer can be cured. Many people have lived long and healthy lives after breast, skin, and many other forms of cancer. These people die from other causes and by any standard, can be considered cured of their cancer. Still what constitutes a cure is illusive. The five-year survival rate for all forms of cancer is 62 percent. Though people who survive for five years after detection cannot be considered cured, this high survival rate illustrates that cancer can be treated even for those with inherited faulty genes.

Medical consultation is essential when considering hormone replacement therapy. For years hormone replacement therapy (HRT) has been prescribed

by medical doctors. Nearly 40 percent of post-menopausal women in the United States have been on HRT (initially estrogen and then a combination of estrogen and progestin) making it the second most prescribed medication in the country. More than 45 million prescriptions were written in the year 2000 accounting for over $1 billion in sales.

The drugs were thought to be effective in reducing symptoms of menopause, preventing loss of bone density, and reducing risk of heart disease. However, it has been known for some time that long-term exposure to estrogen increases risk of some forms of cancer, but depending on individual health risk profiles, doctors chose to prescribe or not prescribe HRT. For many, the benefits were thought to outweigh the risks. A recent large-scale study was stopped prior to its intended finishing date of 2005 because "the overall health risks exceed any benefits" for those using HRT. Results showed that breast cancer risk was higher among those who took HRT, and it was not effective in preventing heart disease. Stroke and pulmonary embolism risk was higher though risk of colon-rectal cancer and osteoporosis was lower among HRT users. Another recent study reported a higher incidence of ovarian cancer among those on long-term HRT compared to those in a placebo group.

HRT is still supported by some experts as a method of relieving symptoms of menopause such as hot flashes, sleep disturbances, fatigue, poor concentration, and disruption of work and recreational activities though other experts have challenged these benefits.

Studies such as those reported here consider group risk rather than individual risk. The risk of increased disease from HRT is relatively small compared to other risk factors. Nevertheless, small risks add up over time. Most experts agree that each case should be considered individually with patient and doctor weighing all risks and benefits before choosing a course of action. For those who do not continue HRT alternate methods of preventing bone loss and reducing post-menopausal symptoms should be discussed with their physician.

Recognizing early warning signals can help reduce the risk of cancer. The acronym CAUTION will help you remember these early warning signs. Look for the following:

C = Changes in bowel or bladder habits
A = A sore that does not heal
U = Unusual bleeding or discharge
T = Thickening or lump in the breast or elsewhere
I = Indigestion or difficulty swallowing
O = Obvious change in a wart or mole
N = Nagging cough or hoarseness

Diabetes

Several classifications of diabetes cause health risk to many individuals. Glucose, a source of energy, is a sugar in the blood. Normally, glucose levels range from 50 to 100 mg per each 100 ml of blood. Diabetes mellitus, typically referred to as diabetes, is a disease that occurs when the blood glucose is chronically high. As many as thirty different reasons exist for high blood sugar. Therefore, diabetes is really many different diseases, not just one. There is no cure for diabetes, but in most cases it can be controlled with proper medication and a healthy lifestyle.

Insulin, a hormone produced by the pancreas, regulates the glucose in the blood. When a person's body fails to produce adequate insulin and the individual needs to take insulin (oral or injection) to regulate blood-glucose levels, he or she is said to have **Type I diabetes.** About 5 percent of all diabetics have Type I diabetes, and this condition is typically diagnosed before the age of thirty.

Type II diabetes is typically non-insulin dependent and can often be controlled with significant lifestyle changes and drugs other than insulin. Nearly 95 percent of all diabetics have Type II diabetes. About 11.1 million diabetics have been diagnosed and another 5.9 million are unaware of their condition. Type II diabetes was referred to as adult onset diabetes in the past because it was a disease that occurred later in life. In the last decade, children and adolescents have begun to develop the disease. This development is closely tied to the epidemic of obesity among youth thought to be caused primarily by excessive calorie intake and sedentary living.

Before people develop Type II diabetes, they almost always have a condition referred to as pre-diabetes. People with this condition have high blood glucose levels but not high enough to be diagnosed as diabetic. This condition was formerly known as impaired glucose tolerance but the name was changed to help focus attention on the seriousness of the problem of this condition. Recent research has shown that pre-diabetes can result in long-term damage to the body similar to diabetes. People who do screening and take steps to control pre-diabetes can delay or even prevent the development of Type II diabetes. A third and relatively rare form of diabetes is referred to as gestational diabetes mellitus. This occurs when high blood-sugar levels occur in pregnant women previously not known to have diabetes. This condition is present in about 3 percent of all pregnancies, can have implications for the fetus, and may or may not result in a diabetes state after pregnancy. Other forms of diabetes are rare.

People have a familial predisposition to Type I and Type II though the predisposition is greater for Type I diabetes. Some people with Type II diabetes do not produce enough insulin to regulate their blood-sugar levels. More commonly they are insensitive to insulin, so the body cannot effectively regulate blood sugar.

 Diabetes and related conditions are a leading cause of death in our society. www.mhhe.com/fit_well/web 24 Click 02. As noted in concept 1, diabetes is the seventh leading cause of death, and is a leading killer in other western nations including Canada. People with diabetes have a shortened life span as well as many short-term and long-term complications associated with the disease. People must recognize their illness because proper medication and changes in lifestyle can greatly reduce the complications of the disease and the death rate associated with it.

African Americans and Native Americans are especially at risk of diabetes. Not only is the death rate higher among these groups but so are the health problems associated with the disease. Unlike heart diseases and cancers for which we have made progress toward national health goals of reducing disease rates, the incidence of diabetes has increased in the last decade.

Diabetes is associated with other health problems. People with diabetes have an increased risk of additional health problems. For example, diabetes is considered to be a risk factor for heart disease and high blood pressure. Diabetics have a higher rate of kidney failure (including the need for kidney transplants and kidney dialysis), a high incidence of blindness, and a high incidence of lower limb amputation. Women with diabetes also have a high rate of pregnancy complications. A national health goal is to increase the rate of diagnosis and to increase the number of diabetics who get regular blood lipid assessments, blood pressure checks, and eye examinations.

Lifestyle changes can help reduce the symptoms and complications associated with diabetes. National health goals for the year 2010 reflect lifestyle changes that can help reduce health problems associated with diabetes.

- Reduce overweight (fatness) in the general population. Reducing body fat is probably the most significant way to reduce the incidence of diabetes in our society.

Insulin A hormone that regulates blood-sugar levels.

Type I Diabetes A chronic metabolic disease characterized by high blood-sugar (glucose) levels associated with the inability of the pancreas to produce insulin; also called insulin-dependent diabetes mellitus (IDDM) or juvenile-onset diabetes.

Type II Diabetes A chronic metabolic disease characterized by high blood sugar, usually not requiring insulin therapy: also called non-insulin dependent diabetes mellitus (NIDDM) or adult-onset diabetes.

- Increase daily physical activity. Regular exercise results in calories expended and is one way to help reduce overfatness. It also helps regulate blood-sugar levels and helps body cells become more sensitive to insulin.
- Reduce dietary fat intake, increase intake of complex carbohydrates, and decrease total calorie intake. Particularly important is the value of a sound diet in reducing body fatness.

There has been some recent progress in increasing daily activity levels, but not for totally sedentary people. Furthermore, there has actually been an increase in the incidence of overweight people over the last decade. Health experts suggest that diabetes is a "big problem that will get bigger in the future." It is considered a wasteful disease because lifestyle changes, possible for most people, could greatly reduce the incidence of Type II diabetes.

Screening for pre-diabetes and diabetes is essential to diagnosis and treatment Early diagnosis resulting from attention to symptoms described previously can expedite treatment. New guidelines recommend screening for pre-diabetes and diabetes using either of two blood tests: a fasting plasma glucose (FPG) test that measures levels of glucose in the blood after an overnight fast, or a two-hour oral **glucose tolerance test** (OGTT) that includes the FPG test but also tests glucose levels two hours after a person drinks a standard glucose solution. Guidelines recommend regular screening beginning at age forty-five. Because African Americans, Hispanics, Asians, American Indians, and Pacific Islanders have especially high risk some experts recommend testing at age thirty or earlier for these groups. Others with diabetes risk factors and those with a BMI over 25 should also consider testing at an earlier age.

Technology Update

People with Type I diabetes take blood samples one or more times a day. The samples are used to test their blood sugar levels to determine when insulin must be taken. To take a blood sample, the skin must be punctured, most commonly on the end of a finger. New technology has now been developed that allows some diabetics to test blood sugar levels without having to draw blood. A special computer watch (Glucowatch) automatically takes a reading through the skin every 20 minutes. The watches are not accessible to all diabetics partly because of their cost. The watches require regular service and parts replacement. With future refinement, this technology may help diabetics more effectively manage the disease without taking blood samples and, for this reason, improve their quality of life.

Once diabetes is recognized, adherence to a treatment program is essential to prevent related conditions. www.mhhe.com/fit_well/web24 Click 03. Controlling weight, eating properly, and performing regular exercise can help prevent the symptoms of Type II diabetes, in particular. In addition to these strategies, adherence to a regular medication schedule and stress management are important. However, if symptoms such as nausea, fatigue, weakness, excessive thirst, and loss of weight occur, as they often do in Type I diabetics, or if blurred vision, numbness of the limbs, and skin or gum infections occur, medical help should be sought. Type I diabetics typically test blood samples regularly and self-administer insulin as needed.

Other Health Threats

Injuries are a major cause of death and suffering. Not only are injuries the fifth leading cause of death among people of all ages, but they also claim more lives than chronic and infectious diseases among people aged forty and younger. The major causes of injuries are shown in Table 3.

Injuries also account for much pain and suffering. Of all hospital stays, one in six results from a nonfatal injury.

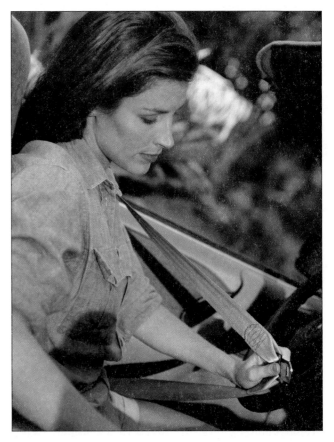

Fastening seat belts saves lives.

Table 3 ► Major Causes of Injuries
• Motor vehicle crashes
• Falls
• Poisoning
• Drowning
• Residential fires

Source: Data from the Public Health Service.

Injury rates are higher among males than females, and they are quite high among ethnic and racial minority groups. In the last decade, the number of deaths caused by unintentional injuries and by work-related injuries has decreased.

Changes in lifestyles can reduce injury rates. A major conclusion of the Public Health Service is that the prevention of injuries requires the combined efforts of many fields, including health, education, transportation, law, engineering, architecture, and safety science.

The second major conclusion of the Public Health Service is that alcohol is "intimately associated" with the causes and severity of injuries. Other lifestyle behaviors are also associated with reducing injury incidence, and some of the steps that can be taken to reduce these injuries are listed in Table 4.

Improved occupational safety could help reduce injury rates. Many of the nation's health goals focus on improving occupational safety, especially among construction, health care (nurses, etc.), farm, transportation, and mine workers. (See Suggested Readings.)

Many mental disorders pose threats to health and wellness. The health goals for the nation identify suicide, schizophrenia, and depression as the most serious mental disorders needing attention. (Though the Public Health Service uses the term mental disorders, they are sometimes called emotional disorders.) Other common mental disorders are panic disorders, alcohol and drug problems, personality disorders, and phobias.

Mental disorders result in loss of life, injury, and inability to function, and they cost the public millions of dollars annually. Nearly one in five adults suffers from a diagnosed mental disorder that limits ability to function effectively and requires special assistance. Depression and other mood disorders affect one in twenty people. These disorders cost $75 billion annually, primarily from loss of productivity. The most serious outcome of mental disorders is suicide (30,000 annually). In the last ten years, progress has been made in reducing suicide.

Table 4 ► Steps to Reduce Injuries
Reduce Motor Vehicle Accidents
• Do not drive while under the influence of alcohol.
• Increase use of shoulder seat belts and air bags.
• Reduce driving speed.
• Use motorcycle helmets.
• Improve safety of off-road vehicles.
• Increase safety programs for pedestrians and cyclists.
• Establish more effective licensing for very young and older drivers.
Improve Home and Neighborhood Environments
• Enact laws requiring new handguns be designed to minimize discharge by children.
• Extend laws requiring sprinkler systems in homes with high risk of fire.
• Increase presence of functional smoke detectors in homes.
• Increase injury education in schools.
• Wear effective face, head, eye, and mouth protection in sports, including helmets for cycling.
• Improve pool and boat safety education.
• Learn cardiopulmonary resuscitation.
• Properly mark poisons and prescription drugs.
• Properly package and store poisons and prescription drugs (childproof).
• Shift to nontoxic fuels for cooking.
• Provide poison education for children and older populations.

Reducing the incidence of suicide and serious injury from suicide attempts is an important national health goal. Suicide attempts are common among all age groups. Women are more likely to attempt suicide than men, but men are 4.5 times more likely to complete a suicide attempt. Among male teenagers, it is the second leading cause of death, and male teenagers with antisocial personality disorders are especially susceptible.

Glucose Tolerance Test A test used to diagnose diabetes. It consists of a blood-sugar measurement following the ingestion of a standard amount of sugar (glucose) after a period of fasting.

Depression is closely associated with suicide, as are alcohol and drug abuse. Inability to cope with stressful life events may contribute to suicide. Examples of precipitating events are divorce, separation, loss of a loved one, unemployment, and financial setbacks.

The best chance for reducing suicides appears to be early detection and treatment of mental disorders such as depression. Professional help should be sought, and as many concerned people as possible should be recruited to help the suicidal individual seek professional assistance. Experts suggest that threats of suicide must be taken seriously.

Depression, a common mental disorder, can usually be treated effectively. www.mhhe.com/ fit_well/web24 Click 04. At some time in life, most people occasionally feel depressed, sad, or blue. This type of depression is usually not a mental disorder. People with clinical depression (classified as a mental disorder) have chronic feelings of guilt, hopelessness, low self-esteem, and dejection. They frequently have trouble sleeping, loss of appetite, lack of interest in social activities, lack of interest in sex, and inability to concentrate.

Among the lifestyle changes that can help relieve symptoms are regular exercise, increased social contact, realistic goal setting, use of stress management techniques (see concept 19), and removing oneself from situations that contribute to depression. These changes, however, may need to be accompanied by professional therapy and/or medication. A major health goal for the year 2010 is to reduce the proportion of people who experience regular sadness or unhappiness.

Sleep disorders can often be helped by lifestyle changes. Sleep disorders, especially insomnia (long-term problems with sleep), can result in depression and other dysfunctions. Physiological problems in the brain can cause sleep disorders, but they are often a result of depression, stress, chronic pain, or abuse of alcohol/drugs. Some sleep disorders require professional help. However, you can take action to prevent insomnia. Examples include creating a healthy sleeping environment, avoiding excessive caffeine or alcohol, exercising regularly, and using stress-management techniques. Establishing a regular routine for sleeping can also be helpful and should include regular sleeping hours and a stress-reduction time before retiring.

Various health threats put the public's health at risk. www.mhhe.com/fit_well/web24 Click 05. The health threats outlined in *Healthy People 2010* are too numerous to be dealt with in depth in this text. More information concerning such health threats as chronic kidney disease, hepatitis, asthma, and arthritis can be found at *Healthy People 2010* website and in the Web Resources section.

Strategies for Action

Self-assessments and regular medical exams can help you determine if you need help with various health problems. Just as the fitness assessments you completed earlier in this book helped you build a profile that will help you improve your fitness, regular self-assessments can help you identify and prevent common health problems. Regular medical exams that include the tests outlined in Table 1 as well as those described in other sections of this concept will help you identify problems that can be treated and cured with early diagnosis. In Lab 24A, you will have the opportunity to assess your cancer risk. In Lab 24B, you will learn to do self-exams to help you resist breast and testicular cancer. Web addresses for self-assessments are provided in Lab 24B.

Staying current with new health information can help you identify and get treatment for health problems. Information about various health problems changes rapidly as new methods of treatment and prevention become available. It is important to learn ways to stay current on health topics. Addresses for websites of reputable health organizations that will help you stay abreast of current information are included in the Web Resources.

Adhering to sound medical advice is important to disease prevention and treatment. Many people in our culture have a fear of disease. Too many avoid medical advice because of this fear. Many of the conditions described in this concept, especially cancer and diabetes, can be managed or cured with early diagnosis and proper treatment. Once a plan of treatment is outlined, it is important to stick with it.

Web Resources

American Cancer Society **www.cancer.org**

American Diabetes Association **www.diabetes.org**

Environmental Protection Agency **www.epa.gov**

Glucowatch Information **www.glucowatch.com**

Healthy People 2010 **www.health.gov/healthypeople**

National Cancer Institute **www.nci.nih.gov**

National Center for Environmental Health
   www.cdc.gov/nceh

National Center for Health Statistics **www.cdc.gov/nchs**

National Institute of Mental Health (NIMH)
   www.nimh.nih.gov

Suggested Readings

Additional reference materials for concept 24 are available at **www.mhhe.com/fit_well/web24 Click 06.**

American Diabetes Association. 2002. The prevention or delay of type 2 diabetes: A position statement. *Diabetes Care* 25:742–749.

Cooper, C. B. 2001. Diabetes mellitus and exercise. *ACSM's Health and Fitness Journal* 5(4):27–28.

Corbin, C. B., and R. P. Pangrazi. (eds.). 1999. *Towards a Better Understanding of Physical Fitness and Activity.* Scottsdale, AZ: Holcomb-Hathaway.

Fletcher, S. W., and G. A. Colditz. 2002. Failure of estrogen plus progestin therapy for prevention. *Journal of the American Medical Association* 288(3):368–371.

National Institutes of Health. 2002. Osteoporosis prevention, diagnosis, and therapy. *NIH Consensus Statements* 17(1):1–45.

Payne, W. A., and D. B. Hahn. 2002. *Understanding Your Health.* 7th ed. St. Louis: McGraw-Hill.

U.S. Department of Health and Human Services. Nov. 2000. *Healthy People 2010.* 2nd ed. With *Understanding and Improving Health and Objectives for Improving Health.* 2 vols. Washington, DC: U.S. Government Printing Office.

Women's Health Initiative Investigators Writing Group. 2002. Risks and benefits of estrogen plus progestin in healthy postmenopausal women. *Journal of the American Medical Association* 288(3):321–333.

 In the News

Recent research has revealed some interesting findings about health threats discussed in this concept. Some of the significant research findings are discussed below.

- **Breast Cancer.** The PAP test, named for its developer George Papanicolaou, resulted in a dramatic reduction in cervical cancer deaths. Two new tests, based on theories developed by Papanicolaou, have been developed to identify breast cancer early. One has now been approved for marketing. The new tests extract sample cells from the milk duct glands in an attempt to identify abnormal cells. While some experts use the new test only for research purposes, others are using it for diagnostic purposes, especially among women of high risk.

- **Colon Cancer.** Previously, we recommended a sigmoidoscopy for those over fifty and those with a family history of colon cancer. The sigmoidoscopy scans the lower part of the large intestine with a video camera to detect precancerous or cancerous polyps. New research suggests that a colonoscopy (a test that scans the entire large intestine) is better because many polyps found by the colonoscopy are not detected by the sigmoidoscopy. Many experts now recommend a colonoscopy (see Table 1) because it is estimated that using this test could save thousands of lives annually.

- **Cardiopulmonary Resuscitation and Heart Attack (CPR).** Together, chest compression and mouth-to-mouth are the components of CPR. A recent study has shown that performing chest compression alone can save the lives of many heart attack victims. While experts do not discourage the use of both components of CPR, the recent study shows that chest compression by itself can dramatically reduce the risk of death among heart attack victims.

Lab 24A: Determining Your Cancer Risk

Name	Section	Date

Purpose: To make you aware of your cancer risk for various types of cancer.

Procedures:

1. Answer the questions in the six-part questionnaire for the various forms of cancer.
2. Record the number of "yes" answers for each form of cancer in the Results section.
3. Use Chart 1 to determine ratings and record the ratings in the Results section.
4. Answer the questions in the Conclusions and Implications section.

Results: Directions: Mark an X over your answer to each question.

Skin Cancer Risk Factor

Do you frequently work or play in the sun for long periods of times?	Yes (X)	No
Do you work or have you worked near industrial exposure (coal mine, radioactivity)?	Yes (X)	No
Do you have a family history of skin cancer?	Yes	No (X)
Do you have fair skin?	Yes	No (X)

Lung Cancer Risk Factor

Do you smoke?	Yes (X)	No
Do you work or have you worked near industrial exposure (coal mine, radioactivity)?	Yes	No (X)
Do you have a family history of cancer?	Yes (X)	No
Do you work in a place that allows smoking, such as a bar, or live in a home with smokers?	Yes (X)	No (X)

Colorectal Cancer Risk Factor

Do you eat poorly, abuse alcohol, or smoke?	Yes (X)	No
Are you African American or over fifty?	Yes	No (X)
Do you have a family history of colon or rectal cancer?	Yes	No (X)
Have you noticed blood in your stool?	Yes	No (X)

Breast Cancer Risk Factor

Do you have a family history of breast cancer?	Yes	No (X)
Are you sedentary, do you eat poorly, or abuse alcohol?	Yes	No (X)
Are you a female over thirty-five who has not had children?	Yes	No (X)
Have you ever detected lumps or cysts in your breasts?	Yes	No (X)

Uterine/Cervical Cancer Risk Factor* (Females)

Do you regularly have bleeding between periods?	Yes	No
Is your body fat level high?	Yes	No
Did you have early intercourse and multiple sexual partners?	Yes	No
Have you had viral infections of the vagina such as HPV?	Yes	No

*Because of the personal nature of several questions, do not record results if turned in to an instructor.

Prostate Cancer Risk Factor (Males)

Do you eat a high-fat or low-fiber diet?	Yes (X)	No
Are you a male over fifty years of age or African American?	Yes	No (X)
Have you have a positive PSA test?	Yes	No (X)
Has a digital rectal exam shown an enlargement of the prostate?	Yes	No (X)

Cancer Type	Score	Rating
Breast	0	
Uterine/cervical (women)*		
Colorectal	1	
Skin	2	
Lung	3	
Prostate (men)	1	

*Do not record results if handed in to an instructor.

Chart 1 ▶ Cancer Risk Ratings

Score	Rating
4	High risk
3	Relatively high risk
2	Lower risk
0–1	Low risk

Conclusions and Implications: In several sentences, discuss the type or types of cancer for which you are at greatest risk and why. Also, discuss the lifestyles you could modify to reduce your risk.

Lab 24B: Breast and Testicular Self-Exams

Name	Section	Date

Purpose: To help you learn to do breast and testicular self-exams.

Procedures:

1. Females should read the procedures for breast self-exams. Note: Males should also be aware of abnormal lumps in their breasts.
2. Males should read the procedures for testicular self-exams.
3. After reading the directions, perform the self-exam.
4. If you find lumps or nodules contact a physician.
5. This procedure should be done monthly. The breast exam is best done a day or two after the end of menstrual flow. For this lab, it can be done at any time.
6. It is not necessary to record your results here. Do answer the questions in the Conclusions and Implications section.

Testicular Self-Exam (Men)

1. Using both hands, grasp one testicle between the thumb and first finger.
2. Roll the testicle gently with the thumb and first finger feeling for lumps or nodules.
3. Examine the other testicle using the same procedure.
4. If you find a lump or nodule consult a physician. Note: A lump or nodule may not be a result of disease but this can only be determined by a physician.
5. For more details concerning a testicular self-exam log onto: www.mhhe.com/fit_well/web24 click 07.

Breast Self-Exam (Women and Men)

1. Lie down on your back. Place a pillow or towel under one shoulder and place the arm overhead.
2. With the opposite hand, gently move the fingers over the breast. Use a circular motion (see picture) to probe for lumps starting in a large circle and continuing to probe in smaller and smaller circles. Examine every part of your breast including your nipple. A band of firm tissue along the lower part of the breast is normal. If you have questions, consult your physician.
3. Finally squeeze each nipple gently between the thumb and first finger. If you notice blood or clear discharge, contact a physician.

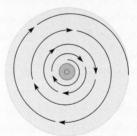

4. For more details concerning a breast self-exam log onto: www.mhhe.com/fit_well/web24 click 08.
5. Repeat on the other breast. If you notice any lumps, report it to a physician.
6. Periodic exams before a mirror can be helpful. With the arms above the head, look for any changes in breast (from your normal). Repeat with the hands on the hips—flex the chest muscles. Again look for any changes from normal.

Conclusions and Implications: In several sentences, discuss the effectiveness of the procedure you performed. Do you think that the directions provided were adequate for you to perform the self-exam effectively? Do you think you will perform this self-exam on a regular basis? What could be done to motivate you and others to do regular self-exams?

Additional Self-Exam Information

Several national health agencies maintain websites that include detailed breast and testicular self- examination information. These sites contain both written and pictorial descriptions of both self- exam procedures. For more information, visit the sites listed below.

American Cancer Society
    www.cancer.org
Mayo Clinic
    www.mayohealth.org
National Cancer Institute
    www.nci.nih.gov

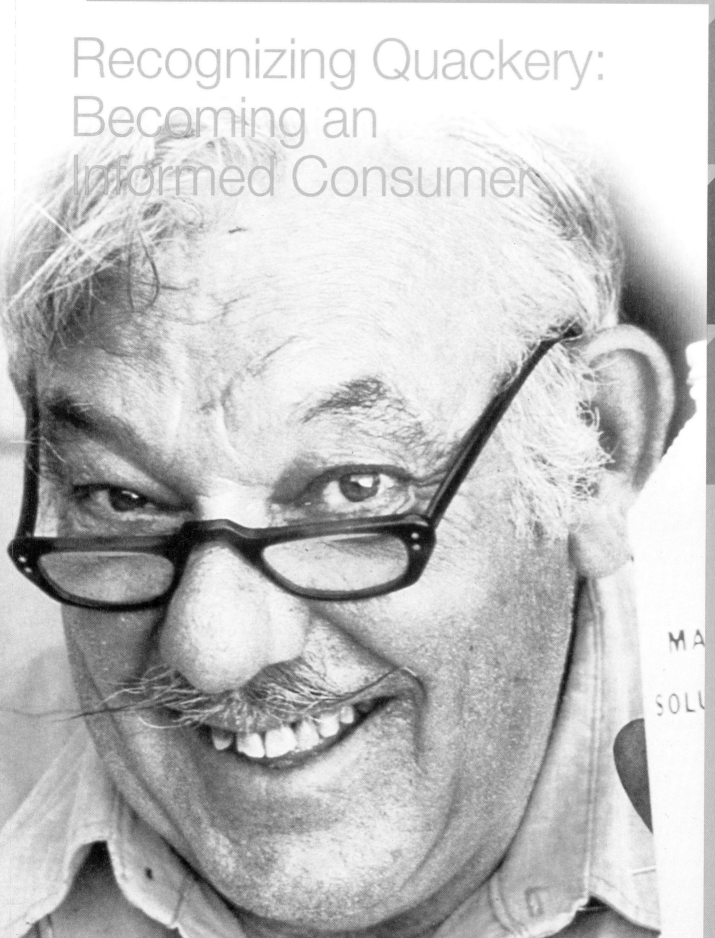

Recognizing Quackery: Becoming an Informed Consumer

"Let the buyer beware" is a good motto for the consumer seeking advice or planning a program for developing or maintaining fitness, health, or wellness.

Health Goals

for the year 2010

- Increase the number of college and university students who receive information on priority health-risk behaviors.

- Improve health literacy and increase access to public health information.

- Increase health communication activities that include research and evaluation.

- Increase adoption and maintenance of appropriate daily physical activity.

- Increase proportion of people who meet national dietary guidelines.

- Promote healthy and safe communities.

People have always searched for the fountain of youth and the easy, quick, and miraculous route to health and happiness. This search often focuses on physical fitness, especially physical activity, nutrition, and weight loss. Unfortunately, our desire for quick and easy solutions has led to as much misinformation as information. For this reason, it is important to seek the truth to protect your health as well as your pocketbooks. This concept discusses some myths and separates fact from fancy.

Becoming an Informed Consumer

Physical activity has many benefits, but it is not a cure-all. Popular books and magazines, television infomercials, and the general media bombard the public with incorrect information about physical activity. The information provided in this book documents the many benefits of physical activity, but it is not a **panacea.** Be suspicious of programs and products that make claims that seem impossible to believe. Consider these general guidelines when making consumer decisions.

- Optimal benefits occur if you select activities from each of the first three levels of the physical activity pyramid.

- Follow the frequency, intensity, and time (FIT) formula for each type of physical activity. Programs that promise complete fitness but do not meet the necessary levels for FIT should be strongly questioned.
- Reject programs that promise total fitness in only a few minutes a week, or promise instant benefits.
- Reject programs that promise instant fat loss or promise increases in the size of glands (e.g., breasts).
- Reject programs that promise changes in size of bony structures (e.g., ankles).
- Reject programs that promise effortless exercise. If it is totally effortless or passive, it is not likely to produce benefits (see section on passive exercise and baths).
- Avoid programs that include dangerous exercises (see concept 12).
- Be sure that a program provides the benefits that are important to you. Some programs may be beneficial for one reason but not for another. For example, Hatha yoga fails to meet some of the claims made for it. It does not help you lose weight, trim inches, strengthen the glands and organs, or cure health problems such as the common cold or arthritis. It can be useful, however, in reducing stress, promoting relaxation, and improving flexibility.
- Be wary of claims for exercise machines and health and fitness clubs that make unrealistic promises (see sections on machines/baths and health clubs).
- Be especially wary of people who make unrealistic promises and stand to gain financially from selling you something.

Getting rid of cellulite does not require a special exercise, diet, cream or device, as some books and advertisements insist. Cellulite is ordinary fat with a fancy name. You do not need a special treatment or device to get rid of it. In fact, it has no special remedy. Fat is fat. To decrease fat, reduce calories and do more physical activity.

Spot reducing, or losing fat from a specific location on the body, is not possible. It is a fallacy. When you do physical activity, calories are burned and fat is recruited from all over the body in a genetically determined pattern. You cannot selectively exercise, bump, vibrate, or squeeze the fat from a particular spot. If you were flabby to begin with, local exercise could strengthen the local muscles, causing a change in the contour and the girth of that body part. But exercise affects the muscles, not the fat on that body part. General aerobic exercises are the most effective for burning fat, but you cannot control where the fat comes off.

Surgically sculpting the body with implants and liposuction to acquire physical beauty will not give you physical fitness and may be harmful. Rather than doing it the hard way, an increasing number of people are having their love handles removed surgically and fake calf and pectoral muscles implanted to improve their physique. Liposuction is not a weight loss technique, but rather a contouring procedure. Like any surgery, it is not without risks. There have been fatalities and there is a risk of infection, hematoma, skin slough, and other conditions.

Muscle implants give a muscular appearance, but they do not make you stronger or more fit. The implants are not really muscle tissue, but rather silicon gel or saline such as that used in breast implants, or a hard substitute. Some complications can occur, such as infection and bleeding, and some physicians believe the calf implant may put pressure on the calf muscles and cause them to atrophy. A better way to improve physique and fitness is proper exercise.

The use of hand weights and wrist weights while walking, running, dancing, or bench-stepping can increase the energy cost but requires caution. Various devices have been marketed for increasing the energy expenditure in activities such as walking, running, and other forms of aerobic exercise. Examples include wrist, arm, or ankle weights and small hand-held weights. Step benches are another device that can be used to increase energy expenditure for aerobic exercise.

The practice of carrying small weights (not more than one to three pounds) while performing aerobic dance, walking, or other aerobic exercise has been found to increase the metabolic cost of the exercise. When the weight is carried, the effect is negligible, but when the arms are pumped (bending the elbow and raising the weight to shoulder height and then extending the elbow as the arm swings down), the energy output can increase enough to make a walk comparable to a slow jog. For the person who does not want to walk or jog faster or farther, it could be an effective way of burning more calories or increasing fitness. Using wrist weights may be better than to carry a weight, since the act of gripping causes an increase in the diastolic blood pressure. Hand weights or wrist weights are more effective than ankle weights because weights that alter your gait pattern can be stressful to the knees. Using weights can be hazardous. Coronary patients and people with high blood pressure should be aware that using weights increases the systolic and diastolic blood pressures. Aerobic dance participants may find it wise to keep the weights below shoulder level if they aggravate the shoulder joint. Anyone with shoulder or elbow joint problems such as arthritis should use weights with caution.

Perhaps a more important consideration is the enjoyment and perception of effort associated with an activity. Walking is a popular activity because it is not especially intense and still offers many health benefits. Though weights can result in more energy expended, if they also make the more intense exercise seem too difficult, adding extra weight may result in decreased interest in performing the activity. Be careful not to make simple tasks seem more difficult than they should be. Doing less intense activity for a longer period of time is better rather than making an activity more intense at the expense of regular participation.

If you are a walker you may want to consider using walking poles. Recent evidence suggests that walking poles (similar to canes, one held in each hand) allow faster and potentially longer walks. Walking poles can also reduce the load on the legs. When you become fatigued, the use of walking poles can result in changes in your walking mechanics. For this reason, it is important to be careful to walk with good form, especially when you get tired. For some people arm work is quite fatiguing. If this is true for you, poles may make walking seem more difficult and reduce your enjoyment of the activity.

The step bench, as used in step aerobics, was designed to increase the intensity of a workout without the high impact of some types of aerobic dance. Small weights can also be used in most forms of aerobic dance activities to increase exercise intensity. Some experts suggest that for step aerobics, weights should be limited to intermediate and advanced exercisers because the bench and the weights provide a double overload. Even for more advanced steppers, it is recommended that weights not exceed 1 to 2 pounds. Up to a point, the aerobic intensity can be increased by adding height to the bench (typically no more than 6 to 8 inches).

Passive Exercise, Passive Devices, and Baths

Passive exercise is not effective in weight reduction, spot reduction, increasing strength, or increasing endurance. **Passive exercise** or devices come in many forms.

- *Rolling machines*—These ineffective wooden or metal rollers, operated by an electric motor, roll up and down the body part to which they are applied. They do not remove, break up, or redistribute fat.

Panacea A cure-all; a remedy for all ills.

Passive Exercise A type of exercise in which no voluntary muscle contraction occurs; some outside force moves the body part with no effort by the person.

- *Vibrating belts*—These wide canvas or leather belts may be designed for the chin, hips, thighs, or abdomen. Driven by an electric motor, they jerk back and forth, causing loose tissue of the body part to shake. They have no beneficial effect on fitness, fat, or figure, and they are potentially harmful if used on the abdomen (especially if used by women during pregnancy, menstruation, or while an IUD is in place). They might also aggravate a back problem.

- *Vibrating tables and pillows*—Some of these quack devices are actually called toning tables. Contrary to advertisements, these passive devices will not improve posture, trim the body, reduce weight, nor will they develop muscle **tonus.** For some people, vibration can help induce relaxation.

- *Continuous Passive Motion (CPM) Tables*—The motor-driven CPM table, unlike the vibrating table, moves body parts repeatedly through a range of motion. Tables are designed to do such things as passively extend the leg at the hip joint, raise the upper trunk in a sit-up-like motion, or rotate the legs while the client lies relaxed. Many of the same false claims are made for it as for the vibrating table. It also claims to remove cellulite, increase circulation and oxygen flow, and eliminate excess water retention. All of these claims are false, but the table might be justified in claiming to maintain the range of motion in certain body parts for people who cannot move themselves. A similar concept is incorporated in small, portable machines used in hospitals and rehabilitation centers to maintain range of motion in the legs of knee surgery patients, maintain integrity of the cartilage, and decrease the incidence of thrombosis. Certainly the normal, healthy person has nothing to gain from using such a device.

- *Motor-driven cycles and rowing machines*—Like all mechanical devices that do the work for the individual, these motor-driven machines are not effective in a fitness program. They may help increase circulation, and some may even help maintain flexibility, but they are not as effective as active exercise. *Nonmotorized cycles and rowing machines* are good equipment for use in a fitness program.

- *Massage*—Whether done by a masseur/masseuse or by a mechanical device, massage is passive, requiring no effort on the part of the individual. It can help increase circulation, induce relaxation, prevent or loosen adhesions, retard muscle atrophy, and serve other therapeutic uses when administered in the clinical setting for medical reasons. However, massage has no useful role in a physical fitness program and will not alter your shape. There is no scientific evidence that it can hasten nerve growth, remove subcutaneous fat, or increase athletic performance. Some athletes (e.g., cyclists) find that it aids in recovery from exercise.

- *Electrical muscle stimulators*—Neuromuscular electrical stimulators cause the muscle to contract involuntarily.

In the hands of qualified medical personnel, muscle stimulators are valuable therapeutic devices. They can increase muscle strength and endurance selectively and aid in the treatment of edema. They can also help prevent atrophy in a patient who is unable to move, and they may decrease spasticity and contracture, but in a healthy person they do not have the same value as exercise. The Federal Trade Commission (FTC) recently filed a false advertising complaint against three firms that market exercise stimulators that promise to build six-pack abs and tone muscles without exercise. These devices, worn over the abdomen, are heavily advertised in infomercials and have been shown to be ineffective and potentially hazardous to health. Electrical stimulators placed on the chest, back, or abdomen can interfere with the normal rhythm of the heart, even for normally healthy people. For those with heart, gastrointestinal, orthopedic, kidney, and other health problems such as epilepsy, hernia, and varicose veins, they can be especially dangerous. These devices are ineffective and potentially harmful for personal use. Also beware of spas and clinics that use these devices and make claims of fitness enhancement for normally healthy people.

- *Weighted belts*—Claims have been made that these belts reduce waists, thighs, and hips when worn for several hours under the clothing. In reality, they do none of these things and have been reported to cause actual physical harm. However, when used in a progressive resistance program, wristlet, anklet, or laced-on weights can help produce an overload and, therefore, develop strength or endurance.

- *Inflated, constricting, or nonporous garments*—These garments include rubberized inflated devices (sauna belts and sauna shorts) and paraphernalia that are airtight plastic or rubberized. Evidence indicates that their girth-reducing claims are *unwarranted*. If exercise is performed while wearing such garments, the exercise, not the garment, may be beneficial. You cannot squeeze fat out of the pores nor can you melt it.

- *Body wrapping*—Some reducing salons, gyms, or clubs advertise that wrapping the body in bandages soaked in a magic solution will cause a permanent reduction in body girth. This so-called treatment is pure quackery. Tight, constricting bands can temporarily indent the skin and squeeze body fluids into other parts of the body, but the skin or body will regain its original size within minutes or hours. The solution is usually similar to epsom salts, which can cause fluid to be drawn from tissue. The fluid is water, not fat, and is quickly replaced. Body wrapping may be dangerous to your health; at least one fatality has been documented.

- *Elastic tights*—These are often worn by athletes such as cyclists for the purpose of decreasing chafing of the skin. Some claims state that the tights help improve venous return and thus recovery from exercise. However, studies have shown that the recovery-response of those who wear tights is no different from those who do not wear them.

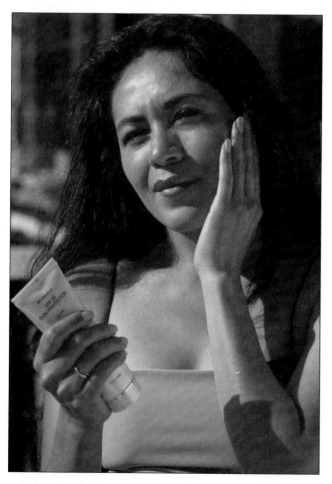 Having a good tan is often associated with being fit and looking good, but getting tanned can be risky business. www.mhhe.com/ fit_well/web25 Click 01. Tanning salons may claim their lamps are safe because they emit only UV-A rays, but these rays can age the skin prematurely and make it look wrinkled and leathery. They may also increase the cancer-producing potential of UV-B rays and cause eye damage. Since there is no warning sign of redness, overdosing can occur. Thirty minutes of exposure to UV-A can suppress the immune system. Tanning devices can also aggravate certain skin diseases. The **Food and Drug Administration (FDA)** advises against the use of any suntan lamp. It is dangerous to use tanning accelerator lotions with the lamps because they can promote burning of the skin. Tanning pills are an even worse choice. They can cause itching, welts, hives, stomach cramps, and

Wearing sunscreen (SPF 15 or higher) is recommended by the American Cancer Society.

diarrhea, and can decrease night vision. Tanning in the sun is also hazardous because it damages the skin, making it age prematurely. It may cause skin cancer. It is best to use products with sun blockers if you must spend long periods in the sun.

Saunas, steam baths, whirlpools, and hot tubs are not effective in weight reduction or in the prevention and cure of colds, arthritis, bursitis, backaches, sprains, or bruises. Baths do not melt off fat; fat must be metabolized. The heat and humidity from baths may make you perspire, but it is water, not fat, oozing from the pores.

The effect of such baths is largely psychological, although some temporary relief from aches and pains may result from the heat. The same relief can be had by sitting in a tub of hot water in your bathroom.

Various baths are potentially dangerous and should be used and maintained properly. The following guidelines/precautions should be considered before using a sauna, steam bath, whirlpool, or hot tub:

- Take a soap shower before and after entering the bath.
- Do not wear makeup or skin lotion/oil.
- Wait at least an hour after eating before bathing.
- Cool down after exercise before entering the bath to avoid overheating.
- Drink plenty of water before or during the bath to avoid dehydration.
- Do not wear jewelry.
- Do not sit on a metal stool; do sit on a towel in the steam or sauna bath.
- Do not bathe alone.
- Do not drink alcohol before bathing.
- Get out immediately if you become dizzy; feel hot, chilled, or nauseous; or get a headache.
- Get approval from your physician if you have heart disease, low or high blood pressure, a fever, kidney disease, or diabetes, are obese or pregnant, or are on medications (especially anticoagulants, stimulants, hypnotics, narcotics, or tranquilizers).
- Prolonged use can be hazardous for the elderly or for children.

Tonus The most frequently misused and abused term in fitness vocabularies. Tonus is the tension developed in a muscle as a result of passive muscle stretch. Tonus cannot be determined by feeling or inspecting a muscle. It has little or nothing to do with the strength of a muscle.

Food and Drug Administration (FDA) A federal agency that recommends and enforces government regulations regarding certain foods and drugs.

- Do not exercise in a sauna or steam bath.
- Skin infections can be spread in a bath; make certain it is cleaned regularly and that the hot tub or whirlpool has proper pH and chlorination.
- Follow these recommendations on temperature and duration of stay:

Sauna: should not exceed 190°F (88°C) and duration should not exceed 10 to 15 minutes.
Steam bath: should not exceed 120°F (49°C) and duration should not exceed 6 to 12 minutes.
Whirlpool/hot tub: should not exceed 100°F (37°C) and duration should not exceed 5 to 10 minutes.

Quacks

You can usually tell the difference between an expert and a quack because a quack does not use scientific methods. www.mhhe.com/fit_well/web25 Click 02. A good example of this fact is seen in a study that attempted to obtain documentation for products claiming to enhance athletic performance. The study found no published scientific evidence existed to support the promotional claims of 42 percent of the products. Thirty-two percent had some scientific documentation but were marketed in a misleading manner, and 21 percent were without any human clinical trials.

Some of the ways to identify quacks, frauds, and rip-offs are to look for these clues:

- They do not use the scientific method of controlled experimentation that can be verified by other scientists.
- To a large extent, they use testimonials and anecdotes to support their claims rather than scientific methods. There is no such thing as a valid testimonial. Anecdotal evidence is no evidence at all.
- They advise you to buy something you would not otherwise have bought.
- They have something to sell.

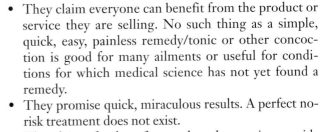

Changing your lifestyle, rather than quick solutions, is the key to health, fitness, and wellness.

- They claim everyone can benefit from the product or service they are selling. No such thing as a simple, quick, easy, painless remedy/tonic or other concoction is good for many ailments or useful for conditions for which medical science has not yet found a remedy.
- They promise quick, miraculous results. A perfect no-risk treatment does not exist.
- The claims for benefits are broad, covering a wide variety of conditions.
- They may offer a money-back guarantee. A guarantee is only as good as the company.
- They may claim the treatment or product is approved by the FDA. Note: Federal law does not permit the mention of the FDA in any way that suggests marketing approval.
- They may claim the support of experts, but the experts are not identified.
- The ingredients or materials in the product may not be identified.
- They may claim there is a conspiracy against them by "bureaucrats," "organized medicine," the FDA, the American Medical Association (AMA), and other experts and governmental bodies. Never believe a doctor who claims the medical community is persecuting him/her or that the government is suppressing a wonderful discovery.
- Their credentials may be irrelevant to the area in which they claim expertise.
- They use scare tactics, such as "If you don't do this, you will die of a heart attack."
- They may appear to be a sympathetic friend who wants to share a new discovery with you.
- They may quote from a scientific journal or other legitimate source, but they misquote or quote out of context to mislead you; they may also mix a little bit of truth with a lot of fiction.
- They may cite research or quote from individuals or institutions that have questionable reputations for scientific truth.
- They may claim it is a new discovery (usually it is said to have originated in Europe). There is never a great medical breakthrough that debuts in an obscure magazine or tabloid. No secret cures or magic formulae have been recognized by the scientific community, a picture on the cover of *Time* magazine, nomination for a Nobel prize, etc.
- The product or organization named is often similar to that of a famous person or creditable institution (e.g., the Mayo diet had no connection with the Mayo Clinic).
- They often sell products through the mail, which does not allow you to examine the product personally. There are no miracle products available only by mail order or from a single source.

You can take some common-sense precautions to avoid being ripped off. The following suggestions can help protect you:

- Read the ad carefully, especially the small print.
- Do not send cash; use a check, money order, or credit card so you will have a receipt.
- Do not order from a company with only a post office box, unless you know the company.
- Do not let high-pressure sales tactics make you rush into a decision.
- Do not order from a company requiring use of an 800 telephone number and a credit card (they may be trying to avoid federal statutes).
- When in doubt, check out the company through your Better Business Bureau (BBB).
- If you have a complaint, write to the company first, but keep a copy of all receipts, checks, and correspondence.
- If that fails, write to the Direct Marketing Association. You may also report to the BBB, postmaster (if it was a mail order), state attorney general, and/or the FTC.

Equipment

The consumer who plans to purchase exercise equipment should keep in mind certain guidelines to get the most for the money. The following suggestions will help you select equipment:

- Unless you are wealthy or just like to collect gadgets, you do not need to buy a lot of exercise equipment. A complete fitness program can be carried out with *no* equipment. If you learn to depend upon equipment, you may eventually feel that you cannot exercise unless you are at home or at a gym.
- If you do not like jogging or swimming, and you hate calisthenics, then the minimal equipment you may want to consider is a bicycle (regular or stationary), treadmill, or rowing machine for cardiovascular fitness; also have a set of weights, pulleys, or isokinetic device for strength and endurance.
- Consult an expert if you want to know the effectiveness of a product. Individuals with college or university degrees in physical education, physical therapy, kinesiotherapy, and kinesiology should be able to give you good advice.
- Buy from a well-established, reputable company that will not disappear overnight and will back up warranties. Avoid mail-order products. If the product is not available in a retail store where it can be examined, you probably should not buy it.
- You get what you pay for. Buying an inexpensive, poorly produced product will result in dissatisfaction in the long run.

Health Clubs

You do not have to join a club, spa, or salon to develop fitness, but if you are considering joining such an establishment, make your choice with care. The consumer should observe these precautions before becoming a member of a club, spa, or salon:

- Do not expect miraculous results as advertised.
- Be prepared to haggle over price and to resist a very hard sell for a long-term contract.
- Choose a no-contract, pay-as-you-go establishment if possible. Otherwise, choose the shortest term contract available.
- Read the fine print of any contract carefully and look for:
  - the interest rate;
  - confession of judgment clauses waiving your right to defend yourself in court;
  - noncancelable clauses;
  - holder-in-due-course doctrines allowing the establishment to sell your contract to a collection agency; and
  - a waiver of the establishment's liability for injury to you on the premises.
- Consult with an independent expert if you have questions about the programs offered by the establishment.
- Do not accept diets, drugs, or food supplements from the club. Your physician will prescribe these if needed.
- You do not have to conform to the program the club suggests for you. Do not perform dangerous exercises, passive exercises, or participate in fraudulent treatments. Choose only those activities that meet the criteria explained in this book.
- Refuse to be pestered by solicitations for new members.
- Make a trial visit to the establishment during the hours when you would normally expect to use the facility to determine if it is open, if it is overcrowded, if the equipment is available, if the attendants are selling

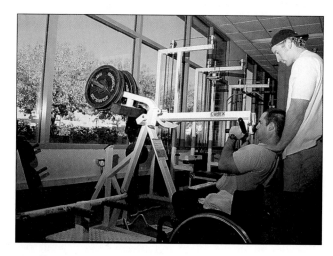

Visit a health club before you join.

rather than assisting, and if you would enjoy the company of the other patrons.

- Determine the qualifications of the personnel, especially of the individual responsible for your program. Is he or she an expert as defined previously?
- Make certain the club is a well-established facility that will not disappear overnight.
- Check its reputation with the Better Business Bureau.
- Investigate the programs offered by the YMCA/YWCA, local colleges and universities, and municipal park and recreation departments. These agencies often have excellent fitness classes at lower prices than commercial establishments and usually employ qualified personnel. For weight loss, investigate franchised clubs, such as Weight Watchers or TOPS, or affiliate with a university or a hospital-based program.

Dietary Supplements

 The burden of proof about the effectiveness of food supplements rests with the consumer. www.mhhe.com/fit_well/web25 Click 03. The passage of the Dietary Supplements Health and Education Act in 1994 shifted the burden of providing assurances of product effectiveness from the FDA to the food supplement industry, which really means it shifted to you—the consumer. Food supplements are typically not considered to be drugs, so they are not regulated. Unlike drugs and medicines, food supplements need not be proven effective or even safe to be sold in stores. To be removed from stores, they must be proven ineffective or unsafe. This leaves consumers vulnerable to false claims. Many experts suggest that quackery has increased significantly since 1994 when the Act was passed.

The act had at least one positive effect. Food supplement labeling must now be truthful and nonmisleading. Claims concerning disease prevention, treatment, or diagnosis must be substantiated in order to appear on the product. Unfortunately, the act did not limit false claims if they are not on the product label. The result has been the removal of claims from labels in favor of claims on separate literature often called third-party literature because the label makes no claims, and the seller makes no written claims (second party). Rather the seller provides claims in literature by other people (third party). The literature is distributed separately from the product, thus allowing sellers to make unsubstantiated claims for products. Also the law does not prohibit unproven verbal claims by sales people. A highly respected medical journal indicates that "alternative treatments should be subjected to scientific testing no less rigorous than that required for advocating unproven and potentially harmful treatments." However, as things currently stand, it is up to the consumer to make decisions about the safety and effectiveness of food supplements so it is especially important to be well informed.

Current legislation does not provide protection to food supplement customers. www.mhhe.com/fit_well/web25 Click 04. Since the Dietary Supplements Health and Education Act was passed in 1994, food supplement sales have doubled (from $8 to more than $16 billion a year). A wide variety of supplements include ergogenic aids, vitamins and minerals, and herbals and botanicals. Ergogenic aids associated with muscle fitness are discussed in concept 12, other ergogenic aids are discussed in concept 14, vitamin and mineral supplements are discussed in concept 18, and herbals and botanicals are discussed here.

Recently the sales of supplements has leveled off, primarily because of the increasing evidence of the danger of some supplements and the evidence showing the ineffectiveness of others. Evidence supports the value of some supplements. As noted earlier in this book, folic acid, calcium, vitamin E, and a daily multiple vitamin supplement can be beneficial for many people. We also know that aspirin can be important for the prevention of heart disease and some forms of cancer, and evidence shows that glucosomine supplements can relieve joint pain for some people. On the other hand, over the past few years, the FDA has received thousands of complaints of adverse events (resulting in approximately 200 deaths). An editorial by *USA Today* newspaper suggests that "troubling side effects mount" and that "putting customers' health at risk is a high price to pay for a free market in diet supplements" (see Suggested Readings). Some of the problems associated with supplements are described in Table 1. Among the adverse effects reported are lead poisoning, nausea, vomiting, diarrhea, abnormal heart rhythm, fainting, impotence, and lethargy. Over a six-year period 2,621 adverse events were reported to the FDA and 184 resulted in death. Also, one study showed that 15 to 20 percent of over 1600 supplements tested included substances that would cause a positive test for drugs banned by sports organizations.

More than one-half of American adults are unaware that food supplements are unregulated by the FDA or any governmental agency. An editorial in *USA Today* offered this comment: "The dirty secret of these unregulated 'natural' products is that their impact can vary widely from one person to another. Dosage strength can be wildly different from brand to brand, even batch to batch. Some can be downright dangerous."

In spite of the problems associated with lack of supplement regulations, a recent study indicates that nearly half of Americans routinely take supplements and slightly more than half believe in the value of the supplements. Interestingly, 44 percent believe that physicians know little or nothing about supplements.

The overwhelming majority (80 percent) believe that the FDA should review the safety of supplements before they are offered for sale. Also more than 60 percent believe that there are not enough rules to insure purity

Table 1 ▶ Problems Associated with Supplements

Problem

Post-surgical problems including bleeding, irregular heart beat, and stroke. Examples: echinacea, ephedra, gingko, kava, St. John's wort, ginsing.

Dangerous interactions with medicines. Examples: ephedra, St. John's wort (interact with birth control pills and HIV pills).

FDA warnings concerning unsubstantiated claims about herbs added to foods such as energy bars and water. Examples: gingko, ginsing, echinacea.

Allergic and other physiological reactions; negative effect on decision making. Example: GHB.

Known ill effects to health. Examples: comfrey (kidneys), kava (liver), ephedra (54 deaths associated with use).

May slow bone mending. Example: Vioxx.

Recalled because of dangerous effects associated with contamination. Examples: PC SPES, Lipokinetix.

Action by the FTC because of deceptive advertisements. Examples: Exercise in a Bottle and Fat Trapper.

Banned by several sporting groups including the International Olympic Committee, NCAA, and NFL. Examples: Steroids, androstendione, ephedra.

Contents may not be what they appear to be and dosage information is unknown. Example: The government does not guarantee contents of supplements and there is little evidence concerning dosage for most supplements.

and accurate dosage amounts. A similar number of adults want more regulation on advertising claims.

USA Today (see Suggested Readings) notes that self-regulation within the industry has not worked well and suggests that the public will have more confidence in supplements "when they know independent experts, not just the hucksters, are watching out for their best interest."

Table 2 presents some questions that should be asked about food supplements. It would be wise to get answers to these questions before you consider using a food supplement.

Fitness Books, Magazines, and Articles

All fitness books do not provide scientifically sound, accurate, and reliable information. Because publishers are motivated by profit and publishing is a highly competitive field, the choice of material to be printed is often selected on the basis of how popular, famous, or attractive the author is, or how sensational or unusual his or her ideas are. Movie stars, models, TV personalities, and even

Olympic athletes are rarely experts in biomechanics, anatomy and physiology, exercise, and other foundations of physical fitness. Having a good figure/physique, being fit, or having gone through a training program does not, in itself, qualify a person to advise others.

If you have read the facts presented in the other concepts, you should be able to distinguish between fact and fiction. To assist you further, however, there are ten guidelines listed in Lab 25A. These might help you evaluate whether or not a book, magazine, or article on exercise and fitness is valid, reliable, and scientifically sound. If the answer to each of the questions is no, then you should be suspicious of the material.

Health Information on the Internet

All Internet websites do not provide scientifically sound, accurate, and reliable information. www.mhhe.com/fit_well/web25 **Click 05.** The development of the Internet (World Wide Web) has made information more and more accessible to the masses. Since 1995, Internet saturation has increased from 9 percent to 66 percent. Nearly three-fourths of teens and young adult computer users seek health information on the Web. Leading topics of information are cancer, diabetes, sexually transmitted diseases, and weight control. A health goal for the nation—as outlined in *Healthy People 2010*—is to increase the proportion of households with access to the Internet with the specific intent of making reliable health information available to as many people as possible. While the development of the Internet has made an almost unlimited amount of health information accessible, it has also been the source of much misinformation, and even fraud.

The FTC is a federal government agency charged with making sure that advertising claims for products are not false or misleading. In an effort to clean up websites, the FTC initiated "Operation Cure-All." As part of this operation, the FTC conducted two "Health Claim Surf Days" during which they identified 800 websites and usenet newsgroups with questionable content. The FTC sent mailers to these sites and 28 percent either removed the claims or the website completely. In spite of the FTC efforts, there is still much health misinformation on the Web, leading one FTC official to suggest that ". . . miracle cures, once thought to have been laughed out of existence, have now found a new medium . . . on the Internet" (see Web Resources).

Another research study randomly selected 400 websites from 27,000 available on four different well-known search engines for a study of cancer. Nearly half had unverified information and 6 percent had major inaccuracies. Clearly, Internet users must be careful in selecting websites for obtaining fitness, health, and wellness information. One of the most useful rules is always get a second opinion.

Table 2 ▶ Questions and Comments about Food Supplements

Questions	Comments
Does the government regulate this product to be sure that it is safe and effective?	Since 1994, food supplements can be sold without proof that they are effective. The government does not test food supplements to ensure effectiveness or safety. The FDA must prove the product to be harmful or ineffective to remove it from the market. It is much harder to prove a product ineffective than to provide evidence that it is effective.
Do claims for the supplement have supporting evidence?	The evidence should be based on research with normal people, not evidence based on a population of subjects who have medical problems or nutritional deficiencies. Third-party information often cites research out-of-context and based on inappropriate studies of atypical, not normal, people.
What are the active ingredients?	If the active ingredient really works, research will show its effectiveness. Of course, if it works, then it is much like a medicine and has similar side effects. Sellers of supplements often suggest the product works, but that it has no side effects that are associated with medicines. Both cannot be true. For example, Cholestin is a variety of red yeast—a natural product. It contains lovastatin, the same active ingredients in medicines for lowering cholesterol. Though the product works, it has now been banned by the FDA as an over-the-counter supplement because it has the same active ingredient as medicine and has the same side effects. The regulation of this product by the FDA has been challenged in the courts by the supplement industry. The decision of the courts will have consequences for future regulation of supplements.
What are the possible side effects and risks of taking the supplement?	As noted above, if a product works as well as a medicine, it probably has the same side effects. If you know the active ingredient, you will know more about the side effects.
Are there possible interactions associated with taking the supplement?	When you take a medicine, you consult a physician or pharmacist about drug interactions. Supplements may interact with other supplements or medicines.
What are the long-term effects of taking the supplement?	Because supplements are not regulated, there has been little research about long-term effects of products. For example, melatonin is a hormone that is used for insomnia. Hormones have strong effects on the body and little is known about melatonin's long-term effects. Consider alternative solutions to long-term use of an unstudied supplement.
Are you sure the product is what it claims to be and that the size of the dose is appropriate?	U. S. Pharmacopeia (USP) is a private nonprofit organization that developed uniform standards for medicines and other health-care products. This organization sets standards for vitamins and minerals to assure quality and purity as well as appropriate size and strength of a standard unit of the product (dose size and strength). When standards are developed, the USP label will ensure that the product is what it says it is. As many as two or three dozen herbal products are currently being evaluated to determine appropriate dose size. Products with the USP label that fail to meet standards will be removed from stores. Without the USP label, you are at the mercy of the company that produces the product. The deaths associated with L-tryptophan, an amino acid supplement, occurred because of contaminants (Peak-X) in the unregulated product.
Who makes the product?	In the absence of regulations, the reputation of the company that makes the product is crucial. Have complaints been made against the company? Have there been health problems with their products? How long has the company been in business? Large pharmaceutical companies are now beginning to sell supplements because of the high profit margin. Using a product from a large drug company is more likely to ensure that a product is what it is supposed to be but it does not ensure that the product is effective.
Is the cost worth the potential benefits?	The costs of dietary supplements are typically quite high. For example, protein supplements may cost as much as $1.00 a gram. The cost per gram in good food such as protein in a chicken breast is typically a few cents per gram. Most experts suggest that even the most effective supplements have relatively small effects at a high cost.
Is the source of your information about the supplement reliable and accurate?	Avoid verbal information about products, especially information from the seller. Be wary of third-party literature or research in obscure journals. Be wary of those who discredit sound medical advice or information from regulatory agencies such as the FDA.

Consult at least two or more sources to confirm information. Getting confirmation of information from non-Web sources is also a good idea. At least one study indicates that many people only consult one source.

You can follow some general rules to help when you use the Web to obtain fitness, health, and wellness information. In general, government websites are good sources that contain sound information prepared by experts and based on scientific research. Government sites will typically include "gov" as part of the address. Professional organizations and universities can also be good sources of information. Organizations will typically have "org" and universities will typically have "edu" as part of the address. However, caution should still be used with organizations because it is easy to start an organization and obtain an "org" Web address. Your greatest trust can be placed in the sites of stable organizations of long standing such as the AMA, the American Cancer Society, the American Heart Association, the American College of Sports Medicine, the National Council against Health Fraud, and the American Alliance for Health, Physical Education, Recreation and Dance, among others listed in this text. The AMA has recently developed extensive guidelines for health information on the Web (see Suggested Readings). The great majority of websites promoting health products have "com" in the title because these are commercial sites that are in business to make a profit. Because they are in business to make a profit, they are more inclined to contain information that is suspect or totally incorrect. Some "com" sites contain good information, for example, those listed at the end of each concept of this book. Nevertheless, it is important to evaluate, with special care, information found at "com" sites. The Tufts University School of Nutrition Science and Policy has developed a website that rates diet and health sites on the Internet. You may want to consult this website (http://navigator.tufts.edu). In Lab 25A, you can rate a website, using a checklist.

When selecting websites for inclusion at the end of each concept of the book, we used the same checklist as in Lab 25A. You will see that a majority of the sites listed are governmental and organizational sites. We do include some commercial sites but with some reservation. What

we see when we evaluate a site may not be what you see when you use the site several weeks or months later. It is important that you evaluate all websites, using the criteria suggested here.

Strategies for Action

  Being a good consumer requires time, information, and effort. **www.mhhe.com/fit_well/ web25 Click 06.** With time and effort, you can gain the information you need to make good decisions about products and services that you purchase. In Lab 25A, you will evaluate an exercise device, a food supplement, a magazine article, or a website. In Lab 25B, you will evaluate a health/wellness or fitness club. Taking the time to investigate a product will help you save money and help you avoid making poor decisions that affect your health, fitness, and wellness. When you are making real decisions about products or services, it is a good idea to begin your investigation well in advance of the day when a decision is to be made. Sales people often suggest that "this offer is only good today." They know that people often make poor decisions when under time pressure, and they want you to make a decision today so that they will not lose a sale.

Web Resources

Agency for Health Care Policy and Research **www.ahcpr.gov**
American Dietetics Association **www.eatright.org**
AMA Health Insight **www.ama-assn.org**
Center for Science in the Public Interest **www.cspinet.org**
Food and Drug Administration **www.fda.gov**
Healthfinder **www.healthfinder.gov**
Medwatch **www.fda.gov/medwatch/**
National Council Against Health Fraud **www.ncahf.org**
Office of Dietary Supplements **http://ods.od.nih.gov**
Quackwatch **www.familyinternet.com/quackwatch/**
Tufts University Nutrition Navigator
   http://navigator.tufts.edu
U.S. Consumer Information Center **www.pueblo.gsa.gov**

Suggested Readings

Additional reference materials for concept 25 are available at **www.mhhe.com/fit_well/web25 Click 07.**

Blendon, R. J. et al. 2001. Americans' views on the use and regulation of dietary supplements. *Archives of Internal Medicine* 161(6):805–810.
Catlin, D. H. et al. 2000. Trace contamination of over-the-counter androstenedione and positive urine test

 ### Technology Update

Medwatch is a website of the FDA. This website provides a variety of consumer information including: safety alerts for drugs, product recall advisories, changes in drug safety labeling, warnings and safety information concerning dietary supplements, and health advisories concerning medical devices. This is an excellent source of information relating to quackery and can be accessed using the URL in the Web Resources.

results for a nandrolone metabolite. *Journal of the American Medical Association* 284(20):2618–2621.

Fairfield, K. M., and R. H. Fletcher. 2002. Vitamins for chronic disease prevention in adults: Scientific review. *Journal of the American Medical Association* 287(23): 3116–3126.

Fletcher, R. H., and K. M. Fairfield. 2002. Vitamins for chronic disease prevention in adults: Clinical applications. *Journal of the American Medical Association* 287(23):3127–3129.

Gugliotta, G. 19 March 2000. Health concerns grow over herbal aids: As industry booms, analysis suggests rising toll in illness and death. *Washington Post* A1+.

Haller, C. A., and N. L. Benowitz. 2001. Adverse cardiovascular and central nervous system events associated with dietary supplements containing ephedra alkaloids. *New England Journal of Medicine* 343(25):1833–1838.

Hutchins, G. M. et al. 2001. Dietary supplements containing ephedra alkaloids. *New England Journal of Medicine* 344(14):1095–1097.

National Council Against Health Fraud. 2000. National surveys produce remarkable findings on alternative health practices and dietary supplement misuse. *NCAHF Newsletter* 23(2):1–4.

National Council Against Health Fraud Newsletter. Published every other month, it contains articles that give objective information about health products and food supplements. NCAHF, P.O. Box 1276, Loma Linda, CA 92354.

Park, R. L. 2000. *Voodoo Science: The Road from Foolishness to Fraud.* New York: Oxford University Press.

Porcari, J. P. 1999. Pump up your walking. *ASCM's Health and Fitness Journal* 3(1):25–29.

Shelton, R. C. et al. 2001. Effectiveness of St. John's Wort in major depression. *Journal of the American Medical Association* 285(15):1978–1986.

USA Today. 15 Apr. 2002. Dietary supplement use: Troubling side effects. *USA Today* 11A.

USA Today. 10 May 2001. Herbal drug bust. *USA Today* A14.

Winker, M. A. et al. 2000. Guidelines for medical and health information sites on the Internet: Principles governing AMA web sites. *Journal of the American Medical Association* 283(12):1600–1606.

 ## In the News

As noted on previous pages, many people use supplements and believe in their value. This update includes information about supplements not reported earlier are discussed here.

- Popular restaurants, including snack bars in health clubs, offer boosts of supplements in smoothies and other health drinks. A boost is a serving of several grams added to the drink. They typically contain one or more of a variety of supplements. For example, a boost may include up to five different supplements in unknown amounts. Most experts indicate that the purchase of a boost is money wasted. Evidence suggests that even the most effective supplements must be taken on a regular basis in appropriate dosage to be effective.

- Even supplements commonly considered to be beneficial such as calcium can be potentially dangerous because current laws do not require that the content of supplements actually contain pure ingredients. A recent study showed that while the majority were lead-free, some nonprescription calcium supplements contain lead, a highly toxic substance.

- The FDA is working on the reclassification of several over-the-counter supplements to make them harder to get and easier to regulate. Substances shown to stimulate muscle growth will be considered for reclassification.

- Although no current evidence of harm exists, USDA advisors are concerned that supplements containing brain and pituitary tissue (common in some body building supplements) may harbor mad cow disease.

- The first short-term study in the United States to study the effectiveness of St. John's Wort showed the supplement to be no more effective than a placebo in preventing depression over an eight-week period.

- Creatine is banned in France and the French Food Safety Agency suggests it may constitute a cancer risk. It is a legal supplement in the U. S. and is not banned by the International Olympic Committee. There is no long-term research to prove or disprove the claims.

- Water is not generally considered a food supplement, but the sale of water has become a big industry. A study by the World Wildlife Fund says that bottled water is no safer and no healthier than tap water in most industrialized nations. Even in less developed countries boiled tap water is a better option because it is safe and much less expensive. This is important because people in these countries have low incomes.

Lab 25A: Practicing Consumer Skills: Evaluating Products

Name		**Section**	**Date**

Purpose: To evaluate an exercise device, a book, a magazine article, a food supplement, or an Internet site.

Procedure:

1. Mark an X in the circle by the product you are evaluating in Chart 1. Choose an exercise device, book/magazine, food supplement, or an Internet site.
2. In the Results section, answer the questions about the product you have chosen to evaluate.
3. Total the marks for the product. The higher the score, the more likely the product is effective.
4. Answer the questions in the Conclusions and Implications section.

Results:

Directions: Place an X by the product you evaluated. Place an X over each true statement (see page 462 for supplements and websites). Provide information about the product in the space provided.

Exercise Device

1. The exercise device requires effort consistent with the FIT formula.

2. The exercise device is safe and the exercise done using the device is safe.

3. There are no claims that the device uses exercise that is effortless.

4. Exercise using the device is fun or is a type that you might do regularly.

5. There are no claims using gimmick words such as "tone," "cellulite," "quick," or "spot fat reduction."

6. The seller's credentials are sound.

7. The product does something for you that cannot be done without it.

8. You can return the device if you do not like it (the seller has been in business for a long time).

9. The cost of the product is justified for the potential benefits.

10. The device is easy to store or you have a place to permanently use the equipment without storing it.

Exercise Device

Name of Device: _____

_____

_____

Description and Manufacturer:

_____

_____

_____

_____

_____

Book or Article

Author(s): _____

_____

_____

Journal Article or Book Title: _____

_____

_____

Journal Name or Name of Publisher:

_____

_____

Date of Publication: _____

_____

_____

Book/Magazine

1. The credentials of the author are sound. He/she has a degree in an area related to the content of the book or magazine.

2. The facts in the article are consistent with the facts described in this book.

3. The authors do not claim "quick" or "miraculous" results.

4. There are no claims about the spot reduction of fat.

5. The author is not selling a product described in the article.

6. Reputable experts are cited.

7. The article does not promote unsafe exercises or products.

8. New discoveries from exotic places are not cited.

9. The article does not rely on testimonials by nonexpert, famous people.

10. The author does not make claims that the AMA, FDA, or other legitimate organization is trying to suppress information.

461

Food Supplement

1. The seller is not the prime source of product information.

2. The seller has been in business for a long time and has a good reputation.

3. There is scientific evidence of product effectiveness.

4. There is clear evidence about the side effects of the active ingredients.

5. The long-term effectiveness and safety of the product are cited.

6. You are sure of the content of the product.

7. You have information that the manufacturer is reputable.

8. The known benefits are worth the cost.

9. There is evidence that you can get benefits from this product that cannot be obtained in good food.

10. There are no claims that use quack words, or claims about conspiracies against the product by reputable organizations.

Food Supplement

Name:_____

_____

_____

Purported Benefit:_____

_____

_____

Manufacturer/Seller:_____

_____

_____

Dose and Active Ingredient:_____

_____

_____

Internet Site

Web Address:_____

_____

_____

Type of Information Provided:_____

_____

_____

Organization or Person Responsible for Information:_____

_____

_____

Internet Site

1. The site does not sell products associated with information provided.

2. The provider is a person, an organization (org), or a governmental agency (gov) with a sound reputation.

3. The site does not use quack words.

4. The site does not try to discredit well-established organizations or government agencies.

5. The site does not rely on testimonials, celebrities, or people with unknown credentials.

6. The site is well regarded by experts, and has a high rating at http://navigator.tufts.edu.

7. The site has a history of providing good information.

8. The site provides complete information that is documented by research.

9. No claims of quick cures or miracle results are made.

10. The site provides information consistent with information provided in this text.

Conclusions and Implications:

☐ Total number of Xs for device, book/magazine, food supplement, or website.

1. In several sentences, give your assessment of the product. Did it score well on the questions? Would you use/buy the product? Explain.

Lab 25B: Evaluating a Health/Wellness or Fitness Club

Name	Section	Date

Purpose: To practice evaluating a health club. (Various combinations of the words *health, wellness,* and *fitness* are often used for these clubs.)

Procedure:

1. Visit a club and pretend to be interested in becoming a member. (Note: Only one or two class members should go to each club to avoid suspicion.)
2. Listen carefully to all that is said and ask lots of questions (without exposing your real motives).
3. Look carefully all around you as you are given the tour of the facilities; ask what the exercises or the equipment does for you or ask leading questions such as, "Will this take inches off my hips?", etc.
4. As soon as you leave the club, rate it using Chart 1. Space is provided for notes in Chart 1.

Chart 1 ▶ Health Club Evaluation Questionnaire

Directions: Place an X over a yes or no answer. Make notes as necessary.	Yes	No	Notes
1. Were claims for improvement in weight, figure/physique, or fitness realistic?	○	○	
2. Was a long-term contract (one to three years) encouraged?	○	○	
3. Was the sales pitch high-pressure to make an immediate decision?	○	○	
4. Were you given a copy of the contract to read at home?	○	○	
5. Did the fine print include objectionable clauses?	○	○	
6. Did they ask you about medical readiness?	○	○	
7. Did they sell diet supplements as a sideline?	○	○	
8. Did they have passive equipment?	○	○	
9. Did they have cardiovascular training equipment or facilities (cycles, track, pool, aerobic dance)?	○	○	
10. Did they make unscientific claims for the equipment, exercise, baths, or diet supplements?	○	○	
11. Were the facilities clean?	○	○	
12. Were the facilities crowded?	○	○	
13. Were there days and hours when facilities were open but would not be available to you?	○	○	
14. Were there limits on the number of minutes you could use a piece of equipment?	○	○	
15. Did the floor personnel closely supervise and assist clients?	○	○	
16. Were the floor personnel qualified experts?	○	○	
17. Were the managers/owners qualified experts?	○	○	
18. Has the club been in business at this location for a year or more?	○	○	

Results:

1. Score the chart as follows:

   A. Give one point for each "no" answer for items 2, 3, 5, 7, 8, 10, 12, 13, and 14 and place the score in the box.

   Total A [ ]

   B. Give one point for each "yes" answer for items 1, 4, 6, 9, 11, and 18 and place the score in the box.

   Total B [ ]

   Total A and B above and place the score in the box.

   Total A and B [ ]

   C. Give one point for each "yes" answer on 15, 16, and 17 and place the score in the box.

   Total C [ ]

2. A total score of 12–15 points on items A and B suggests the club rates at least fair compared to other clubs.
3. A score of three on item C indicates that the personnel are qualified and suggests that you could expect to get accurate technical advice from the staff.
4. Regardless of the total scores, you would have to decide the importance of each item in the questionnaire to you personally, as well as evaluate other considerations such as cost, location, personalities of the clients and the personnel, and so on, to decide if this would be a good place for you or your friends to join.

Conclusions and Implications: In the space below, use several sentences to discuss your conclusion about the quality of this club and whether you think it would fit your needs if you wanted to belong.

Toward Optimal Health and Wellness: Planning for Healthy Lifestyle Change

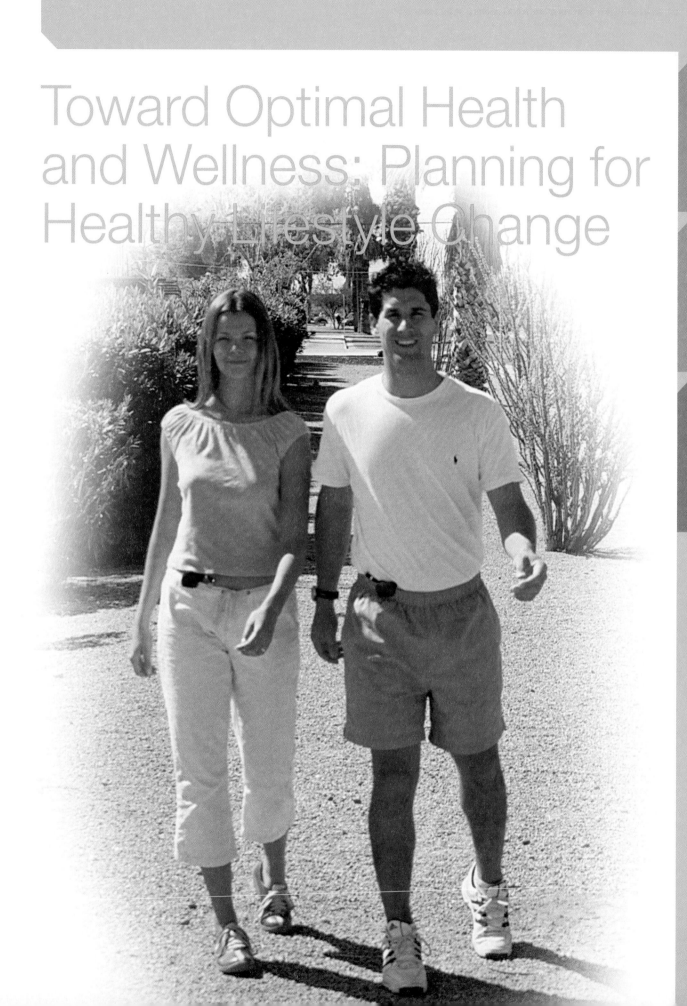

*Using effective self-management techniques that
promote healthy lifestyles can enhance fitness, health,
and wellness for a lifetime.*

Health Goals

for the year 2010

- Increase quality and years of healthy life.

- Increase healthy days.

- Eliminate health disparities.

- Increase adoption and maintenance of appropriate daily physical activity.

- Promote health by improving dietary factors and nutritional status.

- Promote healthy and safe communities.

- Promote availability of high quality health information.

- Increase availability of health care and counseling for mental health problems.

- Avoiding destructive behaviors.

The two primary health goals for the nation for the year 2010 are increasing the quality and years of life and eliminating health disparities so that all people can attain and maintain lifelong fitness, health, and wellness. The focus of this book has been on making priority lifestyle changes such as performing adequate physical activity, eating well, managing stress, and avoiding destructive behaviors. In this concept, you will get information about other factors that can increase quality and years of life including other lifestyle factors, the environment, the health-care system, and hereditary factors. The "Strategies for Action" included at the end of this concept will help you use the self-management skills learned in concept 2 and the self-planning skills learned in concept 5. You will have the opportunity to tie together all of the information in this book so that you can plan for a lifetime of healthy active living.

A Model for Achieving and Maintaining Lifelong Fitness, Health, and Wellness

Many different factors are important to developing lifetime fitness, health, and wellness and some are more in your control than others. In concept 1, you were exposed to a simplified model describing factors important in achieving lifetime fitness, health, and wellness. In this concept, that model (see Figure 1) will be developed in more detail to help you in lifetime planning.

Central to the model are fitness, health, and wellness because these are the states of being (shaded in green and yellow) that each of us wants to achieve. Around the periphery (see Figure 1) are the factors that influence these states of being. Those shaded in blue are the factors over which you have less control (heredity, health-care systems, and environment). Those shaded in red are the factors over which you have greater control (healthy lifestyles and personal actions/interactions).

Heredity (human biology) is a factor over which you have little control. Experts estimate that human biology or heredity accounts for 16 percent of all health problems, including early death. You have already learned that heredity influences each of the different parts of health-related physical fitness including your tendencies to build muscle and to deposit body fat. You also know that each of us reaps different benefits from the same healthy lifestyles based on our hereditary tendencies. Even more important is that predispositions to disease are inherited. For example, some early deaths are a result of hereditary conditions (e.g., congenital heart defects) that are untreatable. Obviously some inherited conditions are manageable (e.g., diabetes) with proper medical supervision and appropriate lifestyles. Heredity is a factor over which we have little control and is, therefore, illustrated in dark blue in Figure 1. Each of us can limit the effects of heredity by being aware of personal family history and making efforts to best manage those factors over which we do have control.

The health-care system effects our ability to overcome illness and improve our quality of life. www.mhhe.com/fit_well/web26 **Click 01.** It is estimated that 10 percent of unnecessary deaths occur

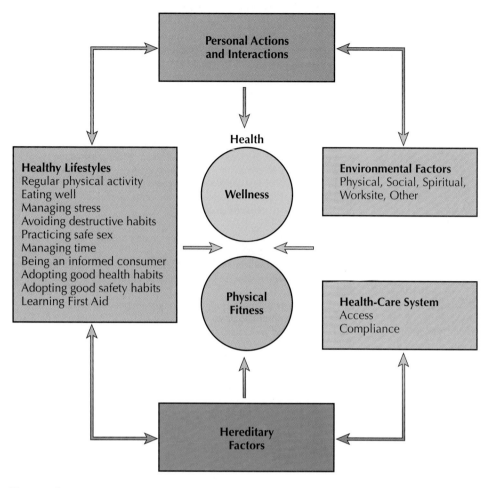

Figure 1 ▶ Factors influencing physical fitness, health, and wellness.

as a result of the health-care system. The quality of life for those who are sick and those who tend to the sick is influenced greatly by the type of medical care received. Access to health care is not equally available to all. A recent study by the Institute of Medicine entitled "Care Without Coverage: Too Little, Too Late" indicates that 18,000 people die unnecessarily in the United States each year because they lack health insurance. Those without health insurance are less likely to be admitted to emergency rooms, less likely to get high-quality medical care, and are at greater risk of complications from illness than those with insurance. Those without insurance often have chronic conditions that go undetected and as a result become untreatable. One of the great health inequities is that those with lower income are less likely to be insured.

Many people fail to seek medical help even though care is accessible. Others seek medical help but fail to comply. For example, they do not take prescribed medicine or do not follow up with treatments. As noted earlier in this book, men are less likely to seek medical advice than women. for this reason treatable conditions sometimes

become untreatable. Once men seek medical care, evidence reveals they get better care than women. Also more of the medical research has been done on men. This is of concern since treatments for men and women often vary for similar conditions.

Wellness as evidenced by **quality of life** is also influenced by the health-care system. Traditional medicine, sometimes referred to as the **medical model,** has focused primarily on the treatment of illness with medicine rather than illness prevention and wellness promotion. Efforts to educate medical and health-care personnel about techniques for promoting wellness have been initiated in recent years. Still it is often up to you (the patient) to find information about health promotion. For example, a patient with risk factors for heart disease might be advised to eat better or to exercise more, but little specific information may be offered.

In Figure 1, the health-care system is colored in a light shade of blue to illustrate the fact that it is a factor over which you may have limited control. There are some things that you can do to assume more control that will be discussed in the strategies for action section of this concept.

Quality of Life A term used to describe wellness. An individual with quality of life can enjoy the activities of life with little or no limitation and can function independently. Individual quality of life requires a pleasant and supportive community quality of life.

Medical Model A term often used to describe the focus of the health-care system on treating illness with medicine with little emphasis on prevention or wellness promotion.

Table 1 ▶ Environmental Factors Influencing Fitness, Health, and Wellness

Physical Environment. Many factors that influence the physical environment interact with each other. Urban sprawl and population growth, for example, are responsible for increased auto travel, and automobiles are the leading source of air pollution. Autos are also a cause of many accidental deaths (safety concern). Air and water pollution results in a variety of health problems and lowered quality of life. Pollution and sanitation problems are associated with population density and are much more likely to cause health problems for low-income people than those in the middle class. Urban sprawl has also been associated with the heat island effect (the increase in temperature in industrial and inner city areas) associated with increases in roadways and rooftops as well as decreased vegetation.

- **Pollution.** Of particular concern is air pollution (increased ozone, hydrocarbons, and particulates). Carbon dioxide is a greenhouse gas that accounts for 80 percent of global warming. Urban sprawl negatively impacts water quantity and quality because water in populated areas is diverted to sewers rather than returning naturally to acquifers. Industrial pollution is another threat to air and water quality. Smoking in public places is a source of pollution.
- **Loss of natural resources.** High gas, oil, and mineral use risks early depletion of resources and can result in disfiguring the landscape and contribute to environmental hazards.
- **Urban sprawl and population growth.** Sprawl reduces opportunities for healthy lifestyles such as walking and biking and increases the need for auto travel. Population growth results in greater housing density and can result in less community and home safety.
- **Sanitation.** Urban growth places great demands on sanitation systems and contributes to land pollution.

Social Environment. A healthy social environment offers opportunities for friendly interactions in a supportive environment. All social environments are not healthy and sometimes you must remove yourself, especially if relationships become abusive. Social environments interact with physical environments. For example, crowded roadways often lead to negative social interactions known as road rage. Drivers with road rage depersonalize other drivers and display behaviors they would not think of under normal circumstances.

- **Sense of community.** Being a part of the greater community is important to social and mental health.
- **Opportunities for personal relationships.** We all need friendly personal interactions. These relationships contribute to all aspects of health and wellness.
- **Family and peer support.** Support by others, especially family members, is important to us all.
- **Time availability.** We tend to take time for what we think is important. Social interactions require that time be spent with other people.
- **Removal from abusive environments.** If relationships become abusive, you may have to remove yourself and others at risk and to seek help of others.

Spiritual Environment. A positive environment provides each person with opportunities to find spiritual fulfillment. Whether interpreted as a belief in a higher power or a personal sense of wholeness associated with something greater than self, spiritual wellness is most likely to occur in a supportive environment (see Column 2). Additional information is presented in the Strategies for Action section of this concept.

- **Opportunities for spiritual development.** Reading spiritual materials, prayer, or meditation, and discussions with others (of similar and dissimilar beliefs) all provide opportunities to clarify and solidify spiritual beliefs.
- **Access to spiritual community.** Finding a community for worship and/or spiritual support has been shown to be comforting and a path to fulfillment for many.
- **Available spiritual leadership.** Like many other life's experiences, spiritual fulfillment may benefit from consultation with those with experience and expertise.

Intellectual Environment. Environments that foster learning and sound critical thinking are important to intellectual wellness. Evidence shows that people with more education are more likely to practice healthy lifestyles, to seek medical help, and to live in healthy environments than those with less education.

- **Access to accurate information.** Whether the source is formal education or self-learning, access to accurate information is essential. Of course, good information is only beneficial if used.
- **Stimulation for effective thinking.** Sometimes, we can become lazy, failing to evaluate information effectively we receive. Seeking environments that stimulate critical thinking (see concept 25) is important.

Work Environment. The work environment is a combination of physical, social, intellectual, and spiritual environments discussed earlier. Work environments are discussed separately because so many people spend so much time at work. Changing the work environment has been shown to be possible with cooperative efforts among workers and management. Many people now consider the perk of a healthy work environment to be as important as more pay.

- **Healthy physical environment.** A healthy work environment includes adequate well-lit pollution free workspace and reasonable work hours.
- **Healthy social environment.** Good relationships with bosses, co-workers, and adequate work breaks are key elements of a healthy social work environment.
- **Opportunity and support for healthy lifestyles.** Many companies now have worksite wellness programs that include opportunities for physical activity and other healthy lifestyle change. Programs that have quality professional leadership have been shown to produce reduced absenteeism, reduced health-care costs, and increased job satisfaction.

Environment Supporting Healthy Lifestyles. When we think of a toxic environment, we often think of a toxic physical environment. In recent years, experts have suggested that environments that reduce opportunities for adopting healthy lifestyle are also toxic. For example, the easy availability of fast food and junk food in vending machines creates a toxic environment for unhealthy eating.

- **Toxic-free environments.** If we are to promote healthy lifestyles at home, work, and school it is important to create environments that encourage active lifestyles. Examples include providing safe open recreational areas and worksite wellness programs.
- **People working together.** Changes designed to promote healthy lifestyles require the efforts of many people. Cooperative efforts by groups with well-defined goals are most likely to be successful.

The environment is a major factor affecting our fitness, health, and wellness. Environmental factors account for nearly one-fourth of all early deaths and affect quality of life in many ways. We do have more control over environmental factors than heredity but they are not totally under our control. For this reason, the environment box is depicted in Figure 1 with a lighter shade of blue than the heredity box.

Some of the more important environmental factors are described in Table 1. You can exert personal control by selecting healthy environments rather than exposing yourself to unhealthy or unsafe environments. This includes your choice of living and work location, as well as the social, spiritual, and intellectual environments. On the other hand, circumstances may make it impossible to make the choices you would prefer. Those who work in cities are typically more exposed to pollution and environmental risks than those who live in rural areas, including the heat island effect described in Table 1. Some suggestions for how you can work to alter the environment in a positive way are discussed later in this concept.

Healthy lifestyles are the greatest contributor to living a long, healthy life. www.mhhe.com/fit_well/web26 Click 02. Estimates show that more than half of early deaths are caused by unhealthy lifestyles. It is for this reason that this book has focused on techniques for changing lifestyles. Lifestyles are depicted in red (Figure 1) because they are much more in your control than the factors previously discussed and depicted in blue.

We have focused on adopting priority healthy lifestyle such as being regularly active, eating well, managing stress, avoiding destructive behaviors, and practicing safe sex because they are all factors over which we have some control and, if adopted, they have considerable impact on

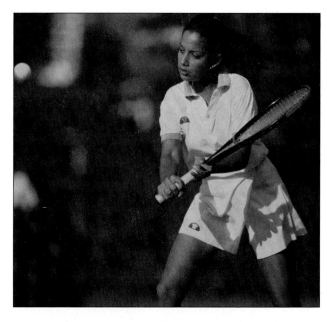

Making one lifestyle change such as becoming more physically active, can lead to other healthy lifestyle changes.

fitness, health, and wellness. Becoming an informed consumer and learning to manage time were also discussed in detail in earlier concepts. Other healthy lifestyles not emphasized in this book are described in Table 2. We hope you will adopt a new way of thinking and that you will use the self-management skills to help you adopt the ten healthy lifestyles depicted in Figure 1.

Personal actions and interactions are under your control and greatly influence your lifetime fitness, health, and wellness. www.mhhe.com/fit_well/ web26 Click 03. In the final analysis, you can learn all about heredity, health care, the environment, and

Table 2 ▶ Other Healthy Lifestyles	
Lifestyle	**Examples**
Adopting good personal health habits. Many of these habits, important to optimal health are considered to be elementary because they are often taught in school or at home at an early age. In spite of their importance, many adults regularly fail to adopt these behaviors.	• **Brushing and flossing teeth** • **Regular bathing and hand washing** • **Adequate sleep** • **Care of ears, eyes, and skin**
Adopting good safety habits. Unintentional injuries cost Canadians about $8.7 billion per year and in the United States the cost of injury and violence is $224 billion a year. Thousands of people die each year and thousands more suffer disabilities or problems that detract from good health and wellness. All accidents cannot be prevented but we can adopt habits to reduce risk. Some examples of accidents and habits that can be changed to reduce accident risk are illustrated in the opposite column.	• **Automobile accidents.** Wear seat belts, avoid using phone while driving, not drinking and driving, and resisting aggressive driving. • **Water accidents.** Learn to swim, learn CPR, wear life jackets while boating, not drinking while boating. • **Others.** Safe storage of guns, use of smoke alarms, safe use of ladders and electrical equipment, proper car, bike, motor cycle maintenance.
Learning first aid. Many deaths could be prevented and the severity of injury could be reduced if those at the site of emergencies were able to administer first aid. Examples of types of first aid that all people should learn are illustrated.	• **Learn cardiopulmonary resuscitation (CPR)** • **Learn the Heimlich maneuver** to assist people who are choking. • **Learn basic first aid**

healthy lifestyles; if you do not use what you learn, it will not help you. You are ultimately responsible for your personal actions. For this reason, we have depicted the box illustrating personal actions and interactions (Figure 1) in red. You can learn about your family history and use the information to limit the negative influence of heredity. You can do research about the health-care system and the environment to minimize the problems associated with them. Perhaps most important of all, you can learn self-management skills to help you in adopting healthy lifestyles.

It has been said that a person who thinks that good health is totally out of personal control is a fool. It has also been said that a person who thinks that he or she is totally in control of personal health is a fool. Both statements have merit. It would seem wise to learn as much about what you cannot control and use that information to make wise decisions.

Your interactions also influence your fitness, health, and wellness. You are not in this world alone. To be sure, your various environments influence you greatly. More important, however, is how you interact in these environments (see Table 1). You have a choice about the environments in which you place yourself, who you interact with in these environments, and how you interact with the environments themselves.

None of us makes perfect decisions all of the time. Sometimes we take actions and make choices with faulty or inadequate information. The more we learn, the less likely we are to repeat mistakes. From a positive point of view, well-informed people are healthier, happier, and more fulfilled than those who are less careful choosing a course of action.

Strategies for Action

Consider Strategies for Taking Advantage of Your Heredity. By now you are well aware that heredity is a factor that affects all aspects of physical fitness as well as your health and wellness. You can use several strategies to overcome negative predispositions and to take advantage of positive ones.

- **Learn about your family history.** If members of your family have had specific diseases or health problems make sure you inform your physician. Investigate to see if the conditions could affect you.

- **Take action to prevent other risk factors for conditions for which you have a predisposition.** For example, if you have a family history of Type II diabetes, you must do regular activity, eat well, and keep your body fat level in the good fitness zone.

- **Take advantage of your hereditary strengths.** Self-assessments can help you see where you have strength and account for weaknesses. Build on your strengths and find ways to compensate for your weaknesses. For example, people who have fewer fast-twitch muscle fibers will probably not be great sprinters but often have more slow-twitch fibers that favor cardiovascular and endurance performances such as distance running.

 Consider Strategies for Using the Health-Care System Effectively. www.mhhe.com/fit_well/ web26 Click 04. Do a self-assessment of your current use of health care (see Lab 26A). Develop a plan using some of the strategies described below (see Lab 26B).

- **Get periodic medical exams.** Do not wait until something is wrong before you seek medical advice. After forty years of age a yearly preventive physical exam is recommended. Younger people should have an exam at least every two years. Mammograms for women and prostate tests (PSA) for men are recommended. Breast and testicular self-exams are important (see concept 24).

- **Get medical insurance.** Find a way to get health insurance. Young people who save money by avoiding the payment of insurance premiums are placing themselves (and families) at risk.

- **Immunize.** Pneumonia and the flu are the sixth leading cause of death. With immunization, death, hospitalization, and loss of healthy days decrease dramatically. Many children go without immunizations that could prevent illness.

- **Identify a regular doctor and a convenient emergency care center.**

- **Become familiar with the symptoms of common medical problems.**

- **If symptoms persist, seek medical help.** Many deaths can be prevented if early warning signs of medical problems are heeded.

- **If medical advice is given, comply.** People commonly stop taking medicine when symptoms stop rather than taking the full amount of medicine prescribed.

- **If you have doubts about medical advice, get a second opinion.**

- **Be cautious when using the Internet for health information.** If you use the Internet for health information, be sure to use reliable websites (see concept 25). Seek information from more than one source.

- **Make your wishes for health care known.** Have a medical power of attorney. This document spells out the treatments you desire in the case of severe illness. Without such a document, your loved ones may not be able to make decisions consistent with your wishes. Be sure that your loved ones have a similar document so that you can help them carry out their wishes.

Consider strategies for improving your environment. Do a self-assessment to determine the quality of your environment (see Lab 26A). Develop a plan for improving your environment using the following practical strategies (Lab 26B).

- **Strategies for improving the physical environment.** Recycle, carpool, use public transportation, safely dispose of hazardous waste, conserve water, use fuel efficient cooling, heating, and appliances, buy environmentally friendly products, do not litter, work with others to seek public policy change, join a zoning board.
- **Strategies for interacting with the physical environment.** Avoid polluted environments such as smoke-filled establishments, choose a living location low in pollution (see Figure 2), keep your home free of pollutants (regularly check filters, avoid use of toxic products), and stay inside on days with high pollution.
- **Strategies for the social environment.** Find a social community that accommodates your personal and family needs, get involved in community affairs including those that affect the environment, build relationships with family and friends, provide support for others so that the support of others will be there for you when you need it, use time-management strategies to help you allocate time for social interactions.
- **Strategies for the spiritual environment.** Pray, meditate, read spiritual materials, participate in spiritual discussions, find a place to worship, provide spiritual support for others, seek spiritual guidance from those with experience and expertise, keep a journal, experience nature, honor relationships, help others.

- **Strategies for the intellectual environment.** Make decisions based on sound information, educate yourself before making choices and decisions, question simple solutions to complex problems, seek environments that stimulate critical thinking.
- **Strategies for the work environment.** Choose a job that has a healthy physical environment including adequate space, lighting, and freedom from pollution (tobacco smoke) as well as a healthy social, spiritual, and intellectual environment and that has a worksite wellness program led by professionals.
- **Strategies for finding an environment that supports healthy lifestyles.** Choose a place to live that is near parks, playgrounds, and that has sidewalks, bike paths, jogging trails, and swimming facilities; join a gym or health club; avoid environments that limit choices to fast food and food with empty calories; find a social environment that reinforces healthy lifestyles.

Consider strategies for adopting healthy lifestyles. As noted earlier in this concept, healthy lifestyles are the greatest contributor to a long and quality life. For this reason, find ways to incorporate each of the health lifestyles (described in Figure 1) into your life plan. The following list includes other strategies you can use to implement healthy lifestyles.

- **Use the six steps to help you plan lifestyle programs.** In concept 5, you learned about six steps in planning a physical activity program. These same six steps (see Table 3) can be used to plan for each of the many healthy lifestyles. The labs at the end of this concept are designed to help you use the six steps in program planning. Labs 26A and 26B relate to a broad range of lifestyles while Lab 26C helps you use the six steps to plan a lifetime physical activity program.

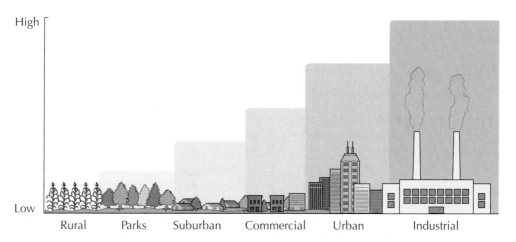

Figure 2 ▶ The effects of urban sprawl and industrial development on the physical environment.

Note: Darker shades reflect greater pollution, greater automobile density, higher temperature (heat effect) and more pavement.

- **Use self-management skills.** Learning and using these self-management skills, discussed in concept 2 and throughout the book, can help you to adopt and maintain healthy lifestyles.
- **Formal steps can become less formal with experience.** Few of us will go through life doing formal fitness assessments every month, writing down goals weekly, or self-monitoring activity daily. However, the more a person does self-assessments, the more he or she is aware of personal fitness status. This awareness reduces the need for frequent testing. For example, a person who does regular heart rate monitoring knows when he or she is in the target zone without counting heart rate every minute. A person who has frequently used skinfold measures to self-assess fatness can develop a good sense of body fatness with less frequent measurements. The same is true of other self-management skills. With experience, you can use the techniques less formally.

Consider Strategies for Taking Action and Benefitting from Interactions. In the end, it is what you do that counts. You can learn everything there is to know about fitness, health, and wellness, but if you do not take action and take advantage of your interactions with people and your environments, you will not benefit (see Figure 1). Some strategies for taking action and interacting effectively are listed below.

- **Collect and evaluate information before you act.** Become informed before you make important decisions. Get information from good sources and consult with others you trust.
- **Plan your actions and interactions.** Use the information in this book to plan your actions. Seek environments that produce positive interactions. People who plan are not only more likely to act but are also more likely to act effectively.
- **Put your plans in action.** Do not put off until tomorrow what you can do today. For good plans to be effective, they must be implemented. Actions and interactions that influence various dimensions of wellness are described in Table 3.
- **Honor your beliefs and relationships.** Actions and interactions that are inconsistent with basic beliefs and that fail to honor important relationships can result in reduced quality of life.
- **Seek the help of others and provide support for others who need your help.** As already noted, support by friends, family, and other significant others can be critical in helping you to achieve fitness, health, and wellness. Seek help for failing and abusive relationships. If your attempts to change meet with failure, do not set yourself up for repeated failure. Get help! Do what you can to be there for others who need your help.

Table 3 ▶ Factors Influencing Wellness

Dimension of Wellness	Influential Factors
Physical wellness	Pursuing behaviors that are conducive to good physical health (being physically active and maintaining a healthy diet).
Social wellness	Being supportive of family, friends, and co-workers and practicing good communication skills.
Emotional wellness	Balancing work and leisure and responding proactively to challenging or stressful situations.
Intellectual wellness	Challenging yourself to continually learn and improve in your work and personal life.
Spiritual wellness	Praying, meditating, or reflecting on life.
Total wellness	Taking responsibility for your own health and happiness.

Most colleges have programs through their health center that provide free, confidential assistance or referral. Many businesses now have Employee Assistance Programs (EAP). The programs have counselors who will help you or your family members find help with a particular problem. The EAP staff are dedicated to help you without revealing personal information to your employer. These programs have a strong record for helping people with problems ranging from small to very serious, such as drug addiction or smoking cessation. Many other programs and support groups are now available to help you change your lifestyle. For example, most hospitals and many health organizations now have hotlines that provide you with referral services for establishing healthy lifestyles.

Consider your personal beliefs and philosophy when making decisions. Though science can help you make good decisions and solve problems, most experts tell you that there is more to it than that. Your personal philosophy and beliefs play a role. Factors to consider are listed below.

- **Clarify your personal philosophy and consider a new way of thinking.** The determination as to whether a person is healthy, fit, or well is often subjective. Many make comparisons to other people, and such comparisons often result in setting personal standards impossible to achieve. Achieving the body fat of a model seen on television is not realistic nor healthy for most people. Expecting to be able to perform like a professional athlete is not something most of us can achieve. It is for this reason that the standards for fitness, health, and wellness in this book are based on health criteria rather than comparative criteria. As you began your study on this book, you were introduced to the HELP philosophy. Adhering to this philosophy can help you adopt a new way of thinking. This philosophy suggests that each person should use health (H) as the basis for making decisions rather than comparisons to others. This is something that everyone (E) can do for a lifetime (L). This allows each of us to set personal (P) goals that are realistic and possible for each person to attain. You may adopt all or parts of this philosophy. Whether you do or do not, you should have a clear idea of your own personal philosophy

The new way of thinking simply allows each of us to be successful on our own terms rather than comparing ourselves to others in ways that make success impossible. As you set personal health, fitness, and wellness goals, consider using a new way of thinking.

- **Allow for spontaneity.** The reliance on science emphasized in this book can help you make good choices. But if you are to live life fully you sometimes must allow yourself to be spontaneous. In doing so, the key is to be consistent with your personal philosophy so your spontaneous actions will be enriching rather than a source of future regret.
- **Believe that you can make a difference.** As noted previously, you make your own choices. Though heredity and several other factors are out of your control, the choices that you make are yours. Believing that your actions make a difference is critical to taking action and making changes when necessary. We hope the information presented in this book helps you make choices that allow you to be fit, healthy, and well for a lifetime.

Web Resources

American College Health Association **www.acha.org**
American Dietetics Association **www.eatright.org**
Health Canada Online **www.hc_sc.gc.ca**
Health Canada-Physical Activity Guide
    www.hc_sc.gc.ca/hppb/paguide
Healthfinder **www.healthfinder.gov**
Healthy People 2010 **www.health.gov/healthypeople**
Mayo Clinic Website **www.mayoclinic.com**
Morbidity and Mortality Weekly Reports **www.cdc.gov/mmwr**
National Institute of Alcohol Abuse and Alcoholism
    www.niaaa.nih.gov
National Institute of Drug Abuse **www.nida.nih.gov**
National Institute of Environmental Health Sciences
    www.niehs.nih.gov
U.S. Consumer Information Center **www.pueblo.gsa.gov**
World Health Organization **www.who.int**

Suggested Readings

 Additional reference materials for concept 26 are available at **www.mhhe.com/fit_well/web26 Click 05.**

American College of Sports Medicine. 2000. *ACSM's Guidelines for Exercise Testing and Exercise Prescription.* 6th ed. Philadelphia: Lippincott, Williams and Wilkins.

Booth, F. W., and M. W. Chakravarthy. 2002. Cost and consequences of sedentary living: New battleground for an old enemy. *President's Council on Physical Fitness and Sports* 3(16):1–8.

Corbin, C. B., and R. P. Pangrazi. 2001. Toward a uniform definition of wellness: A commentary. *President's Council on Physical Fitness and Sports* 3(15):1–8.

Diener, E., R. E. Lucas, and S. Oishi. 2002. Subjective well-being: The science of happiness and life satisfaction. In Snyder, C. R., and Lopez, S. J. *Handbook of Positive Psychology.* New York: Oxford University Press.

Frumkin, H. In press. Urban sprawl and public health. *Public Health Reports* 117.

Institute of Medicine. 2002. *Care Without Coverage: Too Little, Too Late.* Washington, DC: National Academy Press.

Keyes, C. L., and S. J. Lopez. 2002. Toward a science of mental health. In Snyder, C. R., and Lopez, S. J. *Handbook of Positive Psychology.* New York: Oxford University Press.

Pargament, K. I., and A. Manhoney. 2002. Spirituality: Discovering and conserving the sacred. In Snyder, C. R., and S. J. Lopez. *Handbook of Positive Psychology.* New York: Oxford University Press.

Payne, W. A., and D. B. Hahn. 2002. *Understanding Your Health.* 7th ed. St. Louis: McGraw-Hill.

Seward, B. L. 2001. *Health and the Human Spirit.* Boston: Allyn and Bacon.

Snyder, C. R., and S. J. Lopez. 2002. *Handbook of Positive Psychology.* New York: Oxford University Press.

U.S. Department of Health and Human Services. Nov. 2000. *Healthy People 2010.* 2nd ed. With *Understanding and Improving Health and Objectives for Improving Health.* 2 vols. Washington, DC: U.S. Government Printing Office.

World Health Organization. 2000. *World Health Report 2000.* Geneva: World Health Organization.

In the News

According to Dr. Tedd Mitchell, Wellness Director at the Cooper Clinic in Dallas, people give various excuses for not seeing a doctor or getting a regular medical checkup. How would you classify yourself?

- **Gamblers.** These people do not think about their health until a serious problem occurs.
- **Martyrs.** These people are so busy taking care of others that they fail to take care of themselves.
- **Economists.** These people think the cost of preventive exams is too high for the benefits received.
- **Shamans.** These people buy in on the latest health fad and self-diagnose while avoiding regular medical care.

- **Informers.** These people have an ax to grind with health-care professionals and avoid health care for this reason.
- **Queens of Denial** (Cleopatra Syndrome). These people do not believe something could be wrong with them or do not want to know if there is.
- **Busy Bees.** These people feel they are too busy to take the time to get regular medical care.

The Bottom Line: According to Dr. Mitchell, "there is no good reason to avoid your annual visit to the doctor."

Lab 26A: Assessing Factors That Influence Fitness, Health, and Wellness

Name	**Section**	**Date**	

Purpose: To assess the factors that relate to fitness, health, and wellness.

Chart 1 ▶ Assessment Questionnaire: Factors That Influence Fitness, Health, and Wellness

Factor	Very True	Somewhat True	Not True At All	Score
Heredity				
1. I have checked my family history for medical problems.	③	②	①	
2. I have taken steps to overcome hereditary predispositions.	①	②	③	
			Heredity Score =	
Health Care				
3. I have health insurance.	③	②	①	
4. I get regular medical exams and have my own doctor.	③	②	①	
5. I get treatment early, rather than waiting until problems get serious	③	②	①	
6. I carefully investigate my health problems before making decisions.	③	②	①	
			Health-Care Score =	
Environment				
7. My physical environment is healthy.	③	②	①	
8. My social environment is healthy.	③	②	①	
9. My spiritual environment is healthy.	③	②	①	
10. My intellectual environment is healthy.	③	②	①	
11. My work environment is healthy.	③	②	①	
12. My environment fosters healthy lifestyles.	③	②	①	
			Environment Score =	
Lifestyles				
13. I am physically active on a regular basis.	③	②	①	
14. I eat well.	③	②	①	
15. I use effective techniques for managing stress.	③	②	①	
16. I avoid destructive behaviors.	③	②	①	
17. I practice safe sex.	③	②	①	
18. I manage my time effectively.	③	②	①	
19. I evaluate information carefully and am an informed consumer.	③	②	①	
20. My personal health habits are good.	③	②	①	
21. My safety habits are good.	③	②	①	
22. I know first aid and can use it if needed.	③	②	①	
			Lifestyles Score =	
Personal Actions and Interactions				
23. I collect and evaluate information before I act.	③	②	①	
24. I plan before I take action.	③	②	①	
25. I am good about taking action when I know it is good for me.	③	②	①	
26. I honor my beliefs and relationships.	③	②	①	
27. I seek help when I need it.	③	②	①	
			Action/Interaction Score =	

Procedures:

1. Answer each of the questions in the questionnaire on page 475. Consider the information in concept 26 as you answer each question.
2. Calculate scores for heredity (sum items 1 and 2), health care (sum items 3–6), environment (sum items 7–12), lifestyles (sum items 13–22), and actions/interactions (sum items 23–27).
3. Determine ratings for each of the scores using the Rating Chart.
4. Record your scores and ratings in the Results section. Answer the questions in the Conclusions/Implications section.

Factor	Score	Rating
Heredity		
Health Care		
Environment		
Lifestyles		
Actions/Interactions		

Rating Chart

Factor	Healthy	Marginal	Needs Attention
Heredity	6	4–5	below 4
Health Care	11–12	9–10	below 9
Environment	16–18	13–15	below 13
Lifestyles	26–30	20–25	below 20
Actions/ Interactions	13–15	10–12	below 10

In the space below discuss your scores for the five factors (sums of several questions) identified in the questionnaire. Use several sentences to identify specific areas that need attention and changes that you could make to improve.

For any individual item on the questionnaire, a score of one is considered low. You might have a high score on a set of questions and still have a low score in one area that indicates need for attention. In several sentences, discuss actions you could take to make changes related to individual questions (see questionnaire on page 475).

Appendix

Metric

Approximate
to Traditiona

Length

centimeters to

meters to feet:

meters to yard

kilometers to

Mass (Weight)

grams to ounc

kilograms to

Area

square centim

square meters

square meters

Volume

milliliters to f

liters to quart

liters to gallor

Appendi

Metric

Ch

Cla

Hig

Go

Ma

Lo

Cla

Hig

Go

Ma

Lo

Lab 26B: Planning for Improved Fitness, Health, and Wellness

Name	Section	Date

Purpose: To make plans to make changes in areas that can most contribute to improved fitness, health, and wellness.

Procedures:

1. Experts agree that it is best not to make too many changes all at once. Focusing attention on one or two things at a time will produce better results. Based on your assessments made in Lab 26A,, select two areas in which you would like to make change. Choose one from the list related to environments and health care and one related to lifestyle change. Place a check by those areas in Chart 1 in the Results section. Because Lab 26C is devoted to physical activity, it is not included in the list. You may want to make additional copies of this lab for future use in making other changes in the future.

2. Use Chart 2 to determine your Stage of Change for the changes you have identified. Since you have identified these as an area of need it is unlikely that you would identify the stage of maintenance. If you are at maintenance, you could select a different area of changes that would be more useful.

3. In the appropriate locations record the change you want to make related to your environment or health care. State your reasons, your specific goal(s), your written statement of the plan for change, and a statement about how you will self-monitor and evaluate the effectiveness of the changes made. In Chart 3, record similar information for the lifestyle change you identified.

Results:

Chart 1 ▶ Check one in each column.

Area of Change	✔	Area of Change	✔
Health Insurance		Eating Well	
Medical Checkups		Managing Stress	
Selecting a Doctor		Avoiding Destructive Habits	
Physical Environment		Practicing Safe Sex	
Social Environment		Managing Time	
Spiritual Environment		Becoming a Better Consumer	
Intellectual Environment		Improving Health Habits	
Work Environment		Improving Safety Habits	
Environment for Lifestyles		Learning First Aid	

Chart 2 ▶ List the two areas of change identified in Chart 1.

Make a rating using the diagram at the right.

Identified Area of Change	Stage of Change Rating
1.	
2.	

Maintenance — The change has lasted at least six months.

Action — "I have made some short-term changes"

Preparation — "I am getting ready to change."

Contemplation — "I am thinking about a change."

Precontemplation — "I don't want to change."

Note: Some of the areas identified in this assignment relate to personal information. It is appropriate not to divulge personal information to others (including your instructor) if you choose not to. For this reason, you may choose not to address certain problems in this assignment. You are encouraged to take steps to make changes independent of this assignment and to consult privately with your instructor to get assistance.

3. In several sen

Chart 2 ▶ Twelve-Minute Swim Rating Chart (score in meters)

Men (Age)

Classification	17–26	27–39	40–49	50+
High-performance zone	644+	598+	552+	506+
Good fitness zone	552–643	506–597	460–551	413–505
Marginal fitness zone	460–551	414–505	368–459	322–412
Low fitness zone	below 459	below 413	below 367	below 321

Women (age)

Classification	17–26	27–39	40–49	50+
High-performance zone	552+	506+	460+	414+
Good fitness zone	460–551	414–505	367–459	321–413
Marginal fitness zone	367–459	321–413	276–366	230–320
Low fitness zone	below 366	below 320	below 275	below 229

Chart 3 ▶ Isometric Strength Rating Scale (kg)

Classification Men	Left Grip	Right Grip	Total Score
High-performance zone	57+	61+	118+
Good fitness zone	45–56	50–60	95–117
Marginal zone	41–44	43–49	84–94
Low zone	<41	<43	<84

Women			
High-performance zone	34+	39+	73+
Good fitness zone	27–33	32–38	59–72
Marginal zone	20–26	23–31	43–58
Low zone	<20	<23	<43

Suitable for use by young adults between 18 and 30 years of age. After 30, an adjustment of 0.5 of 1 percent per year is appropriate because some loss of muscle tissue typically occurs as you grow older.

Chart 4 ▶ Power Rating Scale

Classification	Men	Women
Excellent	68 cm+	60 cm+
Very good	53–67 cm	48–59 cm
Good	42–52 cm	37–47 cm
Fair	31–41 cm	27–36 cm
Poor	<32 cm	<27 cm

Chart 5 ▶ Reaction Time Rating Scale

Classification	Score in inches	Score in centimeters
Excellent	More than 21"	53+
Very good	19"–21"	48–52
Good	16"–18 3/4"	41–47
Fair	13"–15 3/4"	33–40
Poor	Below 13"	<33

Chart 6 ▶ Speed Rating Scale

Classification	Men Yards	Men Meters	Women Yards	Women Meters
Excellent	24+	22+	22+	20+
Very good	22–23	20–21.9	20–21	18–19.9
Good	18–21	16.5–19.9	16–19	14.5–17.9
Fair	16–17	14.5–16.4	14–15	13–14.4
Poor	<16	<14.5	<14	<13

Calorie Guide to Common Foods

Beverages

Coffee (black)	0
Coke (12 oz.)	137
Hot chocolate, milk (1 cup)	247
Lemonade (1 cup)	100
Limeade, diluted to serve (1 cup)	110
Soda, fruit flavored (12 oz.)	161
Tea (clear)	0

Breads and Cereals

Bagel (1 half)	76
Biscuit (2" × 2")	135
Bread, pita (1 oz.)	80
Bread, raisin ($^1/_2$" thick)	65
Bread, rye	55
Bread, white enriched ($^1/_2$" thick)	64
Bread, whole wheat ($^1/_2$" thick)	55
Bun (hamburger)	120
Cereals, cooked ($^1/_2$ cup)	80
Corn flakes (1 cup)	96
Corn grits (1 cup)	125
Corn muffin ($2^1/_2$" diam.)	103
Crackers, graham (1 med.)	28
Crackers, soda (1 plain)	24
English muffin (1 half)	74
Macaroni, with cheese (1 cup)	464
Muffin, plain	135
Noodles (1 cup)	200
Oatmeal (1 cup)	150
Pancakes (1–4" diam.)	59
Pizza (1 section)	180
Popped corn (1 cup)	54
Potato chips (10 med.)	108
Pretzels (5 small sticks)	18
Rice (1 cup)	225
Roll, plain (1 med.)	118
Roll, sweet (1 med.)	178
Shredded wheat (1 med. biscuit)	79
Spaghetti, plain cooked (1 cup)	218
Tortilla (1 corn)	70
Waffle ($4^1/_2$" × 5")	216

Dairy Products

Butter, 1 pat ($1^1/_2$ tsp.)	50
Cheese, cheddar (1 oz.)	113
Cheese, cottage (1 cup)	270
Cheese, cream (1 oz.)	106
Cheese, Parmesan (1 tbsp.)	29
Cheese, Swiss natural (1 oz.)	105
Cream, sour (1 tbsp.)	31
Frozen custard (1 cup)	375
Frozen yogurt, vanilla (1 cup)	180
Ice cream, plain (prem.) (1 cup)	350
Ice cream soda, choc. (large glass)	455
Ice milk (1 cup)	184
Ices (1 cup)	177
Milk, chocolate (1 cup)	185
Milk, half-and-half (1 tbsp.)	20
Milk, malted (1 cup)	281
Milk, skim (1 cup)	88
Milk, skim dry (1 tbsp.)	28

Milk, whole (1 cup)	166
Sherbet (1 cup)	270
Softserve cone (med.)	335
Whipped topping (1 tbsp.)	14
Yogurt (1 cup)	150

Desserts and Sweets

Cake, angel (2" wedge)	108
Cake, chocolate (2" × 3" × 1")	150
Cake, plain (3" × $2^1/_2$")	180
Chocolate, bar	200–300
Chocolate, bitter (1 oz.)	142
Chocolate, sweet (1 oz.)	133
Chocolate, syrup (1 tbsp.)	42
Cocoa (1 tbsp.)	21
Cookies, plain (1 med.)	75
Custard, baked (1 cup)	283
Doughnut (1 large)	250
Gelatin, dessert (1 cup)	155
Gelatin, with fruit (1 cup)	170
Gingerbread (2" × 2" × 2")	180
Jams, jellies (1 tbsp.)	55
Pie, apple ($^1/_7$ of 9" pie)	345
Pie, cherry ($^1/_7$ of 9" pie)	355
Pie, chocolate ($^1/_7$ of 9" pie)	360
Pie, coconut ($^1/_7$ of 9" pie)	266
Pie, lemon meringue ($^1/_7$ of 9" pie)	302
Sugar, granulated (1 tsp.)	27
Syrup, table (1 tbsp.)	57

Fruit

Apple, fresh (med.)	76
Applesauce, unsweetened (1 cup)	184
Avocado, raw ($^1/_2$ peeled)	279
Banana, fresh (med.)	88
Cantaloupe, raw ($^1/_2$, 5" diam.)	60
Cherries (10 sweet)	50
Cranberry sauce, unsweetened (1 tbsp.)	25
Fruit cocktail, canned (1 cup)	170
Grapefruit, fresh ($^1/_2$)	60
Grapefruit juice, raw (1 cup)	95
Grape juice, bottled ($^1/_2$ cup)	80
Grapes (20–25)	75
Nectarine (1 med.)	88
Olives, green	72
Olives, ripe (10)	105
Orange, fresh (med.)	60
Orange juice, frozen diluted (1 cup)	110
Peach, fresh (med.)	46
Peach, canned in syrup (2 halves)	79
Pear, fresh (med.)	95
Pears, canned in syrup (2 halves)	79
Pineapple, crushed in syrup (1 cup)	204
Pineapple ($^1/_2$ cup fresh)	50
Prune juice (1 cup)	170
Raisins, dry (1 tbsp.)	26
Strawberries, fresh (1 cup)	54
Strawberries, frozen (3 oz.)	90
Tangerine ($2^1/_2$" diam.)	40
Watermelon, wedge (4" × 8")	120

Meat, Fish, Eggs

Bacon, drained (2 slices)	97
Bacon, Canadian (1 oz.)	62
Beef, hamburger chuck (3 oz.)	316
Beef, pot pie	560
Beef steak, sirloin or T-bone (3 oz.)	257
Beef and vegetable stew (1 cup)	185
Chicken, fried breast (8 oz.)	210
Chicken, fried (1 leg and thigh)	305
Chicken, roasted breast (2 slices)	100
Chili, without beans (1 cup)	510
Chili, with beans (1 cup)	335
Egg, boiled	77
Egg, fried	125
Egg, scrambled	100
Fish and chips (2 pcs. fish; 4 oz. chips)	275
Fish, broiled (3" × 3" × $^1/_2$")	112
Fish stick	40
Frankfurter, boiled	124
Ham (4" × 4")	338
Lamb (3 oz. roast, lean)	158
Liver (3" × 3")	150
Luncheon meat (2 oz.)	135
Pork chop, loin (3" × 5")	284
Salmon, canned (1 cup)	145
Sausage, pork (4 oz.)	510
Shrimp, canned (3 oz.)	108
Tuna, canned ($^1/_2$ cup)	185
Veal, cutlet (3" × 4")	175

Nuts and Seeds

Cashews (1 cup)	770
Coconut (1 cup)	450
Peanut butter (1 tbsp.)	92
Peanuts, roasted, no skin (1 cup)	805
Pecans (1 cup)	752
Sunflower seeds (1 tbsp.)	50

Sandwiches
(2 slices of plain bread)

Bologna	214
Cheeseburger (small McDonald's)	300
Chicken salad	185
Egg salad	240
Fish fillet (McDonald's)	400
Ham	360
Ham and cheese	360
Hamburger (small McDonald's)	260
Hamburger, Burger King Whopper	600
Hamburger, Big Mac	550
Hamburger (McDonald's Quarter Pounder)	420
Peanut butter	250
Roast beef (Arby's Regular)	425

Sauces, Fats, Oils

Catsup, tomato (1 tbsp.)	17
Chili sauce (1 tbsp.)	17
French dressing (1 tbsp.)	59
Margarine (1 pat)	50
Mayonnaise (1 tbsp.)	92

Mayonnaise-type (1 tbsp.)	65	Beans, navy (1 cup)	642	Peas, field ($^1/_2$ cup)	90
Vegetable, sunflower, safflower oils		Beans, pork and molasses (1 cup)	325	Peas, green (1 cup)	145
(1 tbsp.)	120	Broccoli, fresh cooked (1 cup)	60	Pickles, dill (med.)	15
		Cabbage, cooked (1 cup)	40	Pickles, sweet (med.)	22
Soup, Ready to Serve (1 cup)		Cauliflower (1 cup)	25	Potato, baked (med.)	97
Bean	190	Carrot, raw (med.)	21	Potato, french fried (8 sticks)	155
Beef noodle	100	Carrots, canned (1 cup)	44	Potato, mashed (1 cup)	185
Cream	200	Celery, diced raw (1 cup)	20	Radish, raw (small)	1
Tomato	90	Coleslaw (1 cup)	102	Sauerkraut, drained (1 cup)	32
Vegetable	80	Corn, sweet, canned (1 cup)	140	Spinach, fresh, cooked (1 cup)	46
		Corn, sweet (med. ear)	84	Squash, summer (1 cup)	30
Vegetables		Cucumber, raw (6 slices)	6	Sweet pepper (med.)	15
Alfalfa sprouts ($^1/_2$ cup)	19	Lettuce (2 large leaves)	7	Sweet potato, candied (small)	314
Asparagus (6 spears)	22	Mushrooms, canned (1 cup)	28	Tomato, cooked (1 cup)	50
Bean sprouts (1 cup)	37	Onions, french fried (10 rings)	75	Tomato, raw (med.)	30
Beans, green (1 cup)	27	Onions, raw (med.)	25		
Beans, lima (1 cup)	152				

Due to space limitations, it is not possible to list the nutrient content of all commercially available foods. You can access many valuable Web-based resources to obtain more detailed lists of foods or complete dietary analyses. The Nutrition Department at Tufts University has developed a webpage called Nutrition Navigators (http://www.navigator.tufts.edu/) that reviews the quality of various nutrition-related websites. The list below highlights a few of the dietary analysis programs that received favorable reviews from the Nutrition Navigator website. These resources are recommended for students interested in learning about the nutrient content of foods not listed in appendices C and D. Directly consulting the Nutrition Navigator site may bring up additional sites that may be useful as well.

Cyberdiet www.cyberdiet.com/

This website, developed by a team of registered dietitians, offers a variety of information about nutrition. The database of commonly used foods (www.cyberdiet.com/ni/htdocs/index.html) can be quickly searched for dietary information. An advantage of this database is that it allows you to search by various categories of foods and quickly view and compare foods in a similar category.

Diet Analysis Website dawp.anet.com/

This diet analysis site lets you enter the foods you've eaten over the course of a day, and then, based on the RDA, reports a complete nutritional review of your diet. Tufts Nutrition Navigator gives this site a rating of "better than most."

Fast Food Finder www.olen.com/food/

This online analysis program, developed with support from the Minnesota Attorney General's Office, allows you to obtain dietary information about nearly all items available from fast food chains.

Nutrition Analysis Tool www.nat.uiuc.edu

This diet analysis program, developed by the University of Illinois Department of Food Science/Nutrition, provides a nutrient analysis of foods by searching foods within the USDA database.

Sante Food Database www.nightcrew.com/sante7000/sante7000_search.cfm

This website program provides a nutrient analysis of over 7,248 foods that are listed in the U.S. Department of Agriculture (USDA) database. The report provides a listing of over twenty-nine nutrients for each food.

Appendix D

Calories of Protein, Carbohydrates, and Fats in Foods*

Food No./Food Choice	Total Calories	Protein Calories	Carbohydrate Calories	Fat Calories
Breakfast				
1. Scrambled egg (1 lg)	111	29	7	75
2. Fried egg (1 lg)	99	26	1	72
3. Pancake (1-6^W)	146	19	67	58
4. Syrup (1 T)	60	0	60	0
5. French toast (1 slice)	180	23	49	108
6. Waffle (7-inch)	245	28	100	117
7. Biscuit (medium)	104	8	52	44
8. Bran muffin (medium)	104	11	63	31
9. White toast (slice)	68	9	52	7
10. Wheat toast (slice)	67	14	52	6
11. Peanut butter (1 T)	94	15	11	68
12. Yogurt (8 oz. plain)	227	39	161	27
13. Orange juice (8 oz.)	114	8	100	6
14. Apple juice (8 oz.)	117	1	116	0
15. Soft drink (12 oz.)	144	0	144	0
16. Bacon (2 slices)	86	15	2	70
17. Sausage (1-link)	141	11	0	130
18. Sausage (1 patty)	284	23	0	261
19. Grits (8 oz.)	125	11	110	4
20. Hash browns (8 oz.)	355	18	178	159
21. French fries (reg.)	239	12	115	112
22. Donut cake	125	4	61	60
23. Donut glazed	164	8	87	69
24. Sweet roll	317	22	136	159
25. Cake (medium slice)	274	14	175	85
26. Ice cream (8 oz.)	257	15	108	134
27. Cream cheese (T)	52	4	1	47
28. Jelly (T)	49	0	49	0
29. Jam (T)	54	0	54	0
30. Coffee (cup)	0	0	0	0
31. Tea (cup)	0	0	0	0
32. Cream (T)	32	2	2	28
33. Sugar (t)	15	0	15	0
34. Corn flakes (8 oz.)	97	8	87	2
35. Wheat flakes (8 oz.)	106	12	90	4
36. Oatmeal (8 oz.)	132	19	92	21
37. Strawberries (8 oz.)	55	4	46	5
38. Orange (medium)	64	6	57	1
39. Apple (medium)	96	1	86	9
40. Banana (medium)	101	4	95	2
41. Cantaloupe (half)	82	7	73	2
42. Grapefruit (half)	40	2	37	1
43. Custard pie (slice)	285	20	188	77
44. Fruit pie (slice)	350	14	259	77
45. Fritter (medium)	132	11	54	67
46. Skim milk (8 oz.)	88	36	52	0
47. Whole milk (8 oz.)	159	33	48	78
48. Butter (pat)	36	0	0	36
49. Margarine (pat)	36	0	0	36

Food No./Food Choice	Total Calories	Protein Calories	Carbohydrate Calories	Fat Calories
Lunch				
1. Hamburger (reg. FF)	255	48	120	89
2. Cheeseburger (reg. FF)	307	61	120	126
3. Doubleburger (FF)	563	101	163	299
4. $^1/_4$ lb. Burger (FF)	427	73	137	217
5. Doublecheese burger (FF)	670	174	134	362
6. Doublecheese baconburger (FF)	724	138	174	340
7. Hot dog (FF)	214	36	54	124
8. Chili dog (FF)	320	51	90	179
9. Pizza, cheese (slice FF)	290	116	116	58
10. Pizza, meat (slice FF)	360	126	126	108
11. Pizza, everything (slice FF)	510	179	173	158
12. Sandwich, roast beef (FF)	350	88	126	137
13. Sandwich, bologna	313	44	106	163
14. Sandwich, bologna-cheese	428	69	158	201
15. Sandwich, ham-cheese (FF)	380	91	133	156
16. Sandwich, peanut butter	281	39	118	124
17. Sandwich, PB and Jelly	330	40	168	122
18. Sandwich, egg salad	330	40	109	181
19. Sandwich, tuna salad	390	101	109	180
20. Sandwich, fish (FF)	432	56	147	229
21. French fries (reg. FF)	239	12	115	112
22. French fries (lg. FF)	406	20	195	191
23. Onion rings (reg. FF)	274	14	112	148
24. Chili (8 oz.)	260	49	62	148
25. Bean soup (8 oz.)	355	67	181	107
26. Beef noodle soup (8 oz.)	140	32	59	49
27. Tomato soup (8 oz.)	180	14	121	45
28. Vegetable soup (8 oz.)	160	21	107	32
29. Small salad, plain	37	6	27	4
30. Small salad, French dressing	152	8	50	94
31. Small salad, Italian dressing	162	8	28	126
32. Small salad, bleu cheese	184	13	28	143
33. Potato salad (8 oz.)	248	27	159	62
34. Cole slaw (8 oz.)	180	0	25	155
35. Macaroni and cheese (8 oz.)	230	37	103	90
36. Taco beef (FF)	186	59	56	71
37. Bean burrito (FF)	343	45	192	106
38. Meat burrito (FF)	466	158	196	112
39. Mexican rice (FF)	213	17	160	36
40. Mexican beans (FF)	168	42	82	44
41. Fried chicken breast (FF)	436	262	13	161
42. Broiled chicken breast	284	224	0	60
43. Broiled fish	228	82	32	114
44. Fish stick (1 stick FF)	50	18	8	24
45. Fried egg	99	26	1	72
46. Donut	125	4	61	60
47. Potato chips (small bag)	115	3	39	73
48. Soft drink (12 oz.)	144	0	144	0

*Notes:
1. FF by a food indicates that it is typical of a food served in a fast food restaurant.
2. Your portions of foods may be larger or smaller than those listed here. For this reason you may wish to select a food more than once (i.e., two hamburgers) or select only a portion of a serving (i.e., divide the calories in half for a half portion).
3. An oz. equals an ounce or 28.35 grams.
4. T = Tablespoon and t = teaspoon.
The principal reference for the calculation of values used in this appendix were the *Nutritive Value of Foods*, published by the United States Department of Agriculture, Washington, D.C., Home and Gardens Bulletin, No. 72, although other published sources were consulted, including Jacobson, M., and S. Fritschner, *The Fast-Food Guide* (an excellent source of information about fast foods), New York, Workman Publishing Company.

Food No./Food Choice	Total Calories	Protein Calories	Carbohydrate Calories	Fat Calories
49. Apple juice (8 oz.)	117	1	116	0
50. Skim milk (8 oz.)	88	36	52	0
51. Whole milk (8 oz.)	159	33	48	78
52. Diet drink (12 oz.)	0	0	0	0
53. Mustard (t)	4	0	4	0
54. Catsup (t)	6	0	6	0
55. Mayonnaise (T)	100	0	0	100
56. Fruit pie	350	14	259	77
57. Cheese cake	400	56	132	212
58. Ice cream (8 oz.)	257	15	108	134
59. Coffee (8 oz.)	0	0	0	0
60. Tea (8 oz.)	0	0	0	0
Dinner				
1. Hamburger (reg. FF)	255	48	120	89
2. Cheeseburger (reg. FF)	307	61	120	126
3. Doubleburger (FF)	563	101	163	299
4. ¼ lb. Burger (FF)	427	73	137	217
5. Doublecheese burger (FF)	670	174	134	362
6. Doublecheese baconburger (FF)	724	138	174	412
7. Hot dog (FF)	214	36	54	124
8. Chili dog (FF)	320	51	90	179
9. Pizza, cheese (slice FF)	290	116	116	58
10. Pizza, meat (slice FF)	360	126	126	108
11. Pizza, everything (slice FF)	510	179	173	158
12. Steak (8 oz.)	880	290	0	590
13. French fried shrimp (6 oz.)	360	133	68	158
14. Roast beef (8 oz.)	440	268	0	172
15. Liver (8 oz.)	520	250	52	218
16. Corned beef (8 oz.)	493	242	0	251
17. Meat loaf (8 oz.)	711	228	35	448
18. Ham (8 oz.)	540	178	0	362
19. Spaghetti, no meat (13 oz.)	400	56	220	124
20. Spaghetti, meat (13 oz.)	500	115	230	155
21. Baked potato (medium)	90	12	78	0
22. Cooked carrots (8 oz.)	71	12	59	0
23. Cooked spinach (8 oz.)	50	18	18	14
24. Corn (one ear)	70	10	52	8
25. Cooked green beans (8 oz.)	54	11	43	0
26. Cooked broccoli (8 oz.)	60	19	26	15
27. Cooked cabbage	47	12	35	0
28. French fries (reg. FF)	239	12	115	112
29. French fries (lg. FF)	406	20	195	191
30. Onion rings (reg. FF)	274	14	112	148
31. Chili (8 oz.)	260	49	62	148
32. Small salad, plain	37	6	27	4
33. Small salad, French dressing	152	8	50	94
34. Small salad, Italian dressing	162	8	28	126
35. Small salad, bleu cheese	184	13	28	143
36. Potato salad (8 oz.)	248	27	159	62
37. Cole slaw (8 oz.)	180	0	25	155
38. Macaroni and cheese (8 oz.)	230	37	103	90
39. Taco beef (FF)	186	59	56	71
40. Bean burrito (FF)	343	45	192	106
41. Meat burrito (FF)	466	158	196	112
42. Mexican rice (FF)	213	17	160	36
43. Mexican beans (FF)	168	42	82	44
44. Fried chicken breast (FF)	436	262	13	161

Food No./Food Choice	Total Calories	Protein Calories	Carbohydrate Calories	Fat Calories
45. Broiled chicken breast	284	224	0	60
46. Broiled fish	228	82	32	114
47. Fish stick (1 stick FF)	50	18	8	24
48. Soft drink (12 oz.)	144	0	144	0
49. Apple juice (8 oz.)	117	1	116	0
50. Skim milk (8 oz.)	88	36	52	0
51. Whole milk (8 oz.)	159	33	48	78
52. Diet drink (12 oz.)	0	0	0	0
53. Mustard (t)	4	0	4	0
54. Catsup (t)	6	0	6	0
55. Mayonnaise (T)	100	0	0	100
56. Fruit pie (slice)	350	14	259	77
57. Cheese cake (slice)	400	56	132	212
58. Ice cream (8 oz.)	257	15	108	134
59. Custard pie (slice)	285	20	188	77
60. Cake (slice)	274	14	175	85
Snacks				
1. Peanut butter (1 T)	94	15	11	68
2. Yogurt (8 oz. plain)	227	39	161	27
3. Orange juice (8 oz.)	114	8	100	6
4. Apple juice (8 oz.)	117	1	116	0
5. Soft drink (12 oz.)	144	0	144	0
6. Donut, cake	125	4	61	60
7. Donut, glazed	164	8	87	69
8. Sweet roll	317	22	136	159
9. Cake (medium slice)	274	14	175	85
10. Ice cream (8 oz.)	257	15	108	134
11. Soft serve cone (reg.)	240	10	89	134
12. Ice cream sandwich bar	210	40	82	88
13. Strawberries (8 oz.)	55	4	46	5
14. Orange (medium)	64	6	57	1
15. Apple (medium)	96	1	86	9
16. Banana (medium)	101	4	95	2
17. Cantaloupe (half)	82	7	73	2
18. Grapefruit (half)	40	2	37	1
19. Celery stick	5	2	3	0
20. Carrot (medium)	20	3	17	0
21. Raisins (4 oz.)	210	6	204	0
22. Watermelon (4" × 6" slice)	115	8	99	8
23. Chocolate chip cookie	60	3	9	48
24. Brownie	145	6	26	113
25. Oatmeal cookie	65	3	13	49
26. Sandwich cookie	200	8	112	80
27. Custard pie (slice)	285	20	188	77
28. Fruit pie (slice)	350	14	259	77
29. Gelatin (4 oz.)	70	4	32	34
30. Fritter (medium)	132	11	54	67
31. Skim milk (8 oz.)	88	36	52	0
32. Diet drink	0	0	0	0
33. Potato chips (small bag)	115	3	39	73
34. Roasted peanuts (1.3 oz.)	210	34	25	151
35. Chocolate candy bar (1 oz.)	145	7	61	77
36. Choc. almond candy bar (1 oz.)	265	38	74	164
37. Saltine cracker	18	1	1	16
38. Popped corn	40	7	33	0
39. Cheese nachos	471	63	194	214

See Note in Appendix C for additional nutrition information on the Web.

Calorie, Fat, Saturated Fat, Cholesterol, and Sodium Content of Selected Fast Food Items

Burger King	calories	total fat	sat. fat	chol.	sodium
Hamburger	320	14	7	45	530
Whopper Jr.	410	23	8	50	520
Whopper	680	39	13	80	940
Chicken sandwich	660	39	11	70	1330
Double cheeseburger	570	34	19	110	1020
Bacon double cheeseburger	780	47	19	105	1390
Double whopper	920	57	22	150	1020
Double whopper with cheese	1020	65	27	170	1460
Fries (small - 2.25 oz)	230	11	60	0	530
Fries (medium - 4 oz)	360	18	10	0	690
Fries (large - 5.5 oz)	500	25	13	0	940
Fries (king - 6 oz)	600	30	16	0	1140
Onion rings (medium - 3.5 oz)	320	16	8	0	460
Onion rings (king - 5.5 oz)	550	27	13	0	N/A
Coca Cola classic (small - 16 oz)	160	0	0	0	N/A
Coca Cola classic (med - 22 oz)	230	0	0	0	N/A
Coca Cola classic (large - 32 oz)	330	0	0	0	N/A
Coca Cola classic (king - 42 oz)	430	0	0	0	N/A
Shake (medium - 14 oz)	460	8	5	30	320
Apple pie	340	14	6	0	470
Sundae pie	310	18	15	10	140

Taco Bell	calories	total fat	sat. fat	chol.	sodium
Chicken fiesta burrito	370	12	4	35	1000
Bean burrito	370	12	4	10	1080
Chili cheese burrito	330	13	5	24	900
Chicken burrito supreme	410	16	6	45	1120
Steak burrito supreme	420	16	6	35	1140
7-layer burrito	520	22	7	25	1270
Grilled stuft chicken burrito	690	29	8	70	1900
Grilled stuft steak burrito	690	30	8	60	1970
Chicken chalupa nacho cheese	350	19	5	25	640
Chicken chalupa baja	400	24	5	40	660
Beef chalupa nacho cheese	370	22	6	25	740
Steak chalupa baja	400	24	6	30	680
Chicken gordita supreme	300	13	5	45	530
Steak gordita supreme	300	14	5	35	550
Beef gordita supreme	300	14	5	35	550
Chicken soft taco	190	7	3	35	480
Beef soft taco	210	10	4	30	570
Steak soft taco	280	17	4	35	630
Taco supreme	260	16	6	40	350
Double decker taco supreme	420	21	8	40	760
Pintos and cheese	180	8	4	15	640
Nachos	320	18	4	5	560
Nachos supreme	440	24	7	35	800
Nachos bell grande	760	39	11	35	1300
Chicken quesadilla	540	30	12	80	1270
Taco salad with salsa	850	52	14	70	2250
Shake (large - 32 oz)	1010	29	19	115	530
Cola (small - 16 oz)	100	0	0	0	10
Cola (medium- 20 oz)	130	0	0	0	10

McDonalds	calories	total fat	sat. fat	chol.	sodium
Hamburger	280	10	4	30	590
Fillet o-fish	470	26	5	50	890
Crispy chicken	550	27	5	50	1180
Cheeseburger	330	14	6	50	830
Quarter pounder	430	21	8	70	840
Big Mac	590	34	11	85	1090
Quarter pounder with cheese	590	30	13	95	1310
French fries (small - 2.5 oz)	210	10	3	0	140
French fries (medium - 5 oz)	450	22	8	0	290
French fries (large - 6 oz)	540	26	9	0	350
French fries (supersize - 7 oz)	610	29	10	0	390
Grilled chicken caesar salad	100	3	2	40	240
Garden salad	100	6	3	75	120
Chef salad	150	8	4	95	740
Caesar dressing	150	13	3	10	400
Thousand island dressing	130	9	2	15	350
Honey mustard	160	11	2	15	260
Coca Cola classic (small - 16 oz)	150	0	0	0	N/A
Coca Cola classic (med - 21 oz)	210	0	0	0	N/A
Coca Cola classic (large - 32 oz)	310	0	0	0	N/A
Coca Cola classic (supersize - 42 oz)	410	0	0	0	N/A
Shake (small -14 oz)	360	9	6	40	230
Hot fudge sundae	340	12	9	30	170
McFlurry	610	22	14	75	250
Shake (large - 32 oz)	1010	29	19	115	530

Wendy's	calories	total fat	sat. fat	chol.	sodium
Grilled chicken sandwich	300	7	2	55	740
Spicy chicken sandwich	410	14	3	65	1280
Chicken breast fillet sandwich	430	16	3	55	750
Chicken club sandwich	470	20	5	65	940
Jr. cheeseburger	310	12	6	45	800
Jr. cheeseburger deluxe	350	16	6	45	800
Jr. bacon cheeseburger	380	19	7	55	870
Classic single with everything	410	19	7	70	920
Big bacon classic	580	30	12	100	1460
Classic double with everything	760	45	19	175	1730
Classic triple with everything	1030	65	29	245	2280
Chicken nuggets	230	16	3	30	470
French fries (small - 3 oz)	270	13	4	0	90
French fries (medium - 5 oz)	420	20	6	0	130
French fries (biggie - 5.5 oz)	470	23	7	0	150
French fries (great biggie - 6.5 oz)	570	27	8	0	180
Plain baked potato	310	0	0	0	30
Chili	210	7	3	30	800
Broccoli and cheese potato	470	14	3	5	470
Bacon and cheese potato	530	17	4	25	820
Cola (small - 16 oz)	100	0	0	0	10
Cola (medium - 20 oz)	130	0	0	0	10
Cola (biggie - 32 oz)	210	0	0	0	20
Frosty (small)	170	4	3	20	100
Frosty (large)	330	8	5	35	200

Values from the Restaurant Confidential by Jacobson and Hurley by the Center for Science in the Public Interest (CPSI). New York: Workman Publishing Company 2002.

Canada's Food Guide to Healthy Eating

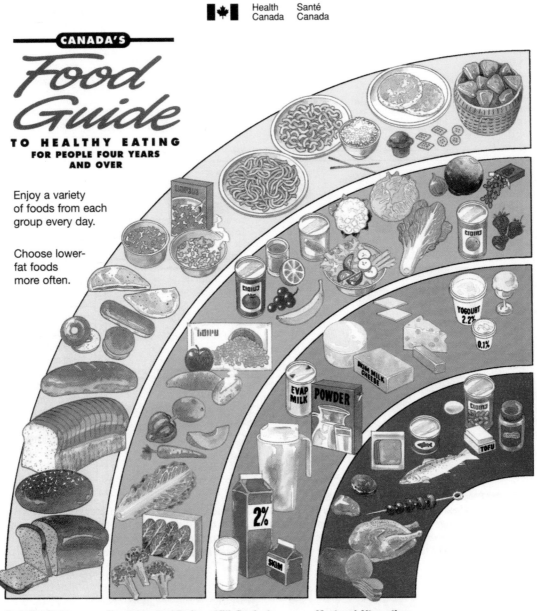

Health Canada / Santé Canada

CANADA'S

Food Guide

TO HEALTHY EATING
FOR PEOPLE FOUR YEARS
AND OVER

Enjoy a variety
of foods from each
group every day.

Choose lower-
fat foods
more often.

Grain Products
Choose whole grain
and enriched
products more often.

Vegetables and Fruit
Choose dark green and
orange vegetables and
orange fruit more often.

Milk Products
Choose lower-fat milk
products more often.

Meat and Alternatives
Choose leaner meats,
poultry and fish, as well
as dried peas, beans
and lentils more often.

Canada

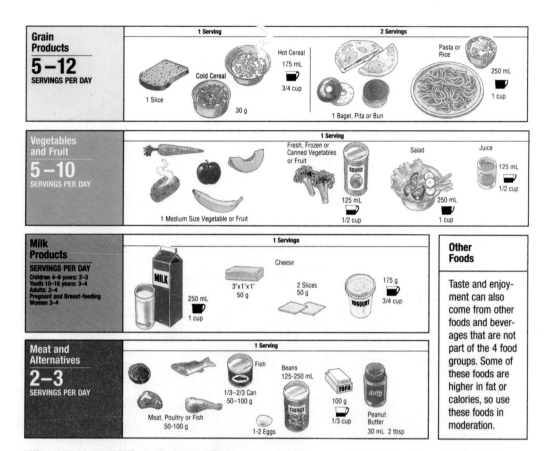

Different People Need Different Amounts of Food

The amount of food you need every day from the 4 food groups and other foods depends on your age, body size, activity level, whether you are male or female and if you are pregnant or breast-feeding. That's why the Food Guide gives a lower and higher number of servings for each food group. For example, young children can choose the lower number of servings, while male teenagers can go to the higher number. Most other people can choose servings somewhere in between.

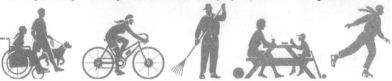

Consult *Canada's Physical Activity Guide to Healthy Active Living* to help you build physical activity into your daily life.

Enjoy eating well, being active and feeling good about yourself. That's VITALIT

© Minister of Public Works and Government Services Canada, 1997
Cat. No. H39-252/1992E   ISBN 0-662-19648-1
No changes permitted. Reprint permission not required.

Selected References

This list includes references new to the fifth edition of Concepts of Fitness and Wellness. *For a complete listing of all references, please go to the Online Learning Center at* **www.mhhe.com/corbin5e.**

Abraham, W. T. et al. 2002. Cardiac resynchronization in chronic heart failure. *New England Journal of Medicine* 346(3): 1845–53.

The Alan Guttmacher Institute. 2001. *Teenagers Sexual and Reproductive Health.* The Alan Guttmacher Institute.

American College of Sports Medicine. 2002. Progression models in resistance training for healthy adults (position stand). *Medicine and Science in Sports and Exercise* 34(2): 364–380.

American College of Sports Medicine, American Dietetics Association, and Dietitians of Canada. 2000. Nutrition and Athletic Performance. *Medicine and Science in Sports and Exercise* 32 (12): 2130–45.

American Council on Education, Center for Policy Analysis. 2002. *Access & Persistence: Findings from 10 Years of Longitudinal Research on Students* Washington, D.C.

American Dietetics Association. *The Health Professional's Guide to Popular Dietary Supplements.* Chicago, IL: American Dietetic Association, 2000.

American Dietetics Association. 2002. Position of the American Dietetics Association: food and nutrition misinformation. *Journal of the American Dietetics Association,* 102(2): 260–69.

American Dietetics Association. 2002. Position of the American Dietetics Association: Weight Management." *Journal of the American Dietetics Association* 102(8): 1145–55.

American Dietetics Association (R. L. Duyff, author). 1998. *The American Dietetic Association's Complete Food and Nutrition Guide.* New York: Wiley.

American Dietetics Association (M. A. Hess, author). 1997. *The Supermarket Guide.* New York: Wiley.

American Dietetics Association (M. Hudnall, author). 1998. *Vitamins, Minerals and Dietary Supplements.* New York: Wiley.

American Dietetics Association (M. Hudnal, author) 1998. *Carbohydrates: What You Need to Know.* New York: Wiley.

Andre-Petersson, L. et al. 2002. Adaptive behavior in stressful situations and stroke incidence in hypertensive men: results from prospective cohort study, men born in 1914 in Malmo, Sweden. *Stroke* 32(8): 1712–20.

Anttila, T. et al. 2001. Serotypes of *Chlamydia trachomatis* and risk for development of cervical squamous cell carcinoma." *JAMA* 285(1): 47–51.

Associated Press. August 15, 2001. "Many Test Late for HIV, Study Suggests." *Arizona Republic.*

Bagnardi, V. et al. 2001. Alcohol consumption and the risk of cancer: a meta-analysis." *Alcohol: Research & Health* 25(4): 263–70.

Baker, F. et al. 2000. Health risks associated with cigar smoking. *JAMA* 284(6): 735–40.

Bar-Or, O. 2000. Juvenile obesity, physical activity, and lifestyle changes. *Physician and Sports Medicine* 28(11): 51+.

Bell, D. G. et al. 2001. Effect of caffeine and ephedrine ingestion on anaerobic exercise performance. *Medicine and Science in Sports and Exercise* 33(8): 1399–403.

Berg, A., and U.S. Preventive Services Task Force. 2001. Screening for chlamydial infection: recommendations and rationale. *American Journal of Preventive Medicine* 20(30): 90–94.

Berland, G. K. et al. 2001. Health information on the internet: accessibility, quality, and readability in english and spanish. *JAMA* 285(20): 2612–21.

Bernardi, L. et al. 2001. Effect of rosary prayer and yoga mantras on autonomic cardiovascular rhythms: comparative study." *British Medical Journal* 323: 1446–49.

Billett, E., and Turner, J. 2001. Phenylethylamine: a possible link to the antidepressant effects of exercise? *British Journal of Sports Medicine.* 35: 342–43.

Blair, S. N. 2001. Guest editorial to accompany physical fitness and activity as separate heart disease risk factors. *Medicine and Science in Sports and Exercise* 33(5): 762–64.

Blair, S. N. et al. 2001. *Active Living Every Day.* Champaign, IL: Human Kinetics.

Blair, S. N., and Jackson, A. S. 2001. A guest editorial to accompany physical fitness and activity as separate heart disease risk factors: a meta-analysis. *Medicine and Science in Sports and Exercise* 33(5): 762–64.

Blanck, H. M. et al. 2001. The use of nonprescription weight loss products: results from a multistate survey." *JAMA* 286: 930–35.

Blendon, R. J. et al. 2001. Americans' views on the use and regulation of dietary supplements. *Archives of Internal Medicine* 161(6): 805–10.

Booth, F. W., and M. W. Chakravarthy. 2002. Cost and consequences of sedentary living: new battleground for an old enemy." *President's Council on Physical Fitness and Sports* 3(16)(2002): 1–8.

Bouchard, C. "Physical Activity and Health: Introduction to the Dose-response symposium." *Medicine and Science in Sports and Exercise* 33(6)(supplement): S347–50.

Brandon, L. J. et al. 2000. Strength training for older adults." *ACSM's Health and Fitness Journal* 4(6): 13–28.

Brehm, B. A. 2000. Maximizing the psychological benefits of physical activity. *ACSM's Health and Fitness Journal* 4(6): 7–11.

Breslau, N. et al. 2001. Nicotine dependence in the United States: prevalence, trends, and smoking persistence. *Archives of General Psychiatry* 58(9): 810–16.

Broocks, A. et al. 1998. Comparison of aerobic exercise, clomipramine, and placebo in the treatment of panic disorder. *American Journal of Psychiatry* 155(5): 603–09.

Browning, K. H. 2001. Hip and pelvic injuries in runners. *Physician and Sports Medicine* 29(1): 23+.

Bryant, C. X. et al. 2001. High-protein, low carbohydrate diets: fact vs. fiction." *Fitness Management* 17(12): 40–45.

Burke, E. et al. 2000. *Long-Distance Cycling: Build the Strength, Skills and Confidence to Ride as Far as You Want.* Emmaus, PA: Rodale Press.

Carver, C. S., and M. F. Scheier, 2002. Optimism. In Snyder, C. R., and S. J. Lopez, *Handbook of Positive Psychology.* New York: Oxford University Press.

Catlin, D. H. et al. 2000. Trace contamination of over-the-counter androstenedione and positive urine test results for a nandrolone metabolite." *JAMA* 284(20): 2618–21.

Cauchon, D. August 24, 2001. Marijuana attains record support. *USA Today.*

Centers for Disease Control and Prevention. 2000. *Measuring Healthy Days.* Atlanta, GA: CDC.

Centers for Disease Control and Prevention. 20001. *HIV/AIDS Surveillance Report* 13(1).

Centers for Disease Control and Prevention. 2002. Trends in cigarette smoking among high school students—United States." *Morbidity and Mortality Weekly Reports* 51(19): 409–12

Centers for Disease Control and Prevention. 2002. Annual smoking-attributable mortality, years of potential life lost, and economic costs—United States." *Morbidity and Mortality Weekly Reports* 51(14): 300–03.

Centers for Disease Control and Prevention. 2001. *Morbidity and Mortality Weekly Report: HIV Testing Among Racial/Ethnic Minorities—United States, 1999.* Atlanta, GA: Centers for Disease Control and Prevention.

Centers for Disease Control and Prevention. 2000. Prevalence of leisure-time physical activity among overweight adults—United States 1998." *Morbidity and Mortality Weekly Report* 49(15): 326–30.

Chintanadilok, J., and D. T. Lowenthal, 2002. Exercise in treating hypertension. *Physician and Sports Medicine* 30(3): 11–28.

Chong, D. L., and S. N. Blair, 2002. "Cardiorespiratory fitness and smoking-related and total cancer mortality in men." *Medicine and Science in Sports and Exercise* 34(5): 735–39.

Chrusch, M. et al. 2001. Creatine supplementation combined with resistance exercise in older men." *Medicine and Science in Sports and Exercise* 33(12): 2111–17.

Colberg, S. R. 2001. Exercise: a diabetes 'cure' for many. *ACSM's Health and Fitness Journal* 5(2): 20–26.

Coleman, E. 2000. AHA dietary guidelines." *Sports Medicine Digest* 22: 133. www.sportsmeddigest.com

Community Epidemiology Work Group. 2001. *Epidemiologic Trends in Drug Abuse, Volume 1: Highlights and Executive Summary.* Bethesda, MD: National Institute on Drug Abuse.

Cooper, C. B. 2001. Diabetes mellitus and exercise. *ACSM's Health and Fitness Journal* 5(4): 27–28.

Corbin, W. R., and K. Fromme. 2002. Alcohol use and serial monogamy as risks for sexually transmitted diseases in young adults. *Health Psychology* 21(3): 229–36.

Cotman, C. W., and C. Engesser-Cesar. 2002. Exercise enhances and protects brain runction. *Exercise and Sport Sciences Reviews* 30(2): 75–79.

Courneya, K. S. 2001. Exercise interventions during cancer treatment. *Exercise and Sports Sciences Reviews* 29(2): 60–64.

Courneya, K. S. et al. 2000. Social support and the theory of planned behavior in the exercise domain. *American Journal of Health Behavior* 24: 300–08.

Couture, C. J., and K. A. Karlson 2002. Tibial stress injuries. *Physician and Sports Medicine* 30(6): 29–36.

Criswell, L. A. et al. 2002. Cigarette smoking and the risk of rheumatoid arthritis among postmenopausal women: results from the Iowa Women's Health Study. *American Journal of Medicine* 112(6): 465–71.

Czikszentmihalyi, M. 2002. Television Addiction Is No Mere Metaphor. *Scientific American*

Dagnone, R. R. et al. 2000. Reduction in obesity and related comorbid conditions after diet-induced weight loss or exercise-induced weight loss in men. *Annals of Internal Medicine* 133(2): 92–103.

Davis, M. et al. 2000. *The Relaxation and Stress Reduction Workbook* (5th ed.). Oakland, CA: New Harbinger.

Dawson, D. A., and B. F. Grant. 1998. Family history of alcoholism and gender: their combined effects on DSM-IV alcohol dependence and major depression. *Journal of Studies on Alcohol* 59(1): 97–106.

Deci, E. L., and R. M. Ryan, (Eds.). 2002. *Handbook of Self-Determination Research.* Rochester, NY: University of Rochester Press.

Derby, C. A. et al. 2000. Modifiable risk factors and erectile dysfunction: can lifestyle changes modify risk?" *Urology* 56(2): 302–06.

Diener, E., R. E. Lucas, and S. Oishi. 2002. Subjective well-being: the science of happiness and life satisfaction. In Snyder, C. R., and S. J. Lopez. *Handbook of Positive Psychology.* New York: Oxford University Press.

DiPietro, L. 1999. Physical activity in the prevention of obesity: current evidence and research issues." *Medicine and Science in Sports & Exercise* 31: S542–46.

Dowling, E. A. 2001. How exercise affects lipid profiles of women." *Physician and Sports Medicine* 29(9): 45–52.

Drezner, J. A., and S. A. Herring. 2001. Managing low back pain. *Physician and Sports Medicine* 29(8): 37–43.

Dufek, J. S. 2002. Exercise variability: a prescription for overuse injury prevention. *ACSM's Health and Fitness Journal* 6(4): 18–23.

Dufour, M. C., F. S. Stinson, and M. F. Caces. 1993. Trends in cirrhosis morbidity and mortality: United States, 1979–1988." *Seminars in Liver Disease* 13(2): 109–25.

Duncan, C. S. et al. 2002. Bone mineral density in adolescent female athletes: relationship to exercise type and muscle strength. *Medicine and Science in Sports and Exercise* 34(2): 286–94.

Durek, E. 2001. The use of exercise in the cancer recovery process. *ACSM's Health and Fitness Journal* 5(1): 6–10.

Edwards, K. J. 2001. Stress, negative social exchange, and health symptoms in university students. *Journal of American College Health* 50(2): 57–80.

Eickhoff-Shemek, J. 2002. Exercise equipment injuries: who's at fault? *ACSM's Health and Fitness Journal* 6(1): 27–30.

Ettinger, W. H., R. Burns, and S. P. Messier. 1997. A randomized trial comparing aerobic exercise and resistance exercise with a health education program in older adults with knee osteoarthritis: the fitness arthritis and seniors trial (FAST). *JAMA* 277(1): 25–31.

Executive Office of the President, Office of National Drug Control Policy. 2001. *The Economic Costs of Drug Abuse in the United States, 1992–1998.* Washington, DC: Office of National Drug Control Policy.

Expert Panel on Detection, Evaluation and Treatment of High Blood Cholesterol in Adults. 2001. Executive summary of the NCEP expert panel on detection, evaluation and treatment of high blood cholesterol in adults. *JAMA* 285: 2486–97.

Fairfield, K. M., and R. H. Fletcher. 2002. Vitamins for chronic disease prevention in adults: scientific review. *JAMA* 287(23): 3116–26.

Fetrow, C. W., and J. R. Avila. 1999. *Professional Handbook of Alternative Medicines.* Springhouse, PA: Springhouse Publications.

Fink, G. (Ed.). 2000. *Encyclopedia of Stress.* San Diego, CA: Academic Press.

Fiore, M. C. et al. 2000. Clinical practice guideline for treating tobacco use and dependence: A U. S. Public Health Service Report. JAMA 283(24): 3244.

Fischer, P. M. et al. 1991. Brand logo recognition by children aged 3 to 6 years: Mickey Mouse and Old Joe the Camel. *JAMA* 266(22): 3145–48.

Fletcher, R. H., and K. M. Fairfield. 2002. Vitamins for chronic disease prevention in adults: clinical applications. *JAMA* 287(23): 3127–30.

Fletcher, S. W., and G. A. Colditz. 2002. Failure of estrogen plus progestin therapy for prevention. *JAMA* 288(3): 368–71.

Food and Nutrition Board Institute of Medicine. 2001. *Dietary Reference Intakes:* Vitamin A, Vitamin K, Arsenic, Boron, Chromium, Copper, Iodine, Iron, Manganese, Moybdenum, Nickel, Silicon, Vanadium, and Zinc. Washington, DC: National Academy Press.

Francis, P. R. et al. 2001. An electromyographic approach to the evaluation of abdominal exercises. *ACSM's Health and Fitness Journal* 5(4): 8–14.

Frank, J. W. et al. 1996. Disability resulting from occupational low back pain. *Spine* 21: 2908–17.

Franklin, B. A. 2001. Lifestyle activity: a new paradigm for exercise prescription. *ACSM's Health and Fitness Journal* 5(4): 33–35.

Frankovich, R. J. et al. 2001. Inline skating injuries. *Physician and Sports Medicine* 29(4): 57–64.

Franks, B. D., E. T. Howley, and Y. Iyriboz. 1999. *The Health Fitness Handbook.* Champaign, IL: Human Kinetics.

Fredrickson, B. L. 2002. Positive emotion. In Snyder, C. R., and S. J. Lopez. *Handbook of Positive Psychology.* New York: Oxford University Press.

Fried, P. et al. 2002. Current and former marijuana use: preliminary findings of a longitudinal study of effects on IQ in young adults. *Canadian Medical Association Journal* 166(7): 887–91.

Friedenreich, C. M. et al. 2001. Relation between intensity of physical activity and breast cancer risk reduction. *Medicine and Science in Sports and Exercise* 33(9): 1538–45.

Friedland, R. P. 2001. Activity and Alzheimers. *Proceedings of the National Academy of Sciences.* 98: 3440–45.

Frumkin, H. In press. Urban sprawl and public health." *Public Health Reports.* (117).

Furr, S. R. 2001. Suicide and depression among college students: a decade later. *Professional Psychology—Research & Practice* 32(1): 97–100.

Gabel, K. A., and R. J. Lund. 2002. Weight loss at a cost: implications of high-protein, low carbohydrate diets. *Journal of Physical Education Recreation and Dance* 73(2)(2002): 18–21.

Gardner, A. W. 2001. Exercise for patients with peripheral artery disease. *Physician and Sports Medicine.* 29(8): 25–36.

Glantz, S. A, & P. Jamieson. 2000. Attitudes toward secondhand smoke, smoking, and quitting among young people. *Pediatrics* 106(6): e82.

Golderberg, L., and P. Twist. 2001. *Strength Ball Training: Sixty-Nine Exercises Using Swiss Balls and Medicine Ball.* Champaign IL: Human Kinetics.

Goodman, W. C. 2002. *The Invisible Woman: Confronting Weight Prejudice in America.* Carlsbad, CA: Gurze Books.

Goran, M. I. et al. 2002. Impaired glucose tolerance in obese children and adolescents. *New England Journal of Medicine* 347(11): 290–92.

Gordon, P. M. et al. 2000. The quantity and quality of physical activity among those trying to lose weight. *American Journal of Preventive Medicine* 18(1): 83–86.

Gotshalk, L. A. et al. 2002. Creatine supplementation improves muscular performance in older men. *Medicine and Science in Sports and Exercise* 34(3): 537–43.

Grant, R. M. et al. 2002. Time trends in primary HIV-1 drug resistance among recently infected persons. *JAMA* 288 (2): 181–88.

Greenfeld, L. A. 1998. *Alcohol and Crime: An Analysis of National Data on the Prevalence Alcohol Involvement in Crime.* Report prepared for the Assistant Attorney General's National Symposium on Alcohol Abuse and Crime, NCJ 168–632. Washington, DC: U.S. Department of Justice.

Haller, C. A., and N. L. Benowitz. 2001. Adverse cardiovascular and central nervous system events associated with dietary supplements containing ephedra alkaloids. *New England Journal of Medicine* 343(25): 1833–38.

Hamrick, N., S. Cohen, and M. S. Rodriguez. 2002. Being popular can be healthy or unhealthy: stress, social network fiversity, and incidence of upper respiratory infection. *Health Psychology* 21(3): 294–98.

Harwood, H. 2000. *Updating Estimates of the Economic Costs of Alcohol Abuse in the United States: Estimates, Update Methods, and Data.* Report prepared by the Lewin Group for the National Institute on Alcohol Abuse and Alcoholism.

Hedelin, R. et al. 2000. Short-term overtraining: effects on performance, circulatory responses, and heart rate variability. *Medicine and Science in Sports and Exercise* 32(8): 1480–84.

Hedelin, R. et al. 2000. Cardiac autonomic imbalance in an overtrained athlete. *Medicine and Science in Sports and Exercise* 32(9): 1531–33.

Herning, R. I. et al. 2001. Marijuana abusers are at increased risk for stroke: preliminary evidence from cerebrovascular refusion data. *Annals of the New York Academy of Sciences* 939: 413–15.

Hockenbury, T., and G. J. Sammarco. 2001. Evaluation and treatment of ankle sprains. *Physician and Sports Medicine* 29(2): 57–64.

Hogg, R. S. et al. 2001. Rates of disease progression by baseline CD4 cell count and viral load after initiating triple-drug therapy. *JAMA* 286(20): 2568–77.

Hohl, C. M. et al. 2001. Polypharmacy, adverse drug-related events, and potential adverse drug interactions in elderly patients presenting to an emergency department. *Annals of Emergency Medicine* 38(6): 666–71.

Hootman, J. M. et al. 2002. Epidemiology of musculoskeletal injuries among sedentary and physically active adults. *Medicine and Science in Sports and Exercise* 34(5): 838–44.

Hoyert, D. et al. 2001. *National Vital Statistics Reports, Deaths: Final Data for 1999*. Hyattsville, MD: Centers for Disease Control and Prevention.

Hunter, G. R. et al. 2001. High-resistance versus variable-resistance training in older adults. *Medicine and Science in Sports and Exercise* 33(10): 1759–64.

Hunter, J. P., and R. N. Marshall. 2002. Effects of power and flexibility training on vertical jump technique. *Medicine and Science in Sports and Exercise* 34(3): 478–86.

Institute of Medicine. 2001. *Clearing the Smoke: Assessing the Science Base for Tobacco Harm Reduction*. Washington, DC: National Academy Press.

Jacobson, M. F., and J. Hurley. 2002. *Restaurant Confidential*. New York: Workman Publishing.

Jebb, S. A., and M. S. Moore. 1999. Contribution of a sedentary lifestyle and inactivity to the etiology of overweight and obesity: current evidence and research issues. *Medicine & Science in Sports and Exercise* 31: S534–41.

Jenkins, D. A. et al. 2002. Glycemic index: overview of implications in health and disease. *American Journal of Clinical Nutrition* 76: 266S–273S.

Jenkins, D. J. A., C. W. C. Kendall, V. Vuksan, et al. 2002. Soluble fiber intake at a dose approved by the U.S. Food and Drug Administration for a claim of health benefits: serum lipid risk factors for cardiovascular disease assessed in a randomized controlled crossover trial." *American Journal of Clinical Nutrition* 75: 834–39.

Johnston, M. I., and J. Flores. 2001. Progress in HIV vaccine development. *Current Opinion in Pharmacology* 1: 504–10.

Jonas, S. 2001. Weighing in on the obesity epidemic: what do we do now? *ACSM's Health and Fitness Journal* 5(5): 7–10.

Juniu, S. 2002. Implementing handheld computing technology in physical education. *Journal of Physical Education, Recreation and Dance* 73(3): 43–48.

Karnath, B. 2002. Smoking cessation. *American Journal of Medicine* 112(5): 399–40.

Katsanos, C. S. et al. 2001. Exercise expenditure relative to perceived exertion: stationary cycling and treadmill walking. 72(2): 176–81.

Katzmarzyk, P. T., and L. C. Cora. 2002. Musculoskeletal fitness and risk of mortality. *Medicine and Science in Sports and Exercise* 34(5): 740–744.

Kayne, S. B., K. Wadeson., and A. MacAdam. 2000. Is glucosamine an effective treatment for osteoarthritis? a meta-analysis. *Pharmaceutical Journal* 265: 759–63.

Kenny, D. T. et al. (Eds.). 2002. *Stress and Health: Research and Clinical Applications*. Amsterdam, Netherlands: Harwood Academic Publishers.

Kesaniemi, Y. A. et al. 2001. Dose-response issues concerning physical activity and health. *Medicine and Science in Sports and Exercise*. 33(6)(supplement): S347–50.

Kestenbaum, R. 2001. *The Ultralight Backpacker: The Complete Guide to Simplicity and Comfort on the Trail*. St. Louis: McGraw-Hill.

Keyes, C. L., and S. J. Lopez. 2002. Toward a Science of Mental Health." In Snyder, C. R., and Lopez, S. J. *Handbook of Positive Psychology*. New York: Oxford University Press.

Khan K. M., T. Liu-Ambrose, M. M. Sran et al. 2002. New criteria for female athlete triad syndrome? As osteoporosis is rare, should osteopenia be among the criteria for defining the female athlete triad syndrome? *British Journal of Sports Medicine* 36(1): 10–13.

King, D. S. et.al. 1999. Effect of oral androstenedione on serum testosterone and adaptations to resistance training in young men: a randomized controlled trial. *JAMA* 281: 2020–28.

King, J. M. 2001. The evolution of strength training equipment. *Fitness Management* July 7: 46–51.

Knudson, D. V., P. Magnusson, and M. McHugh. 2000. Current issues in flexibility fitness. *President's Council on Physical Fitness and Sports Research Digest* 3(10): 1–8.

Krauss, D. 2000. *Mastering Your Inner Game*. Champaign, IL: Human Kinetics.

Krauss R. M. et al. 2000.AHA dietary guidelines revision 2000: a statement for health-care professionals from the nutrition committee of the American Heart Association. *Circulation* 102: 2284–99.

Kruskall, L. J. et al. 2002. Eating disorders and disordered eating—are they the same? *ACSM's Health and Fitness Journal* 6(3): 6–12.

Kubzansky, L. D. et al. 2001. Is the glass half empty or half full? A prospective study of optimism and coronary heart disease in the normative aging study. *Psychosomatic Medicine* 63: 910–16.

Lacey, J. V. et al. 2002. Menopausal hormone replacement therapy and risk of ovarian cancer. *JAMA* 288(3): 334–41.

Larimer, M. E., and J. M. Cronce. 2002. Identification, prevention and treatment: a review of individual-focused strategies to reduce problematic alcohol consumption by college students. *Journal of Studies on Alcohol* Supplement No. 14: 148–63.

Lee, I. M., and S. N. Blair. 2002. Cardiorespiratory fitness and stroke mortality in men. *Medicine and Science in Sports and Exercise*.34(4): 592–95.

Lee, I. M., and R. S. Paffenbarger. 2001. Preventing coronary heart disease. *Physician and Sports Medicine* 29(2): 37–47.

Leinwand, D. October 5, 2000. Ecstasy knockoff blamed in nine deaths in Illinois, Florida." *USA Today*.

Leinwand, D. July 20, 2001. Studies show ecstasy can damage brain." *USA Today*.

Li, R. et al. 2000. Trends in fruit and vegetable consumption among adults in the United States. *American Journal of Public Health* 90: 777–81.

Liebman, B. 2002. Anti-oxidants: no magic bullets. *Nutrition Action Health Letter* 29(3): 1–6.

Locke, E. A. 2002. Setting goals for life and happiness. In Snyder, C. R., and S. J. Lopez. *Handbook of Positive Psychology*. New York: Oxford University Press.

Lonczak, R. D. 2002. Effects of the Seattle social development project on sexual behavior, pregnancy, birth, and sexually transmitted disease outcomes by age 21 years." *Archives of Pediatrics & Adolescent Medicine* 156(5): 438–47.

Long, J., and M. Hodgson. 200. *The Complete Hiker* (2nd ed.). St. Louis: McGraw-Hill.

Lovett, R. 2001. *The Essential Touring Cyclist: A Complete Guide for the Bicycle Traveler* (2nd ed.). St. Louis: McGraw-Hill.

Lovett, R., and P. Petersen. 2000. *The Essential Cross-Country Skier.* St. Louis: McGraw-Hill.

Mackey, R. H. et al. 2002. Correlates of aortic stiffness in elderly individuals: a subgroup of the cardiovascular health study. *American Journal of Hypertension.* 15(1): 16–23.

Maddux, J. E. 2002. Self-efficacy: the power of believing you can. In Snyder, C. R., and S. J. Lopez. *Handbook of Positive Psychology.* New York: Oxford University Press.

Mandelblatt, J. S. et al. 2002. Benefits and costs of using HPV testing to screen for cervical cancer. *JAMA* 287(18): 2372–81.

Manore, M. M. 2002. Carbohydrate: friend or foe? part 1. *ACSM's Health and Fitness Journal* 6(1): 33–35.

Manore, M. M. 2002. Carbohydrate: friend or foe? part 2. *ACSM's Health and Fitness Journal* 6(3): 26–29.

Manwell, L. B. et al. 1998. Tobacco, alcohol, and drug use in a primary care sample: 90-day prevalence and associated factors. *Journal of Addictive Diseases* 17(1): 67–81.

Marcus, B. H. et al. 2000. Physical activity behavior change: issues in adoption and maintenance. *Health Psychology* 19(1): 32–41.

McAlindon, T. 2001. Glusoamine for osteoarthritis: dawn of a new era? *Lancet* 357(9252): 247–53.

McClean, J. A. et al. 2001. Dietary restraint, exercise, and bone density in young women: are they related? *Medicine and Science in Sports and Exercise* 33(8): 1292–96.

McGill, S. M. 2001. Low back stability: from formal description to issues for performance and rehabilitation. *Exercise and Sports Science Reviews* 29(1): 26–31.

McLester, J. R., and P. Bishop. 2000. Comparison of 1 day and 3 days per week of equal-volume resistance training in

experienced subjects. *The Journal of Strength and Conditioning Research* 14(3): 273–81.

Meacham, S. L. et al. 2002. Nutrition suggestions for the cancer survivor. *ACSM's Health and Fitness Journal* 6(1): 6–12.

Medicine and Science in Sports and Exercise. 2001. "Dose-response issues concerning physical activity and health: an evidence-based symposium. *Medicine and Science in Sports and Exercise* 33(6).

Mei, Z., L. M. Grummer-Strawn, and A. Pietrobelli, et al. 2002. Validity of body mass index compared with other body-composition screening indexes for the assessment of body composition in children and adolescents. *American Journal of Clinical Nutrition* 75: 978–85.

Metcalf, L. et al. 2001. Postmenopausal women and exercise for prevention of osteoporosis. *ACSM's Health and Fitness Journal* 5(3): 6–14.

Meyers, J. et al. 2002. Exercise capacity and mortality among men referred for exercise therapy. *New England Journal of Medicine* 346(11): 793–801.

Miller, L. 2000. *Advanced Inline Skating.* St. Louis: McGraw-Hill.

Miller, L. 1998. *Get Rolling: A Beginner's Guide to Inline Skating* (2nd ed.). St. Louis: McGraw-Hill.

MMWR. 2001. Physical activity trends in the US. *Morbidity and Mortality Weekly Reports* 50(9): 166+.

MMWR. 2000. Prevalence of leisure-time and occupational physical activity trends among adults. *Morbidity and Mortality Weekly Reports* 49(19): 20+.

Mondloch, M. V., D. C. Cole and J. W. Frank. 2001. Does how you do depend on how you think you'll do? A systematic review of the evidence for a relation between patients' recovery expectations and health outcomes. *Canadian Medical Association Journal* 165(2): 174–79.

Moreau, K. L. 2001. Increasing daily walking lowers blood pressure in postmenopausal women. *Medicine and Science in Sports and Exercise* 33(11): 1825–31.

Moreno, V. et al. 2002. Effect of oral contraceptives on risk of cervical cancer in women with human papillomavirus infection: the IARC multicentric case-control study." *Lancet* 359(9312): 1085–92.

Morgan, J. F. 2000. From charles atlas to adonis complex: fat is more than a feminist issue. *Lancet* 356: 1372–73.

Mueller, D. 2002. Yoga Therapy. *ACSM's Health and Fitness Journal* 6(1): 18–24.

Murray, R. P. et al. 2002. Longitudinal analysis of the relationship between changes in smoking and changes in drinking in a community sample: the winnipeg health and drinking survey. *Health Psychology* 21(3): 237–43.

Nakamura, J., and M. Csikszentmihilyi. 2002. The concept of flow. In Snyder, C. R., and S. J. Lopez. *Handbook of Positive Psychology* New York: Oxford University Press.

National College Health Assessment. 2000. *NCHA Spring 2000 Reference Group Executive Summary.* Baltimore, MD: ACHA.

National Highway Traffic Safety Administration. 2002. *2001 Early Assessment of Motor Vehicle Traffic Crashes.* Washington, DC: National Highway Traffic Safety Administration, National Center for Statistics and Analyses.

National Institute of Allergy and Infectious Diseases. 2002. *HIV HIV/AIDS Statistics.* Bethesda, MD: National Institutes of Health.

National Institute of Allergy and Infectious Diseases. January 10, 2002. The SMART way to fight AIDS. *NIAID News.*

National Institute of Allergy and Infectious Diseases. 2002. *Treatment of HIV.* Bethesda, MD: National Institutes of Health.

National Institute on Drug Abuse. 2002. *Marijuana Infofax.* Bethesda, MD: NIDA.

National Institute on Drug Abuse. 2001. *Monitoring the Future: National Results on Adolescent Drug Use.* Bethesda, MD: NIDA.

National Institute of Drug Abuse. Revised April 2000. *Research Report-Steroid Abuse and Addiction.* Bethesda, MD: NIDA, 2000, Publication No. 00–3721.

National Institutes of Health. 2002. Osteoporosis prevention, diagnosis, and therapy." *NIH Consensus Statements.* 17(1): 1–45.

National Institutes of Health, National Heart, Lung and Blood Institute. 1998. *Clinical Guidelines for the Identification, Evaluation, and Treatment of Overweight and Obesity in Adults.* Washington, DC: National Institutes of Health. Available at www.nhlbi.nih.gov.

Neiman, D. C. 2000. Exercise soothes arthritis: joint effects. *ACSM's Health and Fitness Journal* 4(3): 20–27.

Nelson, T. F., and H. Wechsler. 2001. Alcohol and College Athletes. *Medicine and Science in Sports and Exercise* 33(1): 43–47.

Nguyen T. T., L. C. Dale, K. von Bergmann, and I. T. Croghan. 1999. Cholesterol-lowering effect of stanol ester in a U.S. population of mildly hypercholesterolemic men and women: a randomized controlled trial. *Mayo Clinic Proceedings* 74(12): 1198–206.

Office of the Surgeon General. 2001. *The Surgeon General's Call to Action: Prevent and Decrease Overweight and Obesity.* Washington, DC: Superintendent of Documents, U.S. Government Printing Office.

Olivaridia, R. et al. 2000. Muscle dysmorphia in male weight lifters. *American Journal of Psychiatry* 157: 1291–96.

Olson, J. 2001. Millennium trails: honor the past, imagine the future. *Journal of Physical Education, Recreation and Dance* 72(1): 23–26.

Otsuka, R et al. 2001. Acute effects of passive smoking on the coronary circulation in healthy young adults. *JAMA* 286: 436–41.

Page, S. January 28, 2002. Date rape drug GHB making inroads in nations club scene. *USA Today.*

Panel on Clinical Practices for Treatment of HIV Infection. 2002. *Guidelines for the Use of Antiretroviral Agents in HIV-Infected Adults and Adolescents.* Washington, DC: Department of Health and Human Services and the Henry J. Kaiser Family Foundation.

Pargament, K. I., and A. Manhoney. 2002. "Spirituality: discovering and conserving the sacred. In Snyder, C. R., and S. J. Lopez. *Handbook of Positive Psychology.* New York: Oxford University Press.

Paterson, R. J. 2000. *The Assertiveness Workbook: How to Express Your Ideas and Stand Up for Yourself at Work and in Relationships.* Oakland, CA: New Harbinger Publications, Inc.

Petricoin, E. F. et al. 2002. Use of proteomic patterns in serum to identify ovarian cancer. *Lancet* 359(9306): 572–579.

Phillips, A. N. et al. 2001. Swiss HIV cohort study: Frankfurt HIV clinic cohort. EuroSIDA study group: HIV ciral load response to antiretroviral rherapy according to the baseline CD4 cell count and viral load. *JAMA* 286(20): 2560–67.

Physician and Sports Medicine. 2002. New formula for estimates of maximal heart rate. *Physician and Sports Medicine* 29(7): 13–14.

Pi Sunyer, F. X. 2002. Glycemic index and disease. *American Journal of Clinical Nutrition* 76: 290S–298S.

Pope, H., and D. Yurgilun-Todd. 1996. The residual cognitive effects of heavy marijuana use in college students. *JAMA* 275(7): 521–27.

Pryor, E. 2000. *Keep Moving: Fitness Through Aerobics and Step* (4th ed.). St. Louis: McGraw-Hill.

Putnam, R. 2000. *Bowling Alone: The Collapse and Revival of the American Community.* New York: Simon & Schuster.

Quittner, J. July 24, 2000. High-tech walking. *Time* 77.

Rabin, B. S. 1999. *Stress, Immune Function, and Health: The Connection.* New York: NY: Wiley-Liss.

Rasmussen, B. B., E. Volpi, D. C. Gore, and R. R. Wolfe. 2000. "Androstenedione does not stimulate muscle protein anabolism in young healthy men. *Journal of Clinical Endocrinology and Metabolism* 85: 55–59.

Reneman, L. et al. 2001. Effects of dose, sex, and long-term abstention from Use on toxic effects of MDMA (ecstasy) on brain serotonin neurons. *Lancet* 358(9296): 1864–69.

Rhodes, R. E. et al. 2002. Extending the theory of planned behavior to the exercise domain. *Research Quarterly for Exercise and Sport* 73(2): 193–99.

Rigotti, N. A., J. E. Lee, and H. Wechsler. 2000. U.S. college students' use of tobacco products: results of a national survey. *JAMA* 284(6): 699–705.

Ritter, J. April 6, 2001. Ads linked to rise in rate of HIV infections. *USA Today.*

Roberts, G. 2001. *Advances in Motivation in Sports and Exercise.* Champaign, IL: Human Kinetics.

Robinson, J. June 11, 2002. Teen's view offers insight into the obesity epidemic. *Gallup Tuesday Briefing.*

Rockwell, J. A. et al. 2001. Creatine supplementation affects muscle creatine during energy restriction. *Medicine and Science in Sports and Exercise* 33(1): 61–68.

Roizen, M. F., and E. A. Stephenson. April 1, 2000. Want to live longer? here's exactly how! *Prevention.*

Rutherford, M. et al. November 13, 2000. Pal power: if friends are gifts we give

ourselves, it's good to be greedy. Hold on to what you've got and grab some more. *Time.*

Rutledge, T. et al. 2002. Psychosocial variables are associated with atherosclerosis risk factors among women with chest pain: the WISE study. *Psychosomatic Medicine* 63(2): 282–288.

Ryan, M. 1999. *Complete Guide to Sports Nutrition.* VeloPress.

Ryan, R. M., and E. L. Deci. 2000. Self-determination theory and the facilitation of intrinsic motivation, social development, and well-being. *American Psychologist* 55: 68–78.

Sacker, I. M., and M. A. Zimmer. 2002. *Dying to Be Thin: Understanding and Defeating Anorexia Nervosa and Bulimia-A Practical, Lifesaving Guide.* New York: Time-Warner Bookmark.

Sanborn C. F., M. Horea, B. J. Siemers et al. 2000. Disordered eating and the female athlete triad. *Clinics in Sports Medicine* 19(2): 199–213.

Schilling, B. K. et al. 2001. Creatine supplementation and health variables. *Medicine and Science in Sports and Exercise* 33(2): 183–188.

Schlosser, E. 2001. *Fast Food Nation: The Dark Side of the All-American Meal.* New York: Houghton Mifflin.

Schmidt, W. D., C. J. Biwer, and L. K. Kalscheuer. 2001. Effects of long- versus short-bout exercise on fitness and weight loss in overweight females. *Journal of the American College of Nutrition* 20(5): 497–501.

Schniffing, L. 2001. Can exercise gadgets motivate patients? *The Physician and Sports Medicine.* 29(1): 15–18.

Schnirring, L. 2001. New formula estimates maximal heart rate. *The Physician and Sports Medicine* 29(7): 13–14.

Schwellnus, M. P. 1999. Skeletal muscle cramps during exercise. *The Physician and Sports Medicine* 27(12): 1019.

Seligman, M. E. P. 2002. Positive psychology, positive prevention, and positive therapy. In Snyder, C. R., and S. J. Lopez. *Handbook of Positive Psychology* New York: Oxford University Press.

Seward, B. L. 2001. *Health and the Human Spirit* Boston: Allyn and Bacon.

Shapiro, S. L. et al. 2002. Meditation and positive psychology. In Snyder, C. R., and S. J. Lopez. *Handbook of Positive Psychology.* New York: Oxford University Press.

Sharp, M. A. et al. 2002. Comparison of the physical fitness of men and women entering the U.S. Army: 1978–1998. *Medicine and Science in Sports and Exercise* 34(2): 356–63.

Shelton, D. L. April 10, 2000. Men avoid physician visits, often do not know whom to see. *AmedNews,* www.amednews.com.

Shepard, R. J. 2001. Exercise in the Heat. *The Physician and Sports Medicine* 29(6): 21–31.

Shiver, J. W. et al. 2002. Replication-incompetent adenoviral vaccine vector elicits effective anti-immunodeficiency-virus immunity. *Nature* 415(6869): 331–35.

Short, K. R., and M. J. Joyner. 2002. Activity, obesity, and Type II Diabetes. *Exercise and Sport Sciences Reviews* 30(2): 51–52.

Sidman, C. L. 2002. Count your steps to health and fitness. *ACSM's Health and Fitness Journal* 6(1): 13–17.

Simon, A. M. et al. 2002. Cyclo-oxygenase-2 function is essential for bone fracture healing. *Journal of Bone and Mineral Research* 17(6): 963–76.

Singletary, K. W., and S. M. Gapstur. 2001. Alcohol and breast cancer: review of epidemiologic and experimental evidence and potential mechanisms. *JAMA* 286(17): 2143–51.

Sinha, R. et al. 2002. Prevalence of impaired glucose tolerance among children and adolescents with marked obesity. *New England Journal of Medicine* 346(4): 802–10.

Skurnick, J. H. et al. 2002. Correlates of nontransmission in U. S. women at high tisk of human immunodeficiency virus type 1 infection through sexual exposure. *The Journal of Infectious Diseases* 185: 428–38.

Slattery, M. L., and J. D. Potter. 2002. Physical activity and colon cancer. *Medicine and Science in Sports and Exercise* 34(6): 913–19.

Smith, J. K. 2001. Exercise and atherogenesis. *Exercise and Sports Sciences Reviews* 29(2): 49–53.

Snyder, C. R. (Ed.). 2001. *Coping with Stress: Effective People and Processes* New York: Oxford University Press.

Snyder, C. R., and S. J. Lopez. 2002. *Handbook of Positive Psychology* New York: Oxford University Press.

Sohn, E. 2002. The hunger artists. *U.S. News and World Report* 132(20): 44–50.

Solowij, N. et al. 2002. Cognitive functioning of long-term heavy cannabis users seeking treatment. *JAMA* 287(9): 1123–31.

Stables, G. J., A. F. Subar, and B. H. Patterson et al. 2002. Changes in vegetable and fruit consumption and awareness among U. S. adults: results of the 1991 and 1997 5-a-day for better health program surveys. *Journal of the American Dietetic Association* 102(6): 809–17.

Sternberg, S. August 17, 2001. Government report on condoms stresses abstinence. *USA Today.*

Sternberg, S. February 27, 2002. New AIDS vaccine appears safe, promising. *USA Today.*

Stevenson, S. W. and E. A. Dudley. 2001. Dietary creatine supplementation and muscular adaptation to resistance overload. *Medicine and Science in Sports and Exercise* 33(8): 1304–10.

St. Joer, S. T. et al. 1999. Dietary protein and weight reduction: a statement for healthcare professionals from the nutrition committee of the Council on Nutrition, Physical Activity and Metabolism of the American Heart Association. *Circulation* 104: 1869–74.

Stoike, P. J. 2001. Automated external defibrillators: purchasing and staff training considerations. *ACSM's Health and Fitness Journal* 5(4): 20–25.

Strauss, R. S., and H. A. Pollack. 2001. Epidemic increase in childhood overweight, 1986–1998. *JAMA* 286(22): 2845–48.

Strote J., J. E. Lee, and H. Wechsler. 2002. Increasing MDMA use among college students: results of a national survey. *Journal of Adolescent Health* 30(1): 64–72.

Substance Abuse and Mental Health Services Administration. 2001. *Summary of Findings from the 2000 National Survey on Drug Abuse.* Washington, DC: U.S. Department of Health and Human Services.

Sundgot-Borgen, J. 2002. The effect of exercise, cognitive therapy, and nutritional counseling in treating bulimia nervosa. *Medicine and Science in Sports and Exercise* 34(2): 190–95.

Sutton, L., and L. Rapport. 2002. Glucosamine: con or cure? *Nutrition* 18: 534–36.

Task Force of the National Advisory Council on Alcohol Abuse and Alcoholism. 2002. *How to Reduce High-Risk College Drinking: Use Proven Strategies, Fill Research Gaps.* Bethesda, MD: National Institutes of Health.

Task Force of the National Advisory Council on Alcohol Abuse and Alcoholism. 2002. *High-Risk Drinking in College: What We Know and What We Need to Learn.* Bethesda, MD: National Institutes of Health.

Tate, D. F., R. R. Wing, and R. A. Winett. 2001. Using internet technology to deliver a behavioral weight loss program. *JAMA* 285: 1172.

Taylor, A. J. et al. 2002. Physical activity and the presence and extent of calcified coronary atherosclerosis. *Medicine and Science in Sports and Exercise.* 34(2): 228–33.

Thompson, P. D. 2001. Cardiovascular risks of wxercise. *The Physician and Sports Medicine* 29(4): 33–47.

Thompson, P. D. 2001. Exercise rehabilitation for cardiac patients. *Physician and Sports Medicine* 29(1): 69–75.

Thompson, S. R., M. M. Weber, and L. B. Brown. 2001. The relationship between Health and Fitness Magazine reading and eating-disordered weight-loss methods among high school girls. *American Journal of Health Education* 32(3): 133–138.

The Tobacco Use and Dependence Clinical Practice Guideline Panel, Staff, and Consortium Representatives. 2000. A clinical practice guideline for treating tobacco use and dependence: a U.S. Public Health Service Report. *JAMA* 283(24): 3244–54.

Townsend, C. 2001. *The Advanced Backpacker: A Handbook of Year-Round, Long-Distance Hiking.* St. Louis: McGraw-Hill.

Townsend, C. 2001. *The Backpacker's Pocketguide.* St. Louis: McGraw-Hill.

Traverso, G. et al. 2002. Detection of APC mutations in fecal DNA from patients with colorectal tumors. *New England Journal of Medicine* 346(5): 311–20.

Turner, J. et al. 2001. Pulmonary complications of HIV infection study group: adverse impact of cigarette smoking on dimensions of health-related quality of life in persons with HIV infection. *AIDS Patient Care & Standards* 15(12): 615–24.

United States Public Health Service Office of the Surgeon General. 2001. *Surgeon General's Call to Action to*

Promote Sexual Health and Responsible Sexual Behavior. Washington, DC: USPHS Office of the Surgeon General.

USA Today. April 15, 2002. Dietary supplement use: troubling side effects. *USA Today,* 11A.

Van Camp S. P., C. M. Bloor, and F. O. Mueller et al. 1995. Nontraumatic sports death in high school and college athletes. *Medicine and Science in Sports and Exercise* 27: 641–47.

Van Loan, M. D. 2001. Do you restrict your food intake? The implications of food restriction on bone health. *ACSM's Health and Fitness Journal* 5(1): 11–14.

Verducci, T. 2002. Totally juiced. *Sports Illustrated* 96(23): 34.

Wardlaw, G. M. 2002. *Contemporary Nutrition* (5th ed.). St. Louis: McGraw-Hill.

Wechsler, H. et al. 2002. Trends in college binge drinking during a period of increased prevention efforts. Findings from four Harvard School of Public Health College alcohol study

surveys: 1993–2001. *Journal of American College Health* 50(5): 203–17.

Westcott, W. L., R. A. Winett, E. S. Anderson et al. 2001. Effects of regular and slow-speed resistance training on muscle strength. *Journal of Sports Medicine and Physical Fitness* 41(2): 154–58.

White, J. 2001. Mixing faith and fitness. *ACSM's Health and Fitness Journal* 5(4): 15–19.

Wieberg, S. August 16, 2001. Survey: schools source of 15–20% of substances. *USA Today.*

Wilde, B. E., C. L. Sidman, and C. B. Corbin. 2002. A 10,000-step count as a physical activity standard for sedentary women. *Research Quarterly for Exercise and Sport* (72)(1): 411–414.

Williams, M. 2002. *Nutrition for Health, Fitness and Sports* (6th ed.). St. Louis: McGraw-Hill.

Williams, P. T. 2001. Physical fitness and activity as separate heart disease risk factors: a meta analysis. *Medicine and Science in Sports and Exercise* 33(5): 754–61.

Wilson, J. et al. 2001. Effects of walking poles on lower-extremity gait mechanics. *Medicine and Science in Sports and Exercise* 33(1): 142–147.

Women's Health Initiative Investigators Writing Group. 2002. Risks and benefits of estrogen plus progestin in healthy postmenopausal women. *JAMA* 288(3): 321–33.

Wong, G., and W. H. Dietz. 2002. Economic burden of obesity in youths aged 6 to 17 years: 1979–1999. *Pediatrics* 109: e81.

World Health Association. 2000. *Obesity: Preventing and Managing the Global Epidemic.* Geneva, Switzerland: World Health Organization. www.who.int.

Zakzanis, K. K. and D. A. Young. 2001. Memory impairment in abstinent MDMA (ecstasy) users: a longitudinal investigation. *Neurology* 56(7): 966–69.

Zvosec, D. L. et al. 2001. Adverse events, including death, associated with the use of 1,4- butanediol. *The New England Journal of Medicine* 344(2): 87–94.

Credits

Photos, Figures, and Tables

Concept 1

CO1: © Bob Winsett/CORBIS; p. 5: © Jim Cummins/Getty Images/Taxi; p. 8 top left: © Charles B. Corbin; p. 8 bottom right: © David Young Wolff/Photo Edit; p. 8 bottom left: © PhotoDisc/Getty Images; p. 8 top right: © Myrleen Cate/Index Stock Imagery; p. 8 middle left: © Bonnie Kamin/Photo Edit; p. 9 top left: © PhotoDisc/Getty Images; p. 9 bottom left: Corel; p. 9: middle top: © Vic Bider/Photo Edit; p. 9 middle bottom: Corel; p. 9 top right: © Kevin Syms/David R. Frazier Photolibrary; p. 12: © Michael Brinson/Index Stock Imagery.

Concept 2

CO2: © Bob Winsett/Index Stock Imagery; p. 24: © BSIP Agency/Index Stock Imagery; p. 26: © Courtesy of Vivonics; p. 29: © Tom McCarthy/PhotoEdit.

Concept 3

CO3: © Charles B. Corbin; p. 36 Table 1: American College of Sports Medicine. *ACSM's Guidelines for Exercise Testing and Prescription* (6th ed.), Philadelphia: Lippencott, Williams, and Wilkins, 2000.

Concept 4

CO4: © Kevin Syms/David R. Frazier; p. 51: © David Young Wolff/Photo Edit.

Concept 5

CO5: © PhotoDisc/Getty Images; p. 62: © PhotoDisc/Getty Images; p. 63: © Jim McGuire/Index Stock Imagery; p. 68: Bob Winsett/CORBIS.

Concept 6

CO6: © John Kelly/Getty Images/The Image Bank; p. 80 Table 2: National Institute for Health. The Sixth Report of the Joint Committee on Detection, Evaluation and Treatment of High Blood Pressure. NIH Publication Number 98-4080, 1997; p. 84: © Charles B. Corbin; p. 85: © Lori Adamski Peek/Getty Images/Stone.

Concept 7

CO7: © Brand X Pictures; p. 94: Cara Sidman; p. 98 left: © David R. Frasier Photolibrary; p. 98 right: © Myrleen Ferguson/Photo Edit.

Concept 8

CO8: © Zefa Visual Media-Germany/Index Stock Imagery; p. 107 Table 1 and Figure 6: Blair, S. N. et al. "Influences of Cardiorespiratory Fitness and Other Precursors on Cardiovascular Disease and All-Cause Mortality in Men and Women." *Journal of the American Medical Association.* 276(3)(1996): 205; p. 108: Bouchard, C. "Heredity and Health-Related Physical Fitness." In Corbin, C. B. and Pangrazi, R. P. *Toward a Better Understanding of Physical Fitness and Activity.* Scottsdale, AZ: Holcomb-Hataway, 1999; p. 111 left: © Charles B. Corbin; p. 111 right: © Mark Ahn; p. 113: Courtesy of Polar®; p. 114 Table 7: Borg, G. "Psychological Bases of Perceived Exertion." *Medicine and Science in Sports and Exercise.* 14(1982):377; p. 117 Chart 1: Adapted from the *One Mile Walk Test* with permission from the author, James M. Rippe, M. D.; p. 117 Chart 2: Data from Kasch, F. W. and Boyer, J. L. *Adult Fitness: Principles and Practices.* Palo Alto, CA: Mayfield Publishing Co., 1968; p. 118–119 Charts 3, 4, and 5: Astrand, P. O. and Rodahl, K. *Textbook of Work Physiology.* St. Louis: McGraw-Hill, 1986; p. 119–120 Charts 6 and 7: Cooper, K. H. *The Aerobics Program for Total Well-Being.* Toronto: Bantam Books, 1982; p. 121 Chart: Borg, G. "Psychological Bases of Perceived Exertion." *Medicine and Science in Sports and Exercise.* 14(1982):377.

Concept 9

CO9: © Paul A. Souders/CORBIS; p. 129: Courtesy of Timex®; p. 132: © Leland Bobbe/Getty Images/Stone; p. 134 top: © Tim Pannell/CORBIS; p. 134 bottom: © Bill Miles/CORBIS; p. 138: © Ken Akers/First Image West.

Concept 10

CO10: © Frank Conaway/Index Stock Imagery; p. 145: © Benelux Press/Getty Images/Taxi; p. 150 Figure 3: Shier, D., Butler, J., and Lewis, R. *Hole's Human Anatomy and Physiology.* (8th ed.) St. Louis: McGraw-Hill, 2002; p. 153 In the News: USA Today Research. Injuries to Major Leagues Skyrocket. *USA Today.* July 8, 2002, page 1C.

Concept 11

CO11: Corel; p. 167 Figure 1: Shier, D., Butler, J., and Lewis, R. *Hole's Human Anatomy and Physiology.* (8th ed.) St. Louis: McGraw-Hill, 2002;

p. 169: ©Sue Benett/Ad Stock; p. 173: © Mark Ahn; p. 177: King, J. M. "The Evolution of Strength Training Equipment." *Fitness Management.* July (2001):46–51; p. 181 & 196: © Charles B. Corbin; .

Concept 12

CO12: © Mark Ahn; p. 123: © Charles B. Corbin

Concept 13

CO13: © Fotografia, Inc./CORBIS; p. 230: © Charles B. Corbin

Concept 14

CO14: © Bohemian Nomad Picturemakers/CORBIS; p. 251: Corel; p. 253: © Richard Hamilton Smith/CORBIS; p. 254: Wilmore, J. H. and Costill, D. L. *Training for Sports and Activity* (2nd ed.). Dubuque, IA: Times Mirror Higher Education, 1988; p. 257: ©PhotoDisc/Getty Images; p. 257: Brittenham, G. "Plyometric Exercise: A Word of Caution." *Journal of Physical Education, Recreation and Dance.* January (1992): 20–23; p. 262: Williams, M. H. "Nutritional Ergogenics and Sports Performance." *PCPFS Research Digest.* 2(10)(1998):1–8; p. 265: Adams, W. et al. *Foundations of Physical Activity.* Champaign, IL: Stipes, 1965, p. 111.

Concept 15

CO15: © Charles B. Corbin; p. 275: © David R. Laurie; p. 277 Table 2: Lohman, T. G., Houtkooper, L. H. and Going, S. B. "Body Fatness Goes High Tech." *ACSM's Health and Fitness Journal.* 1(1)(1998); p. 278: Photo courtesy of Tanita Corporation of America, Inc. Arlington Heights, IL.; p. 280: © Bob Daemmrich/Stock Boston; p. 280 Figure 3: Lee, C.D., Jackson, A. A. and Blair, S. N. "Cardiorespiratory Fitness, Body Composition, and All-Cause and Cardiovascular Disease Mortality in Men." *American Journal of Clinical Nutrition,* 69(3)(1999): 373–380; p. 285 Table 4: Corbin, C. B. and Lindsey, R. *Fitness for Life* (4th ed.). Champaign, IL: Human Kinetics, 2002; p. 291–292 Charts 1 & 2: Baumgartner, T. A. and Jackson, A. S. *Measurement and Evaluation* (5th ed.). Dubuque, IA: Times Mirror, 1995.

Concept 16

CO16: © Jon Riley/Index Stock Imagery; p. 309 Figure 1: Based on information from Manore, M.

M. Vitamin and Minerals. Part II Who needs to supplement? *ACSM's Health and Fitness Journal.* 5(3)(2001): 30; p. 311 Figure 2: United States Department of Agriculture; p. 315: © Corbis; p. 316 Figure 6: Williams, M. *Nutrition for Fitness and Sports* (4th ed.). 1995. St. Louis: McGraw-Hill; p. 319: © Charles B. Corbin; p. 322: © Josh Mitchell/Index Stock Imagery.

Concept 17

CO17: © Mark Ahn; p. 336: © Donna Day/Getty Images/Stone; p. 337: © PhotoDisc/Getty Images.

Concept 18

CO18: © Brian Bailey/Getty Images/Stone; p. 350: © Corbis; p. 350 Table 2: Kanner, A. D. et al. Comparison of Two Modes of Stress Measurement: Daily Hassles and Uplifts Versus Major Life Events." *Journal of Behavioral Medicine.* 4(1)(1981):1–39; p. 355: Adapted from Gallagher, R. "Survey of College Counseling Centers." University of Pittsburgh; p. 356: Sarazon, I. G., Johnson, J. H. and Siegel, J. M. "Assessing the Impact of Life Changes: Development of the Life Experiences Survey." 1978. *Journal of Consulting and Clinical Psychology.* 46(5):932–946.

Concept 19

CO19: © Warren Morgan/CORBIS; p. 365: © Lori Adamski Peek/Getty Images/Stone; p. 370:

© PhotoDisc/Getty Images; p. 371–372 Tables 3 & 4: Burns, D. D. *The Feeling Good Handbook.* New York: Plume Books, 1999; p. 374: Hamrick, N., Cohen, S., & Rodriguez, M. S. 2002. Being popular can be healthy or unhealthy: Stress, social network diversity, and incidence of upper respiratory infection. Health Psychology, 21(3):294–298.

Concept 20

CO20: © Gary Buss/Getty Images/Taxi; p. 386: © Dennis McDonald/Photo Edit; p. 391: Health Canada.

Concept 21

CO21: © PhotoDisc/Getty Images; p. 397 Table 1: Developed by Alaska Chapter of MADD and reprinted in the *Orange County (CA) Chapter Newsletter,* Winter 1989–1990, page 5. Reprinted by permission of MADD/Orange County, CA and MADD/Anchorage, AK. Table 5: National Institute on Alcohol Abuse and Alcoholism. *Alcohol: Getting the Facts.* Bethesda, MD: NIAAA, 2002 (publication 96-4153, 2001 revision).

Concept 22

CO22: © PhotoDisc/Getty Images; p. 412 Figure 22.3: National Institute of Drug Abuse; p. 413: © Richard Hutchings/Photo Edit; p. 411 Figure 2?: Substance Abuse and Mental Health Services

Administration, Summary of Findings from the 2000 National Survey on Drug Abuse. Washington, DC: Department of Health and Human Services, 2001.

Concept 23

CO23: © Eye Wire/Getty Images; p. 424: ©David R. Frazier Photolibrary; p. 426: CDC-Atlanta, GA.

Concept 24

CO24: © Tomas del Amo/Index Stock Imagery; p. 434: ©Larry Mulvehill/Photo Researchers, Inc.; p. 440: ©Yellow Dog Productions/Getty Images/The Image Bank.

Concept 25

CO25: © David R. Laurie; p. 453: © Gary Conner/Index Stock Imagery; p. 454 & 455: © Mark Ahn.

Concept 26

CO26: © Charles B. Corbin; p. 470: ©Amwell/Getty Images/Stone; p. 475: Adapted from: Mitchell, T. "What's Your Excuse?" *USA Weekend.* January 4–6, 2002, page 4.

Index

F